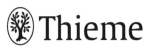

Procedural Dermatology

Volume II: Laser and Cosmetic Surgery

Postresidency and Fellowship Compendium

Yoon-Soo Cindy Bae, MD
Mohs Micrographic Surgeon and Dermatologic Oncologist
Cosmetic and Laser Surgeon
Laser & Skin Surgery Center New York;
Clinical Assistant Professor of Dermatology
New York University Grossman School of Medicine
The Ronald O. Perelman Department of Dermatology
New York, New York, USA

David H. Ciocon, MD
Director of Procedural Dermatology and Dermatologic Surgery
Associate Professor of Medicine
Director of Clinical Operations
Division of Dermatology
Montefiore Medical Center
Albert Einstein College of Medicine
Bronx, New York, USA

314 Illustrations

Thieme
Stuttgart • New York • Delhi • Rio de Janeiro

Library of Congress Cataloging-in-Publication Data is available from the publisher.

Important note: Medicine is an ever-changing science undergoing continual development. Research and clinical experience are continually expanding our knowledge, in particular our knowledge of proper treatment and drug therapy. Insofar as this book mentions any dosage or application, readersmay rest assured that the authors, editors, and publishers have made every effort to ensure that such references are in accordance with **the state of knowledge at the time of production of the book.**

Nevertheless, this does not involve, imply, or express any guarantee or responsibility on the part of the publishers in respect to any dosage instructions and forms of applications stated in the book. **Every user is requested to examine carefully** the manufacturers' leaflets accompanying each drug and to check, if necessary in consultation with a physician or specialist, whether the dosage schedules mentioned therein or the contraindications stated by the manufacturers differ from the statements made in the present book. Such examination is particularly important with drugs that are either rarely used or have been newly released on the market. Every dosage schedule or every form of application used is entirely at the user's own risk and responsibility. The authors and publishers request every user to report to the publishers any discrepancies or inaccuracies noticed. If errors in this work are found after publication, errata will be posted at www.thieme.com on the product description page.

Some of the product names, patents, and registered designs referred to in this book are in fact registered trademarks or proprietary names even though specific reference to this fact is not always made in the text. Therefore, the appearance of a name without designation as proprietary is not to be construed as a representation by the publisher that it is in the public domain. Thieme addresses people of all gender identities equally. We encourage our authors to use gender-neutral or gender-equal expressions wherever the context allows.

Thieme addresses people of all gender identities equally. We encourage our authors to use gender-neutral or gender-equal expressions wherever the context allows.

© 2023. Thieme. All rights reserved.

Georg Thieme Verlag KG
Rüdigerstrasse 14, 70469 Stuttgart, Germany
+49 [0]711 8931 421, customerservice@thieme.de

Cover design: © Thieme
Cover image source: © YummyBuum/stock.adobe.com
Typesetting by TNQ Technologies, India

Printed in Germany by Beltz Grafische Betriebe   5 4 3 2 1

DOI: 10.1055/b000000254

ISBN: 978-3-13-242407-4

Also available as an e-book:
eISBN (PDF): 978-3-13-242408-1
eISBN (epub): 978-3-13-258257-6

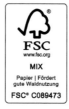

FSC
www.fsc.org
MIX
Papier | Fördert
gute Waldnutzung
FSC® C089473

Contents

17 Procedural Hair Restoration: Platelet-Rich Plasma for Hair Loss and Hair Transplant 193

Benjamin Curman Paul

18 Blepharoplasty, Lower Facelift, and Brow Lift 208

Robert Blake Steele, Rawn Bosley, and Cameron Chesnut

Preface

This volume represents the collective wisdom and experience of experts in our field who pioneered most of the laser and cosmetic treatments available today. Many of them comprise a new generation of thought leaders and innovators who continue to push the boundaries of treatment possibilities and outcomes. The purpose of this compendium is to address any knowledge gaps in the field of cosmetic dermatology among those who have recently completed their training and lack experience and expertise, particularly with respect to the latest developments in cosmetic technology. Hopefully, this compendium will enrich their existing skillsets and serve as an inspiration for developing additional techniques that best serve our patients.

As we are aware from our annual dermatology meetings, our field continues to evolve as we hear of new products and devices. Some persist, while others we never hear about again. Since the best physicians are life-long students, my hope in producing this textbook is to plant a seed from which further knowledge can continuously grow and expand, particularly as our technology continues to evolve.

This volume discusses the most up-to-date developments in cosmetic dermatology, including topics such as soft tissue fillers and botulinum toxin, laser treatment of vascular and pigmented lesions, ablative and nonablative resurfacing, body contouring, tissue tightening, liposuction, and surgical approaches to cosmetic rejuvenation, to name a few. Our authors adopt an approach that is patient-centered and tailored to the patient's needs, concerns, and native anatomy/skin type/functional status. The knowledge we share does not exist in a vacuum and owes heavily to the work of luminaries, both past and present. We are grateful to the investments of time and labor of all our contributing authors, without whom this work would not be possible.

Yoon-Soo Cindy Bae, MD

Contributors

Gee Young Bae, MD
Clinical Professor
Department of Dermatology
Asan Medical Center
Seoul, South Korea

Yoon-Soo Cindy Bae, MD
Mohs Micrographic Surgeon and
    Dermatologic Oncologist
Cosmetic and Laser Surgeon
Laser & Skin Surgery Center New York;
Clinical Assistant Professor of Dermatology
New York University Grossman School of Medicine
The Ronald O. Perelman Department of Dermatology
New York, New York, USA

Leonard J. Bernstein, MD, FAAD
Assistant Clinical Professor
Department of Dermatology
Weill Cornell Medical College – New York
    Presbyterian Hospital
New York, New York, USA

Andreas Boker, MD
Assistant Clinical Professor
Department of Dermatology
NYU School of Medicine
New York, New York, USA

Jordan Borash, MD
Acne Research Fellow
Department of Dermatology
Dermatology Institute of Boston
Boston, Massachusetts, USA

Rawn Bosley, MD
Chesnut MD Cosmetic Surgery Fellowship
Clinic5C
Spokane, Washington, USA

Jeremy A. Brauer, MD
Clinical Associate Professor
The Ronald O. Perelman Department of Dermatology
New York University Grossman School of Medicine
New York, New York, USA

Wilfred Brown, MD, FACS
Plastic and Reconstructive Surgeon
Private Practice
Middlebury, Connecticut, USA

Daniel Callaghan, MD
Mohs Surgeon
Advanced Dermatology and Cosmetic Surgery
Denver, Colorado, USA

Cameron Chesnut, MD, FAAD, FACMS, FASDS
Dermatologic Surgeon
American Academy of Facial Plastic and
    Reconstructive Surgery;
Clinical Assistant Professor
University of Washington School of Medicine
Seattle, Washington, USA

Mitalee P. Christman, MD
Dermatologist
SkinCare Physicians
Chestnut Hill, Massachusetts, USA

Maressa C. Criscito, MD, FAAD
Assistant Professor
Mohs Micrographic Surgery and
    Dermatologic Oncology
The Ronald O. Perelman Department of Dermatology
New York University Grossman School of Medicine
New York, New York, USA

Trina G. Ebersole, MD
Resident Physician
Division of Plastic and Reconstructive Surgery
St. Louis School of Medicine
Washington University
St. Louis, Missouri, USA

Jason Emer, MD, PC
Emerage Medical
West Hollywood, California, USA

Sabrina Guillen Fabi, MD
Goldman, Butterwick, Fitzpatrick, Groff and Fabi
Cosmetic Laser Dermatology
San Diego, California, USA

Amanda Fazzalari, MD
Chief Resident
Department of General Surgery
Stanley J. Dudrick Department of Surgery
Saint Mary's Hospital - Trinity Health of
    New England
Waterbury, Connecticut, USA

Adam Friedman, MD, FAAD
Professor and Chair of Dermatology;
Associate Residency Program Director;
Director of Translational Research;
Director of Supportive Oncodermatology
Department of Dermatology
George Washington School of Medicine and
 Health Sciences
Washington, DC, USA

Daniel P. Friedmann, MD, FAAD
Board-Certified Dermatologist
Westlake Dermatology & Cosmetic Surgery;
Clinical Research Director
Westlake Dermatology Clinical Research Center;
Diplomate of the American Board of Venous and
 Lymphatic Medicine
Austin, Texas, USA

Roy G. Geronemus, MD
Director
Laser & Skin Surgery Center of New York;
Clinical Professor of Dermatology
New York University Medical Center
New York, New York, USA

David J. Goldberg, MD, JD
Medical Director
Skin Laser & Surgery Specialists;
Director
Cosmetic Dermatology and Clinical Research
Schweiger Dermatology Group;
Clinical Professor of Dermatology;
Past Director
Mohs Surgery and Laser Research
Icahn School of Medicine at Mount Sinai
New York City, New York, USA

Samantha Gordon, MD
Dermatologist
Department of Dermatology
Dermatology & Aesthetics
Chicago, Illinois, USA

Emmy M. Graber, MD, MBA
President
Department of Dermatology
The Dermatology Institute of Boston
Boston, Massachusetts, USA

Ezra Hazan, MD
Clinical Instructor
Department of Dermatology
Icahn School of Medicine at Mount Sinai
New York, New York, USA

Rhett A. Kent, MD
Department of Forefront Dermatology
Arlington, Virginia, USA

Hooman Khorasani, MD
Associate Professor
Department of Dermatology
Icahn School of Medicine at Mount Sinai
New York, New York, USA

Margo H. Lederhandler, MD
Mohs Micrographic and Reconstructive Surgeon and
 Dermatologist
Department of Dermatology
Weill Cornell Medicine
New York, New York, USA

Austin Lee, BS
Research and Medical Assistant
New York Cosmetic, Laser, and Skin Surgery
Center
New York City, New York, USA

Monica K. Li, MD, FRCPC, FAAD
Department of Dermatology and Skin Science
University of British Columbia
Vancouver, British Columbia, Canada

Richard L. Lin, MD, PhD
Dermatologist
New York University
New York, New York, USA

Michael B. Lipp, DO, FAAD
SKINAESTHETICA
Redlands, California, USA

Jennifer L. MacGregor, MD
Clinical Professor
Department of Dermatology
Columbia University Medical Center
New York, New York, USA

Margaret Mann, MD
Associate Clinical Professor
Department of Dermatology
Case Western Reserve University
Cleveland, Ohio, USA

Joseph N. Mehrabi, MD
Resident
Maimonides Medical Center
Brooklyn, New York, USA

Vineet Mishra, MD
Associate Professor of Dermatology
Department of Dermatology
University of California San Diego
San Diego, California, USA

Teri N. Moak, MS, MD
Resident Physician
Department of Surgery
Division of Plastic and Reconstructive Surgery
Washington University, Barnes Jewish Hospital
St. Louis, Missouri, USA

Laurel M. Morton, MD
Physician
SkinCare Physicians
Chestnut Hill, Massachusetts, USA

Robert D. Murgia, DO, MA, FAAD
Dermatology and Skin Health
Peabody, Massachusetts, USA

Emily C. Murphy, MD
Resident
Department of Dermatology
George Washington School of Medicine and
    Health Sciences
Washington, DC, USA

Benjamin Curman Paul, MD
Facial Plastic Surgeon
Otolaryngology – Head and Neck Surgery
Lenox Hill Hospital
New York, New York, USA

Deanne Mraz Robinson, MD, FAAD
Assistant Clinical Professor
Department of Dermatology
Yale New Haven Hospital
New Haven, Connecticut, USA

Cameron Rokhsar, MD, FAAD, FAACS
Founder and Medical Director
New York Cosmetic, Laser, and Skin Surgery Center
New York City, New York, USA

Nazanin Saedi, MD
Dermatology Associates of Plymouth Meeting
Plymouth Meeting, Pennsylvania, USA

Jeffrey F. Scott, MD
Assistant Professor
Department of Dermatology
Johns Hopkins School of Medicine
Baltimore, Maryland, USA

Sachin M. Shridharani, MD, FACS
Director
Department of Aesthetic Plastic Surgery
LUXURGERY
New York, New York, USA

Seaver L. Soon, MD
Courtesy Staff Physician
Department of Dermatology
Scripps Green Hospital
La Jolla, California, USA

Robert Blake Steele, MD
Fellow
Department of Facial Cosmetic and
    Mohs Micrographic Surgery
Chesnut Institute of Cosmetic and
    Reconstructive Surgery
Spokane, Washington, USA

Alexa B. Steuer, MD, MPH
Dermatology Resident Physician
The Ronald O. Perelman Department of Dermatology
New York University Grossman School of Medicine
New York, New York, USA

Nina Lucia Tamashunas, BS
Medical Student
School of Medicine
Case Western Reserve University
Cleveland, Ohio, USA

Andrea Tan, MD
Resident
Department of Dermatology
Stony Brook University Hospital
Stony Brook, New York, USA

Grace M. Tisch
LUXURGERY
New York, New York, USA

Jordan V. Wang, MD, MBE, MBA
Medical Research Director
Laser & Skin Surgery Center of New York
New York, New York, USA

Robert Weiss, MD
Former Associate Professor
Department of Dermatology
Johns Hopkins University School of Medicine
Baltimore, Maryland, USA

Lindsey Yeh, MD
B.TOX.BAR
Los Gatos, California, USA

Michael Zumwalt, MD
Dermatologist/Mohs Surgeon
Skin Cancer and Dermatology Institute
Reno, Nevada, USA

1 Nonablative Rejuvenation

Daniel Callaghan and Laurel M. Morton

Summary

Nonablative rejuvenation can be achieved with a number of devices and is successfully used to treat many components of the aging process including texture irregularities, pigment irregularities, and tissue laxity. As the name implies, it does so without ablating the epidermis, which provides a lower potential for side effects and a shorter downtime than ablative lasers. The devices used for nonablative rejuvenation are diverse and include intense pulsed light, lasers in the visible light and mid-infrared spectrums, microneedling, radiofrequency, and photodynamic therapy. This chapter explores these interventions in detail and provides clinicians with a roadmap to be able to select the most appropriate treatment for each unique patient.

Keywords: nonablative rejuvenation, laser, IPL, microneedling, radiofrequency, PDT

1.1 Introduction

"Rejuvenation" is a broad term that describes the process of making the skin appear younger. The aging process, whether it is intrinsic aging programmed by genetics or extrinsic aging due to factors such as the sun, is composed of a number of core features including the following: volume loss, texture irregularities including fine or deep rhytides and acne scars, and pigment irregularities such as telangiectasias, lentigines, or melasma. Today, dermatologists have a widespread number of treatment options available to help rejuvenate their patients' skin. Although this is no doubt beneficial for patients, as everyone ages differently, it can also be overwhelming and challenging to determine which treatment is best suited for each patient.

Despite the vast number of treatment options available, they all function with the same goal, which is to deliver targeted energy or trauma to the skin to either destroy a lesion such as a lentigo or to stimulate collagen remodeling and neocollagenesis. The devices in our rejuvenation armamentarium include intense pulsed light (IPL), lasers, photodynamic therapy (PDT), microneedling, and radiofrequency (RF). IPL devices work by producing incoherent light of multiple wavelengths to deliver energy to the tissue, whereas lasers use specific wavelengths to target chromophores in tissue including melanin, hemoglobin, or water. PDT combines a photosensitizer such as 5-aminolevulinic acid (5-ALA) with light to target actinic keratoses. Microneedling uses physical trauma, whereas RF devices produce heat through electrical impedance. Beyond this, there are some devices that combine the above, such as microneedling and RF. There is a huge variety of treatment options available made by multiple device companies and all with different treatment parameters.

Ablative technologies such as the carbon dioxide laser, either fully or fractionally ablative, produce impressive results and may be considered by some as the "gold standard" for rejuvenation. However, these devices are associated with a number of adverse effects and a prolonged recovery time, which make them unrealistic options for many patients. For this reason, nonablative rejuvenation treatments have become increasingly popular over the years and are the focus of this chapter.

1.2 Modalities Available

1.2.1 Intense Pulsed Light

IPL sources are not lasers but flashlamp devices that produce noncoherent, multiwavelength light at wavelengths between 400 and 1,200 nm. Clinicians can utilize filters that block wavelengths shorter than the selected filter, thereby emitting only longer wavelengths that can penetrate the skin more deeply. Other factors that can be adjusted with IPL include fluence, pulse duration, and frequency of pulses administered. These are selected based on skin type, target, and severity of the target. IPL provides the benefit of minimal downtime. To reduce the risk of side effects, darker skin types should be treated with filters that employ longer wavelengths, longer pulse durations, and conservative fluences, whereas lighter skin types can be treated with a broader range of wavelengths, narrower pulse durations, and higher fluences. The clinical endpoint for IPL is often described as a mild amount of erythema and darkening of ephelides or lentigines, which develop within minutes of a pulse.

A systematic review by Wat et al found that IPL had a strong or moderate indication for the treatment of lentigines, melasma, rosacea, capillary malformations, and telangiectasias.[1] In a split-face study comparing IPL with the 755-nm nanosecond Q-switched (QS) alexandrite, it was demonstrated that IPL was equivalent to QS nanosecond alexandrite for the treatment of solar lentigines, although the QS nanosecond alexandrite was more effective for the treatment of ephelides.[2] Wang et al also evaluated IPL for the treatment of melasma and found that the IPL group experienced 39.8% improvement compared with the control group, which was treated with hydroquinone and sunscreen and had a more modest (11.6%) improvement.[3] Unfortunately, as has been the case with other melasma studies, results did not prove to be consistently sustainable. In a split-face, randomized, blinded trial, IPL was found to be equivalent to the pulsed dye laser (PDL) for the treatment of facial telangiectasias.[4] Additionally, Goldberg and Cutler demonstrated that IPL has some effect at improving facial rhytides.[5]

Several studies have evaluated IPL for "rejuvenation" in general, including the overall treatment of rhytides, skin coarseness, irregular pigmentation, pore size, and telangiectasias. One study, in particular, selected 49 subjects who were treated with a series of four or more full-face treatments at 3-week intervals and found that 100% of subjects reported some degree of satisfaction and 96% would recommend the treatment.[6]

1.2.2 532-nm KTP Laser and 595-nm PDL

Based on the theory of selective photothermolysis, there are a number of devices that use a unique wavelength to target a specific pigmentary defect, typically brown or red. Oxyhemoglobin, which is the chromophore targeted by vascular lasers, has absorption peaks at 542 and 577 nm. Absorption of the laser energy heats the oxyhemoglobin and leads to vessel wall damage. Along with IPL, the other energy-based devices that are most frequently used to treat telangiectasias and facial redness include the 595-nm (and rarely 585-nm) PDL and the 532-nm potassium titanyl phosphate (KTP) laser. Patients can typically expect at least 50 to 90% improvement after a series of one to three treatments with these devices[7] (▶ Fig. 1.1).

When treating telangiectasias or facial erythema, PDL can be used with a fluence and pulse duration above or below the purpura threshold. In a split-face study comparing purpuric to subpurpuric passes, Iyer and Fitzpatrick found a 43.4% reduction in surface area covered by telangiectasias with a single purpuric pass compared with 35.9% on the side treated with four subpurpuric passes. They also reported that purpuric settings may be

required to treat larger caliber vessels.[8] Although it may be slightly less effective, patients typically prefer subpurpuric settings with multiple passes because there are fewer adverse effects and less downtime.[9]

A randomized, split-face study evaluating 20 subjects with Fitzpatrick skin types I to III found that when comparing PDL to IPL, PDL had superior vessel clearance, but there was no significant difference between the effect on irregular pigmentation or skin texture. They did not find any reduction of rhytides with either device.[10]

In addition to treating telangiectasias and facial erythema like the PDL, the 532-nm KTP laser can be used to treat pigmented lesions. In a split-face study evaluating patients with pigment-related photodamaged facial skin who were treated with the 532-nm KTP alone or combined with the 1,064-nm neodymium:yttrium aluminum garnet (Nd:YAG) laser, the KTP alone was found to be safe and effective, but the addition of the 1,064-nm Nd:YAG provided no appreciable clinical difference.[11] In regard to treatment of erythema, a retrospective study of 647 patients treated with the KTP for a number of superficial vascular lesions including but not limited to telangiectasias, spider angiomas, and port-wine stains found that 77.6% of patients at 6 weeks were graded as being "cleared" or having "marked improvement."[12]

When comparing the 595-nm PDL to the 532-nm KTP for the treatment of facial telangiectasias in a split-faced study, it was demonstrated that both devices were highly effective. The authors did find that the 532-nm KTP laser appeared to be more effective but caused more swelling and erythema. Greater erythema has also been observed with the new generation of high peak power KTP devices with spike-free pulses.[13] As the 532-nm KTP has higher melanin absorption and penetrates the skin more superficially, the 595-nm PDL is a safer option for skin of color, but caution must still be exercised when using aggressive fluences.

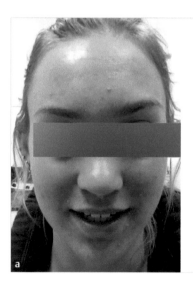
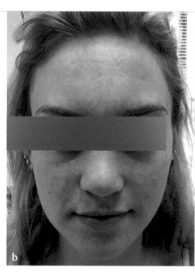

Fig. 1.1 (a) Postinflammatory erythema (PIE) secondary to acne. **(b)** Improvement of PIE after three sessions of pulsed dye laser at monthly intervals using the following parameters: 10 mm, 7.5 J/cm^2, 6 milliseconds. (These images are provided courtesy of Dr. Yoon-Soo Cindy Bae.)

1.2.3 694-nm Ruby Laser

Pigmentary issues are a chief concern of patients and one of the earliest and most obvious signs of photoaging. There are a number of devices that take advantage of the theory of selective photothermolysis and target melanosomes and melanocytes including the 532-nm KTP as previously discussed, the 694-nm QS ruby, 755-nm QS alexandrite, or the 1,064-nm QS Nd:YAG. Because of the higher absorption of the 532-nm wavelength by hemoglobin, treatment of pigmented lesions with the 532-nm wavelength may result in more purpura at lower fluences, compare to longer wavelengths. One study evaluating the QS ruby in 91 Iranian patients with lentigines and Fitzpatrick skin types II to IV found that 59.3% of patients had complete clearance after one treatment, while the remaining had complete clearance by the second treatment.[14] Like many other lasers, the 694-nm ruby laser has also been developed as a fractional laser, and has been reported to be safe and effective at treating infraorbital dark circles as well as melasma.[15,16]

1.2.4 755-nm Alexandrite Laser

The 755-nm alexandrite laser also preferentially targets melanin and is one of the most popular lasers to treat pigmented lesions. QS alexandrite lasers that are used for rejuvenation typically have pulses that are nanosecond in duration and, more recently, picosecond in duration. Melanosomes have a thermal relaxation time of 10 to 100 nanoseconds, and since nanosecond lasers have pulse durations in this range, they have the potential to heat surrounding tissue with a greater risk of adverse effects. Picosecond lasers have pulse durations that are much shorter, which reduces this risk.[17]

The QS nanosecond alexandrite has long been used for the treatment of pigmentary issues, although is more commonly used to treat discrete lesions rather than field treating an entire area (▶ Fig. 1.2a, b). Jang et al studied the treatment of freckles in 197 cases of Asian skin with the QS nanosecond alexandrite and found that more than 76% of freckles were removed with an average of 1.5 treatment sessions with no adverse effects.[18] Another study compared the QS nanosecond alexandrite to the QS nanosecond Nd:YAG for the treatment of benign melanocytic nevi and found that both resulted in significant improvement in the nevi, but the QS nanosecond alexandrite produced slightly better results.[19]

In recent years, QS alexandrite lasers have been developed to deliver pulses in the picosecond range. One randomized, single-blind study evaluating a QS 755-nm picosecond alexandrite laser compared to a nonablative 1,927-nm fractionated thulium laser for the treatment of facial photopigmentation and aging involved 20 females. Investigators found that although both lasers improve facial photopigmentation, the 755-nm QS picosecond alexandrite had statistically significant greater improvement in investigator assessments of photoaging/skin quality and subject satisfaction.[20] Lee et al compared the QS picosecond 755-nm alexandrite to the QS nanosecond 1,064-nm Nd:YAG for the treatment of melasma in 12 Asian patients in a split-faced manner and found that the 755-nm picosecond alexandrite laser had a superior and faster clearance rate.[21]

A more recent innovation is the application of a diffractive lens array to the picosecond 755-nm alexandrite laser. The purpose of the diffractive lens array is to deliver energy as apices of high-fluence regions, which essentially turns it into a fractionated laser that redistributes energy and allows multiple passes to be used to treat an area safely.[22] One 755-nm picosecond alexandrite laser with a diffractive lens array has been shown in multiple studies to be safe and effective for improving facial rhytides and pigmentation.[17,23] It has also been shown to be effective at treating acne scarring, and is thought to be safer in patients with more darkly pigmented skin relative to traditional nonablative fractional resurfacing lasers that target water[22,24] (▶ Fig. 1.3a, b).

1.2.5 1,064-nm Nd:YAG Laser

The 1,064-nm Nd:YAG laser has long been used for nonablative resurfacing and was one of the first devices used for this purpose. Its wavelength is absorbed by water, melanin, and hemoglobin; however, it has a lower affinity for melanin and hemoglobin than lower wavelength

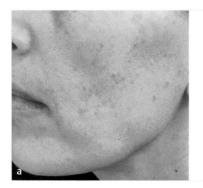
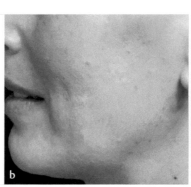

Fig. 1.2 (a) Diffuse cheek lentigines. **(b)** Improvement in lentigines following one treatment with the Q-switched alexandrite 755-nm laser.

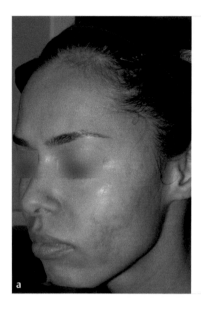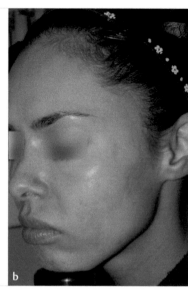

Fig. 1.3 **(a)** Acne scarring and mild dyschromia. **(b)** Improvement in acne scarring and discoloration following four treatments with a picosecond alexandrite 755-nm laser with diffractive lens array. (These images are provided courtesy of Cynosure and Emil Tanghetti, MD.)

lasers. With deeper penetration and lower absorption of melanin, it can be used more safely in darker-skinned patients. For nonablative resurfacing, it is commonly used in QS mode with a nanosecond domain in order to take advantage of the theory of selective photothermolysis, targeting pigmented structures while avoiding damage to the adjacent normal tissue. The QS nanosecond Nd:YAG is often used to treat pigmented tattoos, but it has also been found to be effective in the treatment of rhytides. A pilot study by Goldberg and Whitworth found that 9 of 11 patients treated with the QS nanosecond Nd:YAG periorally or periorbitally for rhytides demonstrated improvement.[25] As with other lasers that improve rhytides, the theory is that a thermal dermal wound leads to collagen shrinking, remodeling, and formation, which has been demonstrated by histology.[26] One study comparing the QS nanosecond Nd:YAG to IPL found that the QS nanosecond Nd:YAG has comparable efficacy for facial rhytides but with fewer side effects.[27] However, a later split-face study comparing IPL to the QS nanosecond Nd:YAG found them to be equally effective at treating skin texture, pore size, and sebum secretion, but the IPL was more effective at treating skin tone beyond the first treatment.[28] In a study involving Asian patients with skin types III to V, the QS nanosecond Nd:YAG was found to improve pore size, sebaceous skin texture, and skin tone.[29]

The long-pulsed 1,064-nm Nd:YAG in the millisecond domain also has a role in rejuvenation. Periorbital reticular veins can make one appear significantly older and are a frequent complaint of patients. One study, which included 17 patients with telangiectasias and periorbital reticular veins, found that there was greater than 75% improvement in 97% of the treated sites. Notably, of the eight periorbital reticular veins that were treated, 100% were found to have essentially 100% resolution.[30]

More recently, the QS nanosecond Nd:YAG has also been developed as a fractional device and has been found to be safe, painless, and modestly effective at treating facial and neck rhytides, with an 11.3% improvement over baseline after two treatments at 2- to 4-week intervals.[31]

1.2.6 Mid-Infrared Wavelength Lasers

Although there are now a number of fractional devices, including the 755-nm alexandrite and the 1,064-nm Nd:YAG, nonablative fractional resurfacing lasers were originally developed in the mid-infrared wavelengths including the 1,550-nm erbium-doped fiber laser, the 1,540-nm erbium glass, the 1,440-nm Nd:YAG, and the 1,565-nm fiber laser. These mid-infrared wavelengths use water as a chromophore, which leads to dermal denaturation and coagulation without tissue ablation. Coagulative microscopic treatment zones (MTZs) created by these lasers are surrounded by normal viable tissue from which new cells are recruited, allowing for faster re-epithelialization and minimal side effects relative to ablative resurfacing.[32]

Nonablative fractional lasers in the mid-infrared wavelengths are typically used to treat mild-to-moderate rhytides and dyspigmentation as well as scars, including acne scarring (▶ Fig. 1.4a, b). Patients usually require a series of five to six treatments, but because the downtime is far shorter than with ablative fractional lasers, these treatments are generally better tolerated with fewer side effects. An advantage to nonablative lasers is their versatility to be used off the face, unlike some ablative lasers (▶ Fig. 1.5a, b). This is because ablative lasers pose a more significant risk of side effects within the face locations due to the paucity of adnexal structures from which tissue regeneration typically originates.

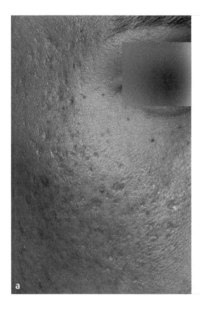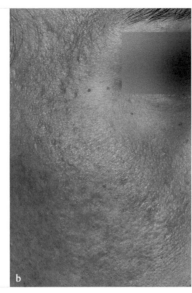

Fig. 1.4 (a) Boxcar acne scarring at the cheek. **(b)** Visible improvement in boxcar acne scarring following five sessions with the FRAXEL 1,550-nm laser. This photograph was taken 3 months following the last treatment. (The copyright images, provided courtesy of Solta Medical Aesthetic Center, and the trademark FRAXEL® are owned by Solta Medical or its affiliates and are used by permission.)

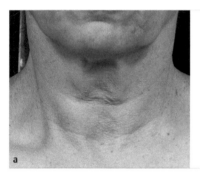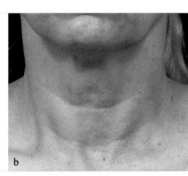

Fig. 1.5 (a) Texture irregularities in neck skin. **(b)** The nonablative fractional devices can be safely used off the face as shown by the improvement of neck skin texture following two treatments with the FRAXEL 1,550-nm laser. (The copyright images, provided courtesy of Solta Medical Aesthetic Center, and the trademark FRAXEL® are owned by Solta Medical or its affiliates and are used by permission.)

The original 1,550-nm erbium-doped fiber fractional laser demonstrated improvements of at least 51 to 75% in photodamage in 73% of patients after three successive treatments administered at 3- to 4-week intervals.[33] Although clinical evidence suggests that there is a skin-tightening effect with these mid-infrared nonablative fractional lasers, definitive histologic evidence is lacking.[34]

Similarly, a study involving 22 individuals with mild-to-moderate periorbital and perioral fine lines revealed gradual clinical and histologic improvement in all patients after three treatments with a 1,540-nm erbium glass laser with minimal side effects.[35] A 1,565-nm erbium-doped fiber nonablative fractional laser also led to a statistically significant decrease in photodamage and rhytides with 16 female subjects receiving three treatments at 4- to 5-week intervals.[36] Lasers in these wavelengths have been found to be safe and effective for rejuvenation in skin of color patients.[37]

Lasers in the mid-infrared spectrum have been demonstrated to be effective for nonablative rejuvenation, and it is reasonable to believe that they are similarly efficacious. One difference in these mid-infrared devices is how they deliver their energy, as some are rolled across the skin, some are stamped, and some utilize nonsequential scanning technology that allows them to be delivered in a single pass in a stamping fashion.

Nonablative fractional lasers at a slightly higher wavelength, such as the 1,927-nm thulium laser, reach a shallower depth and are intended to treat dyschromia and more superficial rhytides (▶ Fig. 1.6a, b). A study by Brauer et al evaluating the use of the 1,927-nm thulium laser found that two treatments for facial photopigmentation produced moderate to marked improvement in overall appearance and pigmentation with high patient satisfaction.[38] It has also been found to be effective for the treatment of melasma.[39] This device is likely safe and effective for the treatment of overall photodamage and pigmentation off of the face, on the neck, chest, arms, and hands[40] (▶ Fig. 1.7a, b).

1.2.7 Photodynamic Therapy

PDT is most commonly used to treat actinic keratoses and superficial nonmelanoma skin cancers. However, the idea of "photodynamic photorejuvenation" was introduced by

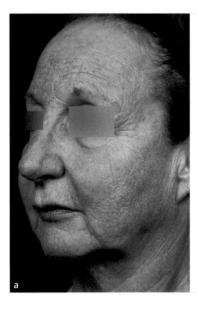
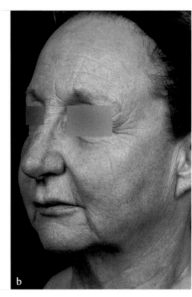

Fig. 1.6 (a) Facial texture and color irregularities due to photoaging. (b) Improvement is seen in both texture and color 1 month following two treatment sessions with the FRAXEL 1,927-nm thulium laser. (The copyright images, provided courtesy of Solta Medical Aesthetic Center, and the trademark FRAXEL® are owned by Solta Medical or its affiliates and are used by permission.)

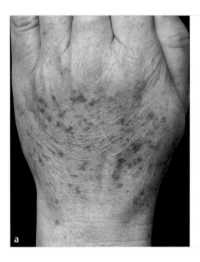
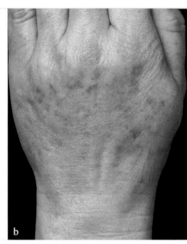

Fig. 1.7 (a) Dorsal hand lentigines. (b) Dorsal hand lentigines, dramatically improved, status post three treatments with the FRAXEL 1,927-nm thulium laser. (The copyright images, provided courtesy of Solta Medical Aesthetic Center, and the trademark FRAXEL® are owned by Solta Medical or its affiliates and are used by permission.)

at least 2002.[41] Using one of two available photosensitizers, 5-ALA or a methyl ester of 5-ALA (MAL), and a light source such as red or blue light-emitting diodes (LEDs), IPL, or PDL, patients can expect significant improvement in actinic keratoses and pigmented lesions (50–90%) and improvement in skin tone, texture, and coarseness with overall cosmetic improvement up to 50 to 80%.[42] It has been estimated that one "PDT-IPL" rejuvenation session may be equivalent to three sessions of IPL alone.[43] For patients who predominantly have actinic keratoses, red or blue LED lights are recommended. However, if the patient has fewer actinic keratoses but more lentigines and telangiectasias, IPL may be more appropriate.

1.2.8 Radiofrequency

RF devices take advantage of the conductivity differences of tissue types to produce heat through electrical impedance. Like resurfacing lasers, RF devices can be subdivided into fractional or nonfractional categories. Further classification includes whether or not the device is monopolar, bipolar, or multipolar, which is determined by the number of electrodes used to create the electric current. RF devices are typically associated with minimal downtime, an excellent safety profile, and minimal discomfort. Traditionally, they have frequently been used for their skin-tightening effect. However, new fractional RF devices are also used to improve rhytides, scars, or epidermal lesions.

Monopolar RF devices are based on the principle of volumetric heating, delivering uniform heat at controlled depths of the deep dermis and subdermal layers, which in turn leads to collagen contraction and remodeling over 4 to 6 months. The goal of this treatment is skin tightening. Contact cooling from a cryogen spray on the treatment tip protects the epidermis. A multicenter study involving 66 patients at three clinical sites demonstrated that at 6 months, 92% of patients had a measurable improvement in facial skin laxity.[44]

More recently, fractional skin resurfacing has been applied to RF devices. These are frequently composed of an array of needles inserted into the skin to serve as electrodes, with little to no impact on the epidermis and an effect centered around the dermis. Devices may employ stationary pins that emit the energy from their tips or combine them with microneedling. In a study looking at the treatment of 12 healthy females with varying degrees of rhytides, hyperpigmentation, or acne redness, a fractional RF device with stationary pins was found to improve both skin texture and pigmentation.[45] A retrospective study of a similar device with stationary pins found that patients being treated for rhytides, hyperpigmentation, or erythema associated with acne vulgaris were highly satisfied 3 months after treatment.[46] In a study with 27 Chinese patients with moderate facial photoaging, a microneedle fractional RF system demonstrated significant improvement in facial photoaged skin after three treatments, which was maintained up to the 6-month mark with mild-to-moderate pain and no adverse effects.[47]

Of note, fractional RF devices may also be made with coated pins to further protect the epidermis and have been shown to be safe to improve skin texture, wrinkles, and acne scars in skin type VI patients.[48] There is little risk of hyperpigmentation as RF heat is not preferentially absorbed by melanin.

1.2.9 Microneedling

Microneedling, also known as percutaneous collagen induction therapy, is a minimally invasive procedure that aims to achieve the same goal of nonablative fractional laser rejuvenation using needles to create microchannels as opposed to light-based energy. It has been used for skin rejuvenation, to treat acne scars or other surgical scars, enlarged pores, rhytides, and dyschromia. Microneedling devices are rolled across the skin and use multiple fine needles to penetrate the skin, which leads to collagen and elastin formation and release of growth factors.[49] A study of 10 female patients treated with two sessions of microneedling on upper lip rhytides showed a 2.3-fold reduction in wrinkle severity using the Wrinkle Severity Rating Scale after 30 weeks.[50] Patients often undergo a series of three to six sessions at biweekly or monthly intervals to achieve optimal improvement.[51]

1.3 Indications

It is not practical to review specific indications for each device on the market. Rather, it is more useful to define the specific components of aging and review which treatment options are best for each indication. Although many devices are studied and reported to treat a number of aspects of rejuvenation, in truth some devices clearly excel for a specific treatment goal.

- Pigmentary issues:
  - Erythema and telangiectasias:
    - 595-nm PDL and 532-nm KTP and IPL.
  - Facial reticular veins:
    - Long-pulsed 1,064-nm Nd:YAG.
  - Hyperpigmentation including lentigines, melasma, and postinflammatory hyperpigmentation (PIH):
    - Discrete hyperpigmented lesions: 532-nm KTP, QS 694-nm Ruby, QS nanosecond 755-nm alexandrite, QS picosecond 755-nm alexandrite, or the QS nanosecond 1,064-nm Nd:YAG.
    - Diffuse hyperpigmentation: 1,927-nm thulium laser, IPL, and picosecond 755-nm alexandrite with diffractive lens array
- Textural issues including fine lines, wrinkles, skin texture, and scarring:
  - Mid-infrared devices in the 1,440- to 1,565-nm wavelengths (though ablative techniques likely remain the gold standard).
  - Microneedling for mild textural complaints.
  - Picosecond 755-nm alexandrite with diffractive lens array, fractional QS 1,064-nm Nd:YAG, and IPL.
- Skin laxity:
  - RF devices typically provide good results in terms of skin tightening (microfocused ultrasound, not discussed in this chapter, can also be utilized).
- Actinic keratoses:
  - PDT with LEDs, IPL, or PDL (these may also address erythema or hyperpigmentation).
  - Nonablative fractional resurfacing devices in the mid-infrared range, particularly the 1,927-nm thulium device.
- Combined pigment and textural concerns:
  - IPL, the mid-infrared nonablative fractional resurfacing lasers including the 1,927-nm devices, the picosecond 755-nm alexandrite with diffractive lens array, and combined microneedling/RF devices.

1.4 Patient Selection, Contraindications, and Preoperative Procedures

1.4.1 Patient Selection

Appropriate patient selection is essential for best results from nonablative rejuvenation procedures. A treatment plan should be uniquely specialized for the individual, taking into account patient goals and expectations, downtime and risk that is acceptable to the patient, expected treatment results, and skin typing.

As discussed, rejuvenation can improve skin discoloration, fines lines, wrinkles, texture, and tone. During a consultation, the physician should ask the patient what issue is bothering him or her. If discoloration is a primary concern, it is important to make a diagnosis for the cause of discoloration. Lentigines and photodamage are likely to respond well to fractional lasers such as a 1,927-nm thulium laser or picosecond fractional array as well as nonfractional light and lasers including IPL and QS 755- and 1,064-nm lasers. On the other hand, if the discoloration is due to PIH, it should be explained that even though the same devices can be employed, this condition can be more difficult to improve with devices alone and adjunctive interventions such as strict photoprotection and bleaching or brightening products may also be useful. Treating physicians should evaluate every patient for melasma. This is a particularly difficult condition to manage as it is frequently exacerbated by laser and light treatment and tends to recur. Many experts forego laser or light devices altogether when treating this condition and opt for bleaching and brightening creams. If lasers are used, it is worth considering a low-fluence QS or picosecond laser, both of which have shown efficacy for melasma with a lower side effect profile.[21,52,53,54] Pre- and/or posttreatment with bleaching agents such as triple combination creams including hydroquinone, tretinoin, and a corticosteroid may also yield better results.[55]

If a patient's concern is regarding fine lines, texture, or acne scarring, lasers that induce more collagen remodeling are preferred options. In particular, infrared devices that utilize wavelengths including but not limited to 1,550 and 1,540 nm have demonstrated improvement in skin texture with a series of treatments.[56,57,58] More recently, fractional visible spectrum picosecond lasers with 532-, 755-, and 1,064-nm wavelengths have also demonstrated improvement of acne scarring.[24,59]

It is also important to manage patient expectations. During the consultation process, they should be informed that, often, multiple sessions are required for ideal results and it is likely that maintenance will be required over time as we continue to age and experience sun exposure and resulting photodamage.

A significant factor in choosing a treatment modality is understanding what a patient is willing to experience with respect to procedure discomfort and healing time. For instance, the infrared nonablative fractional devices, while providing good results, can be more uncomfortable and cause significant erythema, edema, and scaling skin for up to a week. This may not be an option for patients with significant work or social obligations. These patients may be willing to undergo less aggressive procedures at greater frequency. Another consideration is that each laser comes with risks such as infection, hyperpigmentation, or hypopigmentation. Some patients are comfortable with these risks and others are not. Explaining each device's side effect and risk profile is essential so that patients are well educated prior to choosing a treatment plan.

It is important to select individuals that you expect will respond well. For instance, dark discrete lentigines improve more significantly with treatment compared to faint lesions because selective photothermolysis depends on the pigment differential between lesional and normal skin. Conditions with dermal melanin deposition such as certain types of PIH and melasma may not respond well to device monotherapy. Additionally, patients who have deep rhytides and significant volume loss may not notice the incremental change from nonablative collagen remodeling and these patients may be encouraged to seek more aggressive interventions such as ablative resurfacing with adjunctive procedures including neurotoxins and soft-tissue fillers.

Skin typing is extremely important when recommending a treatment. Lower skin type patients (I–II) can safely undergo most rejuvenation procedures. As skin type increases, melanin-targeting devices are more likely to cause PIH or even hypopigmentation, burns, and scarring. This is particularly true for high-energy QS devices. As skin type increases, side effect risk also increases for IPL procedures,[60] though some IPL devices are likely safe in type IV Asian skin.[61] Infrared-range devices, which have less pigment specificity, have been used in all skin types but are more likely to cause hyperpigmentation in darker skin types[62,63] (▶ Fig. 1.8a, b). Rejuvenation interventions that do not employ light or laser energy, such as RF and insulated microneedling devices, are safer in most skin types.

1.4.2 Contraindications

Patients should be evaluated for contraindications at the time of both consultation and treatment. QS devices and IPL must not be used on tanned skin due to risk of burning, scars, and hypopigmentation, which can be permanent. Signs of skin breakdown and active bacterial (i.e., impetigo, cellulitis, or abscess), viral (i.e., herpes simplex virus [HSV] or varicella-zoster virus [VZV]), or fungal (i.e., cutaneous candidiasis) infection are also a contraindication. Another less-encountered contraindication for pigment-specific lasers is a history of oral gold therapy. QS lasers, in particular, can cause iatrogenic chrysiasis, usually a gray discoloration of the skin at the site of laser treatment, in those with a history of systemic gold therapy. It can be difficult to eradicate.

A relative contraindication is active dermatitis and moderate-to-severe acne, particularly when acne is a more likely side effect, such as during fractional nonablation. Melasma or a history of melasma should also be considered a relative contraindication for some devices as the application of many high-energy devices may exacerbate this condition.

Historically, isotretinoin use was considered a contraindication to laser surgery and a waiting period of 6 to 12 months post isotretinoin was recommended. However, there is likely insufficient evidence to support this guideline.[64] In one recent split-face study, patients

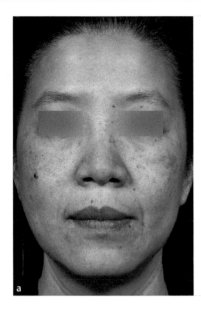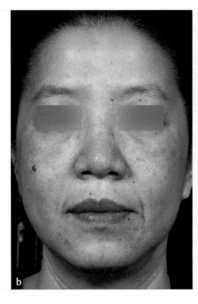

Fig. 1.8 (a) Facial hyperpigmentation seen in Asian skin. **(b)** Improvement in hyperpigmentation following one treatment with the FRAXEL 1,927-nm thulium laser without any evidence of postinflammatory hyperpigmentation. (The copyright images, provided courtesy of Solta Medical Aesthetic Center, and the trademark FRAXEL® are owned by Solta Medical or its affiliates and are used by permission.)

on isotretinoin 10 mg daily had one half of the face treated with 1,550-nm nonablative fractional laser. The laser-treated side had significantly better improvement of comedo count and acne scarring compared to the untreated side without significant adverse events.[65] In another 2017 study of 10 patients, half the face was treated with 3-monthly 1,550-nm nonablative fractional laser treatments 1 month status post isotretinoin use. Wound healing was normal and no keloids or hypertrophic scars were noted on the treatment side.[66] Caution should be taken when treating patients with recent isotretinoin use, but it may not be necessary to wait 6 months.

1.4.3 Preoperative Procedures

Prior to procedures, a patient should be evaluated a final time for contraindications. Consent must be performed, during which time, risks, alternatives, and expectations are reviewed. For any procedure, the face should be cleansed to remove any aesthetic products such as makeup, sunscreen, and moisturizer, and pretreatment photographs and documentation must be completed. The patient may benefit from topical anesthesia for 15 to 60 minutes, depending on the treatment modality. Adopting a laser checklist, which is kept adjacent to every device, is another useful way to ensure that contraindications have been ruled out, appropriate laser settings have been chosen, and necessary protective eyewear is used by all participants.[67]

Additional preoperative protocols can vary between providers. However, several practices should be considered. Patients' with a history of herpes simplex may benefit from prophylaxis with acyclovir or valacyclovir. This is more important during nonablative fractional procedures, but an HSV breakout could occur after any type of

treatment. Bacterial prophylaxis is generally not required prior to nonablative laser procedures. Topical preparations prior to laser treatments are sometimes utilized. As mentioned earlier, the addition of triple combination cream for several weeks prior to treatment may increase the efficacy of treatment, particularly when the goal is improvement of melasma.[55] Plain hydroquinone may also be used. Whether hydroquinone enhances results is slightly controversial as at least one 2018 study of 40 patients (skin types III–V) suggested pretreatment with 2% hydroquinone did not change outcomes for patients treated for photoaging and melasma with the fractional nonablative 1,927-nm device.[68] It is not necessary to stop retinoid products prior to laser procedures, but some patients may find their skin less irritated following treatment if retinoid is discontinued 1 to 2 weeks prior to treatment.

1.5 Techniques

Appropriate technique during laser surgery is essential to achieve best outcomes and to prevent adverse events. Details to consider include organization of the treatment room, appropriate mechanics of delivery, and understanding proper endpoints.

A treatment room should be organized so that the treating physician, assistants, and patient are comfortable and can perform their duties. The laser should be placed appropriately near the examination table so that the laser arm can reach the patient without overstretching device cords, which can cause laser damage, and so that the physician is ergonomically positioned. It is important to keep wavelength-specific laser goggles near the device so that both providers and patients are protected. If multiple lasers are located in one room, goggles should be carefully labeled.

In a majority of cases, lasers are designed to work best when their treatment handpieces are held perpendicular to the skin surface at a specified distance. Since the surface of the face is not flat, it is important that a provider is continuously self-checking to ensure the laser is held appropriately. If a step-off or spacer is present, be sure to keep the recommended distance from the skin's surface. Laser placement that is too close or too far can result in a burn or decreased efficacy. Positioning is also important if the device requires cooling. Dynamic cooling may not work appropriately if the handpiece is not held perpendicularly and contact cooling must, by definition, be in contact with the skin.

Good technique also includes spacing device pulses at appropriate intervals. This varies between devices and a practitioner should be educated about each device he or she utilizes. At times, overlap or pulse stacking is appropriate and in other cases, such as with QS lasers, pulses should never be double stacked. Scanning devices should be applied with a uniform speed and in a consistent manner so that the entire skin surface is treated with a homogenous energy for reliable and even results.

Knowledge of expected treatment endpoints, the initial appearance of tissue following treatment, is important to achieve best results and prevent adverse events. Endpoints vary between devices. QS lasers cause a faint, temporary whitening of target lentigines. When low fluence is used, as with melasma, whitening does not usually occur. Long-pulsed lasers generally do not cause whitening. Wavelengths of 532 and 1,064 nm, when used for lentigines, may also cause purpura or pinpoint petechiae due to concurrent absorption by hemoglobin. IPL causes mild-to-moderate erythema and darkening of lesions, which may be seen within minutes or require hours to appear. Nonablative fractional lasers usually cause mild erythema and edema within minutes. Pinpoint white dots may or may not appear.[69] Petechiae is much less common and if this occurs, the practitioner should carefully review his or her settings.

1.6 Postoperative Instructions

Patients are largely responsible for their postoperative care and it is important to provide careful instructions that describe best behaviors and practices for ideal healing and results. Appropriate care decreases risk of adverse events and speeds improvement of expected side effects. That said, one important benefit of nonablative rejuvenation is that the postoperative period is generally short-lived and side effects are mild including the following: edema, erythema, expected temporary darkening of treated lesions, and occasionally scaling skin or mild desquamation.

Immediate postoperative care is simple for nonablative procedures and should include application of ice for several minutes, which enhances patient comfort and reduces edema. This may be repeated every 1 to 2 hours for up to several days after treatment. The most essential practice is sun avoidance and the use of sunscreen. In most cases, it is reasonable to apply cosmetics 12 to 24 hours following a procedure and it is important to choose moisturizers that are noncomedogenic to prevent an acne breakout following fractional procedures.

In some cases, perioperative medications may be indicated. Completion of a prophylactic antiviral course during nonablative fractional treatments is recommended for patients with a history of HSV. Postsurgical antibiotics can decrease risk of acne in at-risk patients following fractional nonablation.[62] Provider preference may also include the use of topical bleaching agents for melasma. In our practice, we have found that the topical application of an antioxidant serum post procedure and use of a hydrating facial mask also enhance the patient experience.

1.7 Potential Complications and Management

Generally speaking, the risk of serious complications following nonablative laser treatment is low and this is one reason for its popularity. However, adverse events can result and include the following: acneiform eruptions, discoloration (prolonged erythema, hypopigmentation, hyperpigmentation, exacerbation of melasma), infection, and scarring. Importantly, the safety profiles for nonablative laser types vary.

In regard to nonablative fractional treatments, Graber et al reported that 961 1,550-m erbium-doped laser treatments on skin types I to V showed a 7.6% risk of complication.[62] The most common complications were acneiform eruptions (1.87%) and HSV outbreaks (1.77%). Another notable adverse event was PIH with an incidence of 0.26% in skin types I and II and incidences of 2.6% in skin type III, 11.6% in skin type IV, and 33% in skin type V.[62] Mahmoud et al have also reported that the incidence of PIH in skin types IV to VI is significant.[63] Graber et al's study also reported prolonged erythema, prolonged edema, dermatitis, impetigo, and purpura.[62] When considering only darker skin types (III–IV), another retrospective review of 856 treatments demonstrated a similar risk of complication (5.0%), but prolonged erythema (1.8%), PIH (1.1%), and worsening of melasma (0.9%) were more common than HSV breakouts (0.6%) and acneiform eruptions (0.2%).[70] Patients with a history of HSV were given prophylaxis in the latter study.

Acneiform eruptions, more common after fractional treatments,[71] and HSV outbreaks, most common when the perioral area is treated,[71] can be treated with topical or oral antibiotics and antivirals, respectively. These conditions will also resolve naturally. PIH improves on its own but may require many months (mean time to resolution is about 50 days[62]). Use of topical lightening creams, prescription and nonprescription (i.e., hydroquinone, kojic acid, tranexamic acid), may hasten its resolution.

PIH can be a significant adverse effect for patients. It is possible that picosecond lasers may pose a lower risk. Khetarpal et al reported no incidence of PIH in 16 patients with skin types I to III who completed a treatment protocol for picosecond fractional rejuvenation.[17] Another study of patients with skin types III and IV reported no incidence of PIH following 107 treatments with a similar intervention.[72] Even skin types IV to VI can likely safely undergo picosecond rejuvenation, though PIH may still be more likely in this patient group. Haimovic et al treated 56 patients with skin types IV to VI. Six patients developed transient PIH for less than 2 weeks and two patients developed PIH that took several months to resolve (when treated off-face).[73]

Discoloration can be a significant risk for QS lasers and IPL due to their melanin specificity. Higher skin types are unlikely to tolerate certain wavelength lasers such as 532 and 755 nm. In some cases, 1,064 nm may be used in darker skin types due to its deeper penetration. Careful review of manufacturer instructions and communication with other specialists familiar with your device is the best way to determine the most effective and safest treatment parameters.

Hypopigmentation is less common than PIH, but it can be seen with QS lasers. At times, this may be a "relative" hypopigmentation after treatment of lentigines.[71] It has also been reported with the use of low-fluence QS 1,064-nm laser for rejuvenation and melasma in Asian patients.[74,75] The cause for this is unknown, but authors' theorized excessive fluences and phototoxicity to melanocytes were to blame.[74] This hypopigmentation is difficult to treat.

Although bacterial infection following nonablative laser is infrequent, Xu et al reported a series of five patients, who within 1 week of receiving treatment with the 1,550-/1,927-nm fractional laser, developed methicillin-sensitive *Staphylococcus aureus* infections, at least one of which led to systemic sequelae.[76] Signs of bacterial infection may include persistent erythema, erosions, serous drainage, inflammatory papules, and pustules. Pain, fevers, and chills could be present in more serious cases.[76] If an infection is suspected, cultures and empiric antibiotic therapy should be started. Given the rare occurrence of infection, prophylactic antibiotics are likely unnecessary and may increase risk of antibiotic resistance.

Fortunately, scarring is also rare. However, this could potentially occur with any energy device. Risk factors include high fluence, inadequate cooling (when indicated), inappropriate pulse stacking, high repetition rate, and infection.[71]

1.8 Pearls and Pitfalls

1.8.1 Pearls

- Appropriate patient selection is essential for best outcomes. Choosing the modality that will lead to the most success and least risk of complications for a particular patient will create a positive patient–physician relationship. It is important to set reasonable expectations so that patients are satisfied with healing time and results.
- Combination therapy is useful in most patients. In patients who request color and texture improvement, it is common to see early active rhytides or folds and volume loss that are best addressed with botulinum toxin and soft-tissue filler. Tactfully pointing out what can be addressed with laser therapy and what is best improved by other modalities often leads to best patient outcomes.
- Long-term postoperative behaviors can be as important as the short term for best outcomes. Reminding patients to practice sun protection long term and implementing several choice topical preparations such as retinoids, antioxidants, and glycolic acids can lead to longer-lasting results and happier patients.
- Importantly, higher density rather than higher fluence is likely a stronger risk factor for PIH in nonablative fractional treatment.[77]

1.8.2 Pitfalls

- Melasma is frequently a presenting problem for patients. It may be obvious and known to the patient or it may require a physician's diagnosis. Melasma can behave unpredictably and can be exacerbated by higher-energy nonablative treatments. Evaluate each patient carefully for this condition and consider starting with topical bleaching and lightening creams, rather than energy devices, if this is suspected.
- Beware of tanned patients. This can be a particular issue in warmer climates when tans are present year round or after holiday and school breaks when people have been traveling. Often, patients do not realize they are tanned. Therefore, trust your instinct. Compare facial skin (or other skin to be treated) with skin that is not exposed to determine whether a tan is present. In many scenarios, particularly with use of IPL and QS lasers, tanned skin should not be treated.

References

[1] Wat H, Wu DC, Rao J, Goldman MP. Application of intense pulsed light in the treatment of dermatologic disease: a systematic review. Dermatol Surg. 2014; 40(4):359–377

[2] Wang CC, Sue YM, Yang CH, Chen CK. A comparison of Q-switched alexandrite laser and intense pulsed light for the treatment of freckles and lentigines in Asian persons: a randomized, physician-blinded, split-face comparative trial. J Am Acad Dermatol. 2006; 54 (5):804–810

[3] Wang CC, Hui CY, Sue YM, Wong WR, Hong HS. Intense pulsed light for the treatment of refractory melasma in Asian persons. Dermatol Surg. 2004; 30(9):1196–1200

[4] Tanghetti EA. Split-face randomized treatment of facial telangiectasia comparing pulsed dye laser and an intense pulsed light handpiece. Lasers Surg Med. 2012; 44(2):97–102

[5] Goldberg DJ, Cutler KB. Nonablative treatment of rhytids with intense pulsed light. Lasers Surg Med. 2000; 26(2):196–200

[6] Bitter PH. Noninvasive rejuvenation of photodamaged skin using serial, full-face intense pulsed light treatments. Dermatol Surg. 2000; 26(9):835–842, discussion 843

[7] Adamic M, Troilius A, Adatto M, Drosner M, Dahmane R. Vascular lasers and IPLS: guidelines for care from the European Society for Laser Dermatology (ESLD). J Cosmet Laser Ther. 2007; 9(2):113–124

[8] Iyer S, Fitzpatrick RE. Long-pulsed dye laser treatment for facial telangiectasias and erythema: evaluation of a single purpuric pass versus multiple subpurpuric passes. Dermatol Surg. 2005; 31(8, Pt 1):898–903

[9] Woo SH, Ahn HH, Kim SN, Kye YC. Treatment of vascular skin lesions with the variable-pulse 595 nm pulsed dye laser. Dermatol Surg. 2006; 32(1):41–48

[10] Jørgensen GF, Hedelund L, Haedersdal M. Long-pulsed dye laser versus intense pulsed light for photodamaged skin: a randomized split-face trial with blinded response evaluation. Lasers Surg Med. 2008; 40(5):293–299

[11] Negishi K, Tanaka S, Tobita S. Prospective, randomized, evaluator-blinded study of the long pulse 532-nm KTP laser alone or in combination with the long pulse 1064-nm Nd: YAG laser on facial rejuvenation in Asian skin. Lasers Surg Med. 2016; 48(9):844–851

[12] Becher GL, Cameron H, Moseley H. Treatment of superficial vascular lesions with the KTP 532-nm laser: experience with 647 patients. Lasers Med Sci. 2014; 29(1):267–271

[13] Uebelhoer NS, Bogle MA, Stewart B, Arndt KA, Dover JS. A split-face comparison of pulsed 532-nm KTP laser and 595-nm pulsed dye laser in the treatment of facial telangiectasias and diffuse telangiectatic facial erythema. Dermatol Surg. 2007; 33(4):441–448

[14] Sadighha A, Saatee S, Muhaghegh-Zahed G. Efficacy and adverse effects of Q-switched ruby laser on solar lentigines: a prospective study of 91 patients with Fitzpatrick skin type II, III, and IV. Dermatol Surg. 2008; 34(11):1465–1468

[15] Xu TH, Li YH, Chen JZ, Gao XH, Chen HD. Treatment of infraorbital dark circles using 694-nm fractional Q-switched ruby laser. Lasers Med Sci. 2016; 31(9):1783–1787

[16] Jang WS, Lee CK, Kim BJ, Kim MN. Efficacy of 694-nm Q-switched ruby fractional laser treatment of melasma in female Korean patients. Dermatol Surg. 2011; 37(8):1133–1140

[17] Khetarpal S, Desai S, Kruter L, et al. Picosecond laser with specialized optic for facial rejuvenation using a compressed treatment interval. Lasers Surg Med. 2016; 48(8):723–726

[18] Jang KA, Chung EC, Choi JH, Sung KJ, Moon KC, Koh JK. Successful removal of freckles in Asian skin with a Q-switched alexandrite laser. Dermatol Surg. 2000; 26(3):231–234

[19] Rosenbach A, Williams CM, Alster TS. Comparison of the Q-switched alexandrite (755 nm) and Q-switched Nd:YAG (1064 nm) lasers in the treatment of benign melanocytic nevi. Dermatol Surg. 1997; 23 (4):239–244, discussion 244–245

[20] Serra M, Bohnert K, Sadick N. A randomized, single-blind, study evaluating a 755-nm picosecond pulsed Alexandrite laser vs. a non-ablative 1927-nm fractionated thulium laser for the treatment of facial photopigmentation and aging. J Cosmet Laser Ther. 2018; 20 (6):335–340

[21] Lee MC, Lin YF, Hu S, et al. A split-face study: comparison of picosecond alexandrite laser and Q-switched Nd:YAG laser in the treatment of melasma in Asians. Lasers Med Sci. 2018; 33(8):1733–1738

[22] Tanghetti EA. The histology of skin treated with a picosecond alexandrite laser and a fractional lens array. Lasers Surg Med. 2016; 48(7):646–652

[23] Weiss RA, McDaniel DH, Weiss MA, Mahoney AM, Beasley KL, Halvorson CR. Safety and efficacy of a novel diffractive lens array using a picosecond 755 nm alexandrite laser for treatment of wrinkles. Lasers Surg Med. 2017; 49(1):40–44

[24] Brauer JA, Kazlouskaya V, Alabdulrazzaq H, et al. Use of a picosecond pulse duration laser with specialized optic for treatment of facial acne scarring. JAMA Dermatol. 2015; 151(3):278–284

[25] Goldberg DJ, Whitworth J. Laser skin resurfacing with the Q-switched Nd:YAG laser. Dermatol Surg. 1997; 23(10):903–906, discussion 906–907

[26] Goldberg DJ, Silapunt S, DJ G. Histologic evaluation of a Q-switched Nd:YAG laser in the nonablative treatment of wrinkles. Dermatol Surg. 2001; 27(8):744–746

[27] Goldberg DJ, Samady JA. Intense pulsed light and Nd:YAG laser non-ablative treatment of facial rhytids. Lasers Surg Med. 2001; 28(2):141–144

[28] Huo MH, Wang YQ, Yang X. Split-face comparison of intense pulsed light and nonablative 1,064-nm Q-switched laser in skin rejuvenation. Dermatol Surg. 2011; 37(1):52–57

[29] Lee MC, Hu S, Chen MC, Shih YC, Huang YL, Lee SH, MC L. Skin rejuvenation with 1,064-nm Q-switched Nd:YAG laser in Asian patients. Dermatol Surg. 2009; 35(6):929–932

[30] Eremia S, Li CY. Treatment of face veins with a cryogen spray variable pulse width 1064 nm Nd:YAG Laser: a prospective study of 17 patients. Dermatol Surg. 2002; 28(3):244–247

[31] Luebberding S, Alexiades-Armenakas MR. Fractional, nonablative Q-switched 1,064-nm neodymium YAG laser to rejuvenate photoaged skin: a pilot case series. J Drugs Dermatol. 2012; 11 (11):1300–1304

[32] Manstein D, Herron GS, Sink RK, Tanner H, Anderson RR. Fractional photothermolysis: a new concept for cutaneous remodeling using microscopic patterns of thermal injury. Lasers Surg Med. 2004; 34 (5):426–438

[33] Wanner M, Tanzi EL, Alster TS. Fractional photothermolysis: treatment of facial and nonfacial cutaneous photodamage with a 1,550-nm erbium-doped fiber laser. Dermatol Surg. 2007; 33(1):23–28

[34] Kauvar AN. Fractional nonablative laser resurfacing: is there a skin tightening effect? Dermatol Surg. 2014; 40 Suppl 12:S157–S163

[35] Lupton JR, Williams CM, Alster TS. Nonablative laser skin resurfacing using a 1540 nm erbium glass laser: a clinical and histologic analysis. Dermatol Surg. 2002; 28(9):833–835

[36] Friedmann DP, Tzu JE, Kauvar AN, Goldman MP. Treatment of facial photodamage and rhytides using a novel 1,565 nm non-ablative fractional erbium-doped fiber laser. Lasers Surg Med. 2016; 48(2):174–180

[37] Kaushik SB, Alexis AF. Nonablative fractional laser resurfacing in skin of color: evidence-based review. J Clin Aesthet Dermatol. 2017; 10 (6):51–67

[38] Brauer JA, McDaniel DH, Bloom BS, Reddy KK, Bernstein LJ, Geronemus RG. Nonablative 1927 nm fractional resurfacing for the treatment of facial photopigmentation. J Drugs Dermatol. 2014; 13 (11):1317–1322

[39] Polder KD, Bruce S. Treatment of melasma using a novel 1,927-nm fractional thulium fiber laser: a pilot study. Dermatol Surg. 2012; 38 (2):199–206

[40] Polder KD, Harrison A, Eubanks LE, Bruce S. 1,927-nm fractional thulium fiber laser for the treatment of nonfacial photodamage: a pilot study. Dermatol Surg. 2011; 37(3):342–348

[41] Ruiz-Rodriguez R, Sanz-Sánchez T, Córdoba S. Photodynamic photorejuvenation. Dermatol Surg. 2002; 28(8):742–744, discussion 744

[42] Le Pillouer-Prost A, Cartier H. Photodynamic photorejuvenation: a review. Dermatol Surg. 2016; 42(1):21–30

[43] Goldman MP, Atkin D, Kincad S. PDT/ALA in the treatment of actinic damage: real world experience. J Lasers Med Surg. 2002; 14:S:24

[44] Bogle MA, Ubelhoer N, Weiss RA, Mayoral F, Kaminer MS. Evaluation of the multiple pass, low fluence algorithm for radiofrequency tightening of the lower face. Lasers Surg Med. 2007; 39(3):210–217

[45] Hongcharu W, Gold M. Expanding the clinical application of fractional radiofrequency treatment: findings on rhytides, hyperpigmentation, rosacea, and acne redness. J Drugs Dermatol. 2015; 14(11):1298–1304

[46] Ray M, Gold M. A retrospective study of patient satisfaction following a trial of nano-fractional RF treatment. J Drugs Dermatol. 2015; 14 (11):1268–1271

[47] Zhang M, Fang J, Wu Q, Lin T. A prospective study of the safety and efficacy of a microneedle fractional radiofrequency system for global facial photoaging in Chinese patients. Dermatol Surg. 2018; 44(7): 964–970

[48] Battle F, Battle S. Clinical evaluation of safety and efficacy of fractional radiofrequency facial treatment of skin type VI patients. J Drugs Dermatol. 2018; 17(11):1169–1172

[49] Doddaballapur S. Microneedling with dermaroller. J Cutan Aesthet Surg. 2009; 2(2):110–111

[50] Fabbrocini G, De Vita V, Pastore F, et al. Collagen induction therapy for the treatment of upper lip wrinkles. J Dermatolog Treat. 2012; 23 (2):144–152

[51] Alster TS, Graham PM. Microneedling: a review and practical guide. Dermatol Surg. 2018; 44(3):397–404

[52] Kauvar AN. Successful treatment of melasma using a combination of microdermabrasion and Q-switched Nd:YAG lasers. Lasers Surg Med. 2012; 44(2):117–124

[53] Hofbauer Parra CA, Careta MF, Valente NY, de Sanches Osório NE, Torezan LA. Clinical and histopathologic assessment of facial melasma after low-fluence q-switched neodymium-doped yttrium aluminium garnet laser. Dermatol Surg. 2016; 42(4):507–512

[54] Chalermchai T, Rummaneethorn P. Effects of a fractional picosecond 1,064 nm laser for the treatment of dermal and mixed type melasma. J Cosmet Laser Ther. 2018; 20(3):134–139

[55] Jeong SY, Shin JB, Yeo UC, Kim WS, Kim IH. Low-fluence Q-switched neodymium-doped yttrium aluminum garnet laser for melasma with pre- or post-treatment triple combination cream. Dermatol Surg. 2010; 36(6):909–918

[56] Geronemus RG. Fractional photothermolysis: current and future applications. Lasers Surg Med. 2006; 38(3):169–176

[57] Alster TS, Tanzi EL, Lazarus M. The use of fractional laser photothermolysis for the treatment of atrophic scars. Dermatol Surg. 2007; 33(3):295–299

[58] Hedelund L, Moreau KE, Beyer DM, Nymann P, Haedersdal M. Fractional nonablative 1,540-nm laser resurfacing of atrophic acne scars. A randomized controlled trial with blinded response evaluation. Lasers Med Sci. 2010; 25(5):749–754

[59] Bernstein EF, Schomacker KT, Basilavecchio LD, Plugis JM, Bhawalkar JD. Treatment of acne scarring with a novel fractionated, dual-wavelength, picosecond-domain laser incorporating a novel holographic beam-splitter. Lasers Surg Med. 2017; 49(9):796–802

[60] Thaysen-Petersen D, Lin JY, Nash J, et al. The role of natural and UV-induced skin pigmentation on low-fluence IPL-induced side effects: a randomized controlled trial. Lasers Surg Med. 2014; 46(2):104–111

[61] Negishi K, Tezuka Y, Kushikata N, Wakamatsu S. Photorejuvenation for Asian skin by intense pulsed light. Dermatol Surg. 2001; 27(7): 627–631, discussion 632

[62] Graber EM, Tanzi EL, Alster TS. Side effects and complications of fractional laser photothermolysis: experience with 961 treatments. Dermatol Surg. 2008; 34(3):301–305, discussion 305–307

[63] Mahmoud BH, Srivastava D, Janiga JJ, Yang JJ, Lim HW, Ozog DM. Safety and efficacy of erbium-doped yttrium aluminum garnet fractionated laser for treatment of acne scars in type IV to VI skin. Dermatol Surg. 2010; 36(5):602–609

[64] Mysore V, Mahadevappa OH, Barua S, et al. Standard guidelines of care: performing procedures in patients on or recently administered with isotretinoin. J Cutan Aesthet Surg. 2017; 10(4): 186–194

[65] Xia J, Hu G, Hu D, Geng S, Zeng W. Concomitant use of 1,550-nm nonablative fractional laser with low-dose isotretinoin for the treatment of acne vulgaris in Asian patients: a randomized split-face controlled study. Dermatol Surg. 2018; 44(9):1201–1208

[66] Saluja SS, Walker ML, Summers EM, Tristani-Firouzi P, Smart DR. Safety of non-ablative fractional laser for acne scars within 1 month after treatment with oral isotretinoin: a randomized split-face controlled trial. Lasers Surg Med. 2017; 49(10):886–890

[67] Hamilton HK, Dover JS. Using checklists to minimize complications from laser/light procedures. Dermatol Surg. 2014; 40(11):1173–1174

[68] Vanaman Wilson MJ, Jones IT, Bolton J, Larsen L, Fabi SG. The safety and efficacy of treatment with a 1,927-nm diode laser with and without topical hydroquinone for facial hyperpigmentation and melasma in darker skin types. Dermatol Surg. 2018; 44(10):1304–1310

[69] Wanner M, Sakamoto FH, Avram MM, et al. Immediate skin responses to laser and light treatments: therapeutic endpoints—how to obtain efficacy. J Am Acad Dermatol. 2016; 74(5):821–833, quiz 834, 833

[70] Lee SM, Kim MS, Kim YJ, et al. Adverse events of non-ablative fractional laser photothermolysis: a retrospective study of 856 treatments in 362 patients. J Dermatolog Treat. 2014; 25(4):304–307

[71] Al-Niaimi F. Laser and energy-based devices' complications in dermatology. J Cosmet Laser Ther. 2016; 18(1):25–30

[72] Wat H, Yee-Nam Shek S, Yeung CK, Chan HH. Efficacy and safety of picosecond 755-nm alexandrite laser with diffractive lens array for non-ablative rejuvenation in Chinese skin. Lasers Surg Med. 2019; 51 (1):8–13

[73] Haimovic A, Brauer JA, Cindy Bae YS, Geronemus RG. Safety of a picosecond laser with diffractive lens array (DLA) in the treatment of Fitzpatrick skin types IV to VI: a retrospective review. J Am Acad Dermatol. 2016; 74(5):931–936

[74] Chan NP, Ho SG, Shek SY, Yeung CK, Chan HH. A case series of facial depigmentation associated with low fluence Q-switched 1,064 nm Nd:YAG laser for skin rejuvenation and melasma. Lasers Surg Med. 2010; 42(8):712–719

[75] Tian B. The Asian problem of frequent laser toning for melasma. J Clin Aesthet Dermatol. 2017; 10(7):40–42

[76] Xu LY, Kilmer SL, Ross EV, Avram MM. Bacterial infections following non-ablative fractional laser treatment: a case series and discussion. Lasers Surg Med. 2015; 47(2):128–132

[77] Kono T, Chan HH, Groff WF, et al. Prospective direct comparison study of fractional resurfacing using different fluences and densities for skin rejuvenation in Asians. Lasers Surg Med. 2007; 39(4):311–314

2 Ablative Rejuvenation

Mitalee P. Christman and Roy G. Geronemus

Summary

Ablative rejuvenation is still considered the gold standard for nonsurgical treatment of photoaging. Treatment options include both traditional full-field ablative and fractional ablative carbon dioxide and erbium:yttrium aluminum garnet lasers. The ideal candidate has fine static rhytides and appropriate expectations regarding recovery and results. A thorough preoperative consult is performed and antiviral and antibacterial prophylaxis is provided to the patient. A multipronged anesthetic strategy is often necessary for optimal pain management. During the treatment, careful attention is paid to the clinical endpoint of visible wrinkle effacement and total energy delivered to the treatment area. Laser-assisted drug delivery of poly-L-lactic acid, postprocedure peptide serums, and photomodulation might enhance results and patient satisfaction. Close clinical follow-up is warranted to monitor for infectious complications. Recognition of symptoms and signs of other possible complications including erythema, dyspigmentation, and scarring is critical to allow for early intervention. With careful preoperative, intraoperative, and postoperative care, ablative rejuvenation can be a very satisfying and successful procedure.

Keywords: ablative resurfacing, ablative rejuvenation, ablative lasers, resurfacing, carbon dioxide, erbium:YAG

2.1 Introduction

Ablative laser resurfacing is still considered the gold standard for nonsurgical rejuvenation of fine rhytides and photoaging. The spectrum of ablative rejuvenation procedures spans from ablative full-field traditional resurfacing to ablative fractional resurfacing with carbon dioxide (CO_2) and erbium:yttrium aluminum garnet (Er:YAG) lasers. Careful consideration of each patient's goals and lifestyle—along with their skin type, severity of photoaging, depth of rhytides, and scars—informs the ideal treatment for that patient. Once a device is selected, attention to preoperative evaluation, intraoperative technique, and postoperative care will produce reliable clinical results and limit the risk of complications.

Understanding the mechanism and history of ablative lasers requires an understanding of the theory of selective photothermolysis. Briefly, for a laser to treat its target, the wavelength of the laser must be absorbed greatly by the desired chromophore, the pulse duration should be shorter than the thermal relaxation time of the tissue to allow for heat confinement, and the fluence should be sufficient for therapeutic effect while minimizing collateral damage.[1,2] Applying the tenets of this theory for resurfacing the epidermis, the ideal wavelengths target water (the chromophore of the epidermis); the ideal pulse duration is less than 1 millisecond, and the fluence is at least 5 J/cm2—a lower fluence will produce diffuse heating without vaporizing the epidermis.[2] Using sufficient fluence or energy will vaporize the epidermis and produce a zone of residual thermal damage that denatures collagen, triggering neocollagenesis. The size of this zone of residual thermal damage is a function of the laser beam energy and the laser dwell time or pulse duration—the wider the pulse, the greater the thermal damage.

Ablative resurfacing was born in the 1980s with continuous wave (CW) CO_2 lasers. The infrared 10,600-nm CO_2 laser is absorbed by water, vaporizing the epidermis and forming coagulated debris by denaturing collagen and cauterizing small blood vessels in the dermis. Whereas these destructive and hemostatic features of the early CO_2 lasers made them invaluable for the removal of epithelial neoplasms as well as incisional surgery, these same capabilities produced excess thermal injury and an unacceptably high risk of scarring and pigment alteration due to their tissue dwell times being much greater than the thermal relaxation time of the epidermis.

The 1990s saw the introduction of technologies with shorter pulse durations and high peak power and rapidly scanning CW technology, which were relatively safer but still with prolonged recovery time. Initial "superpulsed" high-peak power devices produced high-frequency short pulses (200–1,000 pulses per s) or shuttering of the continuous beam to create a 0.1- to 1-second burst of energy. Subsequent devices either produced a high-energy pulse of 1 millisecond or shorter (ultrapulsed CO_2) or rapidly scanned a CW laser beam so that the tissue dwell time at any individual location was less than 1 millisecond (rapidly scanning CW CO_2). Either of these approaches delivered high energy that allowed penetration of the laser up to a depth of 20 to 30 μm into the skin in a single pass, and the ultrashort pulses ensured that the exposure was shorter than the thermal relaxation time of the epidermis, limiting collateral thermal injury. Further passes with the CO_2 laser produce deeper residual thermal damage that extends about 100 to 150 μm into the dermis and stimulates collagen contracture and skin tightening, clinically translating into improvement of photoaging, rhytides, and scars.[3]

The millennium brought the introduction of the erbium:YAG laser (2,940 nm). This laser has an absorption coefficient for water that is 16 times higher than that of the CO_2 laser. This translates into a lower depth of penetration of about 5 to 15 μm, a narrower zone of residual thermal damage of about 10 to 40 μm leading to a shorter recovery time, albeit at the cost of lower efficacy for neocollagenesis.

Finally, the erbium:yttrium scandium gallium garnet (Er:YSGG) proprietary 2,790-nm wavelength introduced in the late 2000s had an absorption coefficient for water that is about five times that of the CO_2 laser, and was thought to represent a hybrid between CO_2 and Er:YAG in terms of its ratio of penetration to residual thermal damage.[4]

The downtime and complication rates of ablative resurfacing inspired the development of nonablative resurfacing and, in 2004, fractional resurfacing, to minimize risk and improve recovery time. Nonablative resurfacing (Chapter 1) improves wrinkles and photodamage by producing dermal thermal injury while sparing the epidermis; however, multiple treatments are required and the modality is generally considered less effective than ablative resurfacing.[5] Fractional resurfacing thermally ablates microscopic columns of epidermis and dermis in regularly spaced arrays.[6,7] The surrounding tissue is preserved and acts as a reservoir for quicker re-epithelialization and faster healing.[6] This intermediate approach increases efficacy compared to nonablative resurfacing, but with shorter downtime and risks compared to ablative resurfacing.[8] Although high-quality comparative trials are lacking, multiple passes of ablative fractional resurfacing are thought to approach the coverage of traditional full-field resurfacing, and ablative fractional resurfacing has now widely supplanted full-field ablative resurfacing in the therapeutic armamentarium for photoaging.[9]

2.2 Modalities/Treatment Options Available

For the physician wishing to choose a device for ablative rejuvenation, evidence-based selection of a modality is compromised by the quality of data available from uncontrolled studies and a few small randomized controlled trials, and also by the wide variety of criteria used to assess clinical responses among trials. As such, selection of a modality is driven by laser availability, clinical expertise, and patient-specific factors. The differences in the wavelengths available for ablative rejuvenation are detailed in ▸ Table 2.1, and select devices currently available are compared in ▸ Table 2.2. Devices vary based on wavelength, scanning versus stamped delivery, depth of ablation, and extent of thermal injury produced.

2.3 Indications

Ablative resurfacing effectively treats many components of photoaged skin including rhytides, dyspigmentation, elastosis, and actinic damage. Fine rhytides in the periorbital, cheek, and perioral areas can be completely effaced with ablative lasers.[5] In addition to photoaging, other indications for ablative resurfacing include actinic cheilitis, scars, rhinophyma, epidermal nevi, angiofibroma, sebaceous hyperplasia, seborrheic keratoses, adnexal tumors, squamous cell carcinoma in situ, and superficial basal cell carcinoma.

2.4 Patient Selection, Contraindications, and Preoperative Considerations

During the consultation visit, the patient's goals, expectations for the procedure, recovery process and results, contraindications (▸ Table 2.3), preoperative considerations (▸ Table 2.4), and their tolerance for complications should be carefully assessed in addition to their photoaging profile.

Table 2.1 Wavelengths for ablative rejuvenation

Laser	Wavelength	Pulse durations	Ablation threshold	Thermal damage	Comments	Downtime
CO_2	10,600 nm	< 1 ms	5 J/cm^2 (generally 4–10 J/cm^2)	50–80 μm 100 μm	• Greatest effect on dermal collagen remodeling → tightening of mild skin laxity • Relatively higher risk of scarring, dyspigmentation, and prolonged erythema compared to Er:YAG, fractional CO_2 attenuates this risk	10–14 d until re-epithelialization (5–10 d if fractional), followed by weeks to months of erythema
Erbium: YAG	2,940 nm	100–500 μs	0.5 J/cm^2	20 μm	• Requires more passes to ablate similar depth as CO_2 • Reduced thermal damage → less tightening effect • Lower risk for scarring	3–8 d to re-epithelialization
Erbium: YSGG	2,790 nm	200–800 μs	2–3.5 J/cm^2	10 μm with 3 passes	• Proprietary wavelength • Limited comparative data available	About 4 d

Abbreviations: YAG, yttrium aluminum garnet; YSGG, yttrium scandium gallium garnet.

Table 2.2 Specifications of various selected devices available for ablative rejuvenation

Name	Manufacturer	Wavelength (nm)	Laser	Max power (W) or energy delivered	Pulse duration	Spot size	Incisional handpiece	Densities
Fraxel re:pair	Solta	10,600	Fractional CO_2	up to 70 mJ/MTZ (corresponding to a depth of 1.58 mm)	Superpulsed, 0.15–3 ms	135–600 μm	Yes, 0.2 and 2 mm	135-μm handpiece: 3–70% density
Active Fx Ultrapulse	Lumenis	10,600	Fractional CO_2	25–225 mJ (corresponding to ablation depths of 10–300 μm)	Ultrapulsed, 10 μs to 0.9 ms	1.3 mm	Yes, 0.2 and 1 mm	Densities range from 55 to 100%
Deep Fx Ultrapulse	Lumenis	10,600	Fractional CO_2	2.5 to 150 mJ (corresponding to ablation depths from 75 μm to 3.5 mm)	Ultrapulsed, 10 μs to 0.9 ms	120 μm	Yes, 0.2 and 1 mm	Densities range from 1 to 25%
Mixto SX	Lasering	10,600	Fractional CO_2	30 W, 1–480 mJ/spot	Continuous wave, 2.5–16 ms/spot	180 and 300 μm	Yes, 0.3 mm	Densities range from 5 to 40%
CO_2RE	Candela	10,600	Fractional CO_2	1–257 mJ	20 μs to 3 ms	150 and 120 μm	Yes	Light (30–50%), mid (20–40%), deep (1–5%) modes spanning depths of 20–700 μm. Also a fusion mode (mid + deep)
eCO_2	Lutronic	10,600	Fractional CO_2	2–240 mJ	Superpulsed (1–5 ms), ultra-pulsed (40 μs to 1 ms) or continuous wave	120 and 300 μm	Yes, adjustable handpiece from 0.2 to 1 mm	120-μm tip: 1–17% coverage; 300-μm tip: 5–58% density
Smartskin	Cynosure	10,600	Fractional CO_2	1–60 mJ/spot	Superpulsed, 200–2,000 μs	N/A	Yes	0- to 2,000-μm pitch (or distance between scanning spots)
ProFractional XC on Joule platform Contour TRL on Joule platform	Sciton	2,940	Fractional Er:YAG	Up to 400 J/cm^2	Variable	430 μm		Ablation depth of 25–100 μm and treatment density of 5.5, 11, or 22% with or without depth-specific coagulation Up to 800 μm in depth, coagulation up to 130 μm

(Continued)

Table 2.2 (*Continued*) Specifications of various selected devices available for ablative rejuvenation

Name	Manufacturer	Wavelength (nm)	Laser	Max power (W) or energy delivered	Pulse duration	Spot size	Incisional handpiece	Densities
Burane II	Alma	2,940	Er:YAG, fully ablative with standard handpiece, fractional handpiece	1–22 J/cm^2 (max pulse energy: 2.5 J)	350 μs	1–6 mm	No	Fractional handpiece is 7 × 7 pixel
Pearl fractional handpiece on xeo platform	Cutera	2,790	Er:YSGG	<400 mJ/micro-spot	≤1 ms	300 μm	No	4, 8, 12, 16, and 32% density of MTZ
Pearl handpiece (fully ablative) on xeo platform	Cutera	2,790	Er:YSGG	1.5–3.5 J/cm^2	≤1 ms	6 mm	No	Scan size of 30 × 30 mm, densities of 10, 15, and 20%

Abbreviations: YAG, yttrium aluminum garnet; YSGG, yttrium scandium gallium garnet.
Source: Based on Avram MR, Avram MM, Friedman PM. Ablative resurfacing. In: Laser and Light Source Treatments for the Skin. London: JP Medical Ltd.; 2014:82–85. Data verified with companies.

The ideal candidate for ablative resurfacing is a patient with skin types I to III with fine static rhytides, mild laxity if any, and appropriate expectations regarding recovery and results. Many patients' photoaging profiles merit a multi-pronged approach: dynamic rhytides are best targeted with neuromodulators (Chapter 15), telangiectasias are better targeted with vascular lasers, and moderate-to-severe laxity is best treated with plastic surgery procedures—patients who emphasize dissatisfaction with these features should be directed toward these other modalities in combination with ablative resurfacing.

As this procedure calls for considerable logistical planning, we recommend development of a practice-specific preoperative checklist (▶ Table 2.5). Showing patients photographs of the expected recovery and results is critical (▶ Fig. 2.1a–h) for informed consent and patient satisfaction. A variety of pretreatment regimens with glycolic acid, tretinoin, and hydroquinone have failed to reduce postoperative pigmentary alteration; so, we do not recommend these in our practice.[11,12] Antiviral prophylaxis is provided to all patients regardless of history of herpes simplex virus infections.[13,14] Although the evidence for antibacterial prophylaxis is mixed,[15,16] the authors prescribe antibiotics for patients undergoing full-face resurfacing as bacterial superinfection can be devastating in this setting. In the authors' practice, all patients undergoing laser resurfacing are given antiviral prophylaxis with valacyclovir 500 mg twice daily starting from the day prior to the procedure and continuing until re-epithelialization is complete, and all patients are given antibacterial prophylaxis with dicloxacillin 500 mg twice daily for 7 days starting from the day of the procedure. If a patient is on anticoagulation for medical indications, it should be continued as the risks of thromboembolism

Table 2.3 Contraindications for ablative resurfacing

Contraindication	Rationale
History of keloids or abnormal scarring	Greater scar risk
History of radiation therapy Connective tissue diseases such as scleroderma or morphea	Reduction in adnexal structures → absence of bulge stem cells → reduced ability for re-epithelialization
Isotretinoin therapy, concurrent or past 6 mo	Risk of atypical scarring or delayed healing → avoid fully ablative lasers Insufficient evidence to delay fractional ablative lasers during this time[10]
History of facelift or blepharoplasty in the past 6 mo	Altered blood circulation in undermined skin → increased risk of necrosis and scarring
Current cutaneous infection in area to be treated (bacterial or viral)	Potential for local and/or hematogenous spread

Table 2.4 Preoperative considerations for ablative resurfacing

Preoperative consideration	Action
Darker skin phototype (IV or higher)	• Caution regarding postinflammatory pigment alteration • Avoid fully ablative CO_2 resurfacing in favor of Er:YAG or fractional CO_2 • Consider a test area • Consider multiple treatments with nonablative fractional laser using conservative settings in lieu of ablative lasers
Pregnancy/nursing	Delay this elective procedure due to lack of safety data and limitations on treatment of any complications
Psoriasis, vitiligo, lichen planus	Potential for koebnerization → relative contraindication Ask about family history
Nonfacial sites such as neck, hands, chest	High risk of scarring → avoid full-field CO_2 resurfacing, caution with fractional ablative and Er:YAG lasers
Presence of ectropion	Postoperative skin tightening may exacerbate or induce ectropion
Dermatographism	Consider pretreatment with antihistamines
Smoking	Delayed wound healing; avoid smoking before procedure and during postoperative course
Acne	Consider empiric antibiotics if there is recent history of inflammatory lesions
History of herpes simplex virus	Emphasize the importance of compliance with antiviral prophylaxis, which should be offered to all patients
Rosacea	Consider combination with vascular laser; counsel patient to anticipate flare postoperatively

Table 2.5 Preoperative checklist

Presence of static fine rhytides and/or mild laxity

Review of past medical history, medications, and allergies to assess for absence of contraindications or relative contraindications detailed in ▶ Table 2.3 and ▶ Table 2.4

Review of photographs of typical healing process and typical results

Prescription of antiviral and antibacterial prophylaxis:
- Valacyclovir 500 mg twice daily to be started the day prior to the procedure and continued at least 7 d or until re-epithelialization is complete
- Dicloxacillin 500 mg twice daily for 7 d starting from the day of the procedure

Arrangement and documentation of medical risk assessment for intravenous sedation

Informed consent

Clinical photography

Arrangement of postoperative transportation home. Patients undergoing intravenous (IV) sedation will need an escort

Arrangement of home skincare supplies including provision of topical products

Scheduling of procedure and clinical follow-up visits

Provision of postoperative instruction handout

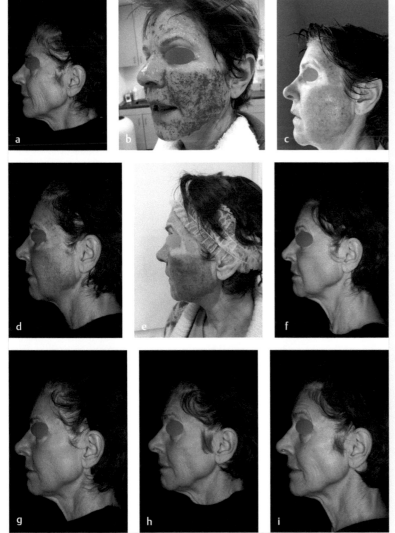

Fig. 2.1 Timeline of treatment and recovery after fractional ablative resurfacing.
(a) Baseline. **(b)** Thirty minutes postoperative appearance. **(c)** Postoperative day 1.
(d) Postoperative day 3. **(e)** Postoperative day 5. **(f)** Postoperative day 7. **(g)** Postoperative day 14. **(h)** Follow-up at 1 month.
(i) Follow-up at 3 months.

outweigh the risks of bleeding, which can be controlled during the procedure.[17]

2.5 Technique

2.5.1 Anesthesia and Pain Management

The discomfort associated with ablative procedures is considerable and a multifaceted anesthetic strategy is imperative for patient comfort especially in full-face procedures. For treatment of individualized cosmetic units, local anesthesia is often sufficient. For very superficial ablative procedures, topical anesthesia may suffice. For full-face procedures, most physicians and patients prefer intravenous (twilight) sedation with an anesthesiologist present for intraoperative monitoring and emergency equipment. In combination with intravenous sedation, the authors use a combination of topical anesthesia with EMLA (lidocaine and prilocaine) cream for 1 hour, followed by sensory nerve blockade using lidocaine 1% with 1:100,000 epinephrine and 1:10 $NaHCO_3$ 8.4%.[18] As the lateral face is not effectively targeted with nerve blocks, a multi-injector needle is used in these areas with a mixture of lidocaine 1% with epinephrine, normal saline, and $NaHCO_3$ in a 5:4:1 ratio. HCO_3 neutralizes the pH of the mixture and decreases the burning sensation during the injection. In the cases where patients opt against intravenous sedation, inhaled nitrous oxide 50%/oxygen 50%[19] is used to further ease the pain of injections.

2.5.2 Intraoperative Safety

The physician and surgical assistants should wear appropriate protection with laser safety glasses, mask, and gloves. The patient should be provided with protective eyewear as well. If treatment will be performed within the orbital rim, lubricated metal ocular shields should be inserted after administration of anesthetic drops. If applicable, the nitrous oxide device should be removed from the room before switching on the laser to limit the risk of ignition. The operative field should be kept clear of flammable materials including alcohol and aluminum chloride.

2.5.3 Operative Technique

Many aspects of the treatment are device dependent; however, some universal treatment principles apply. The topical anesthetic cream is removed and skin dried thoroughly. Hair is secured with a headband and the patient is positioned supine (▶ Fig. 2.2). Intravenous or local anesthetic is administered. The skin is prepped with chlorhexidine and completely dried. Eyelashes and eyebrows are protected with sterile lubricating jelly or a tongue

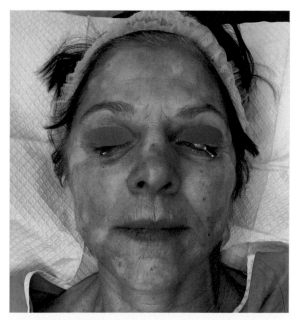

Fig. 2.2 Preoperative positioning with patient supine, headband in place, metal intraocular eye shields in place.

Table 2.6 Example settings for Fraxel re:pair CO_2 ablative fractional resurfacing

	Deeper rhytides	Lighter photodamage followed by PLLA overlay
Rest of face	70 mJ, 50%, 6 passes[a]	70 mJ, 15%, 4 passes[a]
Periocular and perioral	40 mJ, 30%, 4 passes[a] Consider using smaller tip for more precise treatment in hard-to-reach areas	Same as above (no PLLA applied to the periocular area)

Abbreviation: PLLA, poly-L-lactic acid.
[a]Actual number of passes depends on energy goals in ▶ Table 2.7.

depressor. The authors use a fractional CO_2 laser (Fraxel re:pair, Solta Medical Ltd., Hayward, California, United States), which creates microscopic treatment zones with depth of penetration determined by pulse energy. For patients with deep rhytides, we typically use an energy of 70 mJ (corresponding to a depth of 1,580 µm), density of 50% within six passes (▶ Table 2.6); however, importantly, the actual number of passes per cosmetic subunit is determined by energy delivery goals for that subunit. The 135-µm 15-mm tip is used to deliver one nonoverlapping "first pass" over the treatment area. The debris is gently wiped with distilled water–soaked gauze and

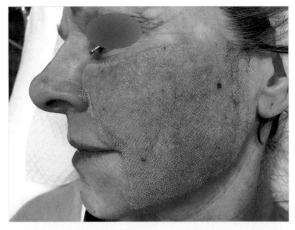

Fig. 2.3 The clinical endpoint is visible effacement of rhytides.

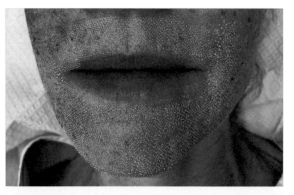

Fig. 2.4 Perioral skin is treated over the vermilion border.

dried to reveal pink partially denatured dermis. Deeper rhytides are stretched with the nondominant hand to ensure complete treatment. Subsequent passes are placed with careful attention to the total energy and the clinical endpoint of visible wrinkle effacement and pinpoint bleeding, indicating the papillary dermis has been reached (▶ Fig. 2.3). Yellow or brown color present after wiping indicates thermal injury and charring, so no further passes should be performed. The perioral and periocular skins are treated with the smaller 135-μm 7-mm tip for more precise energy delivery, using lower settings (40 mJ corresponding to a depth of 1,061 μm, 30% coverage within four passes). Perioral skin is treated over the vermilion border (▶ Fig. 2.4). The transition of the mandible to the neck is also feathered with these lower settings to prevent a sharp demarcation line. Partially desiccated tissue from the final pass is not wiped to serve as a wound dressing. Again, attention to total energy applied to each subunit is critical (▶ Table 2.7) and nonfacial sites such as the hands, neck, and chest especially merit lower energies and lower densities given the prolonged healing time and scar risk. For patients with less severe photodamage, we frequently combine a more superficial resurfacing approach with poly-L-lactic acid (PLLA) overlay (▶ Table 2.6). Immediately after a full-face procedure, the authors apply about 3 mL of a mixture of PLLA prehydrated with 8 mL of diluent 24 hours prior for laser-assisted drug delivery and enhanced neocollagenesis.[20] Although this approach has been described with lower-density ablative fractional treatments, we have also found success applying PLLA after ablation with the higher-density settings described earlier. Finally, sterile gauze soaked in distilled water is applied to the treated area for 10 to 20 minutes for hemostasis and reduction of crust formation (▶ Fig. 2.5). A postprocedure peptide serum is applied[21] and patients are provided with a nonadherent postprocedure face mask. Vital signs are documented.

Table 2.7 Authors' energy goals using Fraxel re:pair CO_2 ablative fractional resurfacing

Location	Energy goals for deeper rhytides (kJ)	Energy goals for lighter photodamage followed by PLLA overlay (kJ)
Each cheek	2–2.5	0.45
Nose and glabella	0.25–0.35	0.1
Upper cutaneous lip	0.3	0.1–0.25
Lower cutaneous lip/chin	0.35–0.5	0.2
Forehead and temples	0.8–1	0.4
Each lower eyelid	0.1–0.2	0.05 (no PLLA on eyelid)
Each upper eyelid	0.1–0.2	0.05 (no PLLA on eyelid)
Neck	1–1.8	0.25 kJ

Abbreviation: PLLA, poly-L-lactic acid.

Once the patients are oriented and ambulatory, they are discharged home with their escort.

2.6 Postoperative Instructions

Patients at the authors' practice are given a postoperative instructions handout (▶ Table 2.8) detailing expectations of recovery and home care instructions. Patients often experience significant swelling and serous exudation in the first 1 to 3 days postoperatively (▶ Fig. 2.1c). Edema is often most severe on postoperative days 2 and 3 and may be managed with ice packs, head elevation, and, if severe,

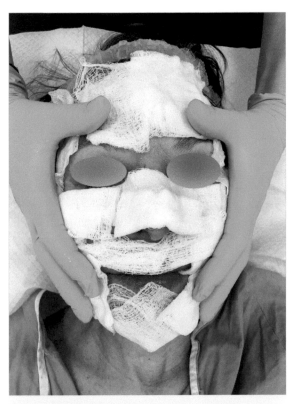

Fig. 2.5 Immediately after treatment, cool compresses made with distilled water are applied to the treatment area for 10 to 20 minutes to reduce crust formation.

Table 2.8 Example postoperative patient counseling

Patient question	Example answer
What should I expect after my laser treatment?	• The treated area may be very red and swollen • Swelling may last for 7 d or longer • Some patients experience redness for 1 mo or longer • You may experience oozing, discomfort, some bleeding, bruising, and crusting of the treated area • You may also experience peeling of the skin on days 3–5 • Postoperative healing varies from patient to patient
How should I take care of the treated area?	• Please use only distilled water until the skin is healed. You may soak the area with distilled water four times a day. You may shower and wash your hair and start using a gentle cleanser and moisturizer 24 h after your procedure • If you have any crusting or bleeding, gently dab the area with a moist gauze, pat dry, and apply gentle moisturizer • Keep the treated area moist at all times—ensure proper healing • Sleep with your head elevated—reduce swelling • You may take acetaminophen as needed for discomfort only
What should I avoid?	• Picking your skin • Wearing sunscreen or makeup until you have physician approval • Abrasive products or exfoliation for at least 4 wk • Direct contact with pets until your skin is healed • Direct or prolonged sun exposure

oral corticosteroids (prednisone 40 mg for 3 days). Cool distilled water compresses are used for wet debridement throughout the first week and reapplied frequently to keep the skin moist, followed by the application of postprocedure ointment or petrolatum or other bland healing ointment. Some physicians advocate for wound dressings for the first 1 to 3 days,[5,22,23] but the authors favor the open approach. Re-epithelialization occurs over 3 to 14 days, depending upon the laser used and the number of laser passes. Topical antibiotics are not routinely prescribed due to the high incidence of allergic contact dermatitis associated with their use. Prophylactic oral antibiotics against gram-positive bacteria are continued for a minimum of 5 days and oral antivirals are continued until re-epithelialization is complete. Acetaminophen may be used for any discomfort. During the first few weeks after the procedure, patients will often complain of pruritus, which is usually self-limited and controlled by antihistamines and mild topical corticosteroids. The authors provide patients with topical products with proprietary peptides[21] to use in the postoperative period, but bland moisturizers may also be used. Patients are scheduled for three follow-up visits with the physician during the first postoperative week to monitor healing, assess for complications, and manage expectations. At these visits, patients may receive a short treatment with intermittent pulsed low-level light-emitting diodes for photomodulation of inflammation and pain.[24,25] Patients may also undergo three facials with an aesthetician to atraumatically remove crusting and improve patient satisfaction in this first postoperative visit.

2.7 Potential Complications and Their Management

Early recognition and management of possible complications (▶ Table 2.9) is critical. Close clinical follow-up during the re-epithelialization process is imperative for this purpose.

Table 2.9 Potential complications and their management

Complication	Origin	Management of patient expectations	Medical management or protective measures
Erythema	Inflammatory response to laser → increased blood flow → erythema	Lasts an average of 1–4 mo 1 mo for Er:YAG 2 mo for CO_2 May last 12 mo posttreatment Flushing with exertion or stress may occur for 12 mo posttreatment	Expectant management Green-tinted makeup Pulsed dye laser
Dyspigmentation	Thermal injury into papillary dermis → intense erythema → resolve with postinflammatory hyperpigmentation mostly in phototypes III–VI (incidence about 36%)[26] Relative hypopigmentation of treated areas relative to photoaged surrounding areas Thermal injury deeper than papillary dermis → delayed postinflammatory hypopigmentation 6–12 mo postoperatively (incidence about 16%)	Usually seen 1 mo after treatment May last several months despite sun protection so treatment should be initiated Difficult to treat	Bleaching agents such as hydroquinone, sun protection May be avoided by treating the entire cosmetic subunit and feathering into surrounding areas Less common with ablative fractional lasers
Acneiform eruptions	Occlusive moisturizers Follicular re-epithelialization	Usually develops in first few weeks postoperatively	Standard acne treatments Manual extraction of milia
Eczematous dermatitis	Impaired barrier in resurfaced skin → increased sensitization to allergens and irritants in predisposed individuals Perioral dermatitis	Usually develops in the first few weeks postoperatively Increases the chances of erythema and postinflammatory hyperpigmentation Possible in predisposed individuals with resurfacing of perioral skin	Emollients Mid-potency topical corticosteroids Doxycycline
Infections	Removal of the skin barrier during resurfacing (epidermis and part of dermis) Presents as persistent or new-onset pain (50%), burning or itching after days 2–3 (33%), excessive yellow exudate or crusting (impetiginization), patchy intense erythema, vesicles, papules, pustules, or areas of "reversal of healing" with new erosions in areas that were previously healed[15,16]	Close clinical follow-up during re-epithelialization is imperative to monitor for infectious complications	Higher risk when more areas are ablated Risk may be minimized with prophylactic antibiotics and appropriate barrier management with topicals Antiviral prophylaxis should be provided to all patients regardless of history given prevalence of activation in patients without a known history of herpes simplex virus Low threshold to obtain bacterial, viral, and yeast cultures; initiate broad antibiotic coverage while awaiting results Consider candidiasis with pruritic intensely erythematous patchy areas
Scarring	More common with a high number of passes or excessively high fluence → excessive thermal damage Harbinger is focal tenderness and/or induration	Early initiation of treatment is key	Topical and intralesional corticosteroids, silicone gel sheeting, pulsed dye laser To minimize risk, consider multiple treatments in lieu of an overly aggressive initial treatment

2.8 Pearls and Pitfalls

The authors' clinical pearls and common pitfalls are as follows.

2.8.1 Pearls

- The key to a satisfied patient is setting appropriate expectations
- The ideal patient has only mild laxity, if any
- Manage discomfort with a multimodal approach including topical anesthesia, local nerve blocks, intravenous sedation, and/or inhaled nitrous oxide
- During treatment, attention to two factors is critical: the clinical endpoint of visible wrinkle effacement and total energy delivered per cosmetic subunit
- Off-facial sites should be treated very conservatively with low total energy, if at all. The authors prefer nonablative fractional lasers for the chest, arms, and dorsal hands
- Close clinical follow-up during the re-epithelialization period is critical
- Enhance results and patient satisfaction with "extras" like laser-assisted drug delivery of poly-L-lactic acid, postprocedure peptide serums, photomodulation, and facials
- Consider augmenting results with neuromodulators and dermal fillers once healed
- It's not all or nothing—consider combining periocular and perioral full-field ablation with fractional ablation on the rest of the face and nonablative resurfacing on the neck and chest
- This is a great skill to learn and practice, so get to know your device

2.8.2 Pitfalls

- Failing to show the patient photographs of the postoperative recovery process and expected results will lead to an unhappy patient
- Attempting to treat moderate or severe laxity that is best treated with a blepharoplasty or facelift will lead to a dissatisfied patient
- "If you pain them, you won't retain them"
- Blindly following company pre-sets without assessing the clinical endpoint and total energy delivered may lead to overtreatment and complications
- Aggressively treating off-facial sites can lead to hypertrophic scarring
- Lack of follow-up may lead to missed diagnoses of infectious complications and a missed opportunity to treat early scarring
- Patients should not feel abandoned during the recovery process, which can be quite significant depending on the depth of ablation
- Relying on only one treatment modality will not produce the same result as a multimodal approach
- Ablating too much body surface area in one treatment is a risk factor for infectious complications
- Do not let your patients miss out on this treatment because you are afraid to offer it

References

[1] Anderson RR, Parrish JA. Selective photothermolysis: precise microsurgery by selective absorption of pulsed radiation. Science. 1983; 220(4596):524–527

[2] Walsh JT, Jr, Deutsch TF. Pulsed CO_2 laser tissue ablation: measurement of the ablation rate. Lasers Surg Med. 1988; 8(3):264–275

[3] Brightman LA, Brauer JA, Anolik R, et al. Ablative and fractional ablative lasers. Dermatol Clin. 2009; 27(4):479–489, vi–vii

[4] Ross EV, Swann M, Soon S, Izadpanah A, Barnette D, Davenport S. Full-face treatments with the 2790-nm erbium:YSGG laser system. J Drugs Dermatol. 2009; 8(3):248–252

[5] Alexiades-Armenakas MR, Dover JS, Arndt KA. The spectrum of laser skin resurfacing: nonablative, fractional, and ablative laser resurfacing. J Am Acad Dermatol. 2008; 58(5):719–737, quiz 738–740

[6] Hantash BM, Mahmood MB. Fractional photothermolysis: a novel aesthetic laser surgery modality. Dermatol Surg. 2007; 33(5):525–534

[7] Manstein D, Herron GS, Sink RK, Tanner H, Anderson RR. Fractional photothermolysis: a new concept for cutaneous remodeling using microscopic patterns of thermal injury. Lasers Surg Med. 2004; 34 (5):426–438

[8] Campbell TM, Goldman MP. Adverse events of fractionated carbon dioxide laser: review of 373 treatments. Dermatol Surg. 2010; 36 (11):1645–1650

[9] Tierney EP, Eisen RF, Hanke CW. Fractionated CO_2 laser skin rejuvenation. Dermatol Ther (Heidelb). 2011; 24(1):41–53

[10] Spring LK, Krakowski AC, Alam M, et al. Isotretinoin and timing of procedural interventions: a systematic review with consensus recommendations. JAMA Dermatol. 2017; 153(8):802–809

[11] Orringer JS, Kang S, Johnson TM, et al. Tretinoin treatment before carbon-dioxide laser resurfacing: a clinical and biochemical analysis. J Am Acad Dermatol. 2004; 51(6):940–946

[12] West TB, Alster TS. Effect of pretreatment on the incidence of hyperpigmentation following cutaneous CO_2 laser resurfacing. Dermatol Surg. 1999; 25(1):15–17

[13] Nestor MS. Prophylaxis for and treatment of uncomplicated skin and skin structure infections in laser and cosmetic surgery. J Drugs Dermatol. 2005; 4(6) Suppl:s20–s25

[14] Metelitsa AI, Alster TS. Fractionated laser skin resurfacing treatment complications: a review. Dermatol Surg. 2010; 36(3): 299–306

[15] Walia S, Alster TS. Cutaneous CO_2 laser resurfacing infection rate with and without prophylactic antibiotics. Dermatol Surg. 1999; 25(11): 857–861

[16] Robertsiii T, Lettieri J, Ellis L. CO_2 laser resurfacing: recognizing and minimizing complications. Aesthet Surg J. 1996; 16(2):142–148

[17] Palamaras I, Semkova K. Perioperative management of and recommendations for antithrombotic medications in dermatological surgery. Br J Dermatol. 2015; 172(3):597–605

[18] Eaton JS, Grekin RC. Regional anesthesia of the face. Dermatol Surg. 2001; 27(12):1006–1009

[19] Brotzman EA, Sandoval LF, Crane J. Use of nitrous oxide in dermatology: a systematic review. Dermatol Surg. 2018; 44(5):661–669

[20] Ibrahim O, Ionta S, Depina J, Petrell K, Arndt KA, Dover JS. Safety of laser-assisted delivery of topical poly-l-lactic acid in the treatment of upper lip rhytides: a prospective, rater-blinded study. Dermatol Surg. 2019; 45(7):968–974

[21] Vanaman Wilson MJ, Bolton J, Fabi SG. A randomized, single-blinded trial of a tripeptide/hexapeptide healing regimen following laser resurfacing of the face. J Cosmet Dermatol. 2017; 16(2):217–222

[22] Batra RS, Ort RJ, Jacob C, Hobbs L, Arndt KA, Dover JS. Evaluation of a silicone occlusive dressing after laser skin resurfacing. Arch Dermatol. 2001; 137(10):1317–1321

[23] Alster TS, Lupton JR. Erbium:YAG cutaneous laser resurfacing. Dermatol Clin. 2001; 19(3):453–466

[24] Avci P, Gupta A, Sadasivam M, et al. Low-level laser (light) therapy (LLLT) in skin: stimulating, healing, restoring. Semin Cutan Med Surg. 2013; 32(1):41–52

[25] Alster TS, Wanitphakdeedecha R. Improvement of postfractional laser erythema with light-emitting diode photomodulation. Dermatol Surg. 2009; 35(5):813–815

[26] Ho C, Nguyen Q, Lowe NJ, Griffin ME, Lask G. Laser resurfacing in pigmented skin. Dermatol Surg. 1995; 21(12):1035–1037

3 Body Contouring

Jennifer L. MacGregor and Amanda Fazzalari

Summary

This chapter highlights the noninvasive body contouring treatment modalities available in the market today. The field of noninvasive body contouring has gained significant popularity and developed rapidly over the past decade, whereas there has been a decrease in the rate of surgical fat reduction. We evaluate the history, clinical evidence, technique, and practice pearls for multiple noninvasive fat reduction technologies, including cryolipolysis, radiofrequency, focused ultrasound, diode laser, low-level laser therapy, and other new modalities. Importantly, appropriate patient selection and counseling of expectations are key to delivering patient satisfaction.

Keywords: noninvasive body contouring, fat reduction, cryolipolysis, radiofrequency, ultrasound, laser, electromagnetic therapy

3.1 Introduction

Noninvasive body contouring is one of the most popular and advancing fields in dermatology. A recent survey from the American Society for Dermatologic Surgery (ASDS) reported noninvasive body contouring made up 57% of cosmetic procedures in 2018, up from 35% in 2014 and 50% in 2016.[1] In addition, when patients were asked to rate what bothers them about their appearance, excess fat ranked first for the sixth year in a row. On the other hand, liposuction procedures were down 30% in 2017 when compared to 2000 according to the American Society of Plastic Surgeons (ASPS) Plastic Surgery Statistics Report.[2] The shift in the treatment of unwanted fat toward more noninvasive measures over traditional surgical fat removal options is largely driven by patient desire to avoid hospitalization, general anesthesia, pain, swelling, scarring, and a prolonged recovery. This demand has led to the development of newer technologies and devices that may serve as a good alternative to traditional surgical therapies in appropriately selected patients.

Noninvasive body contouring can be performed by multiple different modalities, each with distinct biologic effects. In general, these noninvasive devices apply energy externally to the body, selectively inducing changes in the underlying adipocytes. These devices can be categorized based on the type of energy utilized. All of the treatment options available work to achieve the same end goal of adipocyte, or fat cell, apoptosis, and/or necrosis. This chapter will give an overview of and explore the evidence behind the most common noninvasive body contouring devices, including cryolipolysis, radiofrequency (RF), ultrasound (US), diode laser, and low-level laser therapy (LLLT) as well some newer technological advancements.

3.2 Modalities and Treatment Options Available

3.2.1 Cryolipolysis

Introduction

Cryolipolysis is a method of selective removal of fat based on the concept that fat cells are more sensitive to cold temperatures than the surrounding tissue. The concept of cryolipolysis originally derived from the observation of "popsicle panniculitis," a condition in which low temperatures selectively damage subcutaneous fat in the cheeks of young children while leaving skin intact.[3,4] Manstein et al took this observation and evaluated it for the clinical application of reducing areas of unwanted fat.[5] In a preclinical animal study using Yucatan pig models, they determined specific temperatures and exposures needed to trigger adipocyte apoptosis.[5] This preclinical study evaluated the effect of exposure to select cold temperatures of +20 through –7 °C for 10 minutes with histology and serum lipid levels taken at various time points up to 3.5 months. Histologic analysis from this study demonstrated approximately 80% reduction of the upper fat layer of the skin and 40% of the total fat layer thickness at 3.5 months posttreatment.[5] Histology demonstrated that selective cooling leads to an inflammatory response, which declines 90 days after treatment.[5] This initial study suggested that controlled localized surface cooling leads to biologically selective gradual fat loss via apoptosis without damaging the overlying skin.[5]

Similarly, a preclinical porcine study by Zelickson et al reported on the effects of a single session of cryolipolysis of three Yucatan pigs. Histology showed a gradual inflammatory response, or lobular panniculitis, triggered by cold-induced apoptosis that led to an overall reduction in the number of fat cells over a period of 90 days.[6] Gross pathology demonstrated a reduction of the superficial fat layer by 1 cm or 50% at 90 days. US evaluation demonstrated a decrease in the thickness of the subcutaneous fat layer by 0.6 cm or 21% over a 90-day period. Evaluation of lipid levels showed no changes.[6]

A multicenter, prospective, nonrandomized clinical study of 32 subjects treated with cryolipolysis on the flank or back demonstrated an average reduction in fat layer of 22.4% as measured by US 4 months after treatment. No device-related adverse events were reported.[7] Similarly, a small clinical study of 10 subjects who underwent a single treatment of cryolipolysis for 30 to 60 minutes on the flank demonstrated 20.4% reduction in fat thickness measured by US at 2 months and 25.5% at 6 months.[8] Weekly neurologic assessments showed cryolipolysis could result in transient reduction in sensation, which occurred in six of nine subjects. Sensation changes resolved by a mean of 3.6 weeks after treatment. Biopsy showed no long-term changes in the nerves.[8]

These preclinical and clinical results eventually led to the development of the current cryolipolysis device on the market, which was first approved by the U.S. Food and Drug Administration (FDA) in 2010 for the treatment of the flanks, and subsequently has been approved for the abdomen, thighs, upper arms, bra fat, back fat, "banana roll" (under the buttocks at the hip), and submentum. Since its initial approval, several studies have demonstrated the safety and efficacy of cryolipolysis and newly sized/shaped applicators have allowed treatment of various body other body sites.

A subsequent large, retrospective study from Europe of 518 patients with 891 total treatment areas, including flanks, abdomen, back, thighs, knees, and buttocks, demonstrated an average of 23% reduction in fat layer thickness at 3 months based on caliper measurements[9] (▶ Fig. 3.1). Garibyan et al sought to quantify the volumetric reduction of fat in the treated area using three-dimensional (3D) imaging technology and correlating it with caliper measurements. They prospectively evaluated 11 patients treated with a single cycle of cryolipolysis to one randomized flank and took 3D photography before and after 2 months. They found an average fat loss of 56.2 mL for treatment site compared to 16.6 mL in the control site, with a mean absolute difference of 39.5 mL per cycle. This correlated with caliper measurements, which showed an average reduction of treated flank from 45.6 to 38.6 mm, producing approximately 15% reduction of fat loss at 2 months.[10] Overall, 82% of patients were satisfied with the treatment results.[10] These data suggest that a single cryolipolysis treatment may result in about 40 mL of fat volume loss or 15% reduction of the flank at 2 months, which is mild compared to results of liposuction, but still results in significant patient satisfaction.[10] Of note, more fat is likely lost between 2 and 4 months posttreatment but was not measured in this study.

The effect of multiple treatments has also been evaluated. A study looking at Chinese patients in two groups, with group A receiving one treatment session on the abdomen and group B receiving two treatment sessions on the abdomen and flank an average of 3 months apart, demonstrated an average loss of 14.7% in fat layer at 2 months posttreatment using caliper measurements.[11] In addition, they found that increasing the treatment sessions improved the results, with the fat layer reduction rising by 7.2% in the abdomen and 4.3% in the flank 2 months after the last treatment.[11]

The use of cryolipolysis for areas other than the abdomen and flank has also been studied and given FDA approval. A pilot study of 11 subjects using a prototype flat cup vacuum applicator for the treatment of the inner thigh, with the contralateral thigh serving as a control, demonstrated an average of 20% fat reduction, correlating with 3.3-mm reduction, at 16 weeks based on US imaging.[12] Patient surveys revealed 91% patient satisfaction.[12] Similarly, Zelickson et al also demonstrated the efficacy of cryolipolysis using the new flat cup applicator for treating the inner thigh fat. They assessed 45 patients who underwent one treatment session for 60 minutes to bilateral inner thighs and found a 2.8-mm mean reduction in fat layer by US and 0.9-cm mean circumferential reduction in inner thigh fat at the 16-week follow-up.[13] Ninety-three percent of subjects reported being satisfied.[13] The flat cup applicator has also been used successfully for the treatment of arms.[14] A unique conformable-surface panel applicator has been shown to be effective for treatment of outer thigh fat.[15] A prospective, non-randomized, multicenter study of 40 patients demonstrated a 2.6-mm mean reduction in thigh fat thickness based on US data, with 86% patient satisfaction.[15] The submental fat has also been successfully treated with cryolipolysis and gained FDA approval.[16] A multicenter, prospective, open label study evaluated 60 subjects treated with a prototype small-volume vacuum cup applicator (CoolMini applicator, CoolSculpting System, ZELTIQ Aesthetics) in the submental area with a single session for 60 minutes with an optional second treatment at 6 weeks after the initial treatment (▶ Fig. 3.2). US imaging showed mean fat layer reduction of 2 mm, correlating with 20%

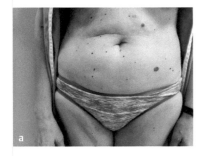 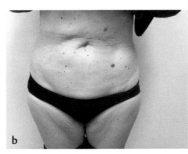

Fig. 3.1 Photograph of lower abdomen treated with one cycle of cryolipolysis showing visible and significant reduction in fat layer with improved contour **(a)** baseline **(b)** 1-month follow-up photograph of flanks treated with one cycle of cryolipolysis. (Procedure and photos courtesy of Dr. Yoon-Soo Cindy Bae at Laser & Skin Surgery Center New York.) (Procedure and photos courtesy of Dr. Yoon-Soo Cindy Bae at Laser & Skin Surgery Center New York.)

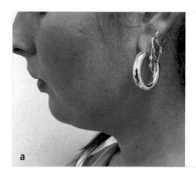
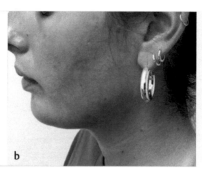

Fig. 3.2 (a, b) Baseline and 1-month post-treatment photographs after one cryolipolysis cycle of submental region with CoolMini applicator. No weight change. (Procedure and photos courtesy of Dr. Yoon-Soo Cindy Bae at Laser & Skin Surgery Center New York.)

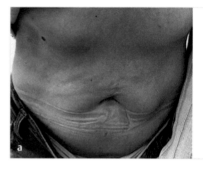
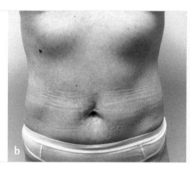

Fig. 3.3 (a, b) Baseline and 1-month follow-up demonstrates visible skin tightening and fat reduction in these baseline and 1-month postcryolipolysis treatment from one cycle to the upper abdomen. (Procedure and photos courtesy of Dr. Yoon-Soo Cindy Bae at Laser & Skin Surgery Center New York.)

reduction, and 83% patient satisfaction.[16] A subsequent study evaluated the safety and efficacy of bilateral overlapping treatments of the submental area in 14 subjects, with about 20% overlap in the center and shorter treatment duration of 45 minutes to treat the entire submental area.[17] The study found significant fat layer reduction, with caliper measurements showing a mean fat layer reduction of 2.3 mm and 3D imaging revealing a mean reduction of fat volume of 4.82 cm³ and fat thickness of 3.77 mm. Ninety-three percent of patients reported being satisfied with treatment.[17]

The modern cryolipolysis device now has newer applicators that offer shorter treatment times while preserving safety and efficacy.[18] The older devices had vacuum suction applicators that treated between two parallel cooling plates for a treatment duration of approximately 60 minutes at a temperature of –10 °C. Newer applicators have been redesigned to contour the cup applicator surface to increase tissue contact with the cooling surface with reduced skin tension, allowing for reduced treatment times of 35 minutes at a lower set temperature of –11 °C.[18] The newer applicators have shown equivalent efficacy with 40% shorter treatment times and increased patient satisfaction due to increased comfort and shorter treatment duration.[18]

Of note, immediate posttreatment manual massage has been shown to enhance the clinical results with cryolipolysis.[19] A study by Boey and Wasilenchuk compared patients receiving 2 minutes of posttreatment massage to a control group receiving standard cryolipolysis treatment only. At 2 months posttreatment, the average fat layer reduction was 68% greater on the massage side, and at 4 months, 21% greater on the massage side.[19] The study used immediate posttreatment manual massage for 1 minute applying a vigorous kneading motion followed by 1 minute of circular massage using the pads of the fingers.[12,19] Posttreatment manual massage is now common practice.

Cryolipolysis has been shown to have durable clinical effects.[20] Two case reports with long-term follow-up data showed continued improvement of treated side after 6 and 9 years.[20]

In addition to subcutaneous fat reduction, cryolipolysis has been observed to be effective for skin tightening.[21,22] A retrospective analysis by Carruthers et al of 464 cryolipolysis treatments revealed notable skin tightening of treatment areas using analysis of clinical photographs (▶ Fig. 3.3). Treatment areas in this study included outer thighs, abdomen, arms, and back. To quantify the changes in skin laxity, investigators and 14 randomly selected patients were asked to fill out surveys. Investigators and patients reported moderate to significant improvement in skin texture and laxity at an average of 2.2 months after treatment.[22] Stevens also have reported data on more than 8,000 cryolipolysis treatments and reported two patients with skin tightening of abdomen and abdomen/flank 4 months after treatment with cryolipolysis.[21] The mechanism for skin tightening has not been clearly elucidated but may be due to dermal thickening and collagen stimulation.[21]

In summary, cryolipolysis for noninvasive body contouring is safe and effective for treatment of unwanted fat in multiple body parts, with the majority of studies showing approximately 20% reduction in fat layer thickness at 3 months posttreatment. Studies suggest that multiple treatment sessions may enhance desired results and effects may be long-lasting. Robust data and consistent, reproducible results have made this technology extremely popular among providers in the medical community.

3.2.2 Radiofrequency

Introduction

Contact and noncontact RF devices have been developed to treat unwanted fat using electromagnetic energy to generate heat in tissue. Fat cells contain electrical dipoles, including positive and negative charges. Alternating electromagnetic fields cause oscillation of the electric dipoles, ultimately generating heat by friction from the movement of atoms and molecules and by the collision of conduction charges with atoms and molecules of the tissue.[23,24] Low-frequency RF waves (at 10^6 Hz) allow deeper penetration of electric field and greater distributions of heat in tissue than higher-frequency energies since the wavelengths are longer.[23] Thus, RF devices offer the opportunity for noninvasive selective heating of relatively large volumes of subcutaneous tissue.

Contact Radiofrequency Devices

Franco et al published a study in 2010 evaluating a noninvasive contact monopolar RF device (Trusculpt, Cutera, Inc., Brisbane, California, United States) to induce thermal damage to fat by creating a controlled electric field that heats fat preferentially.[25] The RF device operated at 1 MHz, a frequency at which the fat has much less attenuation of electric field than skin, and thus, the resultant heat is much greater.[25] The RF device applicator consisted of a multidimensional series of tightly spaced concentric rings that were energized at variable operational frequencies and allowed for uniform heating across the entire surface.[25] The RF applicator also utilized vacuum pressure and continuous cooling to guarantee uniform contact with skin and to further protect the outermost skin layers.[25] The study assessed cell viability of adipocyte cultures in vitro with exposures to various temperatures, ranging 45 to 65 °C for 1, 2, and 3 minutes. They also assessed immediate and delayed tissue response by measuring the clinical temperature in vivo and histology of abdominoplasty patients treated prior to or during surgery for 3 and 22 minutes.[25] The study found that the rate of cell death following exposure to heat in vitro is exponential and dependent on both temperature and length of exposure. They found that exposure to 45 °C for 1 and 3 minutes resulted in 11 and 60% cell death, respectively, whereas exposure to 50 °C for 1 and 2 minutes

resulted in 80 and 84% reduction, respectively.[25] In vivo, the temperature of subcutaneous tissue at 7- to 12-mm depth from the surface increased from 45 to 50 °C, whereas the temperature at the cutaneous level was less than 30 °C during the entire RF exposure. Acute and delayed histologic studies showed normal epidermal and dermal tissues in all biopsies. Whereas subcutaneous tissues were normal acutely, vascular changes started at day 4 and fat necrosis at 4.5- to 10-mm depth was seen starting at day 9. In addition, foamy histiocytes and granulomatous infiltrate were present within the adipose tissue at day 10, suggesting the mechanism of fat reduction as a gradual phagocytic removal of adipocytes. Of note, the lowest temperature threshold for skin damage was found to be 55.6 °C, which resulted in blistering. Temperatures greater than 60 °C were associated with transepidermal necrosis, in-depth burn, and loss of collagen.[25] Therefore, because fat sensitivity to heat is lower than that of skin, selective heating can deliver lethal thermal exposures to fat cells while preserving the overlying skin. The heat-pain threshold, or the lowest heat intensity that is detected as painful by patients, has been found to be at about 43 °C. Franco et al found that although treating adipocytes to 50 °C is safe for the overlying skin, this heat may be too painful for patients, and thus, treating at lower temperatures for longer treatment times would be more clinically applicable.[25] They suggested treating at approximately 45 °C maintained for 5 minutes, with surface skin temperatures at about 43 °C given contact cooling system.[25]

Subsequently, studies found that 2-MHz-frequency RF applicators produce more efficient thermal heating, producing +3 °C increased subdermal temperature as compared to 1-MHz-frequency RF applicators using equivalent settings of 45 °C and equivalent heating times. A small clinical study of seven patients performed by Dr. Bhatia et al and Cutera demonstrated an average of 11% reduction in fat thickness, with up to 24% reduction seen, after a single treatment with 2-MHz monopolar RF device.[26] A newer device has gotten FDA clearance for lipolysis using hands-free monopolar RF device (TruSculpt iD) using up to six 40 cm^2 hands-free handpieces simultaneously at a frequency of 2 MHz, covering up to 300 cm^2 treatment area on the abdomen and flanks in a total of 15 minutes. Clinical results from studies using this device demonstrated average fat reduction of 24%, after a single session with improvements seen 6 to 12 weeks following treatment. Preclinical and clinical data are excellent, but more robust data from a larger number of clinical treatments are needed to ensure these results are durable at longer follow-up durations. In addition, the provider must remain in the room with the patient (even when using a hands-free device) to adjust temperature according to patient comfort and ensure safety.

Noncontact Radiofrequency Devices

Noncontact multipolar RF devices are also available for noninvasive fat reduction. The current device (BLT Vanquish ME, BTL Industries Inc., Boston, Massachusetts, United States) is an operator-independent selective RF field system that heats fat without touching the patient, placed about 1 cm away from the patient. The production of heat induced by rapidly alternating electromagnetic currents that cause oscillation of the dipoles in fat is called "diathermy." The noncontact multipolar RF device utilizes short wave, high-frequency diathermy (27.12 MHz) adapted from devices used in physical therapy for deep heating of tissues.[24] The patented Energy Flow Control (EFC) system automatically tunes the device to selectively deliver energy to the adipose tissue while minimizing risk to skin, muscles, or internal organs.[24] The multipolar broad-field applicator shapes the electromagnetic field around the target area to optimize penetration to the fat layer and to maximize the treatment area. The large panels on this device is useful for targeting larger areas, including abdomen, buttock, and posterior thighs.

The use of this noncontact high-frequency RF device to target adipocytes is based on an in vivo study of porcine models.[24] The study demonstrated that it took 5 minutes to raise adipose tissue temperature to 42 °C and was able to heat adipose tissue to approximately 45 to 46 °C at 10 minutes while safely maintaining skin temperature at 42 °C. Four treatments resulted in 70% reduction of abdominal fat layer and average reduction of fat layer thickness by US of 6.9 mm.[24] Histologic studies demonstrated initial infiltration of foamy macrophages and neutrophil granulocytes with adipose disruption after the second and fourth treatments, whereas epidermal, dermal, and adnexal structures remained unaffected.[24] The terminal deoxynucleotidyl transferase dUTP nick end labeling (TUNEL) method for detecting DNA fragmentation demonstrated an increased apoptotic index (from 13/100 prior to initial treatment to 52/100 following last treatment), suggesting the fat reduction was most likely caused by an apoptotic phenomenon.[24]

The initial human study of noncontact multipolar RF device by Fajkošová et al was a prospective, nonrandomized clinical study evaluating 35 subjects with abdominal fat.[27] Subjects were treated with four 30-minute weekly treatments with Vanquish and found an average decrease in abdominal circumference of 4.93 cm, ranging from 1 to 13 cm.[27] Five subjects showed reduction of ≤ 1 cm, 14 subjects 1 to 4 cm, 9 subjects 4 to 7 cm, 3 subjects 7 to 10 cm, and 4 subjects showed over 10-cm reduction.[27] The best results were associated with subjects having a higher body mass index (BMI). In this initial study, treatment using the Vanquish RF device did not confer documented, reproducible benefit, but there were significant variations in response noted. However, the treatment was well tolerated and safe.[27]

Further studies have corroborated the safety and efficacy of noncontact field RF devices for the treatment of unwanted fat. McDaniel and Samková published a study of 30 females who underwent four weekly 30-minute treatments of bilateral inner and outer thighs (total treatment time of 1 hour) with a noncontact field RF device (BTL Vanquish Flex Applicator, BTL Industries Inc.). At 1 month of follow-up, there was a statistically significant reduction in thigh circumference, with an average circumferential reduction of bilateral thighs of 3.86 cm,[28] with no significant changes in weight. Similarly, Fritz et al performed a study on 40 female subjects treated with four weekly treatments of bilateral inner and outer thighs with the same noncontact field RF device (BTL Vanquish Flex Applicator, BTL Industries Inc.) and found a statistically significant reduction in thigh circumference of 2.43 cm at the 2-week follow-up. The treatment was associated with no pain, discomfort, or adverse events.[29]

Moradi and Palm evaluated an extended treatment protocol, performing four weekly 45-minute treatments using the BTL Vanquish to the abdomen and flanks on 24 subjects. The study demonstrated a statistically significant circumferential reduction of 4.22 cm at the 3-month follow-up visit. Lab tests, including lipids and liver function tests (LFTs), of four subjects remained unchanged at follow-up visits up to 3 months, and no study-related adverse events were reported.[30] Downie and Kaspar utilized magnetic resonance imaging (MRI) on five subjects to demonstrate the results of body contouring using noncontact RF device (BTL Vanquish ME, BTL Industries Inc.). The study found an average reduction of 5.36 mm in fat thickness on MRI at the 1-month follow-up, translating into a significant circumferential reduction.[31]

A long-term follow-up by Fritz and Salavastru collected data on 13 subjects treated with noncontact RF at 4 years after the last treatment. The average waist circumference reduction after the original study was 5.88 cm, and after 4 years, the same subjects had an average reduction of 4.42 cm compared to baseline. The waist circumference reduction was found to be statistically independent of weight change. Thus, the study found that patients preserved an average of 75.2% of the original body contouring effect after 4 years based on waist circumference.[32]

In conclusion, contact and noncontact RF treatments have been shown to have safe and effective results for body contouring. Noncontact RF treatments are associated with more variable results, and more recent data suggest favorable treatment outcome depends on baseline BMI and longer treatment protocol. It should be noted that this device delivers noncontact, operator-independent RF energy to the treatment field, but practitioners do remain in the room with the patient at all times to ensure even heat delivery occurs without surface hot spots that could compromise safety.

3.2.3 Ultrasound

Introduction

Different forms of US have been used to target unwanted fat for years and can broadly be categorized into two categories: low-intensity, low-frequency focused US and high-intensity focused ultrasound (HIFU).[33] In contrast to RF or microwave radiation devices that penetrate tissue deeply but cannot be focused easily, US can penetrate to a selected depth based on frequency and focused precisely using an external transducer.

Nonthermal Low-Intensity Focused Ultrasound

Low-intensity focused US results in mechanical, nonthermal fat reduction. It works by delivering pulsed US waves to deliver concentrated energy at a precise depth below the skin surface, targeting the subcutaneous tissue. The device produces mechanical cell membrane disruption and cavitation of adipocytes without significant temperature elevation (<0.5 °C increase), leading to fat cell lysis with sparing of adjacent blood vessels and nerves.[33]

The Ultrashape Contour I System is a noninvasive low-intensity, low-frequency focused US device currently on the market for fat reduction. It was the first focused US system launched commercially. The device includes an US transducer, a system console, and an external guidance system with real-time video tracking to direct a focused beam of US. The system emits acoustic waves of US energy at a low frequency of approximately ±200 kHz and low intensity of 17.5 W/cm^2 that converge into a confined focal volume up to 15 mm below the skin surface, targeting the subcutaneous fat at a controlled depth.[34,35,36] The video-tracking and guidance system ensures that the treatment is homogeneous throughout the treatment area. In preclinical studies, ex vivo animal skin/fat flaps (porcine) and human abdominoplasty excision specimens demonstrated the safety and efficacy of the Ultrashape system to produce fat cell lysis.[33]

Human clinical studies have further corroborated the safety and efficacy of focused US for fat reduction. Tietalbaum et al demonstrated in a multicenter, controlled clinical trial that a single treatment with Ultrashape Contour I device resulted in a mean reduction of approximately 2.9 mm in skin fat thickness measured at 28 days and approximately 2 cm in the treatment area circumference at 12 weeks after treatment of abdomen, thighs, or flanks.[35] They found that the majority of changes was achieved within 2 weeks and sustained at the 12-week follow-up.[35]

Increased treatment sessions resulted in superior results.[36] Moreno-Moraga et al treated 30 healthy subjects with three treatments at 1-month intervals, with treatment areas including abdomen, inner and outer thighs, flanks, inner knees, and breasts (in males only). This study showed significant reduction in fat thickness, with a mean reduction of 2.28 ± 0.8 cm, and in circumference, with a mean reduction of 3.95 ± 1.99 cm after three treatments.[36]

A subsequent study found that shorter treatment intervals, with three treatment sessions every 2 weeks, had similar results.[34] Treatments were performed in the abdominal region and demonstrated a mean midline circumference reduction of 2.47 cm on day 14 after the first Contour I treatment, 3.51 cm on day 56 (4 weeks after the third treatment), and 3.58 cm on day 112 (12 weeks after the third treatment). The peak midline circumference reduction was 3.12 cm on day 112. A majority of patients (63%) reported a positive change in body contour.[34]

In another large, controlled multicenter clinical study, 150 subjects presenting with excess subcutaneous fat deposits in the abdominal region were randomly assigned to two groups. Group 1 underwent a 4-week control phase before undergoing three abdominal fat reduction treatments at 2-week intervals, while group 2 underwent immediate treatment for a total of three treatment sessions. The study results found a mean reduction in the midline circumference at week 22 of 2.5 ± 2.1 cm in group 1 (12 weeks after the third treatment) and 3.5 ± 2.7 cm in group 2 (18 weeks after the third treatment). In addition, the effect of multiple treatments was found to be cumulative, demonstrating a continued, steady decrease in abdominal circumference after successive treatments and during follow-up up to week 22.[37] These results are consistent with the prior study by Ascher that reported an average of 3.5-cm reduction in circumference after three treatments at 2-week intervals, with a steady decrease in circumference at day 112 of follow-up.[34]

Another study of 46 healthy subjects treated with focused US using the small 12-g transducer on the Ultrashape Contour I V3.1 system for fat reduction in a randomized flank compared with untreated flank found a mean fat thickness reduction of 2.2 mm by US measurement at the 16-week follow-up.[38] Treatment was associated with little or no discomfort.[38]

Further, a combination treatment of focused US and RF may be effective and safe for fat reduction. A study based out of Hong Kong evaluated the use of a second-generation nonthermal focused US device with combined RF handpiece in 17 subjects who underwent three treatments biweekly.[39] The study found statistically significant improvement of abdominal circumference and caliper measurements at 2 weeks post second treatment and follow-up visits.[39]

Another study of 32 Asian patients who underwent three consecutive treatments with combined focused US and RF at 2-week intervals resulted in a statistically significant reduction in mean abdomen circumference of 3.91 cm and fat thickness reduction of 21.4 and 25% of the upper and lower abdomen, respectively, based on MRI measurements.[40] A long-term follow-up study from the same treatment group found no statistically significant change in mean abdominal circumference change over a 1-year follow-up period.[41] These studies suggest the addition of RF treatment before and after focused US may prime the target tissue and enhance the desired results.[40]

Very few comparative studies exist between noninvasive body contouring devices. One study looked to compare the effects of focused US and cryolipolysis on localized abdominal fat.[42] In this study, 60 subjects with BMI > 30 kg/m² were randomly assigned to three groups, using focused US and diet, cryolipolysis and diet, and diet alone. The US device used was the Proslimelt device (Promoitalia, Naples, Italy), 30 to 70 kHz, 45-mm transducer, 3 W/cm², with 30-minute treatment sessions every 2 weeks for 2 months, whereas the Zeltiq (Zeltiq Aesthetics, Pleasanton, California, United States) Cooling Intensity Factor (CIF) 42 for 30 minutes every 2 weeks for 2 months was used for cryolipolysis.[42] The study found that all three groups showed significant improvements in waist circumference and suprailiac skinfold after 2 months, and the US and cryolipolysis treatment groups showed better posttreatment improvement than the diet-only group.[42] There were no statistically significant differences in waist circumference or suprailiac skinfold between the US and cryolipolysis groups.[42] The focused US group found waist circumference reduction of 7.3 cm and skinfold reduction of 5.58 mm, whereas the cryolipolysis group found waist reduction of 6.75 cm and skinfold reduction of 5.3 mm after 2 months.[42] In contrast, the diet group saw a 3.2-cm waist reduction and 2.47-mm skinfold reduction. Of note, there were significant limitations to this comparative study. First, the outcome measurements were crude, as waist circumference measurements are open to error. Second, the focused US device used in this study was different from those available in the United States and treatment protocols used were different from those recommended by the manufacturer. In addition, the follow-up was only 2 months from the last treatment, whereas it has been shown that improvement can be seen up to 3 to 4 months posttreatment with cryolipolysis, thereby underestimating the benefit of cryolipolysis.

In conclusion, low-intensity focused US is a safe and effective method of fat reduction, with most studies consistently demonstrating approximately 3- to 4-cm waist circumference reduction 3 months after three treatments in series.

High-Intensity Focused Ultrasound

In contrast to nonthermal fat reduction, HIFU instead uses focused high-frequency, high-energy US to induce high temperatures and subsequent thermal fat reduction via coagulative necrosis and cell death. At high frequencies (> 2 MHz), US energy is convergent, resulting in focused tissue damage.[43] HIFU applies focused beams of high-power US to ablate targeted tissue and thermally modify collagen through a so-called thermomechanical process. The US energy produces microscopic vibrations and frictional heating at a focal point.[43,44] The rapid heating to a temperature of greater than 56°C in 1 to 2 seconds results in instantaneous thermal coagulative necrosis, causing cell death within the target tissue without affecting overlying skin or surrounding tissues.[45] Given the high precision and reproducibility of tissue ablation, HIFU has been studied for multiple clinical applications, including oncology, neurosurgery, urology, gynecology, and ophthalmology.[45]

A device utilizing HIFU technology (LipoSonix; Medicis Technologies Corporation, Bothell, Washington, United States) has been shown to be safe and effective in the noninvasive reduction of adipose tissue for body contouring.[46] The amount of energy delivered on this HIFU device can be adjusted by varying the peak power and duration of emitted energy. For body sculpting, the thermal HIFU device uses an external transducer rather than a transcutaneous probe, and uses ultrasonic waves at a frequency of 2 MHz with an intensity exceeding 1,000 W/cm² at the focal point of the transducer.[47]

Initial preclinical studies in a porcine model demonstrated that application of HIFU energy at energy levels of 166 to 372 J/cm² generated tissue temperatures approaching 70°C for 1 to 2 seconds at a focal depth of 15 mm, which was sufficient to produce tissue coagulative necrosis of subcutaneous adipose tissue.[48] Adjacent tissue and overlying skin had minimal temperature change. Histological examination demonstrated adipose tissue disruption with well-demarcated borders, consistent with thermomechanical disruption of US energy, and no injury was observed to intervening nerves or arterioles within the path of the HIFU beam.[48] In addition, collagen within the focal zone also showed evidence of contraction and thickening.[48] Pathological specimens demonstrated mild local inflammatory response with gradual resorption of adipose tissue by macrophages via lymphatic vessels.[48] Following treatment, no abnormalities in solid organs or blood parameters, including plasma lipids and LFTs, were observed in the porcine model. Thus, preclinical models demonstrated safe and effective fat disruption and collagen thickening consistent with the thermomechanical properties of focused US.

Subsequently, 3 pilot studies including 152 subjects who presented for elective abdominoplasty were performed with total HIFU energy doses ranging from 47 to 331 J/cm² to evaluate the safety of HIFU prototype device.[44] These studies demonstrated that HIFU effects were limited to the subcutaneous adipose tissue. Histologic specimens revealed well-demarcated disruption of adipocytes in the targeted region at the expected depth, with phagocytosis of released lipids and cellular debris by macrophages occurring after 14 to 28 days. Of note, the removal of lipids and cellular debris occurred gradually over a period of weeks, and healing was 95% complete after 8 to 14 weeks. Thickened collagen consistent with the thermal effects of HIFU was also observed.[44] Changes did not extend into the skin or fascia.[44] There were no significant changes in clinical laboratory parameters, including lipid levels. Adverse events included temporary treatment discomfort, edema, erythema, dysesthesia, and ecchymosis.[44]

A retrospective chart review of 85 subjects who underwent a single HIFU treatment with the LipoSonix system using a mean energy level of 134.8 J/cm^2 and a focal depth of 1.1 to 1.6 cm demonstrated an average waist circumference decrease of 4.6 cm after 3 months.[49]

A larger, randomized sham-controlled trial evaluated 180 patients with subcutaneous abdominal fat ≥ 2.5 cm thick who received HIFU treatment of the anterior abdomen and flanks at three different energy levels with a total of three passes, including 47 J/cm (141 J/cm total), 59 J/cm (177 J/cm), or 0 J/cm (sham control).[46] The study found statistically significant reduction of waist circumference at 12 weeks in the 59 J/cm active treatment group with an average of 2.44-cm reduction.[46] Temporary side effects included mild-to-moderate discomfort, bruising, and edema.[46] Long-term safety data found no reports of scars, burns, or clinically meaningful changes in lipid panel, inflammatory markers, or renal and hepatic function.[47]

A randomized, single-blinded postmarketing study conducted in Canada evaluated 45 subjects who received a single treatment with three passes of HIFU at energy levels of 47 J/cm^2 (141 J/cm^2 total), 52 J/cm^2 (156 J/cm^2), or 59 J/cm^2 (177 J/cm^2) to the anterior abdomen at varying skin depths per pass (1.6, 1.3, and 1.1 cm).[50] This study found that HIFU treatment at all three energy levels and at multiple tissue depths significantly reduced the waist circumference and was generally well tolerated.[50] The mean waist circumference reduction at week 12 of all treatment groups combined was 2.51 cm, with no statistically significant difference between the three energy levels. There was continuous improvement over the three follow-up visits up to week 12.[50] The Global Aesthetic Improvement Scale (GAIS) was rated as improved or much improved in 69 to 86% by patients and 73 to 79% by investigators at week 12. The mean rating of worst pain experienced during the treatment was mild.[50]

Two other postmarketing, multicenter randomized unblinded studies evaluated a single treatment of HIFU (LipoSonix system) of the abdomen or abdomen and flanks using five different treatment protocols with total energy doses ranging between 150 and 180 J/cm^2, with either 30 or 60 J/cm^2 delivered per pass, and with two fixed treatment techniques, grid repeat (GR) and site repeat (SR).[51] In the GR method, each treatment site was treated with a fraction of the total treatment dose by one pass of the single transducer (i.e., 60 of 180 J/cm^2) and passed sequentially through all the treatment sites, before repeating the sequence. In contrast, the SR method

involved treating a single site with multiple passes before moving to the subsequent site. In this study, 118 subjects were treated with one of the five treatment protocols and demonstrated a statistically significant mean reduction of 2.3 cm in waist circumference at 12 weeks for all subjects.[51] The mean reduction in waist circumference was statistically significant for all individual treatment groups, ranging from 1.9- to 3.1-cm reduction at week 12, with no statistically significant differences between the treatment groups in primary endpoint. Waist circumference reductions were seen starting as early as week 4. Patients in the 30 J/cm^2 per pass treatment protocols experienced significantly lower pain scores than the 60 J/cm^2 treatment protocols. This study highlighted that both low-fluence (30 J/cm^2 per pass) and high-fluence (60 J/cm^2 per pass) HIFU treatments delivered in a GR or SR method result in significant abdominal fat reduction of greater than 2 cm, similar to prior studies, with low-fluence treatment groups having better treatment tolerability and higher-fluence groups trending toward greater improvements (not statistically significant).[51]

A study of 12 Chinese patients with adipose thickness of at least 2.5 cm treated with one session of HIFU to the abdomen with total fluence of 150 to 165 J/cm^2 and a mean total fluence of 161 J/cm^2 found statistically significant improvement in waist circumference at 4, 8, and 12 weeks posttreatment. The average decrease of waist circumference was 1 cm at the 12th week follow-up.[52] The study found the higher the total fluence delivered, the larger the decrease in waist circumference.[52] In conclusion, all studies on HIFU to date have consistently demonstrated reduction in abdominal circumference of greater than 2 cm from a single HIFU treatment. It is unclear if increased treatment number would give more significant benefits in fat reduction.

In summary, HIFU is a safe and effective technology for reducing adipose tissue without significant effects on surrounding tissue or blood lipid levels. The majority of studies on the clinical application of HIFU for body contouring demonstrates approximately 1 to 3 cm of waist circumference reduction. However, HIFU has become less popular recently with the advent of nonthermal low-intensity US treatment, which tends to be less painful with similar or superior clinical benefit.

3.2.4 Diode Laser

Based on published studies of absorption spectrum of biologic tissues, fat absorption peaks around 900 to 1,064 nm.[53,54] The 1,060- to 1,064-nm wavelength is efficient at delivering laser energy to the subcutaneous tissue while having low affinity for melanin, making it safe to treat all skin types.[55] This wavelength is also able to penetrate to an appropriate depth to target adipocytes, while being safe to treat darker skin types.[53,56] The concept of direct targeting of adipose tissue by lasers, also known as laser lipolysis, was first pioneered by Apfelberg in 1992, when laser lipolysis was used as an adjunct to traditional surgical liposuction.[57] The preliminary investigation using yttrium aluminum garnet (YAG) optical fiber within the liposuction cannula found no clear benefit and was, thus, not approved by the FDA.[57] Subsequent studies demonstrated that laser-assisted liposuction with direct contact of laser energy at 1,064 nm using an optical fiber with adipose tissue results in adipocyte lysis by thermal damage.[54,55,58,59,60] The U.S. FDA approved the 1,064-nm neodymium:yttrium aluminum garnet (Nd:YAG) laser in October 2006 for surgical incision, excision, vaporization, ablation, and coagulation of all soft tissues for the use in laser-assisted lipolysis.[61] Laser-assisted liposuction led to superior fat reduction, decreased blood loss and ecchymoses, and improved skin tightening as compared to liposuction alone.[54,59,60] Given the success of laser-assisted liposuction, investigators have evaluated fat loss using 1,064-nm Nd:YAG laser lipolysis alone with a 300-μm fiber, without adjunctive liposuction.[61]

For clinical application of laser lipolysis for noninvasive fat reduction, an external device is required. Given that thermal injury is the mechanism of action of laser lipolysis, it is important to minimize risk of overheating the overlying skin.[62] With evidence backed by in vivo and clinical studies, a 1,060-nm diode laser with contact cooling at 15 °C (SculpSure, Cynosure, Inc., Westford, Massachusetts, United States) was the first and only hyperthermic laser FDA cleared in 2015 for noninvasive body contouring of the abdomen, flanks, and thighs with expansion of indication to the submental area in 2017.[63] The current 1,060-nm diode laser device employs four applicator heads joined to create a rectangular zone of thermal radiation of approximately 140 or 35 cm^2 per applicator. Each applicator contains a water-cooled sapphire window that applies direct contact cooling at 15 °C throughout the treatment. Treatment time is set at 25 minutes with power density of 0.9 to 1.4 W/cm^2.[56,64]

The 1,060-nm diode laser leads to injury of the adipocytes through direct heating of the tissue.[63,64] Decorato et al was the first to investigate the histologic and clinical effects of hyperthermic diode laser to adipocytes in the abdominal region. The in vivo study of abdominoplasty patients demonstrated that the 1,060-nm laser device with surface cooling achieved and maintained hyperthermic temperature target of 42 to 47 °C at the subcutaneous adipose tissue level.[64] At this hyperthermic temperature, the lipid bilayer of cell membranes of adipocytes lose their structural integrity, leading to delayed cell death. Hyperthermically damaged adipocytes are removed through the body's natural mechanisms. Histologic studies demonstrate inflammation, followed by macrophage infiltration at approximately 2 weeks posttreatment, with removal of cellular debris completed and new collagen deposition seen at 6 months.[72] Clinical results in six subjects demonstrated average fat reduction of 14, 18, and 18% at 2, 3, and 6 months, respectively.[62] MRI measurements demonstrated 24 and 21% average fat volume reduction at 3 and 6 months, respectively. Blinded photo evaluation showed improvement starting at 1 month posttreatment and maintained at 6 months.[64] Of note, treatment times longer than 30 minutes were associated with a risk of developing palpable nodules in the subcutaneous fat, whereas treatment times less than 20 minutes had minimal effect.[64] The optimal treatment time has been found to be 25 minutes, and the standard power used for this device is 1.1 W/cm^2, which can be adjusted according to patient feedback.[56,64] Initial clinical studies by Decorato found comparable results between hyperthermic laser lipolysis and cryolipolysis in four patients treated on either flank, with 1,060-nm laser leading to 24% reduction in fat volume and cryolipolysis leading to 22% reduction measured by US and MRI.[64]

In a multicenter prospective, randomized controlled study, 49 subjects treated with a single laser treatment to one flank demonstrated statistically significant average fat reduction of 9% at 6 weeks and 14% at 12 weeks posttreatment based on US measurements.[56] The average fat reduction was calculated to be 2.6 mm by US images, and 96% of patients were satisfied with the treatment at week 12. Treatment was generally well tolerated with treatment discomfort the most common adverse event. Other side effects included transient edema and erythema, resolving within 4 to 6 days and tenderness, which resolved within 1 to 2 weeks.[56]

Similarly, a prospective study of 35 subjects who underwent treatment with 1,060-nm laser on the abdomen demonstrated an average reduction in fat layer thickness of 16% (2.65 mm) at 12 weeks posttreatment, with side effects being mild to moderate edema, tenderness, and induration resolving within 1 to 3 weeks posttreatment.[65]

Another study found that fat reduction was maintained at 6 months of follow-up, with mean fat reduction of 4.31 and 2.72 mm of the flanks and abdomen, respectively.[66] Patients may undergo multiple treatment sessions, spaced at least 4 weeks apart, to achieve additional results.[67] Given that this technology is relatively new, additional studies are needed in determining long-term effects of the laser treatment, the efficacy of multiple treatments, and comparative effects to other noninvasive body contouring devices.

3.2.5 Low-Level Laser Therapy

LLLT is defined as the application of low-irradiancy laser light (1–5 W/cm^2) to achieve therapeutic results without thermal effects. LLLT has been used widely in multiple medical fields for the reduction of pain, tissue inflammation, tissue damage, and promotion of wound healing.[68] LLLT was first used as an adjunct to liposuction in 2000.[69] The initial preclinical study by Neira et al used a 635-nm,

10-mW diode laser using a dose that caused no detectable temperature increase in the tissue.[69] LLLT produces transient pores in the cell membrane, releasing stored fat content within the adipocytes and resulting in deflation or "liquefaction" of adipocytes.[69]

LLLT received FDA clearance in 2010. There are multiple LLLT devices currently out on the market.[68] The Zerona Lipolaser (Erchonia Medical, Inc.) works at a wavelength of 635 nm and has four adjustable arms each emitting 17 mW. The Lipo Laser (Mimari, Poland) has six panels measuring 8 × 16 cm that contain 100-mW diodes at a wavelength of 650 nm,[70] whereas the Meridian LAPEX 2000 LipoLaser System (Meridian Medical Inc., Anyang, Korea) is a 635- to 680-nm LLLT device.[71] Treatment may involve six to eight sessions, lasting approximately 20 to 30 minutes per session.[71,72] Clinical studies for LLLT in fat reduction have shown conflicting results.[70,71,72]

A multicenter randomized, placebo-controlled trial of 67 overweight subjects with BMI of 25 to 30 kg/m^2 who were treated with six laser treatments using a 635-nm LLLT with 2.5-mW power device (Zerona lipolaser) over a period of 2 weeks found a mean reduction of 2.5 cm in waist circumference, 2.7 cm across the hip, and 1.6 to 2.1 cm across each thigh compared to baseline.[72] A retrospective study by the same group collected data from 689 patients, demonstrating statistically significant mean circumferential reduction for the waist, hips, and thighs.[73] A second randomized, placebo-controlled trial of 40 subjects who received twice weekly treatments for 4 weeks using 635- to 680-nm LLLT (Meridian LAPEX 2000 lipolaser system, Meridian medical Inc.) found statistically significant cumulative waist circumference reduction of 2.15 cm, with approximately 0.4- to 0.5-cm loss per treatment.[71] In vitro studies showed that LLLT increases fat loss from adipocytes by release of triglycerides, without lipolysis or cell lysis.[71] A more recent randomized split-abdomen controlled study evaluating 24 subjects who underwent six treatments 2 to 3 days apart using 650-nm LLLT did not find a statistically significant reduction of abdominal adipose tissue at 2 weeks posttreatment.[70]

In conclusion, although initial studies suggested LLLT may be an effective body contouring method, the results are conflicting. Although LLLT may still be used among aesthetic centers and spas, it is not favored in the medical and dermatology communities given that early clinical studies have not been reproducible and effects may not be durable.

3.2.6 Newer Treatment Modalities

High-Intensity Focused Electromagnetic Therapy

The majority of noninvasive fat reduction procedures in aesthetic medicine to date primarily target subcutaneous fat, but a novel device using High-Intensity Focused Electromagnetic (HIFEM) therapy pursues body contouring by targeting the underlying musculature, thereby contributing to a firm, toned appearance.[74] HIFEM technology is based on electromagnetic muscle stimulation, which has previously been used for muscle training. The current device (EMSCULPT device, BTL Industries Inc., Marlborough, Massachusetts, United States) has a circular coil that generates an intense alternating magnetic field of up to 1.8 T, which induces a secondary high-magnitude electric current in the underlying tissue, where it interacts with and activates motor neurons. The electromagnetic pulses are delivered at a high frequency, in which muscles are continuously stimulated and prohibited from muscle relaxation, referred to as supramaximal or tetanic contractions.[74]

The clinical effect of HIFEM technology was first studied for this indication in porcine models.[74] Porcine models were treated with a single session of HIFEM for 30 minutes. The initial study determined that the high-frequency oscillating magnetic field affects the motor nerves, causing supramaximal muscle contraction, which leads to increased intracellular concentrations of free fatty acids (FFA). This results in a stress-induced apoptotic response in adipocytes. Histology demonstrated statistically significant increase in fat cell apoptosis with no associated inflammatory response.[74]

A prospective, multicenter, nonrandomized pilot study evaluated 22 subjects treated with HIFEM (EMSCULPT) applied to the abdomen for 30 minutes with a total of four treatment sessions at 2- to 5-day intervals. MRI analysis from this study found a statistically significant average reduction of 18.6% in adipose tissue thickness with 15.4% increase in rectus abdominis muscle thickness and 10.4% reduction in rectus abdominis separation at 2 months posttreatment.[75] MRI data of four selected patients who were followed up at 6 months posttreatment suggest continued improvement in muscles in the long term. Waist circumference measured at the subumbilical level demonstrated an average of 3.8-cm reduction.[75] No adverse events occurred. The only side effect reported was mild muscle soreness 1 day after treatment, which resolved within 24 hours.[75]

Another small clinical study of 19 patients who underwent four treatments on the abdomen with HIFEM for 30 minutes, spaced by 2 to 3 days, demonstrated waist reduction of 4.37 cm at 3 months of follow-up. In addition, about 91% patients reported improvement in abdominal appearance and 92% reported satisfaction with treatment.[76] Muscle fatigue was a frequent side effect that resolved within 12 to 48 hours. No adverse events were reported in this study.[76] The results of these initial clinical studies are promising, and larger, controlled clinical studies are warranted.

In conclusion, HIFEM is a safe and effective device for concurrent improvement in muscle tone and unwanted fat, with temporary muscle fatigue as the most common side effect. Although follow-up of 6 months suggested continued improvement, it is still unclear what maintenance treatment regimen will be required to preserve the initial benefits. Longer follow-up studies for HIFEM are warranted to determine the durability of response, best maintenance regimen, and practicality of long-term use in the clinical setting.

3.3 Indications

Noninvasive body contouring procedures are indicated for the treatment of unwanted localized subcutaneous fats that are resistant to diet and exercise. Noninvasive body contouring is not a substitute for exercise and diet, but can be used as an adjunct. Noninvasive body contouring is not indicated as a treatment of visceral fat or obesity. In general, noninvasive body contouring is safe in all skin types.

Of note, noninvasive body contouring is not a "one-device-fits-all" endeavor. The decision on which noninvasive body contouring device to use is tailored to the needs of each individual patient. Preoperative measurements of fat volume should be employed, including photographs, body weight and circumference measurements, feeling for "pinchable fat," and possibly US measurements to determine the location and depth of fat. The authors frequently quantity fat volume over the anatomical target area to adequately target treatment area/depth by using different devices where appropriate. For example, patients with a small area of pinchable fat localized to the flanks may be good candidates for cryolipolysis. Patients with greater than 2.5 cm subcutaneous fat depth over the general abdomen area may be better candidates for low-intensity focused US, whereas patients with 1- to 1.5-cm fat depth may be better candidates for RF-based treatments.

3.4 Patient Selection, Contraindications, Preoperative Considerations

3.4.1 Patient Selection

Although noninvasive body contouring procedures have been found to be safe and effective in the reduction of subcutaneous fat, it is important to select the appropriate candidates to achieve optimal results. There is no age limitation for noninvasive body contouring procedures mentioned in the literature.[77,78] Noninvasive body contouring procedures are safe in all skin types. The optimal candidate for noninvasive body contouring procedures is relatively fit with localized areas of adiposity, close to ideal body weight and without current large shifts in body weight. Patients should be realistic about their expectations and willing to maintain the results of these

noninvasive procedures post-treatment with a healthy, active lifestyle.[77] Noninvasive procedures are not an indication for obese patients or for visceral fat.[75] Patients should have realistic expectations of mild to modest reduction of localized fat.

Specific considerations depend on the type of treatment. For cryolipolysis, patient should have treatable pockets or bulges of localized fat that fit the applicators available.[78] For best results, a minimum of 2.5 cm of fat should be drawn into the cup,[79] or at least "an inch to pinch" in the target area on initial examination. For US-based fat reduction, the clinician should assess fat thickness, and a minimum of 1.5 cm of fat is generally needed for efficacy. This is because US fat reduction devices focus energy to a depth of 1.5 cm. On the other hand, RF-based treatments can safely target thinner fat layers with penetration depths closer to 1 cm.

3.4.2 Contraindications

General contraindications include pregnancy, cardiac pacemaker or defibrillator, abdominal hernias with abdominal treatments, the presence of malignant tumors within the treatment area, or being medically unwell. Body contouring procedures should not be performed in areas with active dermatitis, severe varicose veins, open or infected wounds, or other cutaneous conditions.[80]

In addition, cryolipolysis is contraindicated in patients with cold-sensitive conditions, including cryoglobulinemia, cold agglutinin disease, paroxysmal cold hemoglobinuria, and cold urticaria.[80] Other relative contraindications cited in the literature include cold sensitivities, like Raynaud's disease, pernio, or chilblains, impaired peripheral circulation in the area to be treated, nerve disorders like diabetic neuropathy, chronic pain, and anxiety disorder.

Contraindications of RF treatments also include the presence of pacemakers, defibrillators, metal implants, or tattoos in the treatment area.

LLLT contraindications included light-sensitizing medications, undergoing photodynamic therapy, or diuretics.

3.4.3 Preoperative Considerations

With all body contouring procedures, it is important to get informed consent, take standardized before-and-after photographs, record baseline and follow-up body weights, and make circumference measurements. Careful assessment and patient education is crucial prior to the procedure. Of note, it is common in our practice to take photos of the treatment both before and at the end of each treatment session to document the immediate tissue effects and the exact treatment area location for future evaluation, treatment, and patient counseling at follow-up.

3.5 Technique

3.5.1 Cryolipolysis

The current FDA-approved cryolipolysis device on the market has cooling panels with or without a vacuum suction, heat extracted according to CIF. The device has multiple system applicators allowing the treatment of numerous body areas, including abdomen, arms, knees, inner thighs, hips, back, axillae, and anterior and lateral submental neck. System applicators including CoolMax, CoolCore, CoolCurve, Coolfit, and CoolMini utilize vacuum suction, whereas CoolSmoothPRO utilizes a surface applicator with three panels and without vacuum. Older devices previously had longer treatment times, but more efficient devices have since come on the market.[18] Previously, standard applicators cooled to –10 °C for 60-minute cycles, but an equivalent protocol using –11 °C for 35 minutes (45 minutes for CoolMax) has been found.[18] In addition, CoolSmooth applicators utilized controlled cooling to –10 °C for 120 minutes, but equivalent current protocol has been found using –13 °C for 75 minutes. Thus, the current device has a range of treatment times depending on the area treated (ranging from 35 mins to 1.15 h). Treatment of multiple areas at once is also safe and effective.[81]

Prior to attaching the system applicator, the treatment area is marked out, cleaned with a treatment wipe, and an adhesive pad is applied for most of the available applicators. The Rayon- and spandex-based adhesive pads are sturdy, withstanding peeling, pulling, and tugging. They have improved adhesions, stabilizing the placement of the applicator on the treatment area. In the case of Coolmini, an applicator gel is applied instead of an adhesive pad to treatment area. Velcro straps and pillows may be used to help support the applicator and the patient comfort during the treatment duration.

After the treatment cycle is over, the treated area should be manually massaged to aid in reperfusion injury and increase efficacy of treatment.[18,82] Other strategies to enhance reperfusion injury may be heating pad, shockwave therapy, topical agents, and/or combination with other energies. The authors recommend taking immediate posttreatment photographs in order to document the posttreatment appearance and exact treatment size for future reference.

3.5.2 Radiofrequency

Treatment with the Trusculpt monopolar RF device typically takes anywhere between 15 and 60 minutes and may require multiple treatments. The treated area does not require a coupling or cooling fluid. The transducer is applied to the treatment area directly over the thin film coating, and there is a feeling of heat or warmth during the treatment. In the newest system, treatment has evolved from operator placed spot treatment applicator to a larger "hands-free" application delivering energy to six-electrode applicators over a single 15-minute treatment cycle. The operator must still be present throughout the entire 15-minute cycle to titrate the electrode temperature based on patient feedback.

The Vanquish system is a contactless RF device that treats unwanted fat in an average of four weekly 30-minute treatments, based on the standard treatment protocol by the manufacturer. It is a hands-free conformable device with a multipolar applicator panel that emits RF. The applicator is placed approximately 1 cm above the skin. The operator adjusts the energy in real time based on patient's feedback and tolerability during the treatment. Thus, despite being "hands free" or contactless, the operator must still be present throughout the entire treatment for safety to ensure that no hot spots or burns occur.

3.5.3 Ultrasound

The Ultrashape Contour I system consists of several subsystems. The main system console and stand contain the computer, which controls the device performance. The therapeutic ultrasonic transducer includes an acoustic contact feedback sensor and delivers the focused US energy. A real-time video tracking and guidance system guides the operator through the treatment in order to focus the energy homogeneously within the designated area.[34] The patient lies supine with arms under the head or at the sides during the treatment with the marked treatment area exposed. Blue drapes are placed outside the treatment area. Supplied colored markers are adhered to the blue drapes, with at least six markers being used for each treatment. A coupling liquid is applied to the skin before and during treatment. The tracking and guidance system allows activation of energy delivery only when the transducer is accurately positioned within the treatment area, and the transducer must be moved over the treatment area until the "end of treatment."[34] Patients typically receive a total of three treatments every 2 weeks.

3.5.4 Diode Laser

The diode laser system is versatile and conformable with nonsuction flat applicators that can be applied in a variety of configurations. Adequate contact of the applicators with the skin is needed, and the total length of treatment is 25 minutes, with 4 minutes to achieve high temperature of 42 to 47 °C, followed by a 31-minute period of cooling/heating cycles. It is the authors' opinion that the provider should remain in the treatment room to monitor the patient for all of the aforementioned heat-based technologies.

3.5.5 Low-Level Laser Therapy

There are multiple types of LLLT currently out on the market with different setups.[68]

3.6 Postoperative Instructions

There is typically no significant downtime for noninvasive body contouring procedures, making it a good alternative to more invasive surgical procedures in appropriately selected candidates. There are also no activity limitations after these noninvasive body contouring procedures.

3.7 Potential Complications and Management

3.7.1 Cryolipolysis

Side effects associated with cryolipolysis are typically minor. Common side effects of cryolipolysis include immediate temporary erythema, bruising, swelling, pain, numbness, and paresthesias.[80] These side effects are generally resolved within a few weeks after treatment.[78] Incidence of postinflammatory hyperpigmentation has been reported to range from 0 to 8.8%,[9,38] with reported cases resolving after a few months.[83] Lipid levels and LFTs are not affected by cryolipolysis.[84] Cryolipolysis has also been associated with delayed-onset pain, characterized by stabbing, burning, or shooting pain, with an incidence of up to 15%.[85] Delayed-onset pain typically has an average onset of 3 days after treatment and lasts an average of 11 days, resolving completely without long-term sequelae.[85] Younger women undergoing abdominal cryolipolysis treatments may be at increased risk for delayed-onset pain.[85] The number of treatment cycles does not impact incidence. The exact etiology of delayed-onset pain is unclear, but hypotheses include ischemic sensory nerve changes and/or enhanced inflammatory response to treatment.[85] The best management strategies have not been studied, but commonly used treatments in our practice are topical anesthesia (lidocaine gel, lidocaine cream, lidocaine patches) and short-term oral medications like gabapentin given at titrated doses.

A published uncommon complication of cryolipolysis includes paradoxical adipose hyperplasia (PAH), characterized by delayed gradual increase of adipose tissue in the treatment area, with onset at about 2 or 4 months posttreatment.[86] The reported incidence in literature varies, initially reported as 1 in 20,000[86] but more recent studies reporting higher incidences closer to approximately 1 in 200 treatments,[86,87,88] suggesting that PAH may be underreported. The mechanism behind PAH is unclear. Hypothesized mechanisms include adipocyte hypertrophy, recruitment of resident or circulating preadipocyte and/or stem cell populations, changes in adipocyte metabolism, or hypoxic injury.[86] Negative pressure suction from the vacuum applicators may stimulate adipocytes, similar to the mechanism of adipose enlargement that has been reported with the BRAVA system used for breast reconstructions.[91] Some authors suggest larger vacuum applicator (CoolMax) may be associated with PAH.[91] The incidence of PAH seems to be higher in males,[86,92] in contrast to females who have increased risk of delayed-onset pain. Pathology of samples have been inconsistent. Jailan et al evaluated areas of PAH using MRI, which showed increase of adipose tissue and histology demonstrating disorganized adipocytes, thickened septa around fat lobules, and increased vascularity.[86] In contrast, Seaman et al evaluated tissue from a female who underwent two sessions of cryolipolysis of the abdomen and flanks. Lipectomy tissue 7 months posttreatment of sites affected by PAH as well as control tissue from the same patient demonstrated decreased viable adipocyte numbers, decreased vascularity, and decreased cells in PAH sample.[87] Management of PAH typically involves surgical correction and liposuction.[89] Recently, a case report on the efficacy of ATX-101 (deoxycholic acid injection) for abdominal PAH was published, with a total of 4.0 mL injected per treatment for a total of three treatment sessions.[93]

3.7.2 Radiofrequency

RF-based treatments are typically well tolerated, and treatments are monitored based on patient feedback. Most common side effects include transient erythema, edema, mild tenderness, and sweating. Posttreatment burns have occurred secondary to cracks or damage to the handpiece electrode or coating. Of note, it is recommended not to use topical or injectable numbing to the treatment area prior to procedure, as patient feedback is important to preventing burns during the treatment.

3.7.3 High-Intensity Focused Ultrasound

HIFU is overall safe and well tolerated. The most commonly reported side effects include procedural pain, temporary postprocedure pain, ecchymosis, swelling, dysesthesia, and erythema.[44,47] Most patients reported mild or moderate pain during the procedure, and all side effects resolve spontaneously.[44,47] Clinical studies found no clinically significant changes in measured safety parameters, including serum lipid levels and LFTs.[46]

3.7.4 Nonthermal Focused Ultrasound

Nonthermal focused US is safe and well tolerated without serious adverse events. Clinical studies found no significant changes in safety parameters, including serum lipid levels, liver markers, pulse oximetry, and liver US.[35] Mild erythema is the most common side effect.[37] Other less common side effects include ecchymosis, dysesthesia during treatment, and blisters.[35]

3.7.5 Diode Laser

Treatment tends to be well tolerated without significant skin damage or significant changes in blood lipid or liver function levels.[56,64] The majority of side effects after diode laser treatment are mild. Most common side effects include treatment discomfort, rating an average of 4 out of 10 in severity.[56] Other less common side effects include transient erythema, edema, blistering, bruising, induration, and subcutaneous nodules.[56] Treatment-related dyspigmentation has not been reported.

3.7.6 Low-Level Laser Therapy

LLLT is well tolerated with low risk of side effects. There have been two reports of skin ulceration with treatment.[70]

3.7.7 High-Intensity Focused Electromagnetic Therapy

HIFEM is a well-tolerated procedure, and treatment is tailored to tolerability. It has been reported that higher BMI patients tend to tolerate higher settings.[75] The most common side effect is mild muscle soreness for the first 24 hours after treatment, which is self-limiting.

3.8 Conclusions

With the trend toward more noninvasive procedures over traditional surgery, the field of noninvasive body contouring has grown significantly. This has led to the development of multiple fat reduction devices currently on the market. The decision relating to which device to use depends on the individual patient's anatomy and the amount, location, and shape of unwanted fat. It also depends on more practical factors, like which devices are available at the practice, practitioner training and expertise, comfort, cost to the patient, and the number of visits and time investment required. Prior to treatment, patients must understand expectations related to durability and proposed maintenance regimens. It is important to counsel that these noninvasive devices take time to see results, usually a period of a few months, and do not result in dramatic fat reduction comparable to surgery. If one treatment modality is not effective for a particular patient, there are alternative modalities. More studies are needed for newer devices to determine if expected results are consistent and durable over the long term, and patients must understand that weight maintenance is paramount to achieving favorable results from noninvasive body contouring.

3.9 Pearls and Pitfalls

Appropriate patient selection and counseling of expectations is crucial to delivering patient satisfaction. It is important to note that none of the above-mentioned noninvasive fat reduction devices will lead to significant weight loss or dramatic results. Obese patients should be recommended to consult with weight reduction specialists or endocrinologists.

In order to record the results of fat reduction treatments, body weight should be measured at baseline and at each follow-up. Standardized photography should be implemented in the practice to document results. Given that most patients may require multiple treatments, photography may be taken outlining the whole treatment area and immediately after treatment to document the exact area treated for follow-up evaluation and treatment.

References

[1] American Society for Dermatologic Surgery. 2018. ASDS Consumer Survey on Cosmetic Dermatologic Procedures. Available at: https://www.asds.net/Portals/0/PDF/consumer-survey-2018-infographic.pdf. Accessed December 15, 2018

[2] American Society of Plastic Surgeons. 2017. Plastic Surgery Statistics Reports. Available at: https://www.plasticsurgery.org/news/press-releases/new-statistics-reveal-the-shape-of-plastic-surgery. Accessed December 15, 2018

[3] Epstein EH, Jr, Oren ME. Popsicle panniculitis. N Engl J Med. 1970; 282(17):966–967

[4] Beacham BE, Cooper PH, Buchanan CS, Weary PE. Equestrian cold panniculitis in women. Arch Dermatol. 1980; 116(9):1025–1027

[5] Manstein D, Laubach H, Watanabe K, Farinelli W, Zurakowski D, Anderson RR. Selective cryolysis: a novel method of non-invasive fat removal. Lasers Surg Med. 2008; 40(9):595–604

[6] Zelickson B, Egbert BM, Preciado J, et al. Cryolipolysis for noninvasive fat cell destruction: initial results from a pig model. Dermatol Surg. 2009; 35(10):1462–1470

[7] Dover JA, Burns J, Coleman S, et al. A Prospective Clinical Study of Noninvasive Cryolipolysis for Subcutaneous Fat Layer Reduction: Interim Report of Available Subject Data. Annual Conference of the American Society for Laser Medicine and Surgery, National Harbor, MD, April 1–5, 2009

[8] Coleman SR, Sachdeva K, Egbert BM, Preciado J, Allison J. Clinical efficacy of noninvasive cryolipolysis and its effects on peripheral nerves. Aesthetic Plast Surg. 2009; 33(4):482–488

[9] Dierickx CC, Mazer JM, Sand M, Koenig S, Arigon V. Safety, tolerance, and patient satisfaction with noninvasive cryolipolysis. Dermatol Surg. 2013; 39(8):1209–1216

[10] Garibyan L, Sipprell WH, III, Jalian HR, Sakamoto FH, Avram M, Anderson RR. Three-dimensional volumetric quantification of fat loss following cryolipolysis. Lasers Surg Med. 2014; 46(2):75–80

[11] Shek SY, Chan NP, Chan HH. Non-invasive cryolipolysis for body contouring in Chinese–a first commercial experience. Lasers Surg Med. 2012; 44(2):125–130

[12] Boey GE, Wasilenchuk JL. Fat reduction in the inner thigh using a prototype cryolipolysis applicator. Dermatol Surg. 2014; 40(9): 1004–1009

[13] Zelickson BD, Burns AJ, Kilmer SL. Cryolipolysis for safe and effective inner thigh fat reduction. Lasers Surg Med. 2015; 47(2):120–127

[14] Wanitphakdeedecha R, Sathaworawong A, Manuskiatti W. The efficacy of cryolipolysis treatment on arms and inner thighs. Lasers Med Sci. 2015; 30(8):2165–2169

[15] Stevens WG, Bachelor EP. Cryolipolysis conformable-surface applicator for nonsurgical fat reduction in lateral thighs. Aesthet Surg J. 2015; 35(1):66–71

[16] Kilmer SL, Burns AJ, Zelickson BD. Safety and efficacy of cryolipolysis for non-invasive reduction of submental fat. Lasers Surg Med. 2016; 48(1):3–13

[17] Bernstein EF, Bloom JD. Safety and efficacy of bilateral submental cryolipolysis with quantified 3-dimensional imaging of fat reduction and skin tightening. JAMA Facial Plast Surg. 2017; 19(5):350–357

[18] Kilmer SL. Prototype CoolCup cryolipolysis applicator with over 40% reduced treatment time demonstrates equivalent safety and efficacy with greater patient preference. Lasers Surg Med. 2017; 49(1):63–68

[19] Boey GE, Wasilenchuk JL. Enhanced clinical outcome with manual massage following cryolipolysis treatment: a 4-month study of safety and efficacy. Lasers Surg Med. 2014; 46(1):20–26

[20] Bernstein EF. Long-term efficacy follow-up on two cryolipolysis case studies: 6 and 9 years post-treatment. J Cosmet Dermatol. 2016; 15 (4):561–564

[21] Stevens WG. Does cryolipolysis lead to skin tightening? A first report of cryodermadstringo. Aesthet Surg J. 2014; 34(6):NP32–NP34

[22] Carruthers J, Stevens WG, Carruthers A, Humphrey S. Cryolipolysis and skin tightening. Dermatol Surg. 2014; 40 Suppl 12:S184–S189

[23] Franco W, Kothare A, Goldberg DJ. Controlled volumetric heating of subcutaneous adipose tissue using a novel radiofrequency technology. Lasers Surg Med. 2009; 41(10):745–750

[24] Weiss R, Weiss M, Beasley K, Vrba J, Bernardy J. Operator independent focused high frequency ISM band for fat reduction: porcine model. Lasers Surg Med. 2013; 45(4):235–239

[25] Franco W, Kothare A, Ronan SJ, Grekin RC, McCalmont TH. Hyperthermic injury to adipocyte cells by selective heating of subcutaneous fat with a novel radiofrequency device: feasibility studies. Lasers Surg Med. 2010; 42(5):361–370

[26] Bhatia A, Maldre L, Kothare A. Subcutaneous Adipose Tissue Reduction Using a Non-Invasive Monopolar Radiofrequency Device: A Case Study with 7 Subjects. Annual Conference of the American Society for Laser Medicine and Surgery, Boston, MA, April 1–3, 2016

[27] Fajkošová K, Machovcová A, Onder M, Fritz K. Selective radiofrequency therapy as a non-invasive approach for contactless body contouring and circumferential reduction. J Drugs Dermatol. 2014; 13(3):291–296

[28] McDaniel D, Samková P. Evaluation of the safety and efficacy of a non-contact radiofrequency device for the improvement in contour and circumferential reduction of the inner and outer thigh. J Drugs Dermatol. 2015; 14(12):1422–1424

[29] Fritz K, Samková P, Salavastru C, Hudec J. A novel selective RF applicator for reducing thigh circumference: a clinical evaluation. Dermatol Ther (Heidelb). 2016; 29(2):92–95

[30] Moradi A, Palm M. Selective non-contact field radiofrequency extended treatment protocol: evaluation of safety and efficacy. J Drugs Dermatol. 2015; 14(9):982–985

[31] Downie J, Kaspar M. Contactless abdominal fat reduction with selective RF™ evaluated by magnetic resonance imaging (MRI): case study. J Drugs Dermatol. 2016;15(4):491–495

[32] Fritz K, Salavastru C. Long-term follow-up on patients treated for abdominal fat using a selective contactless radiofrequency device. J Cosmet Dermatol. 2017; 16(4):471–475

[33] Brown SA, Greenbaum L, Shtukmaster S, Zadok Y, Ben-Ezra S, Kushkuley L. Characterization of nonthermal focused ultrasound for noninvasive selective fat cell disruption (lysis): technical and preclinical assessment. Plast Reconstr Surg. 2009; 124(1):92–101

[34] Ascher B. Safety and efficacy of UltraShape Contour I treatments to improve the appearance of body contours: multiple treatments in shorter intervals. Aesthet Surg J. 2010; 30(2):217–224

[35] Teitelbaum SA, Burns JL, Kubota J, et al. Noninvasive body contouring by focused ultrasound: safety and efficacy of the Contour I device in a multicenter, controlled, clinical study. Plast Reconstr Surg. 2007; 120 (3):779–789

[36] Moreno-Moraga J, Valero-Altés T, Riquelme AM, Isarria-Marcosy MI, de la Torre JR. Body contouring by non-invasive transdermal focused ultrasound. Lasers Surg Med. 2007; 39(4):315–323

[37] Coleman WP, III, Coleman W, IV, Weiss RA, Kenkel JM, Ad-El DD, Amir R. A multicenter controlled study to evaluate multiple treatments with nonthermal focused ultrasound for noninvasive fat reduction. Dermatol Surg. 2017; 43(1):50–57

[38] Gold MH, Coleman WP, IV, Coleman W, III, Weiss R. A randomized, controlled multicenter study evaluating focused ultrasound treatment for fat reduction in the flanks. J Cosmet Laser Ther. 2018; 21(1):1–5

[39] Shek SY, Yeung CK, Chan JC, Chan HH. The efficacy of a combination non-thermal focused ultrasound and radiofrequency device for noninvasive body contouring in Asians. Lasers Surg Med. 2016; 48 (2):203–207

[40] Chang SL, Huang YL, Lee MC, et al. Combination therapy of focused ultrasound and radio-frequency for noninvasive body contouring in Asians with MRI photographic documentation. Lasers Med Sci. 2014; 29(1):165–172

[41] Chang SL, Huang YL, Lee MC, et al. Long-term follow-up for noninvasive body contouring treatment in Asians. Lasers Med Sci. 2016; 31(2):283–287

[42] Mahmoud ELdesoky MT, Mohamed Abutaleb EE, Mohamed Mousa GS. Ultrasound cavitation versus cryolipolysis for non-invasive body contouring. Australas J Dermatol. 2016; 57(4):288–293

[43] Jewell ML, Desilets C, Smoller BR. Evaluation of a novel high-intensity focused ultrasound device: preclinical studies in a porcine model. Aesthet Surg J. 2011; 31(4):429–434

[44] Gadsden E, Aguilar MT, Smoller BR, Jewell ML. Evaluation of a novel high-intensity focused ultrasound device for ablating subcutaneous adipose tissue for noninvasive body contouring: safety studies in human volunteers. Aesthet Surg J. 2011; 31(4):401–410

[45] Ter Haar G. HIFU tissue ablation: concept and devices. Adv Exp Med Biol. 2016; 880:3–20

[46] Jewell ML, Baxter RA, Cox SE, et al. Randomized sham-controlled trial to evaluate the safety and effectiveness of a high-intensity focused ultrasound device for noninvasive body sculpting. Plast Reconstr Surg. 2011; 128(1):253–262

[47] Jewell ML, Weiss RA, Baxter RA, et al. Safety and tolerability of high-intensity focused ultrasonography for noninvasive body sculpting: 24-week data from a randomized, sham-controlled study. Aesthet Surg J. 2012; 32(7):868–876

[48] Jewell ML, Solish NJ, Desilets CS. Noninvasive body sculpting technologies with an emphasis on high-intensity focused ultrasound. Aesthetic Plast Surg. 2011; 35(5):901–912

[49] Fatemi A, Kane MA. High-intensity focused ultrasound effectively reduces waist circumference by ablating adipose tissue from the abdomen and flanks: a retrospective casè series. Aesthetic Plast Surg. 2010; 34(5):577–582

[50] Solish N, Lin X, Axford-Gatley RA, Strangman NM, Kane M. A randomized, single-blind, postmarketing study of multiple energy levels of high-intensity focused ultrasound for noninvasive body sculpting. Dermatol Surg. 2012; 38(1):58–67

[51] Robinson DM, Kaminer MS, Baumann L, et al. High-intensity focused ultrasound for the reduction of subcutaneous adipose tissue using multiple treatment techniques. Dermatol Surg. 2014; 40(6):641–651

[52] Shek SY, Yeung CK, Chan JC, Chan HH. Efficacy of high-intensity focused ultrasonography for noninvasive body sculpting in Chinese patients. Lasers Surg Med. 2014; 46(4):263–269

[53] Jacques SL. Optical properties of biological tissues: a review. Phys Med Biol. 2013; 58(11):R37–R61

[54] Wassmer B, Zemmouri J, Rochon P, Mordon S. Comparative study of wavelengths for laser lipolysis. Photomed Laser Surg. 2010; 28(2): 185–188

[55] Katz B, McBean J. Laser-assisted lipolysis: a report on complications. J Cosmet Laser Ther. 2008; 10(4):231–233

[56] Katz B, Doherty S. Safety and efficacy of a noninvasive 1,060-nm diode laser for fat reduction of the flanks. Dermatol Surg. 2018; 44 (3):388–396

[57] Apfelberg D. Laser-assisted liposuction may benefit surgeons, patients. Clin Laser Mon. 1992; 10(12):193–194

[58] Ichikawa K, Miyasaka M, Tanaka R, Tanino R, Mizukami K, Wakaki M. Histologic evaluation of the pulsed Nd:YAG laser for laser lipolysis. Lasers Surg Med. 2005; 36(1):43–46

[59] Mordon S, Eymard-Maurin AF, Wassmer B, Ringot J. Histologic evaluation of laser lipolysis: pulsed 1064-nm Nd:YAG laser versus cw 980-nm diode laser. Aesthet Surg J. 2007; 27(3):263–268

[60] Badin AZ, Moraes LM, Gondek L, Chiaratti MG, Canta L. Laser lipolysis: flaccidity under control. Aesthetic Plast Surg. 2002; 26(5):335–339

[61] Fakhouri TM, El Tal AK, Abrou AE, Mehregan DA, Barone F. Laser-assisted lipolysis: a review. Dermatol Surg. 2012; 38(2):155–169

[62] Kim KH, Geronemus RG. Laser lipolysis using a novel 1,064 nm Nd: laser YAG. Dermatol Surg. 2006; 32(2):241–248

[63] Schilling L, Saedi N, Weiss R. 1060 nm diode hyperthermic laser lipolysis: the latest in non-invasive body contouring. J Drugs Dermatol. 2017; 16(1):48–52

[64] Decorato JW, Chen B, Sierra R. Subcutaneous adipose tissue response to a non-invasive hyperthermic treatment using a 1,060 nm laser. Lasers Surg Med. 2017; 49(5):480–489

[65] Bass LS, Doherty ST. Safety and efficacy of a non-invasive 1060 nm diode laser for fat reduction of the abdomen. J Drugs Dermatol. 2018; 17(1):106–112

[66] Bass L, Katz B, Doherty P. A Multicenter Study of a Non-Invasive 1060 nm Diode Laser for Fat Reduction of the Flanks and Abdomen: 6-Month Follow-Up. Annual Conference of the American Society for Laser Medicine and Surgery, Boston, MA, March 30–April 3, 2016

[67] Weiss R, McDaniel D, Doherty S, et al. Clinical Evaluation of Fat Reduction Treatment of the Flanks and Abdomen with a Non-Invasive 1060 nm Diode Laser: A Multicenter Study. Annual Conference of the American Society for Laser Medicine and Surgery, Boston, MA, March 30–April 3, 2016

[68] Avci P, Nyame TT, Gupta GK, Sadasivam M, Hamblin MR. Low-level laser therapy for fat layer reduction: a comprehensive review. Lasers Surg Med. 2013; 45(6):349–357

[69] Neira R, Arroyave J, Ramirez H, et al. Fat liquefaction: effect of low-level laser energy on adipose tissue. Plast Reconstr Surg. 2002; 110(3):912–922, discussion 923–925

[70] Jankowski M, Gawrych M, Adamska U, Ciescinski J, Serafin Z, Czajkowski R. Low-level laser therapy (LLLT) does not reduce subcutaneous adipose tissue by local adipocyte injury but rather by modulation of systemic lipid metabolism. Lasers Med Sci. 2017; 32(2):475–479

[71] Caruso-Davis MK, Guillot TS, Podichetty VK, et al. Efficacy of low-level laser therapy for body contouring and spot fat reduction. Obes Surg. 2011; 21(6):722–729

[72] Jackson RF, Dedo DD, Roche GC, Turok DI, Maloney RJ. Low-level laser therapy as a non-invasive approach for body contouring: a randomized, controlled study. Lasers Surg Med. 2009; 41(10):799–809

[73] Jackson RF, Stern FA, Neira R, Ortiz-Neira CL, Maloney J. Application of low-level laser therapy for noninvasive body contouring. Lasers Surg Med. 2012; 44(3):211–217

[74] Weiss RA, Bernardy J. Induction of fat apoptosis by a non-thermal device: mechanism of action of non-invasive high-intensity electromagnetic technology in a porcine model. Lasers Surg Med. 2019; 51(1):47–53

[75] Kinney BM, Lozanova P. High intensity focused electromagnetic therapy evaluated by magnetic resonance imaging: safety and efficacy study of a dual tissue effect based non-invasive abdominal body shaping. Lasers Surg Med. 2019; 51(1):40–46

[76] Jacob CI, Paskova K. Safety and efficacy of a novel high-intensity focused electromagnetic technology device for noninvasive abdominal body shaping. J Cosmet Dermatol. 2018; 17(5):783–787

[77] Meyer PF, Davi Costa E Silva J, Santos de Vasconcellos L, de Morais Carreiro E, Valentim da Silva RM. Cryolipolysis: patient selection and special considerations. Clin Cosmet Investig Dermatol. 2018; 11:499–503

[78] Krueger N, Mai SV, Luebberding S, Sadick NS. Cryolipolysis for noninvasive body contouring: clinical efficacy and patient satisfaction. Clin Cosmet Investig Dermatol. 2014;7:201–205

[79] Afrooz PN, Pozner JN, DiBernardo BE. Noninvasive and minimally invasive techniques in body contouring. Clin Plast Surg. 2014; 41(4):789–804

[80] Ingargiola MJ, Motakef S, Chung MT, Vasconez HC, Sasaki GH. Cryolipolysis for fat reduction and body contouring: safety and efficacy of current treatment paradigms. Plast Reconstr Surg. 2015; 135(6):1581–1590

[81] Klein KB, Bachelor EP, Becker EV, Bowes LE. Multiple same day cryolipolysis treatments for the reduction of subcutaneous fat are safe and do not affect serum lipid levels or liver function tests. Lasers Surg Med. 2017; 49(7):640–644

[82] Sasaki GH, Abelev N, Tevez-Ortiz A. Noninvasive selective cryolipolysis and reperfusion recovery for localized natural fat reduction and contouring. Aesthet Surg J. 2014;34(3):420–431

[83] Adjadj L, SidAhmed-Mezi M, Mondoloni M, Meningaud JP, Hersant B. Assessment of the efficacy of cryolipolysis on saddlebags: a prospective study of 53 patients. Plast Reconstr Surg. 2017; 140(1):50–57

[84] Klein KB, Zelickson B, Riopelle JG, et al. Non-invasive cryolipolysis for subcutaneous fat reduction does not affect serum lipid levels or liver function tests. Lasers Surg Med. 2009; 41(10):785–790

[85] Keaney TC, Gudas AT, Alster TS. Delayed onset pain associated with cryolipolysis treatment: a retrospective study with treatment recommendations. Dermatol Surg. 2015; 41(11):1296–1299

[86] Jalian HR, Avram MM, Garibyan L, Mihm MC, Anderson RR. Paradoxical adipose hyperplasia after cryolipolysis. JAMA Dermatol. 2014; 150(3):317–319

[87] Seaman SA, Tannan SC, Cao Y, Peirce SM, Gampper TJ. Paradoxical adipose hyperplasia and cellular effects after cryolipolysis: a case report. Aesthet Surg J. 2016; 36(1):NP6–NP13

[88] Singh SM, Geddes ER, Boutrous SG, Galiano RD, Friedman PM. Paradoxical adipose hyperplasia secondary to cryolipolysis: an underreported entity? Lasers Surg Med. 2015; 47(6):476–478

[89] Kelly ME, Rodríguez-Feliz J, Torres C, Kelly E. Treatment of paradoxical adipose hyperplasia following cryolipolysis: a single-center experience. Plast Reconstr Surg. 2018; 142(1):17e–22e

[90] Karcher C, Katz B, Sadick N. Paradoxical adipose hyperplasia post cryolipolysis and management. Dermatol Surg. 2017; 43(3):467–470

[91] Stefani WA. Adipose hypertrophy following cryolipolysis. Aesthet Surg J. 2015; 35(7):NP218–NP220

[92] Keaney TC, Naga LI. Men at risk for paradoxical adipose hyperplasia after cryolipolysis. J Cosmet Dermatol. 2016; 15(4):575–577

[93] Ward CE, Li JY, Friedman PM. ATX-101 (deoxycholic acid injection) for paradoxical adipose hyperplasia secondary to cryolipolysis. Dermatol Surg. 2018; 44(5):752–754

4 Cellulite Treatment

Deanne Mraz Robinson and Yoon-Soo Cindy Bae

Summary

Cellulite, which describes the dimpling of the skin that mainly affects the buttocks and posterior thighs of women, affects over 80% of women, but it can negatively impact their quality of life. For this reason, considerable effort has been spent over the years understanding its pathophysiology and establishing effective treatment options. Although innumerable treatment options have been proposed and tested throughout the years, it was only recently that several have emerged that produce durable and reliable results. This chapter will explore these treatment options and will also briefly touch on other methods to improve the overall appearance of the buttocks and posterolateral thighs.

Keywords: cellulite, subcision, Cellfina, Cellulaze, body contouring, Qwo, *Collagenase Clostridium Histolyticum* (CCH), resonic, rapid acoustic pulse technology, Aveli

4.1 Introduction

Cellulite, also known as liposclerosis or edematous fibrosclerotic panniculopathy, refers to the dimpling of the skin that mainly affects the buttocks and posterolateral thighs of women. Although some describe it as a disease, it is of no medical significance and can be seen in 80 to 90% of women after their teens.[1] Cellulite exists across a spectrum and can be made up of either deep, tethered dimples or as shallower, rolling topographic changes, or as a combination of the two. Although it is not pathologic, these textural irregularities can be a great source of distress for those affected by it, analogous to patients who are bothered by textural irregularities on the face, such as wrinkling or acne scarring. In one study, nearly 90% of women stated that having cellulite negatively impacted their quality of life.[2] Although there are a number of different treatment options for textural irregularities on the face, cellulite has proven to be much more challenging to treat. This is not for a lack of effort, as throughout the years there have been a dizzying number of treatment options attempted. The difficulty in treating cellulite stems in part from the differences in anatomy of the buttocks and posterior thighs relative to the rest of the body, as well as a poor grasp of its pathogenesis. Fortunately, as our understanding of the etiology of cellulite has improved recently, so too has our ability to treat it.

Recognizing the pathophysiology of cellulite is crucial to mastering how to treat it, including why some treatment options are successful, whereas many are not. Perhaps the biggest piece of misinformation that exists is that although subcutaneous adipose tissue is a component of cellulite, it is not the only contributing factor. Most physicians who treat cellulite have patients who are extremely fit with healthy body mass indices (BMIs) but who still have cellulite. Furthermore, this can also be illustrated by the fact that cellulite is localized almost entirely to the buttocks and posterior thighs but is rarely found anywhere else, despite adipose tissue being present throughout the body. Certainly, there must be additional factors at play. Rather, cellulite is the result of two major contributing factors including the subcutaneous fat herniating between fibrous connective tissue, as well as fibrous bands that are attached superiorly to the undersurface of the dermis and inferiorly to the deep fascia overlying the muscle. This acts as a tethering cord that pulls the dermis downward.[3] This interplay between the adipose tissue herniating upward and the fibrous septa pulling the skin downward leads to the topographic nodularity and dimpling of the skin that is known as cellulite. Even though we now realize these fibrous septa play a major role in cellulite, we still do not fully understand what leads to the formation of the bands themselves and why they are primarily seen in the buttocks and posterolateral thighs. That said, after extensive research throughout the years, cellulite is now understood to be the result of a complex interplay of a number of factors including microvascular dysfunction and tissue edema, persistent low-grade inflammation, collagen denaturation, tissue laxity, connective tissue fibrosclerosis, and localized adipocyte hypertrophy.[4,5] The fact that cellulite is overwhelmingly found in women and typically emerges around puberty has also led many to postulate hormones are involved.

4.2 Modalities and Treatment Options

Given the difficulty in ascertaining the specific pathophysiology of cellulite, it is understandable that the treatment of cellulite has also proven to be challenging. As there have been so many different treatment options for cellulite over the years, an exhaustive review of everything that has been tried is beyond the scope of this chapter. Broadly put, treatments in the past have targeted a few of the different factors that have been felt to contribute to the formation of cellulite. Specifically, they have focused on diminishing excessive subcutaneous adipose tissue, improve tissue laxity and collagen denaturation, and combat microvascular dysfunction and tissue edema. Treatment options that have targeted excessive subcutaneous adipose tissue include encouraging weight loss, using cryolipolysis, high-intensity focused ultrasound, liposuction, or low-level or high-powered laser therapy. Although these treatments have proven to reduce subcutaneous adipose tissue, because cellulite is not purely a disease of adipose tissue, these treatment options have not consistently reduced the topographic changes that make up cellulite. Treatments that target the microvascular dysfunction and tissue edema that are felt to contribute to the formation of the fibrous bands that make up cellulite that have been investigated include methylxanthines such as caffeine creams, mechanical stimulation (manually or with the use of a device), acoustic wave therapy, or extracorporeal shock wave therapy. These have all failed to consistently improve cellulite, as they are not addressing the fibrous septa and instead are inducing transient edema. Similarly, treatments aimed at improving tissue laxity and collagen denaturation, such as with radiofrequency or infrared light devices, have also failed to demonstrate any improvement as again, they do not address the fibrous septa. All told, two different systematic reviews from 2015, which included 73 and 67 studies, found that none of these treatments demonstrated significant or durable results.[6,7] Part of the reason for the lackluster findings of these reviews is because the studies themselves were largely poorly designed and conducted, and suffered from a number of flaws including small sample sizes, lack of reporting of statistical significance, lack of a control group or randomization, or were nonblinded. Other limitations to these studies were that they used a variety of differing endpoints that were oftentimes subjective or failed to measure a valid indicator of cellulite severity, or lacked follow-up beyond several months. Although there are a number of cellulite severity rating scales, there is a lack of a universally accepted scale.

Although as previously cited, there have been a number of treatment options in the past that have lacked meaningful, lasting results, recently there are a few different treatment options that have produced more impressive, reproducible, and durable results. The similarity between the treatment options that have proven to be successful is that they target the fibrous septa, which as previously discussed are one of the major contributing factors to cellulite. These advances were born out of research by Hexsel et al who treated 232 patients with manual subcision, which aimed to dissect the septa tethering down the skin. They found that 78.87% of patients were satisfied with their improvement in cellulite, while an additional 20.25% were partially satisfied. They also followed these patients for more than 2 years and demonstrated that 9.91% of them maintained their improvement.[8] A more recent study involving 200 women also found that manual subcision, in this case with a specially designed two-sided microsurgical blade, was both safe and effective for treating cellulite.[9]

Based on these favorable results, Cellfina (Ulthera/Merz, Mesa, Arizona, United States) and Cellulaze (Cynosure, Inc., Westford, Massachusetts, United States) were developed to automate or improve upon the subcision process. Although these devices differ in the manner by which they subcise the fibrous septa, they have both been found to produce statistically significant improvement in the appearance of cellulite. Cellfina takes advantage of tissue stabilized-guided subcision (TS-GS) through a vacuum-assisted device, which lifts the affected tissue into a chamber and then releases the fibrous septa with a microblade. This provides both reliable and durable results, which is evidenced in the study by Kaminer et al, which included 45 patients and found that patient satisfaction was 93% at 3 years.[10] No adverse effects or pain were reported at this 3-year follow-up. Notably, to our knowledge, no cellulite study has followed patients longer than this study. Geronemus et al utilized three-dimensional imaging analysis to quantify the changes seen after Cellfina, which demonstrated a 67.4% average improvement in negative volume and 58.4% improvement in the minimum height of dimples.[11] The safety and efficacy of Cellfina was also reproduced in another study involving 53 subjects with moderate-to-severe cellulite.[12] Kaminer has also described a modified technique with Cellfina that can effectively treat mild-to-moderate cellulite.[13] This is significant because all prior studies evaluating Cellfina were treating patients with moderate-to-severe cellulite. For this reason, in the past, patients with mild-to-moderate cellulite may have been told they were not good candidates for the procedure; however, this study demonstrated patients such as these may be successfully treated with this modified technique. Cellfina is cleared by the Food and Drug Administration (FDA) for long-term improvement in the appearance of cellulite on the buttocks and thighs of adult females with no loss of benefit for up to 3 years.

Cellulaze utilizes laser energy to thermally and mechanically subcise fibrous septa as opposed to a blade like Cellfina. It utilizes a long-pulsed side-firing 1,440-nm laser that is inserted subcutaneously to subcise the septa. The thermal energy is also beneficial given the secondary benefit of lipolysis and neocollagenesis, tissue tightening, and dermal thickening. In a 2-year study involving 25 women treated with Cellulaze, independent assessors found that 80% of patients had mild improvement at the 6-month mark, whereas 64% of subjects had sustained mild improvement at 2 years.[14] An additional study involving 57 women revealed there was at least a 1-point improvement in dimple count or contour irregularity in 96% of treated areas at 6 months, which was sustained in 90% of treated areas at 1 year.[14,15] However, there are no studies evaluating Cellulaze past 2 years. Cellulaze is FDA cleared for the improvement in the appearance of cellulite as supported by long-term clinical data for at least 6 months with no observed reduction in treatment benefits up to 9 months of observation. This is in contrast to Cellfina, which is cleared for up to 3 years.

In the summer of 2020, the FDA approved collagenase clostridium histolyticum (CCH) for the treatment of cellulite. CCH is composed of two different collagenases that act to hydrolyze collagen and thereby disrupt collagen structures. This is relevant to cellulite because it can be used as a mechanism to destroy the fibrous septa analogous to Cellfina and Cellulaze. CCH has already been approved for the treatment of several collagen-associated disorders including Dupuytren's contracture and Peyronie's disease. Investigations for the treatment of cellulite demonstrated that it is safe and successful at treating cellulite compared with placebo.[16,17] In the phase 2 study, which was a randomized, double-blind study that included women with moderate or severe cellulite of the buttocks or posterolateral thighs, 357 women were randomized to CCH or placebo. The percentage of women that had either ≥ 2 or ≥ 1 levels of improvement on a validated Cellulite Severity Score was significantly higher in women treated with CCH (10.6 and 44.6%, respectively) versus placebo (1.6 and 17.9%, respectively; $p < 0.001$ for both) at day 71. The most common adverse events were injection site related.[18] More recently, phase 3 data from two studies, which included a total of 845 women receiving up to three treatments with CCH, found that 73.3 and 67.8% of subjects were reported as "Improved," "Very Improved," or "Very Much Improved" in global appearance of their cellulite area as assessed by the Subject Global Aesthetic Improvement Scale in the target buttock at day 71.[19] One potential benefit that CCH has over Cellfina or Cellulaze is that it does not require any post-treatment alterations in physical activity or the use of compressive stockings. Additionally, as it is a quick inject therapy, it may change the current paradigm for meaningful cellulite treatment as the other two available options are procedure based and require anesthesia and some degree of postprocedure care. One potential drawback is that it may require multiple treatments to achieve the desired results, whereas Cellfina and Cellulaze require only a single treatment.

Following on the heels of CCH, the FDA approved the use of rapid acoustic pulse (RAP) technology, Resonic, for the treatment of cellulite. This device uses noninvasive high-frequency sound waves directly onto the cellulite dimples which physically changes the septa that cause cellulite and helps with the appearance of smooth skin. This method only requires one treatment. Due to the noninvasive nature of this technology, patients of all skin types are candidates as there is no risk of postinflammatory hyperpigmentation or hemosiderin staining.[20]

Most recently, another manual subcision device has come to market which utilizes transillumiation at the tip of the device to assist with placement. Study data showed efficacy at day 180 in 20 subjects which was a mean ≥1-point reduction in the CSS (Cellulite Severity Score). In terms of adverse events, investigators reported mild-to-moderate ecchymosis in all subjects and noted a minor self-resolving hematoma, hyperpigmentation, and nodule formation in a smaller subset of subjects. There were no serious AEs.[21]

4.2.1 Putting It All Together

Although we now have several treatment options available to treat the fibrous septa of cellulite, possibly with more on the horizon, this may not be enough to fully satisfy the patient. In the authors' experience, addressing the fibrous septa should be the primary goal when treating cellulite; however, the clinician may need to address other aspects of the posterolateral thighs to make the patient happy. Beyond the dimpling, which is the key feature of cellulite, patients may also have adipose tissue, volume loss, or skin laxity. Treating these may be better classified as body contouring; however, as cellulite is a complex and oftentimes confusing picture, if they are present the majority of patients may also want these to be addressed along with treating any dimpling of the skin. With this in mind, preoperative photographs are important before any treatment because some patients may not appreciate the improvement in dimpling if they are then immediately drawn to these other problem areas such tissue laxity.

Excessive fat can be treated with modalities used to treat adipose tissue on other areas of the body such as cryolipolysis, detergent lipolysis, or liposuction. When there is volume loss, fat transfer, which may be combined with liposuction, has been well described.[22] A biostimulatory filler such as poly-L-lactic acid (PLLA) is also commonly used to improve volume loss; however, multiple treatment sessions may be necessary and this is an off-label indication.[23] Using dilute and hyperdilute calcium hydroxylapatite (CaHA) as another biostimulatory agent to provide volume and tighten the skin is a newer technique that has been described with good results.[24] Treating skin laxity can be attempted with microfocused ultrasound with visualization, radiofrequency (externally or subdermally), or a biostimulatory filler such as PLLA or CaHA.[18] It should be noted that these skin-tightening results can be modest, and patients need to be selected carefully; otherwise, they may be left unhappy.

4.3 Patient Selection

To properly select a patient, it is important to fully understand what it is that bothers the patient. Patients may misunderstand what is actually classified as cellulite, so many present for a consultation where they have excessive adipose tissue, significant laxity, or sagging of the skin with or without actual cellulite. As previously mentioned, these patients may be better suited for an alternative treatment such as body contouring. This is because even if their cellulite is improved after appropriate treatment, the patient may remain unhappy as their specific needs were not addressed. As was previously discussed, issues such as excessive laxity or volume excess or loss can be addressed after the cellulite is addressed, but ultimately it should be established what bothers the patient the most.

When it is understood that it is actually cellulite that is bothering the patient, the next step is ensuring the patient has the proper type of cellulite that will respond best to a treatment such as Cellfina or Cellulaze. Cellulite can present as either deeper lesions, giving the impression of "cottage cheese," or more superficial depressions, which are often described as providing an "orange peel" appearance. Cellfina and Cellulaze traditionally have been thought to provide the optimal results in patients with deeper dimpled or linear depressions, because the fibrous septa that tether these lesions down are easier to localize and provide a more dramatic improvement once treated. However, as previously mentioned, Kaminer et al have since described a modified technique that has been shown to be effective at treating mild-to-moderate cellulite that presents as fine dimpling and rippling, so the experienced clinician may also include these patients as well.[13] Clinical trials for both Cellfina and Cellulaze included patients with skin types I to VI and are safe for all skin types. In patients with dark skin types, particular care should be given regarding photoprotection and minimization of postprocedure bruising as lasting hyperpigmentation and or hemosiderosis can occur.

4.3.1 Contraindications

These procedures are generally contraindicated in patients with coagulation disorders or those on anticoagulant medications. Diabetes, pregnancy, or excessive obesity are also contraindications. Other contraindications include patients with vascular disorders such as phlebitis or vasculitis, vascular fragility, or varicose veins in the area of treatment. Finally, patients with uncontrolled hypertension, those with skin infections or open lesions, or those who have had recent surgery (< 6 weeks) are contraindicated. Caution should be taken in patients with a history of keloidal or hypertrophic scarring as Cellfina and Cellulaze both require small incisional openings into the skin with either the cannula or microblade.

4.3.2 Indications

Cellfina is indicated for long-term improvement in the appearance of cellulite in the buttocks and thigh areas of adult females, with clinical data demonstrating no significant reduction in treatment benefits up to 3 years of observation.

Cellulaze is indicated for improvement in the appearance of cellulite as supported by long-term clinical data for at least 6 months with no observed reduction in treatment benefits up to 9 months of observation.

Qwo is indicated for the treatment of moderate-to-severe cellulite in the buttocks of adult women. Studies show that by day 90 most women had a >1 level improvement in their cellulite after the third treatment.

Resonic is indicated to treat the appearance of cellulite, published results measured at 3 months posttreatment; however, long-term data is soon to be available.

Aveli is indicated for the treatment of cellulite on the buttock and thighs, results measured at 3 months posttreatment.

4.4 Preoperative Instructions

In terms of prepping the patient, it is important to ensure that they have stopped any antiplatelet or anticoagulant medications prior to the procedure. On the day of the procedure, it is crucial to take high-quality pretreatment photographs, which will be instrumental when assessing the patient at follow-up visits. As the dimpling of cellulite is sometimes only revealed in a certain position or with certain lighting, it is important to take these photographs from a number of different positions. Taking at least five photographs including one from directly behind the patient and two from the 45- and 90-degree angles from each direction will allow the clinician to best track these changes. Overhead lighting will allow the cellulite to be visualized fully.

Additionally, some dimples are seen best or accentuated with movement, so dynamic videos of the patient clenching the glutes and or lunging can be particularly helpful.

4.5 Procedure

- Qwo:
  - Markings and preprocedure:
    - With the patient standing, mark the areas to be injected.
    - Adequate photographs should be taken to ensure baseline cellulite is documented.
  - Procedure:
    - Remove the product from the refrigerator and let stand for at least 15 minutes, use only the supplied diluent to reconstitute qwo.
    - With the patient standing, inject CCH subcutaneously, with each injection administered as three 0.1-mL aliquots in three different directions (90 degree perpendicular to the skin surface to inject 0.1mL, then reposition to inject 0.1 mL at a 45-degree angle toward then head, then reposition to inject 0.1 mL at a 45-degree angle toward the foot).
    - Repeat treatment every 21 days for three visits.
  - Immediate postprocedure care:
    - Patient should remain standing for at least 5 minutes after injections.
  - Postprocedure care:
    - Patients should wear compression shorts as often as possible for 1 to 2 weeks. Moderate-to-heavy exercise can resume after 1 week as vigorous exercise prior to that can accentuate bruising.

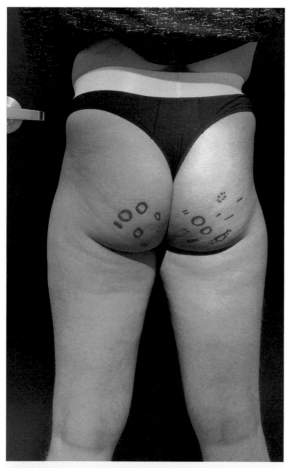

Fig. 4.1 Marking of cellulite dimples with patient standing denoted with representative circles and lines. All dimples were of intermediate depth and to be released at 6-mm depth, hence only one color was used to mark.

encompasses the entirety of the lesion (▶ Fig. 4.1).

– In addition to marking the dimples with the aid of overhead lighting and from different angles, it is useful to have the patient flex their gluteal muscles, which can reveal additional dimples, which are not obvious at rest.

– Photograph the markings: It is prudent to review these marked photographs with the patient prior to the procedure and have them initial the review stating they understand these are the areas that will be treated. This makes it very clear and transparent exactly what areas are and are NOT being addressed with the procedure.

– Position the patient comfortably on their stomach and draped appropriately.

– Prep the patient with an antiseptic scrub.

• Procedure:

○ Assemble the anesthetic delivery system by connecting the 22-gauge needle to the delivery hub. Most patients require small volumes of tumescent fluid, so the authors prefer to prepare 500-mL bags. The on-label anesthetic solution is a 0.1% lidocaine solution with epinephrine. In the authors' experience, a 0.2% lidocaine mixture has been found to be efficacious and well tolerated.

○ Turn on the vacuum and adjust pressure to fully acquire the tissue into chamber and administer 8 mL of tumescent fluid per anesthetic delivery track.

– Repeat this step until all areas are anesthetized. Caution must be given so as not to exceed the total allowable lidocaine volume based on the weight of the patient.

– Wait approximately 20 minutes before starting releases to allow for full epinephrine vasoconstriction.

○ After appropriate dwell time as above, attach the selected release guidance platform to the vacuum tubing.

– Based upon your markings, a depth of 6 or 10 mm can be used. As discussed earlier, for deeper dimples or immediately adjoining lesions, a depth of 10 mm can be used to avoid seromas. For all other releases, 6 mm can be used.

– To optimize results and reduce the risk of seromas and or hematomas, individual releases of lesions/ dimples should be performed. Subcising the least amount of tissue possible will finesse the results and result in less collateral potential tissue damage.

– For the larger oval or circle dimples, which were previously marked with a circle, position the marking into the first treatment window, apply suction, and adjust vacuum to ensure full tissue acquisition. Insert the microblade and move the blade back and forth within the appropriate

○ Potential complications and management:

– Patients may experience bruising; it is important to discuss this with patient prior to the procedure so that the patients are aware.

– Bruising can lead to hemosiderin staining which can be managed with lasers.

• Cellfina:

○ Markings and preprocedure:

– With the patient standing, mark the individual cellulite dimples with a surgical marker. The use of two different colors can be utilized for deeper and shallower lesions as when the patient is prone and after anesthesia, the presence and depth of the dimples will not be able to be discerned. The different colors can be used to correlate to the different depths of release (6 and 10 mm). Additionally, small linear lesion can be marked with a line, and larger oval or circle dimples should be demarcated with a circle that

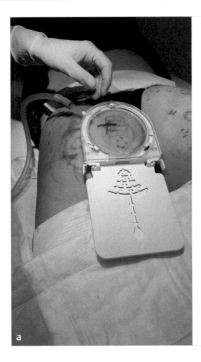 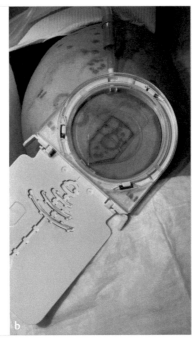

Fig. 4.2 (a, b) P1 rectangular release versus P3 rectangular release. The difference lies in excursion of the cellulite dimple and using the motor module to release only the first track (P1) versus first three tracks (P3).

number of tracks based on the excursion of marking as seen through treatment window (▶ Fig. 4.2).

– For linear lesions, which were marked demarcated with a line, utilize the elegant method as outlined by Kaminer et al. Align the marking with the second treatment window and push the microblade to the second track (▶ Fig. 4.3) and perform release only within this track.

– For lesions smaller than half the second treatment window, an even smaller release can be performed by sweeping the blade back and forth on the side of the track opposite to the lesion.

– For thigh lesions, always align the microblade perpendicular to the dimple of linear depression as releasing the lesions horizontally can result in anetodermic outpouching of subcutaneous adipose tissue.

○ Immediate postprocedure care:

– After the procedure, have the patient sit up and rock back and forth to help express the remaining anesthetic fluid.

– Recleanse the area with an antiseptic cleanser and apply a bland emollient such as petroleum jelly to the entry spots. Cover with nonstick dressings and have the patients wear a medium-strength compression short.

○ Postprocedure care:

– Patients should wear compression shorts as often as possible for 1 to 2 weeks. Moderate-to-heavy exercise can resume after 1 week as vigorous exercise prior to that can accentuate bruising.

○ Potential complications and management:

– Given the mechanism of action, patients should anticipate bruising. Other common adverse events include soreness, tingling, areas of firmness, and/or fluid accumulation. In the pivotal study, these all self-resolved. Additionally, at the 3-year follow-up, there were no reports of sustained pain, treatment effects, or adverse effects.[10,25]

• Cellulaze:

○ Prep and patient positioning:

– Mark the patient in a standing position with a surgical pen. Treatment grids of 5 cm × 5 cm squares should be demarked with dimples and raised areas marked.

– Position the patient comfortably and drape appropriately.

– Prep the patient with an antiseptic scrub.

○ Procedural approach:

– Anesthetize the treatment grids with traditional tumescent anesthesia.

– Using a no. 11 blade, make two to four 1-mm entry point incisions for the laser cannula.

– Introduce the laser cannula and position below the skin surface.

– To treat the raised areas, place the laser cannula in the down position 1 to 2 cm below the dermis and move in a fan-shaped manner.

– To treat the dimples, move the cannula sideways in a fanlike pattern perpendicular to the dimples 3 to 5 mm below the dermis

– For tissue tightening of the dermis, position the fiber 1 to 3 mm below the dermis to heat the 5 cm × 5 cm square.

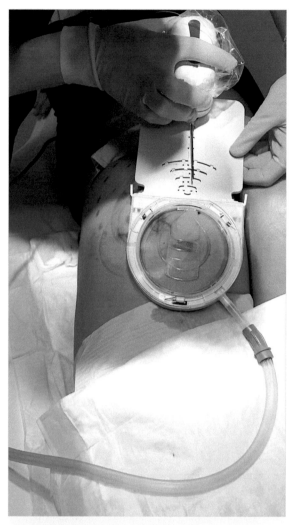

Fig. 4.3 P2 window release. Bypassing the first track with the motor off and releasing only the second track with the microblade for a precise and localized release.

– Remove the fiber and gently massage the treated areas toward the incision site to gently remove any liquefied adipocytes.
  ○ Immediate postprocedure care:
  – After the procedure, the treatment areas should be cleaned and bandaged with compression dressings.
  ○ Rehabilitation and recovery:
  – Patients should wear compression garments for 2 to 3 weeks.
  ○ Potential complications and management:
  – The most common adverse effects are all mild and include discomfort, bruising, swelling, and numbness, which can be managed with over-the-counter-pain medications, pressure, and icepacks, all of which typically resolve within 3 months, and a multicenter study of 57 patients found no adverse events reported at 12 months.[26,27]

– Exudative collections or seromas may rarely be observed and may require intermittent aspiration.
• Resonic:
  ○ Prep and patient positioning:
  – Mark the patient in a standing position with a surgical pen. It may be easier to number the markings to keep track of treated areas.
  – Position the patient comfortably and drape appropriately. Provide noise-cancelling devices or ear plugs to the patient and assistant.
  – Prep the patient with ultrasound gel and hydrocolloid pad.
  ○ Procedural approach:
  – Place the handpiece directly on the hydrocolloid pad which should be on the dimple to be treated.
  – Gently move the handpiece around the treating dimple for 1 minute. Afterward, treat again so each dimple gets 2 minutes of treatment.
  ○ Immediate postprocedure care:
  – After the procedure, the treatment areas should be cleaned.
  ○ Postprocedure care:
  – None.
  ○ Potential complications and management:
  – The most common adverse effects are all mild and include erythema and swelling which can be managed with over-the-counter pain medications, pressure, and icepacks.

4.6 Pearls and Pitfalls

Planning is paramount for success in both Cellfina and Cellulaze cases. Proper identification of the fibrous septa that are contributing to the dimpled appearance of the skin is integral as their release will result in an aesthetically pleasing outcome. Alternatively, releasing all fibrous septa in a given area will not enhance results but will increase the risk for sequela such as hematomas, seromas, and resulting dyspigmentation. Thus, focusing on the pathologic septa is the key to success.

When treating the thighs with Cellfina, remember that coexisting vascular disease can exist and can be common. There is risk of acute bleeding and resulting hemosiderosis if subscision is performed in an area of vascular fragility or varicose veins. As such, the authors suggest using a handheld vein finder, such as AccuVein, to help clarify if venous structures exist in a potentially treated area.

Bruising is a common side effect after treatment with CCH. Therefore, it is important to caution patients with bleeding abnormalities or those who are currently taking antiplatelet or anticoagulant therapy.

Finally, if persistent hyperpigmentation or hemosiderosis does occur postprocedure, interventions such as continued strict photoprotection and the use of fractionated picosecond Alexandrite or Nd:YAG laser treatments, can be helpful for the clearance of lasting hyperpigmentation.[28]

References

[1] Emanuele E. Cellulite: advances in treatment: facts and controversies. Clin Dermatol. 2013; 31(6):725–730

[2] Soares JLM, Miot HA, Sanudo A, Bagatin E. Cellulite: poor correlation between instrumental methods and photograph evaluation for severity classification. Int J Cosmet Sci. 2015; 37(1):134–140

[3] Nürnberger F, Müller G. So-called cellulite: an invented disease. J Dermatol Surg Oncol. 1978; 4(3):221–229

[4] Omi T, Sato S, Kawana P. Ultrastructural assessment of cellulite morphology: clues to a therapeutic strategy? Laser Ther. 2013; 22(2): 131–136

[5] de la Casa Almeida M, Suarez Serrano C, Rebollo Roldán J, Jiménez Rejano JJ. Cellulite's aetiology: a review. J Eur Acad Dermatol Venereol. 2013; 27(3):273–278

[6] Zerini I, Sisti A, Cuomo R, et al. Cellulite treatment: a comprehensive literature review. J Cosmet Dermatol. 2015; 14(3):224–240

[7] Luebberding S, Krueger N, Sadick NS. Cellulite: an evidence-based review. Am J Clin Dermatol. 2015; 16(4):243–256

[8] Hexsel DM, Mazzuco R. Subcision: a treatment for cellulite. Int J Dermatol. 2000; 39(7):539–544

[9] Amore R, Amuso D, Leonardi V, et al. Treatment of dimpling from cellulite. Plast Reconstr Surg Glob Open. 2018; 6(5):e1771

[10] Kaminer MS, Coleman WP, III, Weiss RA, Robinson DM, Grossman J. A multicenter pivotal study to evaluate tissue stabilized-guided subcision using the cellfina device for the treatment of cellulite with 3-year follow-up. Dermatol Surg. 2017; 43(10):1240–1248

[11] Brauer J, Christman M, Bae Y-SC, et al. Three-dimensional analysis of minimally invasive vacuum-assisted subcision treatment of cellulite. J drugs dermatology. 2018;17(9):960

[12] Geronemus RG, Brauer JA, Kilmer SL, et al. An observational study of the safety and efficacy of tissue stabilized-guided subcision to improve the appearance of cellulite. Ski J Cutan Med. 2017; 1(3.1):81

[13] Ibrahim O, Haimovic A, Lee N, Kaminer MS. Efficacy using a modified technique for tissue stabilized-guided subcision for the treatment of mild-to-moderate cellulite of the buttocks and thighs. Dermatol Surg. 2018; 44(10):1272–1277

[14] DiBernardo B, Sasaki G, Katz BE, Hunstad JP, Petti C, Burns AJ. A multicenter study for a single, three-step laser treatment for cellulite using a 1440-nm Nd:YAG laser, a novel side-firing fiber, and a temperature-sensing cannula. Aesthet Surg J. 2013; 33(4):576–584

[15] DiBernardo BE, Sasaki GH, Katz BE, Hunstad JP, Petti C, Burns AJ. A multicenter study for cellulite treatment using a 1440-nm Nd:YAG wavelength laser with side-firing fiber. Aesthet Surg J. 2016; 36(3): 335–343

[16] Goldman MP, Sadick NS, Young L, Kaufman GJ, Smith T, Tursi JP. Phase 2a, randomized, double-blind, placebo-controlled dose-ranging study of repeat doses of collagenase clostridium histolyticum for the treatment of edematous fibrosclerotic panniculopathy (cellulite). J Am Acad Dermatol. 2015; 72(5):AB19–AB19

[17] Dagum AB, Badalamente MA. Collagenase injection in the treatment of cellulite. Plast Reconstr Surg. 2006; 118(4):53

[18] Sadick NS, Goldman MP, Liu G, et al. Collagenase Clostridium histolyticum for the treatment of edematous fibrosclerotic panniculopathy (cellulite): a randomized trial. Dermatol Surg. 2019; 45(8):1047–1056

[19] Endo Pharmaceuticals Inc. Endo Announces Positive Results from Phase 3 Studies of Collagenase Clostridium Histolyticum (CCH) in Patients with Cellulite. Available at: http://investor.endo.com/news-releases/news-release-details/endo-announces-positive-results-phase-3-studies-collagenase. Accessed April 14, 2019

[20] Tanzi E, Capell C, Robertson D. Improvement in the appearance of cellulite and skin laxity resulting from a single treatment with acoustic subcision: findings from a multicenter pivotal clinical trial. Lasers Surg Med. 2022;54(1):121–128

[21] Stevens G, Kaminer M, Fabi S, Fan L. Study of a new controlled focal septa release cellulite reduction method. Aesthet Surg J. 2022

[22] Coleman KM, Pozner J. Combination therapy for rejuvenation of the outer thigh and buttock: a review and our experience. Dermatol Surg. 2016; 42 Suppl 2:S124–S130

[23] Mazzuco R, Sadick NS. The use of poly-L-lactic acid in the gluteal area. Dermatol Surg. 2016; 42(3):441–443

[24] Goldie K, Peeters W, Alghoul M, et al. Global consensus guidelines for the injection of diluted and hyperdiluted calcium hydroxylapatite for skin tightening. Dermatol Surg. 2018; 44 Suppl 1:S32–S41

[25] Kaminer MS, Coleman WP, III, Weiss RA, Grossman J. Tissue stabilized-guided subcision for the treatment of cellulite: A multicenter pivotal study with two-year follow-up. Dermatol Surg. 2016; 42(10):1213–1216

[26] DiBernardo BE, Sasaki GH, Katz BE, Hunstad JP, Petti C, Burns AJ. A multicenter study for cellulite treatment using a 1440-nm Nd:YAG wavelength laser with side-firing fiber. Aesthet Surg J. 2016; 36(3): 335–343

[27] DiBernardo BE. Treatment of cellulite using a 1440-nm pulsed laser with one-year follow-up. Aesthet Surg J. 2011; 31(3):328–341

[28] Wu DC, Goldman MP. Successful treatment of chronic venous stasis hyperpigmentation of the lower limbs with the picosecond alexandrite laser. Dermatol Surg. 2018; 44(6):881–883

5 Skin Laxity: Microneedling

Jordan V. Wang, Joseph N. Mehrabi, and Nazanin Saedi

Summary

Skin tightening has become a common reason for patients to seek cosmetic treatment. In addition to intrinsic aging, many other environmental and physical stressors can negatively impact the skin's structure and clinical appearance. Over time, levels of collagen and elastin in the skin can decrease as the skin loses its optimal architecture, which can manifest as fine lines, wrinkles, roughness, dullness, dryness, and laxity. Microneedling, radiofrequency microneedling, and other laser and energy-based modalities can be utilized to improve the appearance of fine lines, wrinkles, and skin laxity.

Keywords: skin laxity, aesthetics, skin tightening, microneedling, dermatology

5.1 Introduction

In addition to intrinsic aging, facial skin is particularly vulnerable to environmental stressors that can negatively influence its appearance. Excessive exposures to ultraviolet radiation, pollution, smoke, chemicals, and trauma can lead to an abundance of cellular injury. Repetitive damage to the deoxyribonucleic acid (DNA) of skin cells, especially by reactive oxygen species, can contribute to an accumulation of damage that can be harmful to protein maturation, cellular function, and normal physiology.[1,2,3,4] Over time, the skin can also slowly lose its natural elasticity and firmness due to the breakdown of collagen and elastin. This is paired with a reduction in fibroblasts and a decreased ability to repair itself through the formation of new collagen.

The clinical effects of aging and environmental stressors can be quite striking. Facial skin can demonstrate fine lines and wrinkles, dyspigmentation, thinning, roughness, coarseness, and decreased elasticity. Laxity of the facial skin is common, which can manifest itself as overt sagging in the latter and more severe stages. Oftentimes, skin laxity is a major complaint of patients who seek aesthetic procedures. Therefore, it is important for physicians to recognize skin laxity and become acquainted with the various treatment modalities that support skin tightening and overall facial rejuvenation.

5.2 Treatment Options

For the treatment of skin laxity, many options are currently available for patients. Newer options are also seemingly released every year, so it is important for practitioners to keep up to date with the latest and most recent technology and devices. In this chapter, we will cover microneedling and radiofrequency (RF) microneedling specifically. Other options will be briefly mentioned in the end and are also covered elsewhere in this book, including nonablative lasers (Chapter 1), ablative lasers (Chapter 2), and contouring devices (Chapter 3), which can include RF energy and ultrasound technology among other modalities.

5.3 Microneedling

Microneedling, also known as percutaneous collagen induction (PCI) therapy, has been used to safely and effectively treat skin laxity.[5,6] Microneedling creates columns of physical injury using tiny needles that penetrate the skin surface.[7] They can vary in their depth of penetration, which can be controlled by the practitioner. After initial injury, the damaged collagen gets removed by the body's natural processes, and new growth and remodeling subsequently occurs.[8] These processes are stimulated by an upregulation of local growth factors and activation of fibroblasts, which support neocollagenesis, neoelastogenesis, and neovascularization of the tissue.[9] Overall, skin tightening ensues as collagen and elastin remodeling occurs.

Microneedling generally comes in two basic forms, including traditional manual rollers and automated pens.[10] The dermal rollers generally contain needles of fixed length between 0.5 and 3.0 mm, which can vary between the different rollers. The depth of needle penetration can be sensitive to the amount of pressure and technique of the practitioner. In comparison, the automated pens utilize disposable tips that can be cycled at various selected frequencies. In contrast to the rollers, the depth of needle penetration is not as user dependent with these devices. The automated pen is generally preferred in practice due to increased ease of use and improved control of the depth and density of the needles during treatment.

5.4 Radiofrequency Microneedling

Recently, RF microneedling has experienced increased popularity. These specialized needle tips can deliver thermal energy localized to a targeted depth.[10] The needles can be either insulated or noninsulated based on the device and manufacturer, which can help better control the amount and location of heat that is being released. The addition of thermal energy to the needles compared to traditional microneedling serves to increase the amount of controlled damage to the tissue, which can ultimately allow for increased collagen remodeling with each treatment. By adjusting the depth of needle penetration with each successive pass, the physician can layer the thermal energy to allow for maximal coagulation and injury to the dermis. Each RF microneedling device is inherently different from that of a different manufacturer, and they are not interchangeable. Similar settings from each manufacturer does not produce the same histologic and clinical effects, nor does altering them in the same way. The combination of microneedling with RF can offer greatly enhanced skin tightening compared to traditional microneedling.

5.5 Indications

Although it was initially introduced for skin rejuvenation, microneedling has many indications other than for skin laxity. Other common indications include atrophic scars, acne scars, posttraumatic and burn scars, acne, rosacea, alopecia, hyperhidrosis, stretch marks, melasma, actinic keratoses, and topical drug delivery. However, there is still conflicting evidence in the literature on its utility as well as a paucity of larger clinical trials. As with the majority of cosmetic treatments, multiple treatments are generally required to treat these indications. A series of treatments typically includes three to six treatment sessions to achieve the desired clinical outcomes.

5.6 Patient Selection

Selecting the appropriate patient for microneedling is crucial for treatment success and also for patient satisfaction. For the treatment of skin laxity, patients should have mild-to-moderate skin laxity in order to experience the most benefit. More significant and severe skin laxity may be better treated with surgical options, including facelifts. For patients who desire greater improvement with less treatment sessions, RF microneedling may be indicated.

An important factor to consider is the skin tone of the patient. Those with darker skin tones tend to have an increased risk of postprocedural pigmentary changes and postinflammatory hyperpigmentation. This is important to remember when treating skin of color and also to remind patients prior to the procedure in order to offer full disclosure of potential risks and expected outcomes. When using RF microneedling, insulated needle tips may decrease the risk of these events, as the epidermis and superficial dermis can be protected from direct thermal energy.

There are few contraindications for microneedling. It is important not to treat actively infected areas, which should be adequately treated prior to initiation of therapy. For patients who have a history of herpes simplex infections or cold sores located in or around the area to be treated, periprocedural antiviral therapy using valacyclovir or acyclovir is recommended. It is also worthwhile to inquire about a patient's history of hypertrophic scars and keloids, as there is a risk that treatments may exacerbate present lesions or even create new ones. Caution has also been recommended in those with scleroderma, collagen vascular diseases, clotting disorders, immunosuppression, and ongoing chemotherapy or radiation therapy.

During the preoperative period, multiple photographs should be taken of the proposed area to be treated with microneedling. This can help demonstrate to the patient pre- and posttreatment effects to allow for an accurate comparison. Prior to treatment, the patient should wash the area using a gentle cleanser in order to remove any impurities from the skin surface. Intradermal or topical numbing products can be used, such as topical combination benzocaine, lidocaine, and tetracaine or topical lidocaine. If topical agents are used, care must be taken to wipe them off completely. Before starting treatment, alcohol pads or antiseptic cleaner should be used to clean the skin surface again.

5.7 Technique

After appropriate preparation of the skin surface, the skin can be treated with the microneedling device (▶ Fig. 5.1). For the automated pens, a thin layer of a gliding solution is first applied to the treated area. This can allow the pen to more easily move across the skin surface without catching on the skin. The skin should also be pulled taut in order to help with this. The pen is then moved across the skin as the needles oscillate at the selected frequency. For RF microneedling systems, no gliding solution is needed (▶ Fig. 5.2). The needles do not oscillate but penetrate and retract on command. Therefore, it is important to allow the needles to fully retract before moving the device in order to prevent dragging of the skin and causing unintended damage to the skin surface.

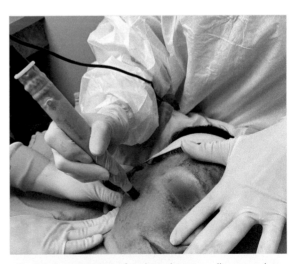

Fig. 5.1 Demonstration of traditional microneedling procedure with automated microneedling pen.

In both types of microneedling, the device should be kept perpendicular to the skin surface to allow for penetration of the needles at a 90-degree angle to the skin. This can ensure adequate needle penetration and controlled damage. Multiple passes, at least two or three, are typically required for treatment. For each pass, a different direction is preferred in order to prevent striping. With each subsequent pass, the depth of needle penetration can be adjusted to allow for layering of the damage to the dermis, which can be especially helpful in RF microneedling. Certain areas of the face, such as the cheeks, can tolerate deeper depths as opposed to other more sensitive and thin-skinned areas, such as the forehead. For traditional microneedling, the treatment endpoint is typically pinpoint bleeding of the area. However, treatment can be more intense in areas that require aggressive treatment. For RF microneedling, the coagulation from the RF can prevent visualization of bleeding, so it is important to fully recognize and understand the treatment settings that are being used.

5.8 Postoperative Instructions

Postoperative instructions for patients begin with a thorough education and discussion on postprocedural expectations. It is important for patients to fully understand what will happen to their skin as it heals over the next several hours to days (▶ Fig. 5.3). Directly following microneedling, patients can expect that the treated areas will look and feel like a moderate sunburn. The skin can feel dry and tight, and it can be sensitive to stimuli. There may be mild inflammation and swelling from the treatment, which typically subsides within several hours. After several days following treatment, the skin may start to flake and peel. Patients should be advised to not pick or scrub the skin when this occurs. For minimal-to-moderate discomfort, patients can take acetaminophen as needed. Excessive bleeding, bruising, or swelling and significant postprocedural pain are not typical. Patients should be advised to seek immediate medical attention if these symptoms are experienced or if they have any concern for possible infection of the area.

It is also essential that patients understand the process of skin tightening. This can help control patient expectations for the procedure, which should in turn increase patient satisfaction. Patients should expect an initial increase in skin tightening within several weeks, but the majority of improvement is expected to take several months to occur. The benefit in the initial period is most

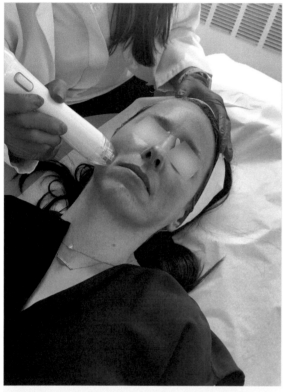

Fig. 5.2 Demonstration of radiofrequency microneedling procedure.

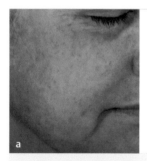
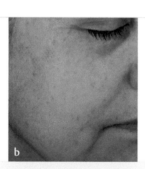
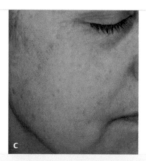
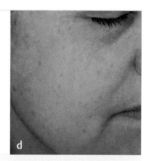

Fig. 5.3 Female subject following radiofrequency microneedling at **(a)** immediate posttreatment, **(b)** 2 days posttreatment, **(c)** 5 days posttreatment, and **(d)** 7 days posttreatment demonstrating postprocedural downtime and healing. (These images are provided courtesy of Dr. Jordan V. Wang and Dr. Roy Geronemus.)

likely from acute disruption of collagen and remodeling of the epidermis. During the subsequent months, new collagen is still continuing to be synthesized and remodeled from the initial stimulation during the procedure. A period of about 3 to 6 months is suggested as the typical timeline for when a patient can expect to visualize maximal or near-maximal improvements following treatment.

Aftercare instructions for most procedures for skin laxity, including microneedling, are relatively simple for patients to follow. They should avoid any harsh chemicals or products while the treated skin is healing. Only a very gentle over-the-counter cleanser and lukewarm water should be used to clean the skin for the next week. Harsh scrubs and brushes, including electronic facial brushes, should be avoided for the next couple of weeks. Gentle moisturizers should be used to aid in skin healing and recovery. Products that contain alpha hydroxyl acids or retinol should be avoided, since these may cause additional irritation in the highly sensitive skin. Patients should avoid cosmetic makeup right after the procedure. These products have the potential to penetrate any channels caused by microneedling and produce irritation. However, it should be noted that there remains debate on whether microneedling actually creates channels in the skin. Patients should refrain from using anti-inflammatory medications, such as ibuprofen, for at least 1 week. It is also very important to avoid prolonged exercise for up to 48 hours and direct sunlight for extended periods of time directly following procedures. Regular application of a broad-spectrum sunscreen that contains physical blockers is also recommended to avoid any issues with pigmentation.

Products that contain hyaluronic acid or similar collagen-stimulating peptides may offer benefit in restoring and regenerating the skin following treatment. Any microneedling-induced physical columns of injury in the skin may allow for deeper penetration to the dermis of these essential proteins and peptides. Again, there still remains controversy on whether microneedling can actually create these channels. If so, microneedling may enhance topical drug delivery. Otherwise, it also has the potential to push topicals into the skin. For this reason, only products designed for dermal application should be used directly before or after microneedling. Caution should be advised when using periprocedural topical products, especially those that contain vitamin C, since reports have demonstrated facial granulomas to occur.[11] It is believed that topical products can introduce immunogenic particles into the dermis and potentiate local or systemic hypersensitivity reactions.

5.9 Potential Complications

Various postoperative complications are possible following microneedling treatments. The most common are temporary swelling, bleeding, bruising, and postoperative pain. These typically resolve within minutes to several hours. More serious complications can include infection, pigmentary changes, and scarring. Patients who present with increasing postprocedural pain, swelling, and drainage, especially when out of proportion to what is expected, should be evaluated in the clinic for possible infection. Although bacterial infections are much more common, viral infections can also occur. Affected areas can be swabbed for bacterial culture or viral polymerase chain reaction (PCR) studies.

Suspected bacterial infections can initially be treated with a broad-spectrum antibiotic that covers both *Staphylococcus* (methicillin-resistant and methicillin-sensitive strains) and *Streptococcus* species until the bacterial culture becomes available. Targeted antibacterial therapy is then more appropriate. Of viral infections, herpes simplex is the most common. In suspected cases of herpetic infections, oral courses of valacyclovir or acyclovir can be started for a duration of at least 1 week. Close observation is necessary in order to ensure proper healing and to decrease the risks of the infection spreading and permanent scarring. Practitioners should remain available to these patients to improve patient outcomes and satisfaction.

Postprocedural pigmentary changes and scarring can also be encountered. Most instances of dyspigmentation are typically temporary, such as postinflammatory hypo- and hyperpigmentation. In these cases, reassurance to the patient is often all that is required. However, pigmentary issues may last for up to several months or even longer, especially in skin of color. If severe or persistent, skin-lightening topicals, such as hydroquinone, or low-powered lasers to target postinflammatory hyperpigmentation can be utilized with close patient follow-up. When scarring occurs, patients should be reassured that this can be a possible and unfortunate outcome but that they will be closely managed to ensure that the scarring will be improved. On some occasions, this can mean using alternate treatment modalities to improve the appearance of the scars, such as those detailed in Chapter 6. It is important to maintain a positive and close patient–physician relationship during these cases.

5.10 Other Modalities

Multiple other technologies have also been employed to treat skin laxity, including ultrasound, RF, and thermomechanical fractional injury (TMFI). All of these involve the use of heat to thermally induce collagen contraction, neocollagenesis, and dermal remodeling, which subsequently leads to skin tightening.

Ultrasound devices emit vibrational acoustic energy, which is absorbed by the tissue to contract the collagen fibers.[12,13] Ultrasound technology can include microfocused and high-intensity focused ultrasound. Microfocused ultrasound delivers low-intensity pulses into the deep reticular dermal and subdermal layers of the skin,

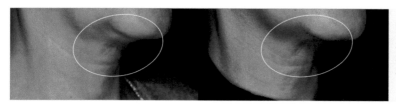

Fig. 5.4 Female subject at baseline and 3 months of follow-up after single treatment with synchronous ultrasound parallel beam technology (Sofwave). (This image is provided courtesy of Dr. Roy Geronemus.)

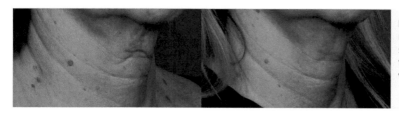

Fig. 5.5 Female subject at baseline and 3-month follow-up after single treatment with synchronous ultrasound parallel beam technology (Sofwave). (This image is provided courtesy of Dr. Arielle Kauvar.)

which disrupts the local architecture and stimulates its distensibility and elasticity.[14] In contrast, high-intensity focused ultrasound focuses heat to the deeper layers of the skin to reach the deep dermis, subdermal connective tissue, and the fibromuscular layer. The goal of this modality is to cause targeted microcoagulation to stimulate collagen remodeling.[15] A newer technology utilizes high-intensity, high-frequency, parallel ultrasound beams (Sofwave, Yoqneam, Israel) that bypass the epidermal layer and direct the thermal damage to depths of 0.5 to 2 mm, while avoiding injury to deeper anatomic structures. This technology has been demonstrated to be effective, safe, and well-tolerated (▶ Fig. 5.4, ▶ Fig. 5.5). For ultrasound devices, topical anesthesia is typically required prior to administration, and the improvements are not typically seen until weeks to months following treatment. Modest tightening and improvement in skin laxity are expected with ultrasound therapy among those who respond[15] using the older modalities. Transient posttreatment side effects can include erythema, purpura, edema, and postinflammatory pigmentation. Serious complications have uncommonly been reported, including scarring, necrosis, motor nerve paresis, and palpable subcutaneous nodules.

RF is frequently marketed for skin tightening and cutaneous rejuvenation. RF devices generate heat in the tissue by generating an alternating electrical current to stimulate collagen remodeling. Monopolar devices have been the most traditionally studied, which have been found to produce mild-to-moderate improvement in most patients.[16] Immediate results can be observed, whereas more dramatic improvements are typically seen months after treatment.[17] Bipolar and multipolar RF devices have multiple electrodes, which can produce different electric fields.[18,19] No significant differences in skin tightening have been observed in trials comparing the monopolar, bipolar, and multipolar technologies.[19,20] However, it is believed that monopolar treatments have the potential to deliver energy deeper and produce deeper effects. Topical

anesthetics are required prior to treatment, and transient side effects include pain, erythema, edema, and postinflammatory hyperpigmentation. Scarring and nodules are rare, yet more severe, side effects. Although multiple treatments are advised in order to maximize improvement, a single treatment may suffice for modest improvements in skin laxity.

TMFI is a relatively new nonablative skin rejuvenation method that combines thermal energy with motion.[21] This device (Tixel, Novoxel, Netanya, Israel) focuses thermal energy on a titanium tip with a grid of pyramids, which, when heated, is pulsed to contact the skin surface and coagulate the tissue. This subsequently creates micro-craters by processes of evaporation and desiccation. Thermal heat transfer using TMFI does not involve any mechanical penetration deeper than the epidermis. In one study, most patients experienced mild-to-moderate improvement in skin laxity and facial rhytides after two to three treatment sessions at 3- to 5-week intervals.[22] Topical anesthetic may be used, but is not always required, prior to treatment, and postprocedural downtime is minimal at 1 to 5 days. Transient postprocedural events include erythema and rarely postinflammatory hyperpigmentation if aggressive settings are administered.

5.11 Pearls and Pitfalls

The most important things to remember with microneedling are to select appropriate patients and to manage their expectations accordingly. Ensure to select patients with mild-to-moderate skin laxity, who would benefit from microneedling procedures as compared to more aggressive treatments or surgical interventions, such as facelifts. Maintaining expectations is crucial to ensuring increased patient satisfaction and retention. The skin type of the patient should also be taken into consideration in order to adequately discuss the risks of pigmentary changes and scarring.

When performing traditional microneedling, it is important to have an adequate amount of gliding gel and not too much. In addition, manual traction on the surrounding skin can help prevent the device from catching on the treated skin. Both of these techniques can improve patient comfort and outcomes. During treatment, the device should be held directly perpendicular to the skin, and multiple directions should be used with each pass to avoid striping.

For RF microneedling, it is important to treat each patient using a similar technique in order to ensure the expected outcome. It has been suggested that interpractitioner techniques may be significantly different, which can account for different outcomes even when using similar devices and settings. Using similar settings between different devices may also produce different outcomes, so practitioners should exercise caution. When treating skin of color, utilizing insulated needle tips, when available, may help reduce the increased risk of pigmentary changes and scarring.

References

[1] Tobin DJ. Introduction to skin aging. J Tissue Viability. 2017; 26(1): 37–46

[2] Cui H, Kong Y, Zhang H. Oxidative stress, mitochondrial dysfunction, and aging. J Signal Transduct. 2012; 2012:646354

[3] Nkengne A, Bertin C. Aging and facial changes: documenting clinical signs, part 1: clinical changes of the aging face. Skinmed. 2013; 11 (5):281–286

[4] Mokos ZB, Ćurković D, Kostović K, Čeović R. Facial changes in the mature patient. Clin Dermatol. 2018; 36(2):152–158

[5] Hou A, Cohen B, Haimovic A, Elbuluk N. Microneedling: a comprehensive review. Dermatol Surg. 2017; 43(3):321–339

[6] Ramaut L, Hoeksema H, Pirayesh A, Stillaert F, Monstrey S. Microneedling: Where do we stand now? A systematic review of the literature. J Plast Reconstr Aesthet Surg. 2018; 71(1):1–14

[7] Harris AG, Naidoo C, Murrell DF. Skin needling as a treatment for acne scarring: an up-to-date review of the literature. Int J Womens Dermatol. 2015; 1(2):77–81

[8] Fabbrocini G, Fardella N, Monfrecola A, Proietti I, Innocenzi D. Acne scarring treatment using skin needling. Clin Exp Dermatol. 2009; 34 (8):874–879

[9] Alster TS, Graham PM. Microneedling: a review and practical guide. Dermatol Surg. 2018; 44(3):397–404

[10] Puiu T, Mohammad TF, Ozog DM, Rambhatla PV. A comparative analysis of electric and radiofrequency microneedling devices on the market. J Drugs Dermatol. 2018; 17(9):1010–1013

[11] Soltani-Arabshahi R, Wong JW, Duffy KL, Powell DL. Facial allergic granulomatous reaction and systemic hypersensitivity associated with microneedle therapy for skin rejuvenation. JAMA Dermatol. 2014; 150(1):68–72

[12] Fabi SG. Noninvasive skin tightening: focus on new ultrasound techniques. Clin Cosmet Investig Dermatol. 2015; 8:47–52

[13] MacGregor JL, Tanzi EL. Microfocused ultrasound for skin tightening. Semin Cutan Med Surg. 2013; 32(1):18–25

[14] Kwan KR, Kolansky Z, Abittan BJ, Farberg AS, Goldenberg G. Skin tightening. Cutis. 2020; 106(3):134–137, 139, E1

[15] Friedman O, Isman G, Koren A, Shoshany H, Sprecher E, Artzi O. Intense focused ultrasound for neck and lower face skin tightening a prospective study. J Cosmet Dermatol. 2020; 19(4):850–854

[16] Polder KD, Bruce S. Radiofrequency: Thermage. Facial Plast Surg Clin North Am. 2011; 19(2):347–359

[17] Boisen J, Alkul S, Malone CH, Munavalli G. Perioral volumization using a temperature controlled fractionated radiofrequency device. J Cosmet Dermatol. 2021

[18] Alexiades-Armenakas M, Dover JS, Arndt KA. Unipolar versus bipolar radiofrequency treatment of rhytides and laxity using a mobile painless delivery method. Lasers Surg Med. 2008; 40(7):446–453

[19] Sadick NS, Nassar AH, Dorizas AS, Alexiades-Armenakas M. Bipolar and multipolar radiofrequency. Dermatol Surg. 2014; 40 Suppl 12:S174–S179

[20] Alexiades M. Laser and light-based treatments of acne and acne scarring. Clin Dermatol. 2017; 35(2):183–189

[21] Elman M, Fournier N, Barnéon G, Bernstein EF, Lask G. Fractional treatment of aging skin with Tixel, a clinical and histological evaluation. J Cosmet Laser Ther. 2016; 18(1):31–37

[22] Daniely D, Judodihardjo H, Rajpar SF, Mehrabi JN, Artzi O. Thermomechanical fractional injury therapy for facial skin rejuvenation in skin types II to V: a retrospective double-center chart review. Lasers Surg Med. 2021:(e-pub ahead of print)

6 Scar Treatments

Daniel P. Friedmann, Michael Zumwalt, and Vineet Mishra

Summary

Numerous safe and effective therapies for improving scar appearance are currently available. Treatment paradigms, however, vary significantly between scar types, with hypertrophic, atrophic, and burn scars benefiting from different combination therapies. This chapter presents a detailed overview of these varying treatment approaches to scars.

Keywords: pulsed dye laser, intense pulsed light, nonablative fractional laser resurfacing, ablative fractional laser resurfacing, bipolar fractional radiofrequency, hypertrophic scar, keloid scar, atrophic acne scar

6.1 Introduction

Scars are the end result of intrinsic cutaneous wound repair pathways that can have significant aesthetic, physical, and psychosocial implications for patients. Numerous safe and effective therapies for improving scar appearance are currently available, with the ideal single or combination of modalities dependent on the type of scar being treated.

6.2 Indications

6.2.1 Hypertrophic Scars

Hypertrophic scars are thought to arise from abnormal fibroblast activation, leading to an excessive collagen deposition confined within the borders of the initial injury.[1] Collagen types I and III are both overexpressed, with greater type III collagen deposition compared to normal scars.[2] Early hypertrophic scars may be erythematous, painful, and pruritic, but they do have a tendency to become asymptomatic and flatten slowly over time without treatment.

6.2.2 Keloids

Unlike hypertrophic scars, keloids extend beyond the original injury borders and can progressively enlarge with time. Dark-skinned individuals are much more susceptible, with a 6 to 16% incidence in African populations.[2] Commonly affected areas for these potentially pruritic, painful, or hyperesthetic lesions include the chest, back, and earlobes.

6.2.3 Atrophic Acne Scars

Although acne scarring may also be hypertrophic or keloidal, 80 to 90% of cases present as atrophic lesions due to abnormal collagen deposition following severe, prolonged dermal and subcutaneous inflammation.[3] Three subtypes of atrophic acne scars exist: ice pick, boxcar, and rolling (▶ Fig. 6.1). Ice pick scars are 1 to 2 mm and have a well-demarcated margin, extending precipitously into the deep dermis. Boxcar scars are 2 to 4 mm and round or quadrilateral in shape, with well-demarcated margins and shallow-to-moderate depth. Rolling scars are often greater than 4 mm and can be tethered to underlying subcutaneous tissue, leading to an undulating appearance with a rolled scar edge. Acne scarring must be differentiated from postinflammatory erythema or postinflammatory hyperpigmentation (PIH) secondary to acne, which are both self-limited and influenced by Fitzpatrick skin type (FST), with PIH more common in FST III to XI.

6.2.4 Other Scars

Surgical and traumatic scars can be hypertrophic or atrophic. Burn scars can present as tight, bandlike, contracted hypertrophic scarring that is painful, pruritic, and can limit joint range of motion, leading to true functional impairment.

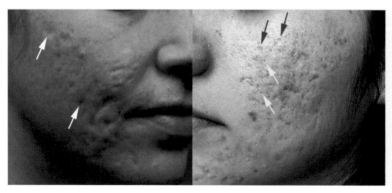

Fig. 6.1 Atrophic acne scarring subtypes include rolling (*white arrows*), boxcar (*blue arrows*), and ice pick (*yellow arrows*).

6.3 Treatment Options

6.3.1 For Hypertrophic and Keloid Scars

Intralesional Injection Therapy

Intralesional injections are considered first-line therapy for the treatment of hypertrophic (▶ Fig. 6.2) and keloid scars, with response rates ranging from 50 to 100%, albeit

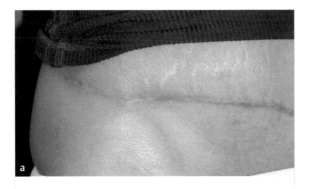

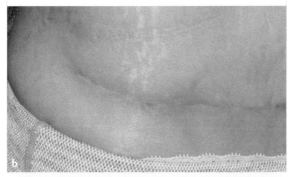

Fig. 6.2 Hypertrophic erythematous surgical scar of the lower abdomen before (a) and after (b) 4 monthly sessions with 1,550-nm nonablative fractional laser resurfacing (35–40 mJ, 14–23%, eight passes) and intralesional injections of 5-fluorouracil (5-FU) 50 mg/mL mixed in 0.9% normal saline (0.1–0.3 mL 5-FU/1 mL total solution, with the last session adding 0.1 mL of triamcinolone 10 mg/mL to the mixture). (These images are provided courtesy of Sabrina G. Fabi, MD, Cosmetic Laser Dermatology, San Diego, California, United States.)

with a recurrence rate of 9 to 50%.[4] Corticosteroid (e.g., triamcinolone) injections inhibit cell proliferation and transforming growth factor-β1 (TGF-β1) expression, whereas 5-fluorouracil (5-FU) is a chemotherapeutic agent that inhibits TGF-β1 and type I collagen gene expression, as well as induces cell cycle G2 arrest and apoptosis of keloidal fibroblasts.[5]

Vascular Light and Laser Devices

Reducing scar erythema dramatically improves overall scar appearance (▶ Fig. 6.3). Although it commonly resolves within 12 months, erythema can persist in a subset of patients past 1 year postinjury.[6] Selective photothermolysis of hemoglobin allows for permanent thermal damage of scar blood vessels while sparing surrounding cutaneous structures.

Pulsed dye laser (PDL; 585–595 nm) and potassium titanyl phosphate (KTP) laser (532 nm; also known as a frequency-doubled neodymium:yttrium aluminum garnet [Nd:YAG] laser) can reduce erythema in surgical, acne, and burn scars by targeting peaks in the oxyhemoglobin absorption spectrum. In an investigator-blinded study of 22 subjects with erythematous and/or hypertrophic acne scars, hemifaces treated with PDL had a 67.5 to 72.5% improvement after one to two sessions, respectively, compared to untreated sides.[7] Keaney and colleagues evaluated PDL versus KTP in a split-scar study of 20 subjects. Improvement in surgical scar erythema was similar between sides at 12 weeks following three sessions.[8] Intense pulsed light (IPL) devices emit incoherent, noncollimated, polychromatic light in the 500- to 1,200-nm range (with a peak at 600 nm) produced by a filtered, xenon flashlamp light source that targets both oxyhemoglobin and deoxyhemoglobin. IPL has been found to improve the appearance of hypertrophic and keloid scars by decreasing scar erythema, height, and hardness.[9]

Radiation Therapy

Radiation therapy (RT; e.g., X-ray, brachytherapy, or electron beam) has been used for treatment-refractory hypertrophic and keloid scars. Radiation inhibits blood vessel formation and decreases fibroblast proliferation, leading to decreased collagen production. It can be used

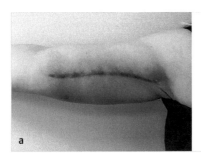
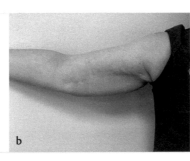

Fig. 6.3 Erythematous surgical scar of the arm before (a) and after (b) four sessions using pulsed dye laser (10 mm, 6 ms, 7.5 J/cm²). (These images are provided courtesy of Dr. Yoon-Soo Cindy Bae.)

as a monotherapy for keloids but is more commonly performed within 24 to 48 hours after keloid excision.[10] A review of 72 studies revealed that recurrence risk decreases from 37 to 22% when RT is combined with surgical excision, compared to monotherapy.[11]

Excision

Excision alone of hypertrophic and keloid scars is not recommended due to the recurrence rate of 45 to 100%.[12] Keloid excision with adjuvant therapy (intralesional triamcinolone/5-FU or RT) is most commonly used for exophytic keloids, like those seen on earlobes from ear piercing (▶ Fig. 6.4).

6.3.2 For Atrophic Scars

Subcision

Discrete rolling acne scars and traumatic or surgical atrophic scars can be treated with subcision, a percutaneous method of severing the fibrotic strands that tether depressed scars to underlying subcutaneous tissue using a sharp needle or blunt cannula.[13] Alam and colleagues[14] showed that subcision improved acne scar appearance by approximately 50%, with 90% of subjects reporting improvement.

Soft-Tissue Fillers

A wide variety of soft-tissue fillers are currently commercially available, with the ability to improve atrophic scars (e.g., traumatic, surgical, or rolling acne scars) by restoring lost volume and stimulating localized collagen production. Hyaluronic acid and calcium hydroxylapatite fillers are excellent volumizers and have been shown to improve acne scarring.[15,16] However, poly-L-lactic acid (PLLA) and polymethyl methacrylate (PMMA) microsphere biostimulatory fillers are often preferred, given the ability of these microparticles to induce marked local fibroblast proliferation and neocollagenesis, leading to gradual, progressive, and long-lasting augmentation. Multiple trials of PLLA for rolling acne scarring have reported significant improvement maintained up to 4 years posttreatment.[17,18,19] PMMA is approved by the Food and Drug Administration for correction of moderate-to-severe, atrophic, distensible facial acne scars, with results shown to last up to 5 years (▶ Fig. 6.5).[20] A recent study of distensible atrophic acne scars found that

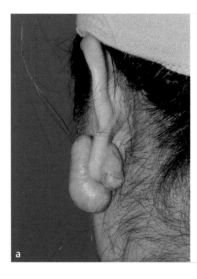
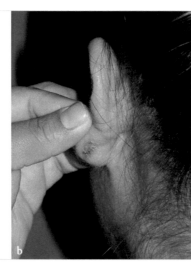

Fig. 6.4 Before (a) and 1 year following (b) excision of a large earlobe keloid excision with adjuvant 10,600-nm CO_2 ablative laser resurfacing (1-mm focused tip, 50 mJ, 1 W), followed by intralesional injections of 5-fluorouracil (5-FU) 50 mg/mL mixed in triamcinolone 10 mg/mL (0.1-mL 5-FU/1 mL total solution) every 3 months.

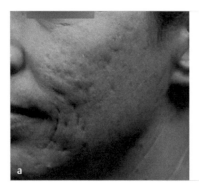
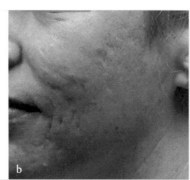

Fig. 6.5 Before (a) and after (b) a single session of sequential polymethylmethacrylate microsphere soft-tissue filler (two syringes) with subcision using a 27-gauge needle, followed by 10,600-nm CO_2 ablative fractional laser resurfacing (27.5 mJ, 30–40% density, 300 Hz) for rolling and boxcar acne scarring, respectively.

microneedling combined with PMMA led to greater clinical improvement than microneedling alone.[21]

Microneedling

Microneedling (or percutaneous collagen induction therapy) is a process by which skin is repeatedly punctured with a perpendicular array of needles, with the resulting dermal–epidermal wounds inducing collagen production that is safe for all skin types.[22] Treatment can be performed by either a manual fixed-needle roller drum (0.5–1.5 mm) or a reciprocating electric motor-driven pen (0.5–2.5 mm). The latter are more commonly utilized due to their variable (and greater) operating speed and penetration depth, disposable needle tips, low consumable cost, and ability to limit treatment to small focal areas.[22] Rolling and boxcar acne scarring are likely to demonstrate far greater improvement with microneedling than ice pick scars.[22,23]

Fractional Radiofrequency

Bipolar fractional radiofrequency (BFR) devices are chromophore independent and utilize an array of electrode pins or insulated (to noninsulated) needles to deliver energy. The latter, known as microneedle fractional radiofrequency (MFR), bypasses the epidermis in order to generate precise, variable-depth (0.5–3.5 mm) dermal microcoagulation zones at the needle tips. Neocollagenesis is thus maximized compared to conventional microneedling while minimizing epidermal damage. Studies have demonstrated the safety and efficacy of MFR for acne scarring in all skin types with minimal downtime.[24,25] A randomized-controlled split-face study comparing MFR with electrode pin BFR showed that MFR led to significantly greater improvement in boxcar and ice pick scarring.[26]

Nonablative Fractional Laser Resurfacing

Instead of producing confluent thermal damage, nonablative fractional laser resurfacing (NAFR) creates columnar microscopic thermal wounds (microthermal treatment zones [MTZs]) that stimulate collagen production, sparing intervening tissue and leaving up to a maximum of 95% of the skin uninvolved.[27] Many patients find it easier to have a noninvasive minimal-downtime procedure like NAFR, despite more marginal and delayed results that require multiple treatment sessions to see substantial improvement, and remain hesitant about or are unable to undergo ablative fractional laser resurfacing (AFR), which is associated with greater discomfort, side effects, a week-long downtime, and an intense postoperative regimen. The safety and efficacy of NAFR for improving the appearance of Mohs surgical scars,[28] traumatic scars,[29] and boxcar acne scars[30] have been reported.

Ablative Fractional Laser Resurfacing

AFR with a 10,600-nm carbon dioxide (CO_2) laser creates MTZs similar to that of NAFR, but ablates the stratum corneum, producing a greater zone of thermal coagulation around the columnar wounds (▶ Fig. 6.6). AFR was found to have efficacy similar to fully ablative CO_2 and erbium laser modalities and superior to 1,550-nm NAFR in a retrospective study of 58 Asian subjects.[31] AFR has also been shown to improve atrophic surgical, traumatic, and burn scars, with AFR able to improve erythema, thickness, pliability, and contractures in the latter.[32,33]

CROSS Technique or Punch Removal

Ice pick acne scars respond extremely well to focal application of 70 to 100% trichloroacetic acid (TCA), a procedure known as chemical reconstruction of skin scars (CROSS). Atrophic acne scars treated with 70% TCA CROSS technique every 2 weeks led to greater than 50% improvement in 66% of subjects, with 81% of subjects feeling satisfied or very satisfied with treatment.[34] Another option for removal of ice pick scars is physical removal with a 1- or 1.5-mm punch biopsy instrument.[35]

6.3.3 For Other Scars
Surgical Revision

Surgical revision may be the best treatment option for surgical scars that have widened due to tension, developed an

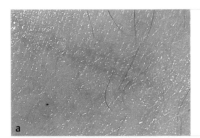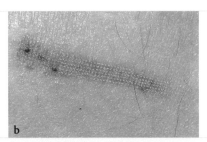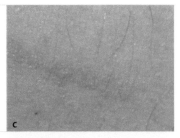

Fig. 6.6 Before (a), immediately after (b), and 3 months following (c) a single treatment of a dyspigmented linear traumatic scar with 10,600-nm ablative fractional laser resurfacing (25 mJ, 5% density, 300 Hz). (These images are provided courtesy of Dr. Daniel P. Friedmann.)

area of bulging on one side of a depressed scar (i.e., trap-door deformity), or that have residual redundant tissue at each end (i.e., standing cone deformity). Nevertheless, the revision should be delayed for at least several months postsurgery, allowing for maximal scar maturation.

A Z-plasty creates two triangular flaps along a linear line that are then transposed across each other, resulting in a rotated and lengthened scar. Given this transposition, the greater the angle utilized, the longer the length of the resulting scar (e.g., 25 and 75% lengthening with a 60- and 30-degree angle, respectively).[36] On the other hand, W-plasties and geometric broken line closures do not lengthen scars, but break them up into multiple, less noticeable subunits.[36]

Dermabrasion

Prior to the advent of fractional ablative and nonablative laser technology, dermabrasion was the mainstay of scarring treatment. Today, manual dermabrasion is used primarily to improve contour and color match between skin grafts or raised, dyspigmented surgical incision lines and normal surrounding skin.[36]

6.4 Pretreatment Considerations

Contraindications to scar treatment include active localized bacterial or fungal infection within the treatment area or chronic immunosuppression.[22] Active pregnancy and breastfeeding are also reasons to delay treatment. A 3- to 7-day course of oral antiviral prophylaxis (valacyclovir 500 mg orally twice a day) should be started 1 day prior to treatment of perioral scars with microneedling and NAFR in patients with a history of cold sores (herpes simplex virus reactivation) and in all patients before perioral treatment with AFR. An oral antibiotic (doxycycline 100 mg orally twice a day for 10 days) and antifungal (fluconazole 150 mg orally for 1 day) should be considered when treating extensive areas of scarring, especially on the face, starting the day before treatment.

Patients with FST III to VI ought to be on topical hydroquinone 4% every night at bedtime or triple combination therapy (e.g., hydroquinone 4%, fluocinolone 0.01%, tretinoin 0.05%) every night at bedtime for at least 4 weeks prior to microneedling, NAFR, and AFR, but it is not required prior to BFR. Smoking significantly impairs wound healing and should be avoided between 2 weeks before and until 2 weeks after any surgical (subcision or punch removal) or resurfacing procedure. Given the overall limited injury produced, over-the-counter and prescription topicals need not be stopped prior to any treatment but should likely be held for up to 1 week posttreatment to minimize irritation.

Realistic expectations, risks, and alternatives must be discussed prior to start of therapy. It is important to emphasize that results can be achieved, albeit slowly and gradually over multiple treatment sessions.

6.4.1 Subcision

Appropriate patient selection for subcision treatment is very important. For acne scarring, subcision should only be used for rolling acne scars and is ineffective for ice pick or boxcar lesions.[14] Given that the vast majority of acne scarring patients have more than one subtype, if not all three, combination therapy is almost always mandatory. Patients must be advised that they are likely to need multiple sessions for optimal results from subcision.

6.4.2 Soft-Tissue Filler

Patients with a history of autoimmune disease may be at greater risk of excessive and unpredictable inflammatory sequelae from filler injection such as granulomas. A history of psoriasis or vitiligo should be ruled out, since they may koebnerize with treatment. Genetic conditions, acquired diseases, or medications that may predispose patients to bleeding and infections must also be ruled out. Any nonessential medications or supplements that increase bleeding risk should be stopped if possible at least 7 days prior to any injectable treatment.

Although allergy to the PMMA product is extremely rare, skin testing for the bovine collagen vehicle component of PMMA is recommended 1 month prior to treatment. A small bleb (0.1 mL) of vehicle is injected intradermally in the anterior forearm and evaluated by the patient for signs of erythema and induration.

6.4.3 Vascular Light and Laser Devices

Utmost caution should be taken when using IPL or laser devices to treat darker skin types—or lighter skin types with recent significant sun exposure, tanning, or sunless tanner use—due to the increased risk of epidermal injury. Tan patients should follow strict sun protection for at least 1 month prior to therapy.

6.5 Treatment Techniques and Protocols

Multiple procedures are commonly performed at the same visit, in order to achieve optimal results by targeting different aspects of acne scarring pathophysiology and to combine treatments into one period of downtime. A deep-to-superficial approach is ideal. For hypertrophic scars, treatment should start with intralesional therapy, followed by PDL, and ending with resurfacing. Likewise, for atrophic scars (e.g., acne scarring), therapy should begin with subcision, followed by soft-tissue filler, resurfacing, and focal destruction of ice pick scars.

For most procedures, application of a topical anesthetic for 30 to 60 minutes is sufficient, with the authors finding that compounded 23% lidocaine/7% tetracaine in a plasticized base produces the most rapid anesthesia (albeit with greater cutaneous vasodilation and irritation). Supplemental forced cold air (5 °C) can also be extremely helpful. For subcision and fractionated ablative laser resurfacing, subcutaneous infiltration with 0.1 to 1% lidocaine with epinephrine is often necessary. Intralesional/superficial lidocaine injections should be avoided immediately prior to nonablative or ablative laser resurfacing, given that lidocaine can potentiate the thermal sensitivity of cell cycle active skin cells[37] and increase the potential for focal ulceration.[38] Intraocular metal eye shields should be used in the rare instance that a scar of eyelid skin within the orbital rim is to be treated.

For all procedures, treatment areas are prepped with 70% isopropyl alcohol immediately pretreatment. Topical chlorhexidine or hypochlorous acid solution is also used prior to filler.

6.5.1 Intralesional Injection Therapy

Given a randomized-controlled study by Alexandrescu and colleagues[5] showing far greater keloid softening and size reduction with combination 5-FU/triamcinolone than with triamcinolone alone, and a meta-analysis[39] confirming fewer side effects and greater improvement in hypertrophic scar and keloid height and subject satisfaction with the combination 5-FU/triamcinolone is now the standard of care. Our standard mixture is 0.9 mL of 5-FU (50 mg/mL) with 0.1 mL of triamcinolone. Although the initial concentration of triamcinolone for markedly indurated or exophytic scars off the face is 20 to 40 mg/mL, initial treatment of facial scars is performed with triamcinolone 5 to 10 mg/mL. Concentration of the triamcinolone should then be reevaluated at each visit. As a scar flattens, it should be reduced by 5 to 10 mg/mL increments to minimize the risk of atrophy; on the other hand, if a scar shows no change, it should be increased by 5 to 10 mg/mL.

It is always best to inject 0.05 to 0.1 mL aliquots, with the number of aliquot injections depending on the size of the scar. The endpoint after injection is minimal blanching. Care should be taken to inject directly into scar, rather than into the underlying tissue, in order to eliminate the risk of subcutaneous atrophy.

6.5.2 Subcision

Although an 18- to 21-gauge beveled, triangular-tipped hypodermic needle has been widely touted as the best instrument for subcision, a recent study found that subcision with a blunt cannula was more effective and led to greater subject satisfaction than with a needle.

The areas to be subcised are circled with a permanent black or blue marker, injected with local anesthesia (1% lidocaine with epinephrine). After 15 to 20 minutes, allowing for maximal vasoconstriction from the epinephrine, the needle or cannula is introduced parallel to the skin surface. It is common to feel increased resistance when advancing immediately underneath a tethered scar. Multiple fanning motions are performed under the scar at the deep dermal to superficial subdermal level, which may produce a light snapping sound or sensation as the fibrous band is severed. This leads to bleeding, clot reorganization, and eventual long-term fibrosis that helps efface the depressed area.[40] Holding the needle or cannula with a needle driver provides optimal control.[40]

6.5.3 Soft-Tissue Filler

PLLA patients receive treatment every 4 to 6 weeks for a minimum of three sessions. Each vial of PLLA is reconstituted at least 24 hours prior to treatment in 7 mL of bacteriostatic water, with an additional 1 mL of 1% lidocaine added immediately prior to use. The 8-mL suspension is then stirred vigorously and drawn up into 3-mL syringes with 1-inch 26-gauge needles. The needle is inserted parallel to the skin under the most depressed portion of the scar, with small retrograde injections performed in a fanning pattern until the scar surface is flush with the surrounding skin.[17]

PMMA requires no reconstitution and is commercially available in a 0.8-mL syringe. Retrograde linear threading technique in a crosshatching pattern by means of a 26- or 27-gauge needle is ideal, with avoidance of overcorrection.[20]

6.5.4 Vascular Light and Laser Devices

PDL can be used for scars at either purpuric or nonpurpuric settings (▶ Fig. 6.7). Pulse durations less than 6 milliseconds can produce purpura secondary blood vessel rupture, whereas longer pulse durations do not. Although both can lead to improvement, nonpurpuric settings (10-mm spot size, 0.45-ms pulse duration, and 3.5 J/cm²) may be more beneficial for surgical scars.[32]

IPL can be performed on Caucasian patients with a 560-nm cutoff filter, 10- to 15-millisecond delay, and initial fluences of 15 to 18 J/cm². Fluence may be increased by 10 to 20% with subsequent treatments, based on clinical response, until an optimal energy density is achieved. Treatment of darker FSTs (III–IV) requires longer delays between pulses (20–50 ms) and/or higher cutoff filters (590 nm) that aid in sparing epidermal melanin.

6.5.5 Microneedling

Microneedle depth should be adjusted based on scar depth, with thicker scars requiring 1.5 to 2.5 mm, whereas

1.0 to 1.5 mm may be sufficient for atrophic scars.[22] A gliding solution (e.g., hyaluronic acid–based product, normal saline, or platelet-rich plasma) is applied immediately pretreatment when using a microneedling pen. With the microneedling pen held perpendicular to the skin surface, multiple passes are performed with a combination of vertical, horizontal, and circular motions until an endpoint of skin erythema, edema, and pinpoint bleeding is achieved. Sterile saline or bacteriostatic water is then used to clean the area.

6.5.6 Fractional Radiofrequency

For both BFR and MFR treatments, the treatment tip must be firmly pressed against the skin to ensure proper skin contact (electrodes) or puncturing (needles), respectively. If inadequate pressure is applied with MFR, the needles insufficiently penetrate the skin, leading to epidermal damage. Three passes are made with slight overlap at different treatment depths, producing microcoagulation zones at various dermal layers for maximal efficacy. The endpoint is erythema, edema, and focal pinpoint bleeding. Like microneedling and NAFR, BFR should be performed every 4 weeks for a minimum of three sessions.

6.5.7 Nonablative Fractional Laser Resurfacing

The aggressiveness of treatment is dependent on the microbeam pulse energy, which controls the depth of penetration, and density, which is often displayed as a percentage of skin or as spots per square centimeter. For stamping handpieces, the amount of overlap between pulses can further titrate treatment intensity. Energy settings with both NAFR and AFR should be adjusted based on the degree of atrophy or hypertrophy being treated. Atrophic boxcar scars may do well with 25 to 45 mJ, whereas hypertrophic scars easily benefit from 60 mJ or more. Studies have shown that low-density NAFR (14% coverage) may produce better outcomes than high-density NAFR (26% coverage) for linear hypertrophic surgical scars.[33]

6.5.8 Ablative Fractional Laser Resurfacing

Deep penetration of laser energy at a low density may produce the best results and limit adverse events for surgical scars (▶ Fig. 6.8). Atrophic boxcar acne scarring can

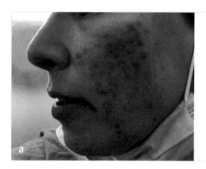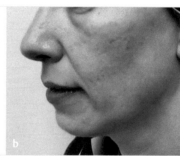

Fig. 6.7 Erythematous acne scars before (a) and after (b) three sessions every 4 weeks with a combination of 1,550-nm nonablative fractional laser resurfacing (70 mJ, 65%, four passes) and 595-nm pulsed dye laser (10 mm, 6 ms, 7.5 J/cm^2). (These images are provided courtesy of Dr. Yoon-Soo Cindy Bae.)

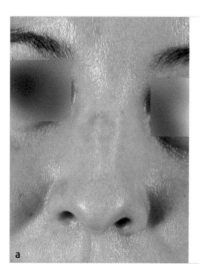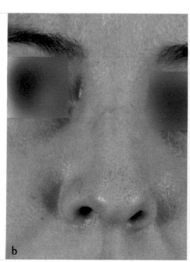

Fig. 6.8 Erythematous traumatic scar of the nasal dorsum before (a) and after (b) a single treatment session with sequential 595-nm pulsed dye laser (10 mm, 0.45 ms, 3.5 J/cm^2, three stacked pulses) and 10,600-nm CO_2 ablative fractional laser resurfacing (25 mJ, 5% density, 350 Hz).

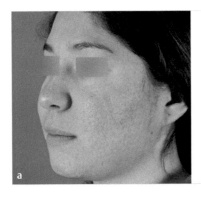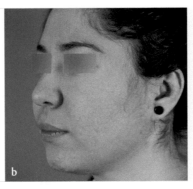

Fig. 6.9 A 27-year-old Hispanic woman with extensive boxcar acne scarring, before **(a)** and after **(b)** a single treatment with 10,600-nm ablative fractional laser resurfacing with 60 mJ, 40% coverage, and eight passes (5.75 kJ total). Triple combination therapy cream with hydroquinone 4%, fluocinolone 0.01%, and tretinoin 0.05% was used for 4 weeks pretreatment.

benefit from pulse energies of 20 to 45 mJ (depending on the device) and densities between 10 and 40% using multiple low-density randomly overlapping passes (▶ Fig. 6.9). Unlike microneedling and NAFR, AFR can produce lines of demarcation between treated and untreated areas, thereby requiring feathering of settings into the periphery of the scar. Off the face, more conservative fluences (15–25 mJ, depending on the device) and densities (a maximum of 10%) should be used, given the greater susceptibility of laser-induced scarring compared to the face.[41]

6.5.9 CROSS Technique or Punch Removal

A sterile wooden applicator is dipped 70 to 100% TCA and then applied to the scars for several seconds until a white frost is seen. CROSS can be performed monthly for up to three to four treatments for best results. Punch removal is performed with a 1-mm (less often 1.5-mm) disposable punch biopsy instrument and often requires injection of 1% lidocaine with epinephrine immediately pretreatment. it may require significantly fewer treatment sessions than CROSS but at the expense of greater downtime. If performed with a resurfacing procedure, the CROSS technique or punch removal should be performed before AFR or after any less invasive resurfacing.

6.6 Postoperative Instructions

Any area treated with a light or laser device, microneedling, radiofrequency, or nonablative laser resurfacing should be protected with a broad-spectrum, light zinc oxide sunscreen during the day, avoiding intense sunlight for the subsequent 7 to 10 days.

6.6.1 Intralesional Injection Therapy

Repeat injections are performed at 4- to 6-week intervals until the scar is flat to the surrounding skin. No special care of the area is required posttreatment.

6.6.2 Subcision

Hemostasis is achieved with manual pressure immediately posttreatment. Intermittent ice application for the first 24 hours is recommended. Mild puncture site bleeding or oozing is common for the first 24 hours, and ecchymosis and edema can persist for up to 1 week postprocedure. Cosmetic outcome should be evaluated at 4 to 8 weeks, at which point resubcision can be performed.

6.6.3 Soft-Tissue Filler

Although firm massage immediately following implantation of PLLA and PMMA, and during the short-term follow-up period, has been recommended to potentially decrease the rate of papule or nodule formation,[42] one study found no papules or nodules despite a complete absence of postprocedure massage.[18]

6.6.4 Ablative Fractional Laser Resurfacing

Proper follow-up and aftercare are vitally important for optimal healing and minimizing infection risk during re-epithelialization. Immediately following the procedure, the patient begins spraying antibacterial and antifungal hypochlorous acid solution and then applying petrolatum, at least four times per day until the area is healed over (approximately postoperative day 6). The area should be washed no more than twice a day and protected from the sun at all times. Once the skin has healed over (approximately postoperative day 6–7), the hypochlorous acid and petrolatum applications can stop, and the patient transitions to a moisturizer pro re nata (PRN) and a mid-potency topical steroid (fluocinolone 0.01%) cream twice a day to decrease erythema. The patient returns to the office on day 3, day 7, 1 month, and 4 months postprocedure.

6.6.5 CROSS Technique or Punch Removal

The treated lesions should be covered with petrolatum at least twice a day until fully healed, approximately 5 to 7 days posttreatment.

6.7 Potential Complications and Management

The majority of adverse events following procedures for scarring are typically mild, technique or procedure related, and transient, resolving within hours to days posttreatment. They include erythema, edema, pain, tenderness, induration, and ecchymosis. The risk of bacterial or fungal infection is extremely rare with many of these procedures, only becoming significant (albeit still low risk) with ablative fractionated laser resurfacing and dermabrasion.

6.7.1 Intralesional Injection Therapy

Although local adverse events from intralesional corticosteroids include dermal atrophy, telangiectasias, hypopigmentation, and ulceration, the use of appropriate concentrations of combination 5-FU/triamcinolone with correct injection technique over multiple sessions minimizes that risk.

6.7.2 Subcision

Subcision should be avoided (or performed with utmost care) in the temporal fossa or mid-mandible in order to avoid accidental injury of the temporal and marginal mandibular branches of the facial nerve, respectively. Indurated papules to small nodules may arise at treatment sites and are self-limited, typically resolving over days to weeks posttreatment.

6.7.3 Soft-Tissue Filler

Posttreatment adverse events such as visible or palpable subcutaneous nodules and delayed granuloma formation, once a significant problem with PLLA, have been minimized with proper product preparation and meticulous injection technique.[43]

6.7.4 Vascular Light and Laser Devices

Less common adverse events following IPL include scattered crusting or short-term (< 2 months) dyspigmentation. Blistering and persistent dyspigmentation are uncommon and likely to be a direct result of excessive overlapping, exorbitant fluences, poor epidermal cooling, and/or insufficient delay between sequential pulses.[44] Regardless,

scarring is exceedingly rare. IPL is generally avoided in the hair-bearing skin of the scalp or the male beard area since it is also a hair removal device.

With PDL, cryogen cooling helps limit epidermal thermal injury that results from melanin absorption of 585- to 595-nm laser energy in darker FSTs, but PIH and crusting are still possible. The use of IPL in FST IV to VI, however, is best avoided.

6.7.5 Microneedling, Fractional Radiofrequency, and Nonablative Laser Resurfacing

NAFR has the advantage of being able to stimulate collagen production with minimal injury to the epidermis, reducing the risk of PIH and prolonged erythema compared to AFR or fully ablative laser therapy. The most common side effects encountered with NAFR are erythema and edema that resolve 3 to 5 days posttreatment.[45] The use of conservative treatment densities can significantly decrease the risk of PIH and dyschromia in Asian or darker skin patients.[46,47] Nevertheless, microneedling or BFR further decreases the risk of these adverse events, making them arguably far better options for patients with FST III to VI.

6.7.6 Ablative Fractional Laser Resurfacing

Although higher risk than NAFR, AFR has a decreased risk of persistent erythema, PIH, and scarring, as well as a faster period of re-epithelialization (1 week) than fully ablative laser therapy.[31] Possible complications from AFR also include acneiform eruptions, milia formation, and infection (0.3–2.0% risk).[48] Postoperative infection is one of the most common causes of scarring.[48]

6.7.7 CROSS Technique or Punch Removal

Care must be taken to not drip the high concentration TCA solution on surrounding skin or nearby areas (e.g., chest or neck), which could lead to inadvertent scarring. Both TCA and punch removal produce a very small scar, with the goal being that the resulting lesion will be flat instead of a deep ice pick shape.

6.7.8 Dermabrasion

The most common complications of dermabrasion include prolonged postoperative erythema and milia formation. Reactivation of herpes simplex virus has been seen postoperatively. Worsening scarring is uncommon and results from overlying an overly aggressive treatment causing a deep dermal injury.

6.7.9 Radiation Therapy

Acute adverse events include erythema, edema, desquamation, ulceration, and necrosis. Longer-term RT side effects include skin pigmentation changes, atrophy, erythema, and telangiectasias.[10]

6.8 Pearls and Pitfalls

Atrophic acne scarring usually exhibits a mixture of lesion types, which makes combination therapy essential. Soft-tissue filler, subcision, laser resurfacing, and CROSS technique or punch removal can all be performed in the same session to target rolling, boxcar, and ice pick scars, respectively.

Less is often more. Scars may actually demonstrate greater improvement with lower fractional laser densities and nonpurpuric PDL treatment parameters.

Microneedling, nonablative laser resurfacing, BFR, and fractionated picosecond laser energy delivery can all resurface superficial skin in darker skin type patients with low risk of dyspigmentation.

PLLA and PMMA microsphere biostimulatory fillers may be preferable compared to hyaluronic acid fillers for rolling acne scars due to their far longer duration of action.

A blunt cannula may be more effective and lead to less complications than a needle for subcision of rolling acne scars.

A 90/10 mixture of 5-FU (50 mg/mL) and triamcinolone (10 mg/mL) is highly effective for reducing the height and thickness of hypertrophic and keloid scars, and it also reduces the risk of steroid-induced atrophy.

References

[1] Gauglitz GG, Korting HC, Pavicic T, Ruzicka T, Jeschke MG. Hypertrophic scarring and keloids: pathomechanisms and current and emerging treatment strategies. Mol Med. 2011; 17(1–2):113–125

[2] Alster TS, Tanzi EL. Hypertrophic scars and keloids: etiology and management. Am J Clin Dermatol. 2003; 4(4):235–243

[3] Fabbrocini G, Annunziata MC, D'Arco V, et al. Acne scars: pathogenesis, classification and treatment. Dermatol Res Pract. 2010; 2010:893080

[4] Wang XQ, Liu YK, Qing C, Lu SL. A review of the effectiveness of antimitotic drug injections for hypertrophic scars and keloids. Ann Plast Surg. 2009; 63(6):688–692

[5] Alexandrescu D, Fabi S, Yeh LC, Fitzpatrick RE, Goldman MP. Comparative results in treatment of keloids with intralesional 5-FU/kenalog, 5-FU/verapamil, enalapril alone, verapamil alone, and laser: a case report and review of the literature. J Drugs Dermatol. 2016; 15 (11):1442–1447

[6] Bond JS, Duncan JAL, Mason T, et al. Scar redness in humans: how long does it persist after incisional and excisional wounding? Plast Reconstr Surg. 2008; 121(2):487–496

[7] Alster TS, McMeekin TO. Improvement of facial acne scars by the 585 nm flashlamp-pumped pulsed dye laser. J Am Acad Dermatol. 1996; 35(1):79–81

[8] Keaney TC, Tanzi E, Alster T. Comparison of 532 nm potassium titanyl phosphate laser and 595 nm pulsed dye laser in the treatment of erythematous surgical scars: a randomized, controlled, open-label study. Dermatol Surg. 2016; 42(1):70–76

[9] Erol OO, Gurlek A, Agaoglu G, Topcuoglu E, Oz H. Treatment of hypertrophic scars and keloids using intense pulsed light (IPL). Aesthetic Plast Surg. 2008; 32(6):902–909

[10] Cheraghi N, Cognetta A, Jr, Goldberg D. Radiation therapy for the adjunctive treatment of surgically excised keloids: a review. J Clin Aesthet Dermatol. 2017; 10(8):12–15

[11] Mankowski P, Kanevsky J, Tomlinson J, Dyachenko A, Luc M. Optimizing radiotherapy for keloids: a meta-analysis systematic review comparing recurrence rates between different radiation modalities. Ann Plast Surg. 2017; 78(4):403–411

[12] Juckett G, Hartman-Adams H. Management of keloids and hypertrophic scars. Am Fam Physician. 2009; 80(3):253–260

[13] Orentreich DS, Orentreich N. Subcutaneous incisionless (subcision) surgery for the correction of depressed scars and wrinkles. Dermatol Surg. 1995; 21(6):543–549

[14] Alam M, Omura N, Kaminer MS. Subcision for acne scarring: technique and outcomes in 40 patients. Dermatol Surg. 2005; 31(3):310–317, discussion 317

[15] Halachmi S, Ben Amitai D, Lapidoth M. Treatment of acne scars with hyaluronic acid: an improved approach. J Drugs Dermatol. 2013; 12 (7):e121–e123

[16] Dierickx C, Larsson MK, Blomster S. Effectiveness and safety of acne scar treatment with nonanimal stabilized hyaluronic acid gel. Dermatol Surg. 2018; 44 Suppl 1:S10–S18

[17] Beer K. A single-center, open-label study on the use of injectable poly-L-lactic acid for the treatment of moderate to severe scarring from acne or varicella. Dermatol Surg. 2007; 33 Suppl 2:S159–S167

[18] Sadove R. Injectable poly-L: -lactic acid: a novel sculpting agent for the treatment of dermal fat atrophy after severe acne. Aesthetic Plast Surg. 2009; 33(1):113–116

[19] Sapra S, Stewart JA, Mraud K, Schupp R. A Canadian study of the use of poly-L-lactic acid dermal implant for the treatment of hill and valley acne scarring. Dermatol Surg. 2015; 41(5):587–594

[20] Karnik J, Baumann L, Bruce S, et al. A double-blind, randomized, multicenter, controlled trial of suspended polymethylmethacrylate microspheres for the correction of atrophic facial acne scars. J Am Acad Dermatol. 2014; 71(1):77–83

[21] Biesman BS, Cohen JL, DiBernardo BE, et al. Treatment of atrophic facial acne scars with microneedling followed by polymethylmethacrylate-collagen gel dermal filler. Dermatol Surg. 2019; 45(12):1570–1579

[22] Alster TS, Graham PM. Microneedling: a review and practical guide. Dermatol Surg. 2018; 44(3):397–404

[23] Harris AG, Naidoo C, Murrell DF. Skin needling as a treatment for acne scarring: an up-to-date review of the literature. Int J Womens Dermatol. 2015; 1(2):77–81

[24] Chandrashekar BS, Sriram R, Mysore R, Bhaskar S, Shetty A. Evaluation of microneedling fractional radiofrequency device for treatment of acne scars. J Cutan Aesthet Surg. 2014; 7(2):93–97

[25] Cho SI, Chung BY, Choi MG, et al. Evaluation of the clinical efficacy of fractional radiofrequency microneedle treatment in acne scars and large facial pores. Dermatol Surg. 2012; 38(7, Pt 1):1017–1024

[26] Min S, Park SY, Yoon JY, Suh DH. Comparison of fractional microneedling radiofrequency and bipolar radiofrequency on acne and acne scar and investigation of mechanism: comparative randomized controlled clinical trial. Arch Dermatol Res. 2015; 307 (10):897–904

[27] Fisher GH, Geronemus RG. Short-term side effects of fractional photothermolysis. Dermatol Surg. 2005; 31(9, Pt 2):1245–1249, discussion 1249

[28] Pham AM, Greene RM, Woolery-Lloyd H, Kaufman J, Grunebaum LD. 1550-nm nonablative laser resurfacing for facial surgical scars. Arch Facial Plast Surg. 2011; 13(3):203–210

[29] Vasily DB, Cerino ME, Ziselman EM, Zeina ST. Non-ablative fractional resurfacing of surgical and post-traumatic scars. J Drugs Dermatol. 2009; 8(11):998–1005

[30] Chrastil B, Glaich AS, Goldberg LH, Friedman PM. Second-generation 1,550-nm fractional photothermolysis for the treatment of acne scars. Dermatol Surg. 2008; 34(10):1327–1332

[31] You HJ, Kim DW, Yoon ES, Park SH. Comparison of four different lasers for acne scars: resurfacing and fractional lasers. J Plast Reconstr Aesthet Surg. 2016; 69(4):e87–e95

[32] Nouri K, Elsaie ML, Vejjabhinanta V, et al. Comparison of the effects of short- and long-pulse durations when using a 585-nm pulsed dye laser in the treatment of new surgical scars. Lasers Med Sci. 2010; 25 (1):121–126

[33] Lin JY, Warger WC, Izikson L, Anderson RR, Tannous Z. A prospective, randomized controlled trial on the efficacy of fractional photothermolysis on scar remodeling. Lasers Surg Med. 2011; 43:265–272

[34] Agarwal N, Gupta LK, Khare AK, Kuldeep CM, Mittal A. Therapeutic response of 70% trichloroacetic acid CROSS in atrophic acne scars. Dermatol Surg. 2015; 41(5):597–604

[35] Field LM. Punch techniques, acne scarring, and resurfacing. Dermatol Surg. 2001; 27(2):219–220

[36] Cerrati EW, Thomas JR. Scar revision and recontouring post-Mohs surgery. Facial Plast Surg Clin North Am. 2017; 25(3):463–471

[37] Raff AB, Thomas CN, Chuang GS, et al. Lidocaine-induced potentiation of thermal damage in skin and carcinoma cells. Lasers Surg Med. 2019; 51(1):88–94

[38] Chuang GS, Manstein D, Tannous Z, Avram MM. Ulceration of mature surgical scars following nonablative fractional photothermolysis associated with intralesional lidocaine injections. Dermatol Surg. 2012; 38(11):1879–1881

[39] Ren Y, Zhou X, Wei Z, Lin W, Fan B, Feng S. Efficacy and safety of triamcinolone acetonide alone and in combination with 5-fluorouracil for treating hypertrophic scars and keloids: a systematic review and meta-analysis. Int Wound J. 2017; 14(3): 480–487

[40] AlGhamdi KM. A better way to hold a Nokor needle during subcision. Dermatol Surg. 2008; 34(3):378–379

[41] Avram MM, Tope WD, Yu T, Szachowicz E, Nelson JS. Hypertrophic scarring of the neck following ablative fractional carbon dioxide laser resurfacing. Lasers Surg Med. 2009; 41(3):185–188

[42] Narins RS. Minimizing adverse events associated with poly-L-lactic acid injection. Dermatol Surg. 2008; 34 Suppl 1:S100–S104

[43] Bartus C, William Hanke C, Daro-Kaftan E. A decade of experience with injectable poly-L-lactic acid: a focus on safety. Dermatol Surg. 2013; 39(5):698–705

[44] Wat H, Wu DC, Rao J, Goldman MP. Application of intense pulsed light in the treatment of dermatologic disease: a systematic review. Dermatol Surg. 2014; 40(4):359–377

[45] Graber EM, Tanzi EL, Alster TS. Side effects and complications of fractional laser photothermolysis: experience with 961 treatments. Dermatol Surg. 2008; 34(3):301–305, discussion 305–307

[46] Yoo KH, Ahn JY, Kim JY, Li K, Seo SJ, Hong CK. The use of 1540 nm fractional photothermolysis for the treatment of acne scars in Asian skin: a pilot study. Photodermatol Photoimmunol Photomed. 2009; 25(3):138–142

[47] Chan HH, Manstein D, Yu CS, Shek S, Kono T, Wei WI. The prevalence and risk factors of post-inflammatory hyperpigmentation after fractional resurfacing in Asians. Lasers Surg Med. 2007; 39(5):381–385

[48] Shamsaldeen O, Peterson JD, Goldman MP. The adverse events of deep fractional CO(2): a retrospective study of 490 treatments in 374 patients. Lasers Surg Med. 2011; 43(6):453–456

7 Pigmented Lesion Removal

Monica K. Li

Summary

Laser and light-based technologies are one of many modalities for treating both congenital and acquired pigmented lesions. This chapter focuses on and presents updated, evidence-based practices and clinical pearls using laser and light-based interventions safely and effectively for various benign epidermal, dermal and mixed pigmentary dermatoses. Strategies on patient selection, technique, and discussion of pre- and postprocedure care to optimize treatment outcomes are discussed. Key considerations in treating benign pigmented lesions in skin of color are summarized. Pearls and pitfalls using laser and light-based treatments are reviewed to support the clinician in managing patient expectations and results.

Keywords: benign pigmented lesions, pigmentation, laser, melasma, ephelides, postinflammatory hyperpigmentation, melanin

7.1 Introduction

Patients seek removal of both congenital and acquired pigmented lesions irrespective of skin phototypes. Physicians must first distinguish pigmented lesions that are potentially malignant from benign. Any clinically or dermoscopically suspicious pigmented lesion warrants a skin biopsy for a definitive diagnosis before further aesthetic treatment.

Laser and light treatment is one modality of many for treating benign pigmented lesions. These lesions are classified based on where melanin is deposited: epidermal, dermal, or mixed. Epidermal pigmented lesions include café au lait macules (CALMs), lentigines, seborrheic keratoses, and ephelides. Examples of dermal and mixed pigmented lesions include melasma, Becker's nevus, postinflammatory hyperpigmentation (PIH), drug-induced hyperpigmentation, nevus of Ota and nevus of Ito, and Hori's nevus (acquired bilateral nevus of Ota-like macules or ABNOM). Such classification is important as it determines the selection of wavelength and device, and subsequent safety and effectiveness of the treatment.

Melanin has a wide energy absorption spectrum permitting the effective use of various laser and light treatments emitting visible and near-infrared wavelengths (250–1,200 nm) to target pigment.[1] The theory of selective photothermolysis forms the basis for energy absorption by the target chromophore while minimizing collateral tissue damage.[2] For benign pigmented lesions, optimal selection of the laser or light modality can avoid nonspecific thermal injury to surrounding tissue, which will minimize the risk of dyspigmentation and scarring.[1]

7.2 Modalities/Treatment Options

Energy devices used to treat benign pigmented lesions can be categorized into either pigment-targeting lasers or intense pulsed light (IPL). Intracellular melanosomes selectively absorb wavelengths emitted in the green, red, or near-infrared spectrum.[1] Although various wavelengths have been used, current standard pigment-targeting lasers include quality- or Q-switched (QS) nanosecond lasers, fractional nonablative or fully ablative lasers, and picosecond lasers. Specifically, QS ruby laser (QSRL; 694 nm), QS neodymium:yttrium aluminum garnet laser (QS Nd:YAG, 532 and 1,064 nm), QS alexandrite laser (QSAL; 755 nm), and picosecond domain lasers (primarily PS 532 and 755 nm and picosecond alexandrite laser [PSAL] 785 or 1,064 nm) have been used safely and effectively for treating benign pigmented lesions. A more recent pigment-targeting laser used to treat skin of color is the 650-microsecond Nd:YAG 1,064-nm laser, for managing melasma and PIH.[3,4] Various IPL (515–1,200 nm) devices have also produced effective treatments.

There are two laser principles that correlate with the evolution of technology for treating pigmented lesions. First, QS lasers deliver energy pulses in nanoseconds (ranging from 3-50 nanoseconds), which is considerably shorter than the thermal relaxation time of melanosomes at about 100 nanoseconds.[1] Hence, QS lasers are considered safe and effective for the treatment of pigmented lesions because they deliver energy within a time frame that confines injury to targeted melanosomes while limiting damage to surrounding structures. This reduces the potential risk of posttreatment dyspigmentation.[1,5] Second, although energy absorption of melanin decreases as the wavelength increases, deeper tissue penetration is achieved with a longer wavelength.[6] A laser with a longer wavelength (such as QS Nd:YAG 1,064 nm) can therefore be used to treat pigmented lesions in darker skin phototypes, lessening epidermal damage and subsequent risk of PIH while still targeting melanin.[6,7]

In recent years, picosecond domain lasers have emerged as devices that can be used effectively for tattoo removal[8] and similarly for melanin reduction.[9,10,11] The advantage of picosecond lasers is its ability to produce greater focal photomechanical effect and higher peak temperature but with reduced thermal effects on surrounding skin.[12] These characteristics are achieved as picosecond lasers deliver pulse durations at least 10 times shorter than QS devices.[13] Thus, lower fluences can be used to target melanin in pigmented lesions.[14] With reduced epidermal injury and PIH, improved potential adverse effects with picosecond laser treatments is favorable and of clinical relevance, particularly for darker skin patients.

Beyond laser, select benign cutaneous pigmentary concerns can be treated using topical, oral and physical modalities that are outside the scope of this chapter. Consistent photoprotection and diligent sunscreen use are essential management strategies. Notably, treatments for melasma and PIH include various topical skin-lightening agents (such as hydroquinone, tretinoin, arbutin, azelaic acid, tranexamic acid, and kojic acid), oral tranexamic acid, and chemical peels.[15,16,17,18,19] Varied success has been reported with use of these options alone or in combination with laser treatments, particularly recognizing the often recalcitrant nature of melasma.

7.3 Indications/Uses

7.3.1 Epidermal Pigmented Lesions

Lentigines

Multiple treatments are often required for lentigines, particularly for darker skinned individuals, due to the need for more conservative parameters. Conventionally, carbon dioxide (CO_2), argon, long-pulsed alexandrite laser, QS lasers including QS Nd:YAG, QSRL, and QSAL, and IPL have demonstrated effectiveness at treating

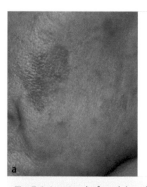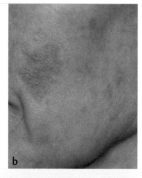

Fig. 7.1 Lentigo before **(a)** and after **(b)** one treatment with 785 nm picosecond laser, 4 J/cm², spot size of 2 mm, pulse rate of 1 Hz.

lentigines.[1,6,10,13,20,21,22,23,24,25] The use of picosecond lasers has recently emerged as the preferred approach for these pigmented lesions (▶ Fig. 7.1).[9,10,12,13,26,27]

Previous studies of conventional laser modalities for treating lentigines reported a high incidence of adverse effects such as PIH, ranging from 10 to 47%.[13] Chan et al reported the use of long-pulsed 532-nm Nd:YAG (2-mm spot size, 6.5–8 J/cm² fluence, and 2-millisecond pulse duration) to effectively treat lentigines in Asian patients with reduced risk of PIH.[23] Negishi et al used a picosecond Nd:YAG laser (532 nm, 750 picoseconds, average 0.35 ± 0.06 J/cm² fluence, 3- to 4-mm spot size, and 0- to 1-Hz pulse rate) for removing lentigines, supported by histologic evidence, in those with Fitzpatrick skin types III and IV.[13] A 5-grade percentage improvement scale was used to evaluate pigment clearance, with melanin index measured objectively using a reflectance spectrophotometer. PIH in the study was described to be less than 5%, with 93% of lentigines demonstrating over 75% clearance after a single treatment (▶ Fig. 7.2).[13]

Ephelides

Clinically similar to lentigines, ephelides typically darken in the summer months and appear during early childhood. Previously reported lasers used effectively to treat ephelides include QSAL and QS Nd:YAG devices.[24,28] Ho et al evaluated four different pigment-specific lasers targeting ephelides in Chinese patients, and found improvement with the long-pulsed dye laser (PDL), QS Nd:YAG and long-pulsed potassium titanyl phosphate (KTP) lasers, but no significant results with the long-pulsed alexandrite laser.[24] Improvement of pigmentation was evaluated using a 4-point visual analog scale.

More recently, picosecond lasers have demonstrated effectiveness at treating ephelides, particularly in Asian patients. Kung et al used a 532- and a 1,064-nm picosecond laser (400-mJ fluence, 450-picosecond pulse duration), and reported at least 50% clearance of treated lesions after an average of one treatment session (▶ Fig. 7.3).[12] Pigment clearance was evaluated using a 5-grade percentage improvement scale. PIH was observed in 4.8%, compared to up

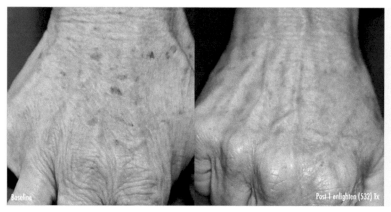

Fig. 7.2 Lentigines at baseline and 1 month following one treatment with a picosecond 532-nm laser. (This image is provided courtesy of Jeffrey TS Hsu, MD, Oak Dermatology, Itasca, Illinois, United States.)

to 25% with QS lasers as described by the authors, and blistering in 6.5% following treatment.[12] However, Yang et al showed a PSAL (average fluence of 4.4 J/cm²) producing comparable and safe clinical outcomes as a QSAL (average fluence of 6.92 J/cm²) for treating freckles in Chinese patients.[29] Lesion clearance rate was assessed comparing the number of the lesions before and after treatment as seen on standardized photographs, with examination by reflectance confocal microscopy of ephelides treated in 4 of 20 patients.

Café au Lait Macules

Current evidence shows variable recurrences following laser treatments of CALMs and patches.[6] Histologically, CALMs are comprised of basilar hyperpigmentation.[6] Common laser modalities used in the past included PDL, copper vapor, QSRL, QSAL, QS Nd:YAG, and erbium-doped YAG (Er:YAG) garnet lasers.[5,30,31,32,33,34,35]

Alster et al described in the mid-1990s the effective use of PDL for CALMs,[35] as well as its safety on a patient with Fitzpatrick skin type V.[33] Kagami et al reported transient bleaching with subsequent repigmentation when using the QSAL for these lesions, irrespective of the number of treatments.[32] Clinical responses to QSAL treatment were evaluated using a 5-grade percentage improvement scale by two independent observers. Other publications overall show that only one-third of treated cases achieve complete or near-complete clearance, with recurrences of 24% occurring at an average of 4 months.[6,30,36] Chan and Kono suggested and demonstrated that a long-pulsed ruby laser cleared CALMs possibly due to increased injury to follicular melanocytes.[37] In recent years, there is growing literature on the use of picosecond lasers for treating CALMs. Artzi et al described 15 patients with skin photo-types II to IV with lightening of CALMs using a PS 532-nm Nd:YAG laser (0.8–1.6 J/cm² fluence, 4- to 5-mm spot size) after an average of 2.47 (range: 1–4) treatments.[38] Two patients, however, had partial recurrences of their pigmented lesions (time interval to recurrence was not reported).[38] Evaluation of treated lesions used a 5-grade percentage improvement scale determined through baseline and follow-up standardized photographs.

Seborrheic Keratoses and Dermatosis Papulosa Nigra

Seborrheic keratoses, and clinically similar dermatosis papulosa nigra appearing in darker skin types, have been treated with CO_2, alexandrite, diode, 1,064-nm QS Nd:YAG, KTP, and various fractionated lasers (▶ Fig. 7.4).[39,40,41,42,43,44] CO_2 lasers were first reported for effective clearance of these lesions.[42] A 2018 publication of a retrospective study by Alegre-Sanchez et al illustrated potential of the PSAL (4.07 J/cm² fluence, 2.5-mm spot size) for treating seborrheic keratoses.[10] Patients with skin types I to III were

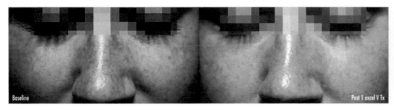

Fig. 7.3 Ephelides at baseline and 1 month following one treatment with a short-pulsed 532-nm laser. (The image is provided courtesy of Jeffrey TS Hsu, MD, Oak Dermatology, Itasca, Illinois, United States.)

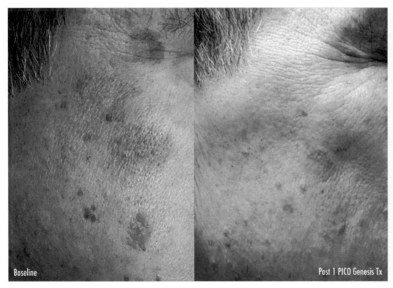

Fig. 7.4 Seborrheic keratoses at baseline and 1 month following one treatment using a 532- and 1,064-nm picosecond laser. (These images are provided courtesy of Jeffrey TS Hsu, MD, Oak Dermatology, Itasca, Illinois, United States.)

treated with two to four treatment sessions, and showed a clearance of 65% of their lesions. Clinical outcomes determined by photographs were evaluated using a 5-grade percentage improvement scale on all patients. However, further study is needed as only four patients were reported.[10]

7.3.2 Dermal or Mixed Pigmented Lesions

Melasma

The multifactorial pathogenesis of melasma, along with its chronicity and recurrences, is often more effectively managed using multimodal approaches. Prior to laser therapy, providing patient education on strict photoprotection and consistent sunscreen use, along with trials of topical skin-lightening agents, constitute prudent initial and first-line management steps. Chemical peels may be considered but should be performed by an experienced clinician. Oral tranexamic acid is a promising option as monotherapy or in combination with topical or laser interventions.[45,46,47]

Laser treatment of melasma alone may be challenging as it can worsen the condition or cause PIH. QSRL,[48] QS Nd:YAG,[49,50] QSAL,[51,52] CO_2,[51,52] and Er:YAG[53,54] have all been described for the treatment of melasma. IPL is another modality for managing melasma.[55,56,57,58] However, the use of IPL produces not only modest outcomes but also a modest recurrence rate unless aggressive topical therapy is used for maintenance up to 12 months posttreatment.[15]

Additionally, nonablative fractionated resurfacing treatments such as the 1,550-nm erbium-doped fiber[59,60,61] and the 1,927-nm thulium fiber lasers[62,63,64] have both been shown to improve melasma. Assessment of responses to laser treatments is commonly determined using the melasma area severity index (MASI). Overall, with the use of topical lightening agents, nonablative fractional laser (NAFL) treatments appear to provide a more durable response compared to IPL and QS interventions.[15] Triple therapy cream consisting of hydroquinone, retinoid, and corticosteroid has been reported to be an effective topical adjunctive option when used with NAFL treatments.[65,66] Tourlaki et al observed marked (>75%) and moderate (51–75%) improvement in MASI scores in 67 and 21% of study subjects, respectively, with the combination of fractional 1,540-nm erbium glass laser treatments and a triple therapy cream.[65] While melasma often recurs with all NAFL treatments, this tends to occur between 3 and 6 months, compared to earlier than 3 months with IPL and QS devices.[15] Given its fractionated output, NAFL treatments may produce more harmonized outcomes by being able to blend melasma with surrounding unaffected skin.[15] Ultimately, fractional laser settings will vary depending on skin phototype and type of melasma being treated, with consideration to use lower densities in darker skinned patients to reduce the risk of postprocedure PIH.[67,68]

In recent years, various wavelengths of picosecond laser devices have been shown to be safe and effective for treating melasma, due to their greater photomechanical effects and reduced thermal impact on surrounding skin.[11,12,16,69,70] The latter advantage in picosecond lasers when compared to conventional QS ones may underlie reduced risk and high rates of PIH following treatment of melasma.[15] Hence, there may be promise of more consistent and predictable results with the use of picosecond lasers for the treatment of melasma.

Nevus of Ota and Nevus of Ito

QS lasers including QSRL, QS Nd:YAG, and QSAL have been described as safe and effective treatments for this nevus type.[71,72,73,74,75,76] The use of picosecond domain lasers have also emerged as an encouraging treatment option for both nevus of Ota[9,26,77,78] and nevus of Ito,[9] although further studies are needed.

Ohshiro et al evaluated a group of six patients, of which two were recalcitrant nevi of Ota unresponsive to QSRL, with five treated using a PSAL (2.5- to 4-mm spot size, 2.83–5.26 J/cm^2 fluence).[78] Treatment sessions ranged from one to three. Erythema was most commonly described following treatment. Fair to excellent clinical improvement was observed of the treated lesions, with transient hyperpigmentation occurring in three patients followed by improvement to complete resolution at 3 months of follow-up.[78] A 5-grade percentage improvement score was used to determine the degree of pigment clearance.

Further work by Ge et al of 53 patients with nevus of Ota demonstrated greater clearance of treated lesions using PSAL when compared to QSAL.[79] In this study, treatment parameters of the PSAL were 2.0- to 4-mm spot size, 1.59 to 6.37 J/cm^2 fluence, and 5-Hz frequency. On average, 5.26 treatment sessions, with each treatment delivered at 12-week intervals, were performed using the PSAL. Complete to excellent clearance of nevus of Ota were reported at the final follow-up visits, conducted up to 3 months after the last treatment session.[79] Evaluation of pigment clearance following laser treatment was determined with standardized photographs using a 5-point percentage improvement score. The authors suggested that longer treatment intervals may optimize clinical outcomes in nevus of Ota specifically among Asian patients while reducing risk of pigmentary complications.[79]

Hori's Nevus (Acquired Bilateral Nevus of Ota-Like Macules)

Conventionally, QS lasers have been used to treat ABNOM and include QS Nd:YAG, QSRL, and QSAL.[80,81,82,83,84] However, high fluences and more than 10 treatment sessions may be needed to achieve favorable clinical outcomes.[85] Unfortunately, QS laser treatments for ABNOM are often associated with high rates of PIH, ranging from 75 to

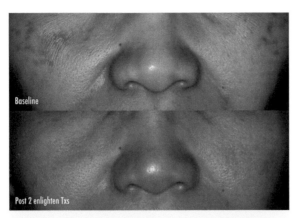

Fig. 7.5 Hori's nevus at baseline and 1 month following two treatments using a 532- and 1,064-nm picosecond laser. (These images are provided courtesy of Jeffrey TS Hsu, MD, Oak Dermatology, Itasca, Illinois, United States.)

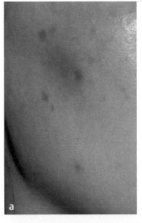
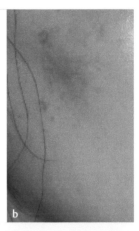

Fig. 7.6 Postinflammatory hyperpigmentation (a) before and (b) after two treatments with 1,064 and 785 nm picosecond laser.

87%,[28,84] attributed possibly to greater presence of perivascular melanocytes in lesions.[86]

Recent use of picosecond lasers shows promise for the treatment of ABNOM (▶ Fig. 7.5).[12,85,86] In a randomized, split-face comparative study evaluating the efficacy of PSAL versus QSAL, ABNOM treated with the former (2- to 2.5-mm spot size, 4.07–6.37 J/cm² fluence, 2.5-Hz pulse rate, and single pass without overlapping) showed significantly better clearance.[86] Evaluation of pigment clearance was determined using standardized photographs 6 months after the final treatments, with a 4-point percentage improvement scale. Adjunctive topical therapies were not used in the study. On the side treated with the picosecond laser, patients experienced significantly less transient side effects including pain and scabbing, and underwent a shorter recovery time.[86]

Becker's Nevus

QS lasers, including QSRL and QSAL, the Er:YAG laser, and the 1,550-nm fractional erbium-doped fiber laser, have been described to improve pigmentation within Becker's nevus.[5,87,88,89,90] Of the QS lasers, QSRL appears to be slightly more effective.[6] An advantage of using long-pulsed ruby and alexandrite lasers is reduction in hair density within the pigmented lesion.[88,90] In the report by Nanni and Alster, the average of three manual hair counts within a 3 cm² area within three representative areas of the nevus was used to determine the effectiveness of hair removal.[90] A few reports of cases suggest that the PSAL[9,10,26] can be used effectively to treat the lesion, but larger, prospective studies are needed.

Postinflammatory Hyperpigmentation

Laser treatments used for PIH target the deposition of hemosiderin or melanin. Fractional 1,550-nm erbium-doped fiber laser,[91,92] 1,064-nm QS Nd:YAG,[93] 1,927-nm nonablative fractional laser,[94] and 755-nm picosecond alexandrite[95] have been described to improve PIH (▶ Fig. 7.6). The challenge of using lasers for PIH is the risk of worsening it; if so, an alternative combination approach is often necessary involving consistent photoprotection, topical lightening agents, and/or chemical peels. Varied success, however, has been reported with the use of topical retinoids, hydroquinone, corticosteroids, dermabrasion, and chemical peels.[96,97,98] When lasers are used, it is prudent to perform test spots and observe for 6 to 8 weeks prior to laser treatment of the entire affected area.

Treating PIH using lasers presents additional challenges in darker skin phototypes due to the risk of developing it. In a large study of 61 patients specifically evaluating Fitzpatrick skin types IV to VI, Bae et al demonstrated that low-energy, low-density nonablative fractional 1,927-nm laser is a safe and effective intervention for improving PIH in this population.[94] A fixed fluence of 5 mJ, fixed spot size of 140 μm, depth of 170 μm, and 5% coverage were used as treatment parameters, with no adjunctive topical interventions.[94] Clinical outcomes were evaluated using photographs and a percentage scale, with improvement reported between 40 and 57%. Studies supportive of using nonablative diode fractional 1,927-nm laser, as well as short-pulsed and picosecond options, evaluated a much smaller group of patients.[9,95,99]

Oral tranexamic acid to prevent PIH following laser treatments of various dermatoses has shown heterogeneous results.[16,18,19] Although it is promising for melasma management when used via oral, topical, and intradermal routes,[45,46,100,101] oral tranexamic acid did not appear to be effective at preventing PIH after QSRL[18] or QS 532-nm Nd:YAG treatments.[19] However, Rutnin et al dermoscopically demonstrated that oral tranexamic acid significantly improved PIH clearance after 6 weeks of use at

1,500 mg/d.[19] Interestingly, intradermal tranexamic acid showed potential where a single dose (50 mg/mL) reduced the risk of PIH development after QS 532-nm Nd:YAG laser treatment of solar lentigines.[102] The effect of oral tranexamic acid used adjunctively with laser interventions for managing PIH remains to be further studied.

Drug-Induced Hyperpigmentation

Various lasers have been used to treat minocycline-induced hyperpigmentation. Many are case reports describing improvement largely with QSAL,[103,104,105] QS Nd:YAG[106] and QSRL,[107] and recently PSAL.[108,109]

Alster and Gupta published the largest series to date of six patients with minocycline-induced hyperpigmentation involving the face and legs, treated with QSAL (6.5–8.5 J/cm^2 fluence, 3-mm spot size, 50-millisecond pulse duration).[103] Complete resolution of the pigmentation was achieved after three to five treatments spaced 2 months apart, with no vesiculation, dyspigmentation, or scarring observed.[103] Treatment effectiveness was determined by clinical observations of complete pigment resolution.

Comparisons of QS technologies with the PSAL have also been reported.[108, 109] In two cases, the PSAL was shown to produce clearance of the pigmentation without prolonged PIH when compared to the QSRL[108] and QS Nd:YAG laser.[109] The degree of pigment clearance was determined with clinical observation.

7.4 Patient Selection/Contraindications/Preoperative Care

Prior to laser treatment of pigmented lesions, obtaining a thorough medical history, including current medications and potential allergies such as to topical anesthetic, is warranted.

Any pigmented lesion suspicious of malignancy requires a definitive diagnosis. One component of the medical history includes inquiring about medical conditions that interfere with QS lasers (e.g., prior systemic gold therapy for managing rheumatoid arthritis). Aside from fully ablative resurfacing and ablative fractionated lasers, the most recent literature supports not delaying laser treatments in patients taking isotretinoin or have taken isotretinoin within the past 6 months when clinically appropriate.[110,111,112] Ultimately, the value of time and other modalities to treat benign pigmented lesions are additional factors to consider when deciding management steps with the patient.

7.5 Patient Selection for Laser Treatment of Pigmented Lesions

It is prudent to avoid treating patients with an acute tan acquired 1 month prior to laser treatment due to increased

Table 7.1 Patient selection considerations for laser treatment of pigmented lesions

Screening	Contraindications
• Have you taken isotretinoin in the past? When was it last used? • Have you had cold sores or herpes infection in the planned treatment area? • Have you developed keloids or abnormal scarring in the past from injury or surgery? • Are there travel plans where a tan may develop? Do you use tanning beds or a sunless tanner?	• Pigmented lesion suspicious of malignancy • Nonadherence with post-laser care • Isotretinoin use within at least the past 6 mo[a] • Unrealistic patient expectations

[a]Particularly for fully ablative or ablative fractionated lasers.

risk of PIH. Patients should be instructed to not use self-tanners 1 week before laser treatment for pigmented lesions. Tinted sunscreen and sunless tanning products must be removed to avoid inadvertent absorption of laser energy and subsequent burn risk. Caution needs to be exercised for patients with a history of keloid scarring, particularly with ablative resurfacing laser interventions. Other important considerations are outlined in ▶ Table 7.1. Patients should be educated that typically a series of treatments are required when treating pigmented lesions, and often, complete clearance is not possible.

Oral antiviral agents should be administered in patients undergoing ablative resurfacing laser treatments and as prophylaxis for those with a history of herpes labialis undergoing nonablative procedures. Patients should be instructed to avoid direct and intentional sun exposure at least 2 weeks prior to and after laser treatments. The diligent use of broad-spectrum sunscreen, using a physical blocker for those with sensitive skin, is advised. Particularly for darker skin phototypes and those with a history of PIH, "priming" the skin with topical lightening agents is commonly practiced. Topical agents used alone or in combination have included azelaic acid, retinoids, hydroquinone, tranexamic acid, kojic acid, ascorbic acid, and corticosteroids.

Additional prelaser care should include a detailed outline of the procedure and postcare instructions, reinforced by written handouts provided for the patient. Informed consent must be reviewed and obtained. Baseline standardized photography should be taken prior to treatment, with photographs obtained prior to each treatment in the series recommended. All individuals in the treatment room should wear wavelength-specific eye protection, with the eye protection applied to the patient even prior to calibration of the device. To ensure optimal eye safety when treating nevus of Ota involving periorbital or eyelid skin, metal corneal shields must be used, and should be inserted by the laser physician. The practice of universal precautions such as protective masks and smoke evacuators constitutes good clinical routine and sound safety measures.

7.6 Technique

It is important to apply general laser principles when treating benign pigmented lesions to achieve safe and effective clinical outcomes. Given the ever-growing number of laser and light devices on the market, it is impossible to outline specific parameters for all of them. However, there are approaches to laser techniques that should be considered (▶ Table 7.2).

Selection of conservative parameters performed on test spots is highly recommended to reduce potential risk of PIH or worsening of the targeted skin condition, particularly given greater prevalence of pigmentary aging changes in darker skinned individuals.[113,114] The selection of energy densities, spot size, frequency, and pulse duration where applicable will depend on the patient skin type and treatment response. However, choosing a lower frequency provides better control of laser delivery to avoid pulse stacking or excessive overlapping of pulses particularly for focal pigmented lesions. In general, laser and light handpieces should be held perpendicular to and in contact with the skin so that wavelengths are delivered consistently and evenly. For elevated pigmented lesions

such as seborrheic keratoses, some authors proposed separating the laser from the lesion surface by 3 to 5 cm to concentrate most of the delivered energy to the superficial layers of the epidermis for subsequent localized injury.[10] Pulse stacking and overlapping should generally be avoided to prevent heat bulking and excess injury to the skin. Expected clinical findings observed focally and immediately after treatment vary depending on the device used. Generally, conservative laser irradiation produces slight immediate whitening of the pigmented lesion with partial whitening seen within the treated area. When assertive settings are delivered, immediate complete whitening of the pigmented lesion can be appreciated.[13,20,115] Whitening is transient and typically disappears within 5 to 20 minutes.[115] In the author's experience, for epidermal pigmented lesions, light frosting or slight darkening is a typical clinical endpoint (▶ Fig. 7.7). Focal mild edema of the treated lesion may also be seen. For dermal pigmented lesions, immediate, denser epidermal whitening of the lesion is a typical response. Mild petechiae within the treated lesion are sometimes observed. Beyond adjusting laser parameters, achieving appropriate clinical treatment endpoints is often operator dependent and subjective based on experience.[115]

After clinical endpoints are achieved, topical corticosteroids can be applied with sunscreen afterward. Light desquamation, typically lasting 1 week, can be managed with petrolatum or other bland ointments. Results are typically seen beginning 3 to 4 weeks after treatments, and patients should be educated on this to manage expectations. If lesions demonstrate a premature plateau in response, even after parameters are adjusted, the use of a different device may be warranted. If lesions repigment, conservative measures using topical lightening agents, photoprotection and watchful waiting for 3 to 4 months should be considered before further laser interventions.

7.7 Postoperative Instructions

General principles for postlaser care apply in the treatment of pigmented lesions. Products that may irritate the skin, such as exfoliating agents, astringents, and topical retinoids, should be typically avoided for 1 week after treatment. Strict photoprotection is advised for 1 month

Table 7.2 General principles on techniques

1. Perform representative test spot(s), particularly in darker skinned individuals, if uncertain about clinical endpoints or potential adverse effects
2. Watch carefully for clinical endpoint to avoid overly assertive treatment
3. Use the lowest fluence possible to achieve the desired clinical outcomes
4. Laser parameters in darker skinned individuals:
   a) Longer pulse duration
   b) Longer wavelength
5. Optimize cooling during treatment sessions
6. Use conservative parameters in initial treatment session and adjust accordingly in subsequent visits if appropriate

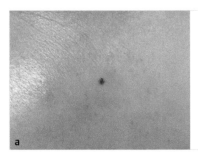
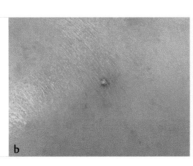

Fig. 7.7 (a, b) Light frosting as an immediate clinical endpoint to indicate treatment response, following use of a picosecond laser.

afterward irrespective of skin phototype to minimize the risk of postinflammatory dyspigmentation. Appropriate and adequate use of sunscreen, with minimum sun protection factor 30 and with broad-spectrum properties, is part of standard postlaser care. Physical sunblock containing titanium or zinc oxide may be considered given transient skin sensitivity following laser treatments. The application of ice packs helps reduce transient erythema, edema, and discomfort for the patient and can be used immediately after treatment. Makeup can be used, but gentle cleansing is required to avoid further irritation of the skin or premature sloughing of possible scabs and scales. Patient education should include expected healing time of treated pigmented lesions; as seen with general wound-healing principles, facial sites typically recover faster due to its vascularity when compared to the extremities.

In darker skinned patients, various interventions to reduce PIH following laser and light treatments have been reported, though with variable success. Judicious use of short-term topical corticosteroids to mitigate inflammation can further reduce the potential risk of dyspigmentation following laser treatment. Mid-potency corticosteroids, such as betamethasone valerate, may be applied once to twice daily for 3 to 7 days after the treatment, depending on the device used and degree of inflammation. Other topical corticosteroid formulations have been used and described in different studies particularly for the treatment of lentigines and ephelides.[13,24,115] Although oral tranexamic acid has been used for its depigmentation effects, it does not appear to prevent PIH following QSRL treatment[18] or QS 532-nm Nd:YAG treatment[19] of facial lentigines.

The use of more ablative technologies to treat pigmented lesions may require additional postcare to reduce potential PIH. Topical antibiotic ointments as well as compounded formulations consisting of hydroquinone, tretinoin, topical corticosteroid, kojic acid, α-hydroxy acid, vitamin C, and/or azelaic acid have been used for this purpose.[116,117] Pretreatment, however, does not appear to be beneficial at lessening PIH; glycolic acid or hydroquinone was not shown to provide preventative benefits following CO_2 laser resurfacing.[118]

7.8 Potential Complications

The combination of proper patient section, pre- and postcare, and laser parameters to achieve appropriate clinical treatment endpoints all contribute to the reduction of laser complications. Laser treatment of pigmented lesions, similar to laser treatments in general, may result in potential adverse effects such as dyspigmentation, scarring, and infection (▶ Table 7.3). In the author's practice, patients are typically followed up by phone 1 week after treatment, and offered in-person appointments 4 to 6 weeks for reassessment and to update photos. Patients should be educated on potential signs and symptoms following laser treatments when medical attention should

Table 7.3 Potential complications of treating benign pigmented lesions using lasers

- Dyspigmentation, including postinflammatory hyperpigmentation and hypopigmentation
- Scarring
- Infection
- Prolonged erythema
- Prolonged edema
- Recurrent herpes labialis
- Acneiform eruptions

be urgently sought, so that management of complications can be instituted as soon as possible.

PIH is of particular concern in darker skinned individuals due to both physiologic and external (laser) factors unique to this population. The spectrum of skin phototypes differs in the amount and epidermal distribution of melanin. Those with darker skin have larger melanocytes that produce more melanin, which are dispersed more extensively, to provide greater natural photoprotection.[119] However, melanin-rich skin also presents with greater risk of PIH that may be triggered after laser treatments.[13,20,21] Specifically, the risk of PIH correlates to the degree of inflammation and disruption of the dermal–epidermal junction depending on the laser type and parameters used. Hence, dedicated efforts to optimize epidermal cooling during the procedure, to use the lowest fluence possible, to not stack pulses, and to adhere diligently to postlaser care all reduce inflammation and risk of potential adverse sequelae.

7.9 Pearls and Pitfalls

Laser treatment of benign pigmented lesions can be rewarding for both the clinician and the patient. However, it needs to be reiterated that any suspicious pigmented lesion based on clinical and/or dermoscopic features must be biopsied prior to laser treatment. Reevaluation for possible malignant transformation within a treated and improved pigmented lesion may be warranted if there are recurrences or atypical changes observed.

Many pigmented lesions have multifactorial etiologies. As such, a multimodal approach, including the use of lasers, is often needed to optimize clinical outcomes in real-world practice. For example, the management of melasma may involve topical lightening and other pigment-targeting cosmeceutical agents, chemical peels, and rigorous photoprotection, along with intermittent series of laser treatments depending on disease course. A combination treatment approach is more effective, and for many patients more affordable, when targeting a chronic, potentially lifelong benign skin condition. Clinicians should be knowledgeable and proficient with options beyond lasers to best serve the needs of their patients.

Choosing conservative laser parameters when initiating treatment for pigmented lesions can reduce potential adverse effects, particularly in darker skinned individuals. Asians, for instance, have been observed to show pigmentary changes at earlier ages, and at greater incidences than skin wrinkling.[113,114,120] However, darker skin phototypes including Asians are also at higher risk of PIH. Setting expectations for patients, that the treatment series is a process and pigmented lesions often are improved but not completely removed and may recur, is a key communication point.

Patient education during the process, beginning at the consultation visit, will reduce the risk of immediate and delayed postprocedure complications, as well as maintenance of clinical results. Without thorough counseling, patients may have a false perception that a lightened pigmented lesion will remain lightened, irrespective of their sun exposure. A further pitfall is that inadequate photoprotection, and not necessarily the laser treatment itself during the postoperative process, may trigger PIH. Hence, the practice of rigorous sun safety measures should be emphasized as a non-negotiable commitment from the patients who choose to undergo treatment of their pigmented lesions.

There is a growing armamentarium of options reflecting advances in laser science to safety and effectively treat patients with benign pigmented lesions. Previous limitations, particularly for darker skinned individuals due to increased potential for dyspigmentation from thermal effects, can be reduced with the judicious use of newer technologies such as picosecond lasers. There is promise of more refined and consistent outcomes with new wavelengths and speeds in laser delivery. For the laser surgeon and patient, the future is certainly bright.

References

[1] Shah S, Alster TS. Laser treatment of dark skin: an updated review. Am J Clin Dermatol. 2010; 11(6):389–397

[2] Anderson RR, Parrish JA. Selective photothermolysis: precise microsurgery by selective absorption of pulsed radiation. Science. 1983; 220(4596):524–527

[3] Roberts WE, Henry M, Burgess C, Saedi N, Chilukuri S, Campbell-Chambers DA. Laser treatment of skin of color for medical and aesthetic uses with a new 650-microsecond Nd:YAG 1064 nm laser. J Drugs Dermatol. 2019; 18(4):s135–s137

[4] Burgess C, Chilukuri S, Campbell-Chambers DA, Henry M, Saedi N, Roberts WE. Practical applications for medical and aesthetic treatment of skin of color with a new 650-microsecond laser. J Drugs Dermatol. 2019; 18(4):s138–s143

[5] Tse Y, Levine VJ, McClain SA, Ashinoff R. The removal of cutaneous pigmented lesions with the Q-switched ruby laser and the Q-switched neodymium: yttrium-aluminum-garnet laser. A comparative study. J Dermatol Surg Oncol. 1994; 20(12):795–800

[6] Polder KD, Landau JM, Vergilis-Kalner IJ, Goldberg LH, Friedman PM, Bruce S. Laser eradication of pigmented lesions: a review. Dermatol Surg. 2011; 37(5):572–595

[7] Anderson RR, Margolis RJ, Watenabe S, Flotte T, Hruza GJ, Dover JS. Selective photothermolysis of cutaneous pigmentation by Q-switched Nd: YAG laser pulses at 1064, 532, and 355 nm. J Invest Dermatol. 1989; 93(1):28–32

[8] Ross V, Naseef G, Lin G, et al. Comparison of responses of tattoos to picosecond and nanosecond Q-switched neodymium: YAG lasers. Arch Dermatol. 1998; 134(2):167–171

[9] Levin MK, Ng E, Bae Y-SC, Brauer JA, Geronemus RG. Treatment of pigmentary disorders in patients with skin of color with a novel 755 nm picosecond, Q-switched ruby, and Q-switched Nd:YAG nanosecond lasers: a retrospective photographic review. Lasers Surg Med. 2016; 48(2):181–187

[10] Alegre-Sanchez A, Jiménez-Gómez N, Moreno-Arrones ÓM, et al. Treatment of flat and elevated pigmented disorders with a 755-nm alexandrite picosecond laser: clinical and histological evaluation. Lasers Med Sci. 2018; 33(8):1827–1831

[11] Jo DJ, Kang I-H, Baek JH, Gwak MJ, Lee SJ, Shin MK. Using reflectance confocal microscopy to observe in vivo melanolysis after treatment with the picosecond alexandrite laser and Q-switched Nd:YAG laser in melasma. Lasers Surg Med. 2018; 7:1–7

[12] Kung K-Y, Shek SYN, Yeung CK, Chan HHL. Evaluation of the safety and efficacy of the dual wavelength picosecond laser for the treatment of benign pigmented lesions in Asians. Lasers Surg Med. 2019; 51(1):14–22

[13] Negishi K, Akita H, Matsunaga Y. Prospective study of removing solar lentigines in Asians using a novel dual-wavelength and dual-pulse width picosecond laser. Lasers Surg Med. 2018; 50(8):851–858

[14] Saedi N, Metelitsa A, Petrell K, Arndt KA, Dover JS. Treatment of tattoos with a picosecond alexandrite laser: a prospective trial. Arch Dermatol. 2012; 148(12):1360–1363

[15] Trivedi MK, Yang FC, Cho BK. A review of laser and light therapy in melasma. Int J Womens Dermatol. 2017; 3(1):11–20

[16] Lee MC, Lin YF, Hu S, et al. A split-face study: comparison of picosecond alexandrite laser and Q-switched Nd:YAG laser in the treatment of melasma in Asians. Lasers Med Sci. 2018; 33(8):1733–1738

[17] Sarkar R, Arora P, Garg KV. Cosmeceuticals for hyperpigmentation: what is available? J Cutan Aesthet Surg. 2013; 6(1):4–11

[18] Kato H, Araki J, Eto H, et al. A prospective randomized controlled study of oral tranexamic acid for preventing postinflammatory hyperpigmentation after Q-switched ruby laser. Dermatol Surg. 2011; 37(5):605–610

[19] Rutnin S, Pruettivorawongse D, Thadanipon K, Vachiramon V. A prospective randomized controlled study of oral tranexamic acid for the prevention of postinflammatory hyperpigmentation after Q-switched 532-nm Nd:YAG laser for solar lentigines. Lasers Surg Med. 2019; 51(10):850–858

[20] Chan HH, Alam M, Kono T, Dover JS. Clinical application of lasers in Asians. Dermatol Surg. 2002; 28(7):556–563

[21] Chan H. The use of lasers and intense pulsed light sources for the treatment of acquired pigmentary lesions in Asians. J Cosmet Laser Ther. 2003; 5(3–4):198–200

[22] Kawada A, Shiraishi H, Asai M, et al. Clinical improvement of solar lentigines and ephelides with an intense pulsed light source. Dermatol Surg. 2002; 28(6):504–508

[23] Chan HH, Fung WK, Ying SY, Kono T. An in vivo trial comparing the use of different types of 532 nm Nd:YAG lasers in the treatment of facial lentigines in Oriental patients. Dermatol Surg. 2000; 26(8):743–749

[24] Ho SGY, Chan NPY, Yeung CK, Shek SY, Kono T, Chan HHL. A retrospective analysis of the management of freckles and lentigines using four different pigment lasers on Asian skin. J Cosmet Laser Ther. 2012; 14(2):74–80

[25] Vachiramon V, Panmanee W, Techapichetvanich T, Chanprapaph K. Comparison of Q-switched Nd: YAG laser and fractional carbon dioxide laser for the treatment of solar lentigines in Asians. Lasers Surg Med. 2016; 48(4):354–359

[26] Chan JC, Shek SY, Kono T, Yeung CK, Chan HH. A retrospective analysis on the management of pigmented lesions using a picosecond 755-nm alexandrite laser in Asians. Lasers Surg Med. 2016; 48(1):23–29

[27] Vachiramon V, Iamsumang W, Triyangkulsri K. Q-switched double frequency Nd:YAG 532-nm nanosecond laser vs. double frequency Nd:YAG 532-nm picosecond laser for the treatment of solar lentigines in Asians. Lasers Med Sci. 2018; 33(9):1941–1947

[28] Wang C-C, Chen C-K. Effect of spot size and fluence on Q-switched alexandrite laser treatment for pigmentation in Asians: a randomized, double-blinded, split-face comparative trial. J Dermatolog Treat. 2012; 23(5):333–338

[29] Yang Y, Peng L, Ge Y, Lin T. Comparison of the efficacy and safety of a picosecond alexandrite laser and a Q-switched alexandrite laser for the treatment of freckles in Chinese patients. J Am Acad Dermatol. 2018; 79(6):1155–1156

[30] Somyos K, Boonchu K, Somsak K, Panadda L, Leopairut J. Copper vapour laser treatment of café-au-lait macules. Br J Dermatol. 1996; 135(6):964–968

[31] Kilmer SL, Wheeland RG, Goldberg DJ, Anderson RR. Treatment of epidermal pigmented lesions with the frequency-doubled Q-switched Nd:YAG laser. A controlled, single-impact, dose-response, multicenter trial. Arch Dermatol. 1994; 130(12):1515–1519

[32] Kagami S, Asahina A, Watanabe R, et al. Treatment of 153 Japanese patients with Q-switched alexandrite laser. Lasers Med Sci. 2007; 22 (3):159–163

[33] Alster TS, Williams CM. Café-au-lait macule in type V skin: successful treatment with a 510 nm pulsed dye laser. J Am Acad Dermatol. 1995; 33(6):1042–1043

[34] Alora MB, Arndt KA. Treatment of a café-au-lait macule with the erbium:YAG laser. J Am Acad Dermatol. 2001; 45(4):566–568

[35] Alster TS. Complete elimination of large café-au-lait birthmarks by the 510-nm pulsed dye laser. Plast Reconstr Surg. 1995; 96(7):1660–1664

[36] Kim HR, Ha JM, Park MS, et al. A low-fluence 1064-nm Q-switched neodymium-doped yttrium aluminium garnet laser for the treatment of café-au-lait macules. J Am Acad Dermatol. 2015; 73(3):477–483

[37] Chan HHL, Kono T. The use of lasers and intense pulsed light sources for the treatment of pigmentary lesions. Skin Therapy Lett. 2004; 9 (8):5–7

[38] Artzi O, Mehrabi JN, Koren A, Niv R, Lapidoth M, Levi A. Picosecond 532-nm neodymium-doped yttrium aluminium garnet laser-a novel and promising modality for the treatment of café-au-lait macules. Lasers Med Sci. 2018; 33(4):693–697

[39] Schweiger ES, Kwasniak L, Aires DJ. Treatment of dermatosis papulosa nigra with a 1064 nm Nd:YAG laser: report of two cases. J Cosmet Laser Ther. 2008; 10(2):120–122

[40] Katz TM, Goldberg LH, Friedman PM. Dermatosis papulosa nigra treatment with fractional photothermolysis. Dermatol Surg. 2009; 35 (11):1840–1843

[41] Kundu RV, Joshi SS, Suh KY, et al. Comparison of electrodesiccation and potassium-titanyl-phosphate laser for treatment of dermatosis papulosa nigra. Dermatol Surg. 2009; 35(7):1079–1083

[42] Fitzpatrick RE, Goldman MP, Ruiz-Esparza J. Clinical advantage of the CO_2 laser superpulsed mode. Treatment of verruca vulgaris, seborrheic keratoses, lentigines, and actinic cheilitis. J Dermatol Surg Oncol. 1994; 20(7):449–456

[43] Culbertson GR. 532-nm diode laser treatment of seborrheic keratoses with color enhancement. Dermatol Surg. 2008; 34(4):525–528, discussion 528

[44] Mehrabi D, Brodell RT. Use of the alexandrite laser for treatment of seborrheic keratoses. Dermatol Surg. 2002; 28(5):437–439

[45] Minni K, Poojary S. Efficacy and safety of oral tranexamic acid as an adjuvant in Indian patients with melasma: a prospective, interventional, single-centre, triple-blind, randomized, placebo-control, parallel group study. J Eur Acad Dermatol Venereol. 2020; 34 (11):2636–2644

[46] Wu S, Shi H, Wu H, et al. Treatment of melasma with oral administration of tranexamic acid. Aesthetic Plast Surg. 2012; 36(4):964–970

[47] Shin JU, Park J, Oh SH, Lee JH. Oral tranexamic acid enhances the efficacy of low-fluence 1064-nm quality-switched neodymium-doped

yttrium aluminum garnet laser treatment for melasma in Koreans: a randomized, prospective trial. Dermatol Surg. 2013; 39(3, Pt 1):435–442

[48] Yoshimura K, Sato K, Aiba-Kojima E, et al. Repeated treatment protocols for melasma and acquired dermal melanocytosis. Dermatol Surg. 2006; 32(3):365–371

[49] Suh KS, Sung JY, Roh HJ, Jeon YS, Kim YC, Kim ST. Efficacy of the 1064-nm Q-switched Nd:YAG laser in melasma. J Dermatolog Treat. 2011; 22(4):233–238

[50] Cho SB, Kim JS, Kim MJ. Melasma treatment in Korean women using a 1064-nm Q-switched Nd:YAG laser with low pulse energy. Clin Exp Dermatol. 2009; 34(8):e847–e850

[51] Angsuwarangsee S, Polnikorn N. Combined ultrapulse CO_2 laser and Q-switched alexandrite laser compared with Q-switched alexandrite laser alone for refractory melasma: split-face design. Dermatol Surg. 2003; 29(1):59–64

[52] Nouri K, Bowes L, Chartier T, Romagosa R, Spencer J. Combination treatment of melasma with pulsed CO_2 laser followed by Q-switched alexandrite laser: a pilot study. Dermatol Surg. 1999; 25(6):494–497

[53] Manaloto RMP, Alster T. Erbium:YAG laser resurfacing for refractory melasma. Dermatol Surg. 1999; 25(2):121–123

[54] Wanitphakdeedecha R, Manuskiatti W, Siriphukpong S, Chen TM. Treatment of melasma using variable square pulse Er:YAG laser resurfacing. Dermatol Surg. 2009; 35(3):475–481, discussion 481–482

[55] Figueiredo Souza L, Trancoso Souza S. Single-session intense pulsed light combined with stable fixed-dose triple combination topical therapy for the treatment of refractory melasma. Dermatol Ther (Heidelb). 2012; 25(5):477–480

[56] Li YH, Chen JZS, Wei HC, et al. Efficacy and safety of intense pulsed light in treatment of melasma in Chinese patients. Dermatol Surg. 2008; 34(5):693–700, discussion 700–701

[57] Wang CC, Hui CY, Sue YM, Wong WR, Hong HS. Intense pulsed light for the treatment of refractory melasma in Asian persons. Dermatol Surg. 2004; 30(9):1196–1200

[58] Goldman MP, Gold MH, Palm MD, et al. Sequential treatment with triple combination cream and intense pulsed light is more efficacious than sequential treatment with an inactive (control) cream and intense pulsed light in patients with moderate to severe melasma. Dermatol Surg. 2011; 37(2):224–233

[59] Lee HS, Won CH, Lee DH, et al. Treatment of melasma in Asian skin using a fractional 1,550-nm laser: an open clinical study. Dermatol Surg. 2009; 35(10):1499–1504

[60] Rokhsar CK, Fitzpatrick RE. The treatment of melasma with fractional photothermolysis: a pilot study. Dermatol Surg. 2005; 31(12):1645–1650

[61] Katz TM, Glaich AS, Goldberg LH, Firoz BF, Dai T, Friedman PM. Treatment of melasma using fractional photothermolysis: a report of eight cases with long-term follow-up. Dermatol Surg. 2010; 36(8):1273–1280

[62] Lee HM, Haw S, Kim JK, Chang SE, Lee MW. Split-face study using a 1,927-nm thulium fiber fractional laser to treat photoaging and melasma in Asian skin. Dermatol Surg. 2013; 39(6):879–888

[63] Niwa Massaki ABM, Eimpunth S, Fabi SG, Guiha I, Groff W, Fitzpatrick R. Treatment of melasma with the 1,927-nm fractional thulium fiber laser: a retrospective analysis of 20 cases with long-term follow-up. Lasers Surg Med. 2013; 45(2):95–101

[64] Polder KD, Bruce S. Treatment of melasma using a novel 1,927-nm fractional thulium fiber laser: a pilot study. Dermatol Surg. 2012; 38 (2):199–206

[65] Tourlaki A, Galimberti MG, Pellacani G, Bencini PL. Combination of fractional erbium-glass laser and topical therapy in melasma resistant to triple-combination cream. J Dermatolog Treat. 2014; 25 (3):218–222

[66] Kroon MW, Wind BS, Beek JF, et al. Nonablative 1550-nm fractional laser therapy versus triple topical therapy for the treatment of melasma: a randomized controlled pilot study. J Am Acad Dermatol. 2011; 64(3):516–523

[67] Sherling M, Friedman PM, Adrian R, et al. Consensus recommendations on the use of an erbium-doped 1,550-nm

fractionated laser and its applications in dermatologic laser surgery. Dermatol Surg. 2010; 36(4):461–469

[68] Kaushik SB, Alexis AF. Nonablative fractional laser resurfacing in skin of color: evidence-based review. J Clin Aesthet Dermatol. 2017; 10 (6):51–67

[69] Choi YJ, Nam JH, Kim JY, et al. Efficacy and safety of a novel picosecond laser using combination of 1064 and 595 nm on patients with melasma: a prospective, randomized, multicenter, split-face, 2% hydroquinone cream-controlled clinical trial. Lasers Surg Med. 2017; 49(10):899–907

[70] Chalermchai T, Rummaneethorn P. Effects of a fractional picosecond 1,064 nm laser for the treatment of dermal and mixed type melasma. J Cosmet Laser Ther. 2018; 20(3):134–139

[71] Shimbashi T, Hyakusoku H, Okinaga M. Treatment of nevus of Ota by Q-switched ruby laser. Aesthetic Plast Surg. 1997; 21(2):118–121

[72] Kono T, Chan HHL, Erçöçen AR, et al. Use of Q-switched ruby laser in the treatment of nevus of Ota in different age groups. Lasers Surg Med. 2003; 32(5):391–395

[73] Geronemus RG. Q-switched ruby laser therapy of nevus of Ota. Arch Dermatol. 1992; 128(12):1618–1622

[74] Chan HH, Leung RSC, Ying SY, et al. A retrospective analysis of complications in the treatment of nevus of Ota with the Q-switched alexandrite and Q-switched Nd:YAG lasers. Dermatol Surg. 2000; 26 (11):1000–1006

[75] Alster TS, Williams CM. Treatment of nevus of Ota by the Q-switched alexandrite laser. Dermatol Surg. 1995; 21(7):592–596

[76] Kono T, Nozaki M, Chan HH, Mikashima Y. A retrospective study looking at the long-term complications of Q-switched ruby laser in the treatment of nevus of Ota. Lasers Surg Med. 2001; 29(2):156–159

[77] Chesnut C, Diehl J, Lask G. Treatment of nevus of Ota with a picosecond 755-nm alexandrite laser. Dermatol Surg. 2015; 41(4):508–510

[78] Ohshiro T, Ohshiro T, Sasaki K, Kishi K. Picosecond pulse duration laser treatment for dermal melanocytosis in Asians: a retrospective review. Laser Ther. 2016; 25(2):99–104

[79] Ge Y, Yang Y, Guo L, et al. Comparison of a picosecond alexandrite laser versus a Q-switched alexandrite laser for the treatment of nevus of Ota: a randomized, split-lesion, controlled trial. J Am Acad Dermatol. 2020; 83(2):397–403

[80] Ee HL, Goh CL, Khoo LSW, Chan ESY, Ang P. Treatment of acquired bilateral nevus of Ota-like macules (Hori's nevus) with a combination of the 532 nm Q-switched Nd:YAG laser followed by the 1,064 nm Q-switched Nd:YAG is more effective: prospective study. Dermatol Surg. 2006; 32(1):34–40

[81] Cho SB, Park SJ, Kim MJ, Bu TS. Treatment of acquired bilateral nevus of Ota-like macules (Hori's nevus) using 1064-nm Q-switched Nd:YAG laser with low fluence. Int J Dermatol. 2009; 48(12):1308–1312

[82] Manuskiatti W, Sivayathorn A, Leelaudomlipi P, Fitzpatrick RE. Treatment of acquired bilateral nevus of Ota-like macules (Hori's nevus) using a combination of scanned carbon dioxide laser followed by Q-switched ruby laser. J Am Acad Dermatol. 2003; 48(4):584–591

[83] Polnikorn N, Tanrattanakorn S, Goldberg DJ. Treatment of Hori's nevus with the Q-switched Nd:YAG laser. Dermatol Surg. 2000; 26 (5):477–480

[84] Lam AY, Wong DS, Lam LK, Ho WS, Chan HH. A retrospective study on the efficacy and complications of Q-switched alexandrite laser in the treatment of acquired bilateral nevus of Ota-like macules. Dermatol Surg. 2001; 27(11):937–941, discussion 941–942

[85] Wong THS. Picosecond laser treatment for acquired bilateral nevus of Ota-like macules. JAMA Dermatol. 2018; 154(10):1226–1228

[86] Yu W, Zhu J, Yu W, Lyu D, Lin X, Zhang Z. A split-face, single-blinded, randomized controlled comparison of alexandrite 755-nm picosecond laser versus alexandrite 755-nm nanosecond laser in the treatment of acquired bilateral nevus of Ota-like macules. J Am Acad Dermatol. 2018; 79(3):479–486

[87] Glaich AS, Goldberg LH, Dai T, Kunishige JH, Friedman PM. Fractional resurfacing: a new therapeutic modality for Becker's nevus. Arch Dermatol. 2007; 143(12):1488–1490

[88] Choi JE, Kim JW, Seo SH, Son SW, Ahn HH, Kye YC. Treatment of Becker's nevi with a long-pulse alexandrite laser. Dermatol Surg. 2009; 35(7):1105–1108

[89] Trelles MA, Allones I, Moreno-Arias GA, Vélez M. Becker's naevus: a comparative study between erbium: YAG and Q-switched neodymium:YAG; clinical and histopathological findings. Br J Dermatol. 2005; 152(2):308–313

[90] Nanni CA, Alster TS. Treatment of a Becker's nevus using a 694-nm long-pulsed ruby laser. Dermatol Surg. 1998; 24(9):1032–1034

[91] Katz TM, Goldberg LH, Firoz BF, Friedman PM. Fractional photothermolysis for the treatment of postinflammatory hyperpigmentation. Dermatol Surg. 2009; 35(11):1844–1848

[92] Rokhsar CK, Ciocon DH. Fractional photothermolysis for the treatment of postinflammatory hyperpigmentation after carbon dioxide laser resurfacing. Dermatol Surg. 2009; 35(3):535–537

[93] Cho SB, Park SJ, Kim JS, Kim MJ, Bu TS. Treatment of post-inflammatory hyperpigmentation using 1064-nm Q-switched Nd:YAG laser with low fluence: report of three cases. J Eur Acad Dermatol Venereol. 2009; 23(10):1206–1207

[94] Bae YC, Rettig S, Weiss E, Bernstein L, Geronemus R. Treatment of post-inflammatory hyperpigmentation in patients with darker skin types using a low energy 1,927 nm non-ablative fractional laser: a retrospective photographic review analysis. Lasers Surg Med. 2020; 52(1):7–12

[95] Lee YJ, Shin HJ, Noh TK, Choi KH, Chang SE. Treatment of melasma and post-inflammatory hyperpigmentation by a picosecond 755-nm alexandrite laser in Asian patients. Ann Dermatol. 2017; 29(6):779–781

[96] Burns RL, Prevost-Blank PL, Lawry MA, Lawry TB, Faria DT, Fivenson DP. Glycolic acid peels for postinflammatory hyperpigmentation in black patients. Dermatol Surg. 1997; 23(3):171–175

[97] Bulengo-Ransby SM, Griffiths CE, Kimbrough-Green CK, et al. Topical tretinoin (retinoic acid) therapy for hyperpigmented lesions caused by inflammation of the skin in black patients. N Engl J Med. 1993; 328(20):1438–1443

[98] Taylor SC, Burgess CM, Callender VD, et al. Postinflammatory hyperpigmentation: evolving combination treatment strategies. Cutis. 2006; 78(2) Suppl 2:6–19

[99] Brauer JA, Alabdulrazzaq H, Yoon-Soo Bae C, Geronemus RG. LLLT fractional 1927 nm for facial skin resurfacing (JDD, 2015).pdf. J Drugs Dermatol. 2015; 14(11):1262–1267

[100] Taraz M, Niknam S, Ehsani AH. Tranexamic acid in treatment of melasma: a comprehensive review of clinical studies. Dermatol Ther (Heidelb). 2017; 30(3):1–8

[101] Sharma R, Mahajan VK, Mehta KS, Chauhan PS, Rawat R, Shiny TN. Therapeutic efficacy and safety of oral tranexamic acid and that of tranexamic acid local infiltration with microinjections in patients with melasma: a comparative study. Clin Exp Dermatol. 2017; 42(7):728–734

[102] Sirithanabadeekul P, Srieakpanit R. Intradermal tranexamic acid injections to prevent post-inflammatory hyperpigmentation after solar lentigo removal with a Q-switched 532-nm Nd:YAG laser. J Cosmet Laser Ther. 2018; 20(7–8):398–404

[103] Alster TS, Gupta SN. Minocycline-induced hyperpigmentation treated with a 755-nm Q-switched alexandrite laser. Dermatol Surg. 2004; 30(9):1201–1204

[104] Nisar MS, Iyer K, Brodell RT, Lloyd JR, Shin TM, Ahmad A. Minocycline-induced hyperpigmentation: comparison of 3 Q-switched lasers to reverse its effects. Clin Cosmet Investig Dermatol. 2013; 6(2):159–162

[105] Green D, Friedman KJ. Treatment of minocycline-induced cutaneous pigmentation with the Q-switched Alexandrite laser and a review of the literature. J Am Acad Dermatol. 2001; 44(2) Suppl:342–347

[106] Greve B, Schönermark MP, Raulin C. Minocycline-induced hyperpigmentation: treatment with the Q-switched Nd:YAG laser. Lasers Surg Med. 1998; 22(4):223–227

[107] Friedman IS, Shelton RM, Phelps RG. Minocycline-induced hyperpigmentation of the tongue: successful treatment with the Q-switched ruby laser. Dermatol Surg. 2002; 28(3):205–209

[108] Sasaki K, Ohshiro T, Ohshiro T, et al. Type 2 minocycline-induced hyperpigmentation successfully treated with the novel 755 nm picosecond alexandrite laser: a case report. Laser Ther. 2017; 26(2): 137–144

[109] Barrett T, de Zwaan S. Picosecond alexandrite laser is superior to Q-switched Nd:YAG laser in treatment of minocycline-induced hyperpigmentation: a case study and review of the literature. J Cosmet Laser Ther. 2018; 20(7–8):387–390

[110] Waldman A, Bolotin D, Arndt KA, et al. ASDS guidelines task force: consensus recommendations regarding the safety of lasers, dermabrasion, chemical peels, energy devices, and skin surgery during and after isotretinoin use. Dermatol Surg. 2017; 43(10):1249–1262

[111] Spring LK, Krakowski AC, Alam M, et al. Isotretinoin and timing of procedural interventions: a systematic review with consensus recommendations. JAMA Dermatol. 2017; 153(8):802–809

[112] Prather HB, Alam M, Poon E, Arndt KA, Dover JS. Laser safety in isotretinoin use: a survey of expert opinion and practice. Dermatol Surg. 2017; 43(3):357–363

[113] Chung JH. Photoaging in Asians. Photodermatol Photoimmunol Photomed. 2003; 19(3):109–121

[114] Larnier C, Ortonne JP, Venot A, et al. Evaluation of cutaneous photodamage using a photographic scale. Br J Dermatol. 1994; 130 (2):167–173

[115] Negishi K, Akita H, Tanaka S, Yokoyama Y, Wakamatsu S, Matsunaga K. Comparative study of treatment efficacy and the incidence of post-inflammatory hyperpigmentation with different degrees of irradiation using two different quality-switched lasers for removing solar lentigines on Asian skin. J Eur Acad Dermatol Venereol. 2013; 27(3):307–312

[116] Goldman MP. The use of hydroquinone with facial laser resurfacing. J Cutan Laser Ther. 2000; 2(2):73–77

[117] Rigopoulos D, Gregoriou S, Katsambas A. Hyperpigmentation and melasma. J Cosmet Dermatol. 2007; 6(3):195–202

[118] West TB, Alster TS. Effect of pretreatment on the incidence of hyperpigmentation following cutaneous CO_2 laser resurfacing. Dermatol Surg. 1999; 25(1):15–17

[119] Kaidbey KH, Agin PP, Sayre RM, Kligman AM. Photoprotection by melanin: a comparison of black and Caucasian skin. J Am Acad Dermatol. 1979; 1(3):249–260

[120] Chung JH, Lee SH, Youn CS, et al. Cutaneous photodamage in Koreans: influence of sex, sun exposure, smoking, and skin color. Arch Dermatol. 2001; 137(8):1043–1051

Suggested Readings

Peltzer K, Pengpid S, James C. The globalization of whitening: prevalence of skin lighteners (or bleachers) use and its social correlates among university students in 26 countries. Int J Dermatol. 2016; 55(2):165–172

Hamed SH, Tayyem R, Nimer N, Alkhatib HS. Skin-lightening practice among women living in Jordan: prevalence, determinants, and user's awareness. Int J Dermatol. 2010; 49(4):414–420

Taylor A, Pawaskar M, Taylor SL, Balkrishnan R, Feldman SR. Prevalence of pigmentary disorders and their impact on quality of life: a prospective cohort study. J Cosmet Dermatol. 2008; 7(3):164–168

Ladizinski B, Mistry N, Kundu RV. Widespread use of toxic skin lightening compounds: medical and psychosocial aspects. Dermatol Clin. 2011; 29 (1):111–123

8 Lasers and Light Devices for Hair Removal

Maressa C. Criscito, Margo H. Lederhandler, and Leonard J. Bernstein

Summary

Laser hair removal is a commonly sought treatment for hypertrichosis or unwanted hair. This chapter reviews the various types of methods to remove unwanted hair as well as the principles behind using laser modalities for hair removal. Finally, a review of how to optimally treat patients is covered.

Keywords: laser hair removal, unwanted hair, hypertrichosis

8.1 Introduction

As excessive and unwanted body hair remains a common concern for many patients, the achievement of permanent or semi-permanent hair removal has been an optimal goal for over a century. Physicians have attempted to achieve permanent hair removal with the employment of electrolysis, initially for the treatment of trichiasis, as early as the 19th century.[1] However, with the development of laser technology in recent years, the field of hair removal has vastly expanded. Laser hair removal (LHR) has revolutionized the field of hair removal due to the ability to selectively target and destroy hair follicles, resulting in long-lasting hair removal, decreasing operator dependency, and reducing potential side effects as compared to other hair removal methods.[2,3] However, despite these advantages, safe and effective LHR requires that the operator has a basic level of understanding of hair anatomy, growth, and physiology, together with a thorough understanding of laser–tissue interactions, all of which are reviewed herein.

8.2 Mechanism of Action

Introduced by Anderson and Parrish in 1983, the theory of selective photothermolysis has revolutionized the field of lasers based on the concept of selectively targeting a particular chromophore based on its absorption spectra and size.[4] The theory of selective photothermolysis describes the phenomenon in which energy is delivered at a wavelength well absorbed by the target within a time period that is less than or equal to the thermal relaxation time of the target. Utilizing this theory, Grossman et al selectively targeted melanin in hair follicles and sparing the surrounding skin using normal-mode, long-pulsed ruby lasers to achieve long-term hair removal, with preliminary studies using the ruby laser revealing the ability to induce a growth delay and permanent hair removal in some individuals.[5] These early results inspired countless others to investigate various wavelengths and laser–tissue interactions in the pursuit of hair removal using laser and light devices.[5,6,7,8]

In 1996, the Food and Drug Administration (FDA) approved the first hair removal laser system and since then, the field has grown tremendously to include multiple lasers and light sources marketed for the treatment of unwanted or excessive hair in both the clinical and, more recently, home environments. The ability to selectively target and destroy hair follicles using laser- and light-assisted devices has led to more long-lasting hair removal and decreases the potential side effects compared to other hair removal methods. Importantly, devices widely in use today mitigate risk of epidermal and superficial dermal injury by employing cooling technology (cold spray, cold air, or cold contact windows). As laser technology continues to advance, the ability for treatments to have long-lasting results, produce minimal discomfort, and be available for all skin phototypes and hair colors broadens as well.

8.2.1 Hair Anatomy and Physiology

The pilosebaceous unit, which consists of the hair follicle and sebaceous glands, serves many roles in the homeostasis of the skin and acts as a source of epithelial cells during wound healing. The hair follicle can exist in two different phenotypes, terminal hairs and vellus hairs. Terminal hairs include androgen-independent hair (eyebrows, eyelashes) and androgen-dependent hairs (scalp, beard, chest, axilla, and pubic region). These hairs are typically long (>2 cm), thick (>60 μm in diameter), pigmented, and tend to extend more than 3 mm deep into the subcutis. Vellus hairs, on the other hand, cover a large portion of the remainder of the body and are short (<2 cm), thin (<30 μm in diameter), often not pigmented, and extend just 1 mm into the dermis.

The hair follicle is composed of three anatomic units: the infundibulum, isthmus, and inferior segments. The infundibulum consists of the region of the hair follicle from the orifice of the follicle to the entrance of the sebaceous duct. The epithelium of the infundibulum is contiguous with the epidermis. The isthmus is located between the opening of the sebaceous duct and immediately above the insertion of the arrector pili muscle at the "bulge." The inferior aspect of the isthmus contains the bulge area of the hair follicle, which is located at the insertion of the arrector pili muscle and extends downward to form the hair bulb at its base during the anagen phase of hair growth.

The hair bulb, which is composed of matrix cells and melanocytes, is the deepest portion of the hair follicle that surrounds the dermal papilla. The dermal papilla contains the neurovascular structure that supplies the hair matrix. The various layers of the hair follicle are formed by the differentiation of matrical cells and include (from outer to inner layers) the outer root sheath, the inner root sheath (composed of the Henle layer, the Huxley layer, and the cuticle), and the three layers of the hair shaft (the cuticle, cortex, and medulla).

The bulge is contiguous with the outer root sheath and provides the insertion point for the arrector pili muscle. It also marks the bottom of the permanent portion of hair follicles. Importantly, the cells within the bulge area and the surrounding follicular cells have stem cell properties, such as multipotency and high proliferative capacity, allowing for the ability to regenerate not only hair follicles but also sebaceous glands and epidermis.[9]

Hair follicles are self-renewing structures and reconstitute themselves throughout the hair cycle. Hair follicles can be subdivided into the permanent and nonpermanent portions, with the upper and middle portion of the follicle being permanent and the lower region being nonpermanent, regenerating with each hair cycle. The follicular bulge forms the most inferior aspect of the permanent follicular structure. Hair undergoes a cyclic growth pattern that includes three phases: anagen, catagen, and telogen. Anagen is the period of active growth and the duration of anagen varies greatly based on anatomic site, accounting for the varying length of hair growth in each body site. Hair lengthening is a result of the outward migration caused by differentiation of bulbar matrix cells, leading to the hair shaft and inner root sheath. The catagen phase is a transition period that follows anagen and lasts approximately 2 to 4 weeks. During this time, the bulbar portion of the hair follicle undergoes degradation through apoptosis. The apoptosis allows for follicle regression with a shortening in length, with a more superficial placement of the hair bulb. Following catagen is the telogen phase, which is the last in the hair cycle and is marked by a period of inactivity lasting 2 to 4 months. The hair cycle continues with new hair growth resuming in a new anagen phase as the cycle repeats itself.

Differentiation of stem cells allows for the regeneration of the hair follicle. Mounting research has demonstrated that keratinocyte stem cells reside in and around the bulge area of the hair follicle, and migrate downward with anagen hair growth.[9] Additional studies have described the role of immature adipocytes during the activation of hair growth, in which adipocyte precursors induce the progression of the follicle from telogen to anagen, further affecting follicular cycling and communicating with follicular stem cells.[10]

The final length of the hair depends on the duration of the anagen phase, which varies depending on body site (▶ Table 8.1). Body sites with long hair, such as the scalp, have a long anagen phase. In contrast, body sites with short hair have a short anagen phase and a long telogen phase. In adults, the hairs of the scalp and body are not synchronous and occur at various stages of growth.

Table 8.1 Hair growth

Body site	Telogen duration (mo)	Anagen duration (mo)
Scalp	3–4	35–40
Upper lip	1–2	3–4
Axillae	3–4	3–6
Suprapubic/genitals	3–4	3–6
Lower limbs	5–6	4–5

Thus, the continuous shedding of telogen hairs and renewal of anagen hairs allow for a steady state of hair density.

Melanin pigmentation within keratinocytes of the hair fiber is what determines hair color. The hair melanin is produced by melanocytes located in the hair bulb epithelium. The density of bulbar melanocytes is greater than that in the epidermis, with approximately 1 melanocyte to 4 basal keratinocytes in the upper hair bulb compared with 1:10 in the basal layer of the epidermis. There are two types of melanin present in the hair: eumelanin (brown–black pigment) and pheomelanin (yellow–red pigment). Fire-red hair contains the highest levels of pheomelanin, whereas other hair colors contain melanocytes with eumelanosomes. Melanogenic activity is closely linked to the hair cycle, with melanogenesis occurring within the early part of the anagen phase of the hair cycle and ceasing with the onset of catagen.

8.3 Hair Removal Methods

8.3.1 Traditional Treatment Modalities

Prior to the introduction of lasers, numerous treatment modalities were utilized to achieve the cosmetic and functional goal of removing or minimizing the appearance of hair. For one, cosmetic procedures, such as bleaching, are used to reduce the pigmentation in an exposed hair shaft, diminishing the appearance of unwanted hair. Additional techniques that produced temporary hair removal options include mechanical hair removal methods as well as chemical depilatories (▶ Table 8.2). In fact, with the exception of electrical epilation, or electrolysis, these techniques have produced only temporary solutions.

Shaving is considered the most popular method of mechanical hair removal and involves the removal of hair above the surface of the skin. Although it is considered a simple mechanical method of hair removal, this modality requires frequent and regular use in order to maintain a desired clinical appearance. Importantly, the act of shaving or trimming does not lead to increased hair length, width, or density, a common misconception. Associated

Table 8.2 Physical methods of hair removal

Short-term methods of hair removal
• Mechanical
• Waxing
• Tweezing
• Threading
• Shaving
• Trimming
• Sugaring
• Chemical
• Depilatory

Long-term methods of hair removal
• Electrical
• Electrolysis
• Photothermal
• Lasers/light devices

Fig. 8.1 Pseudofolliculitis barbae with postinflammatory hyperpigmentation resulting from shaving.

complications of shaving include irritation, superficial abrasions, and pseudofolliculitis barbae (▶ Fig. 8.1).

Mechanical epilation involves the removal of the entire hair shaft and includes methods such as tweezing, waxing, threading, abrasives, sugaring, and the use of mechanical devices. Unlike shaving, epilation causes repetitive trauma to the hair follicle, potentially leading to matrix damage and finer hair growth over time. However, these modalities tend to be painful and require sufficient hair growth prior to effective repeat removal. Potential associated complications include postinflammatory dyspigmentation, folliculitis, pseudofolliculitis barbae, thermal injury, and scarring. Importantly, mechanical epilation should be used with caution in patients on systemic or topical retinoids due to the potential for excessive epidermal injury.

Chemical depilation involves the removal of the hair shaft, including the external projection from the skin surface as well as a small portion within the upper infundibulum. Chemical depilatories commonly contain thioglycolates, such as sodium thioglycolate or calcium thioglycolate, which work by disrupting disulfide bonds of hair keratin, causing hair breakage.[11] Although effective for temporary hair removal, adverse reactions to these agents include skin irritation, allergic contact dermatitis, and pseudofolliculitis barbae.

Permanent hair removal was first attempted in 1886 by electrosurgical epilation, also known as electrolysis.[12] Through electrolysis, a fine needle is inserted into a hair follicle, allowing for an electrical current to damage and eventually destroy the hair follicle.[16] Two types of electrolysis exist and include galvanic (direct current electrolysis) and thermolysis (alternating current electrolysis). While both forms of electrolysis can provide permanent hair removal, the process is highly operator dependent, with an efficacy of 30 to 40% for destroying individual hair follicles noted. Furthermore, the process has been noted to be tedious, time-consuming, costly, and painful, providing an impractical means of hair removal of large surface areas or extensive involvement. Potential risks associated with electrolysis include postinflammatory dyspigmentation, ice pick scarring, and the possibility for infection due to the transmission of bacterial or viral particles.[13]

At present, there are three ways to slow down hair growth: decrease anagen phase, delay the onset of anagen, or prolong the telogen phase. Although pharmacological prolongation of the telogen phase or anagen onset is not possible, the reduction in anagen phase is possible, most notably through the use of eflornithine hydrochloride 13.9% cream. Eflornithine hydrochloride 13.9% cream was first approved by the FDA in August 2000 and considered the first topical prescription treatment for the reduction of unwanted facial hair in women. It acts as an irreversible inhibitor of ornithine decarboxylase (ODC), an enzyme abundantly expressed in the proliferating bulb cells of anagen follicles and which is necessary for the biosynthesis of cationic polyamides, which are crucial for cell growth. Topical application of eflornithine hydrochloride 13.9% cream is effective in slowing hair growth temporarily and should be combined with other hair removal practices. It is classified as a pregnancy category C agent and has associated side effects of stinging, burning, tingling, acne, and folliculitis at the treatment site.

Medical management may also be considered in an attempt to slow or repress hair growth. The goal of these therapies includes the suppression of ovarian or adrenal androgen secretion or the blockage of androgen effects on the hair follicle. Systemic medications include cyproterone acetate, flutamide, spironolactone, and finasteride. The addition of an oral contraceptive may also be considered if serum testosterone concentration is elevated, although antiandrogen therapy is considered to be the most efficient.[14] Importantly, the use of systemic medications provides only partial and temporary hair loss and is associated with significant side effects, which often warrant frequent monitoring.

The advent of lasers has revolutionized the field of hair removal, and lasers have been demonstrated to be more effective, faster, and produce a longer-lasting result compared to mechanical or chemical epilation techniques. Prior to the development of lasers, electrolysis had been the mainstay for long-term hair removal. However, in a comparative study by Görgü et al, the alexandrite laser revealed clearance rates of 74% for LHR of treated sites compared to 35% of those areas treated with electrolysis at 6 months after the initial treatment. Additionally, the treatment duration for the laser was 60 times shorter than that of electrolysis and was felt to be less painful from the patient perspective.[15] Thus, the use of lasers for epilation remains the mainstay of therapy for LHR.

8.4 Preoperative Assessment and Preparation

Prior to treatment, a pretreatment consultation is necessary to determine eligibility. A thorough history and physical examination are necessary for treatment success (▶ Table 8.3). Patient and physician expectations must be fully defined before treatment initiation. Importantly, treatment risks and benefits must be thoroughly reviewed and informed consent should be obtained.

8.4.1 Medical History

A review of the patient's past medical history should include the presence of a familial pattern of excess hair growth or the presence of any underlying medical conditions. If an underlying medical condition is suspected, a workup should be obtained prior to treatment to evaluate for the potential etiology and improve the outcome of laser therapy. Additional inquiries should include a past history of herpes simplex virus (HSV), previous systemic gold therapy, or the recent use of oral retinoids. A past

Table 8.3 Preoperative assessment

Medical history
• Familial hair growth patterns
• Menstrual cycle (in women)
• Herpes simplex infections
• Recurrent skin infection
• Isotretinoin use
• Oral gold therapy
• Previous laser/light therapy
• Recent suntan or exposure to tanning beds
• Underlying endocrine disorders
• Koebnerizing dermatologic disorder
• Hypertrophic or keloidal scarring

Physical examination
• Skin phototype
• Hair density
• Hair color
• Hair coarseness
• Presence of vellus hairs

Patient expectations
• Pain management
• Posttreatment effects on skin
• Erythema
• Edema—perifollicular
• Hair shaft discharge/char
• Need for multiple treatments
• Risks of procedures

history of HSV at or near the treatment site requires prophylactic antiviral therapy. A patient with a past history of gold therapy should not be treated due to the risk of cutaneous chrysiasis, a discoloration of the skin that is noted to occur abruptly after laser interaction with skin that contains gold salts, which has been reported to occur with various laser wavelengths.[17,18] Furthermore, the use of oral retinoids in the recent past may raise concern regarding the higher risk of hypertrophic/keloid scarring following laser treatment. Although the risks are evident with mechanical dermabrasion and fully ablative laser procedures, a recent consensus statement has demonstrated that there is insufficient evidence to support delaying LHR for patients currently on, or having recently completed (within the past 6 months), isotretinoin based on extensive review of the existing literature that has revealed no adverse effects.[19,20,21,22]

At present, there lacks research on the safety and efficacy of LHR in pregnant patients. However, whether the patient is pregnant should be inquired upon prior to treatment. Although patients who are pregnant are not precluded from treatment with LHR, the use of topical anesthetic agents should be avoided during pregnancy and lactation in the postpartum period to avoid toxicity to the fetus or infant. Treatment should also be avoided or proceeded with caution in patients taking photosensitizing medications or those with underlying photosensitizing conditions such as lupus erythematosus or koebnerizing conditions such as psoriasis. Finally, documentation of past hair removal treatment modalities, including method, frequency, date of last treatment, and response, is essential.

8.4.2 Physical Examination

When performing the physical examination, the patient's hair color and skin tone should be noted, as these features will significantly influence the success of the treatment, appropriate laser settings, and potential side effects. The ideal candidate for LHR would have lighter skin phototype (Fitzpatrick skin types I and II) with dark terminal hair. Less ideal candidates are those with darker skin phototypes (Fitzpatrick skin types III and VI) and lighter hair phenotype. Importantly, patients with darker skin phototypes (Fitzpatrick skin types V and VI) may have an increased risk of side effects due to the significant increase in competing epidermal melanin if care is not taken with selection of laser and settings.

Patients with blond, gray, red, or white hair are poor candidates due to reduced melanin chromophore content in the hair shafts. Furthermore, the presence of vellus hairs in the treatment field may preclude the use of laser/light devices. For one, the risk of paradoxical hypertrichosis increases significantly when blonde, fine-textured vellus hairs are irradiated with laser/light energy. The lack of melanin in vellus hairs additionally leads to poor absorption of the light energy, leading to only a minor thermal effect on these hairs, which may induce differentiation of vellus hairs to terminal hairs. Although this effect is often seen along the jawline and neck of women, there have been reports of this effect in men as well.

Preoperative examination should also note the presence or absence of a tan, as a tan in all skin phototypes increases the risk of epidermal injury. If an active tan is present or there is recent sun exposure, laser treatment should be postponed until the tan fades or use of a longer-wavelength device, such as the 1,064-nm neodymium:yttrium aluminum garnet (Nd:YAG) laser should be considered in order to avoid potential side effects such as dyspigmentation. Patients should be instructed to avoid excessive sun exposure for a month before and during the entire treatment course. Documentation of existing tattoos, nevi, and scars within treatment areas is critical in managing treatment outcome. Patients with numerous lentigines should be aware that LHR might result in permanent removal of these.

8.4.3 Patient Expectations

Treatment Discomfort

Prior to treatment, patients should be counseled that the procedure may induce a degree of discomfort. Topical anesthetics may be utilized prior to treatment to minimize the discomfort. Importantly, patients should be discouraged from applying topical anesthetic creams without direction from their physician, as the application of large quantities over a large surface area may lead to significant toxicity and even death.[23] The use of cold air blowers may also be used during LHR treatment to add a significant degree of comfort and distraction to the patient. However, this technique should not be used with laser devices that utilize a dynamic cooling device, as the blowing air will disrupt the coolant flow to the skin and may prevent adequate epidermal protection.

Treatment Effects

Expected posttreatment findings include perifollicular edema, erythema, acneiform eruptions, and charred hair stubble, and patients should be made aware of all of these effects prior to treatment. Perifollicular edema has a variable duration, ranging from a few minutes to 1 to 2 days. However, if treating body sites with very dense and coarse hairs, perifollicular edema may last for up to 1 week after treatment. While cool compresses and ice may be used to hasten its regression, the use of topical corticosteroids can help minimize the perifollicular edema and aid in patient comfort. Acneiform eruptions are transient and can be treated with standard acne regimens.

Treatment Outcomes

Prior to treatment, patients must fully understand the risks and benefits of the procedure, as well as the long-term results. Establishing realistic goals prior to initiation of treatment is paramount. Patients should be aware that although LHR offers a method to significantly delay hair growth, there are a wide range of outcomes with LHR and multiple treatments are often necessary to result in finer hair growth. Temporary hair loss is achievable for most patients through the induction of catagen and telogen. However, long-term hair loss is strongly correlated with a patient's characteristics, such as hair color and skin phototype, as well as treatment parameters. In fact, hair loss in patients with blond, red, gray, or white hair can be maintained by treatment at approximately 3-month intervals. In general, a 20 to 30% hair loss has been observed with each treatment when effective fluences are used in patients with fair skin and dark hair. With the use of lower fluences, as are necessary for Fitzpatrick skin types III or greater, the percentage of hair loss is decreased, and complete permanent hair removal is unlikely. Treatment risks for all patients include blistering, ulceration, scar formation, folliculitis or acne flare, dyspigmentation, increased hair growth, poor to no response, and recurrence. These risks should be addressed before each treatment and informed consent should be obtained.

8.5 Mechanisms of Laser Hair Removal

8.5.1 Specific Laser Systems

Selective photothermolysis underlies the mechanism of LHR as this theory enables selective targeting of pigmented hair follicles by utilizing the melanin of the hair shaft as a chromophore. Although the ideal targets for LHR should be the follicular stem cells, these cells do not contain an appreciable amount of melanin or other chromophores that may serve as a target. Instead, the hair shaft and matrix both contain melanin, which is targeted by LHR therapies. Importantly, the extended theory of selective photothermolysis is the keystone to LHR, as diffusion of heat from the chromophore to the desired target of destruction occurs, allowing for follicular stem cells to be damaged by heat diffusion from the hair shaft or the matrix cells.[16]

The first laser-assisted hair removal device was marketed in 1996 and included the use of a Q-switched (QS) Nd:YAG laser in conjunction with a topical black carbon compound that was applied and massaged into the follicular openings after mechanical removal of the hair with waxing techniques. Since then, the FDA has approved numerous laser and light sources, which do not require additional carbon-based compounds for their use, which will be outlined later (▶ Table 8.4).

Neodymium:Yttrium Aluminum Garnet Laser

The use of QS Nd:YAG laser treatment was initially reported by Goldberg et al. They found that the use of laser epilation, followed by the application of a suspension of carbon mineral oil resulted in hair growth reduction for up to 6 months.[24] From this, it was speculated that filling the empty follicle with a carbon-containing substance acted as an energy-absorbing chromophore. Later studies comparing the use of QS Nd:YAG laser in the absence of the carbon solution indicated that laser irradiation alone also provided a significant delay in hair

growth. Importantly, whereas the QS Nd:YAG laser is capable of treating darker skin types and inducing delayed regrowth, these systems do not produce long-term or permanent hair removal.

On the contrary, long-pulsed 1,064-nm Nd:YAG lasers have deeply penetrating wavelengths and reduced melanin absorption at this wavelength, which requires the use of higher fluences for adequate follicle injury. Although this laser is not as effective in treating patients with lighter hair, it is safe and effective and is the treatment of choice for patients with Fitzpatrick skin types V and VI and for those patients with lighter skin types who happen to be tanned.[25,26,27]

Ruby Laser

The ruby laser emits light at a wavelength of 694 nm and was the first laser to demonstrate both temporary and permanent hair reduction. Grossman et al first reported selective injury to hair follicles using ruby laser pulses delivered through a cold sapphire lens to minimize epidermal injury.[5] In 13 individuals with fair skin and brown or black hair, high-fluence ruby laser pulses (6-mm spot size, fluences of 20–60 J/cm^2, and pulses of 0.27-millisecond duration) induced a hair growth delay lasting 1 to 3 months in all patients. Long-term follow-up of 7 of the 13 patients after 1 or 2 years revealed permanent hair loss only in the shaved areas at all fluences, with skin sites treated with the highest fluence (60 J/cm^2) revealing the greatest hair loss. Since then, multiple studies have further demonstrated that the ruby laser is safe and effective, with the hair growth delay consistent with the induction of telogen. For those individuals who demonstrated permanent hair loss, a reduction in large terminal hairs, an increase in small velluslike hairs, and a decrease in average hair shaft diameter without the presence of fibrosis were noted.[6,8,28,29]

Although the ruby laser is an effective method of hair removal, there are significant dose-related side effects associated with its use. The high epidermal melanin absorption may result in epidermal injury, leading to acute vesiculation, crusting, or pigmentary change. While these events may be observed with any laser system, they more frequently occur with the ruby laser due to its shorter wavelength and greater melanin absorption leading to injury to the epidermis. Use of the ruby laser should be avoided in patients with a history of persistent postinflammatory hyperpigmentation, tanned skin, or in individuals with Fitzpatrick skin type III or greater. Thus, this laser is best used on patients with lighter skin phototypes (I–II).

Alexandrite Laser

The alexandrite laser is a red light laser system, similar to the ruby laser but with a longer wavelength at 755 nm. The longer wavelength of the alexandrite allows for a slightly greater depth of penetration, allowing for a lower

Table 8.4 Laser and light sources used for hair removal

Laser/light source	Wavelength (nm)
Long-pulsed Ruby	694
• EpiLaser	
• EpiTouch	
Long-pulsed Alexandrite	755
• Arion	
• EpiCare	
• Harmony	
• GentleLASE/Max	
• Apogee	
• Elite/Elite MPX	
• PhotoGenica	
• Lutronic clarity 2	
Diode	800–810
• Apex-800	
• F1 Diode	
• Soprano	
• MeDioStar	
• LightSheer Duet	
• SLP1000	
Long-pulsed Nd:YAG	1,064
• Acclaim 7000; Smartepil II	
• LightPod Neo	
• Harmony	
• GentleYAG/GentleMax	
• CoolGlide Classic, Excel, XEI, Vantage	
• Lyra	
• Mydon	
• Profile	
• Softlight	
• Lutronic clarity 2	
Intense pulsed light source	400–1,200
• Estelux Y, Estelux R, Estelux Rs, Medilux Y, Medilux R	
• PhotoLight	

(Continued)

Table 8.4 *(Continued)* Laser and light sources used for hair removal

Laser/light source	Wavelength (nm)
• Prolite	
• Prowave	
• Quadra Q4	
• Elite MPX	
• Eclipse SmoothCool	
• Lumenis One	
• Spectraclear	
Fluorescent pulsed light	615–920
• OmniLight	
Photothermal	400–1,200
• SkinStation	
Optical energy combined with RF electrical energy	580–980
• Aurora DS, DSR	
Diode combined with RF electrical energy	800
• Polaris DS	

risk of epidermal damage due to the slightly lower melanin absorption at this wavelength. Treatment efficacy of the alexandrite laser varies with the anatomic location, pulse duration, and number of treatments. Using the average fluences of 30 to 40 J/cm^2, the efficacy rates of a 3-millisecond alexandrite laser ranges between 60 and 70% after a mean of 5.6 treatments.[30] Importantly, the alexandrite laser has been well established for hair removal in Fitzpatrick skin phototypes I to VI.[28,29,30] However, great care must still be taken when utilizing this laser in the darker skin phototypes including the use of longer pulse durations and lower fluences.

Diode Laser

The introduction of the diode laser (800–810 nm) further added to the LHR armamentarium, as these lasers are less costly to produce, reliable, and compact in size. These lasers reside at the far end of the visible light spectrum and at the near end of the infrared spectrum. They have longer pulse durations and a longer wavelength, allowing for the treatment of Fitzpatrick skin phototypes I to V due to a lower absorption of epidermal melanin. In an early study of the diode laser, a 25% hair count reduction was noted throughout the 20-month follow-up period. Additional long-term results (> 12 months) suggest that the pulsed 800-nm diode laser is as effective as the long-pulsed ruby laser in the removal of terminal hairs.[31,32,33]

A limitation of the traditional diode lasers is the small spot size, the need for higher fluences, and associated discomfort. However, modifications to the diode laser over time have included larger spot size and vacuum-assisted suction. In a study by Ibrahimi and Kilmer, the use of an 800-nm long-pulsed diode laser with a large spot size (22×35 mm), lower average fluences of 10 to 12 J/cm^2, and vacuum-assisted suction demonstrated hair clearance of 54% at 6 months and 42% at 15 months following three treatment sessions.[34] The larger spot size was found to provide similar results with lower fluence, decreasing the risk of potential side effects.[31,32,33] The vacuum-assisted suction brought the hair follicle closer to the epidermal surface, allowing for lower effective fluence, and was also found to decrease treatment discomfort. Braun also sought to address patient comfort using the diode laser and found that while efficacy was similar, perception of treatment discomfort was lower for the low-fluence, multiple-pass in-motion technique compared to a high-fluence, single-pass diode laser.[35]

Intense Pulsed Light

Intense pulsed (nonlaser) light (IPL) sources emit noncoherent, multiwavelength energy within a spectrum that ranges from 500 to 1,200 nm and may be used for hair removal. Filters are placed to cut off undesired wavelengths and target specific chromophores, allowing for more selective treatment. For instance, shorter wavelengths are used for Fitzpatrick skin types I and II for maximal energy delivery, while they are blocked for Fitzpatrick skin types III and darker to avoid excessive epidermal heating. The efficacy of IPL for LHR has been demonstrated in several studies, with one study highlighting a 33% reduction in hair growth after two treatments at 6 months (615-nm filter for Fitzpatrick skin types I and II or 645-nm filter for Fitzpatrick skin types III and above; 2.8- to 3.2-millisecond pulse duration for three pulses with thermal relaxation intervals of 20–30 milliseconds).[36] Importantly, comparative studies of IPL versus other lasers (long-pulsed alexandrite and Nd:YAG) have demonstrated the superiority of laser devices for hair removal.[37,38] Additionally, a disadvantage of IPL systems is that most devices use large rectangular spots, creating difficulty in the treatment of convex or concave hair-bearing areas.

The use of combination treatment with IPL and radiofrequency (RF) has also been explored.[39,40] For one, Sadick and Shaoul investigated the long-term photoepilatory effect of electro-optical synergy (ELOS) technology, which combines an IPL source (680–908 nm) with a bipolar RF device. The goal of this combination modality is to decrease the optical energy to a level safe for all phototypes while using the RF heating to compensate for the lower light energy. An average clearance rate of 75% at 18

months was demonstrated when patients were treated over four sessions with IPL fluences of 15 to 26 J/cm^2 and RF energy of 10 to 20 J/cm^3. On histologic evaluation, thermal damage to hair follicles with vacuolar degeneration was identified.[40] In a separate study by Sochor et al comparing a similar device to both a diode laser and an IPL alone, it was found that the combined IPL and RF device and the diode laser had similar efficacy, both of which were significantly better than the IPL alone.[41] As RF is pigment blind, it was thought that the combined technology of IPL and RF would lead to the successful treatment of light hair phenotypes. However, subsequent evaluations failed to demonstrate any significant long-term hair removal for lighter hair phenotypes.

Microwave Technology

A microwave-based hair removal system was approved by the FDA in 1999 for the removal of unwanted hair in all body sites except the face. The system works by sending pulses of microwave energy to the skin in conjunction with a coolant spray. To date, however, there are no published data available regarding the safety or efficacy of this device.

8.6 Preoperative Preparation for Laser Hair Removal

Treatment can be initiated after consultation and after the risks and benefits of LHR are reviewed. An informed consent should be signed by each patient on the day of service. Preoperative photographs are recommended to monitor patient progress.

Pretreatment instructions should include strict sun avoidance for 6 weeks prior to treatment and daily use of a broad-spectrum sunscreen throughout the treatment course. For patients with skin phototype III or greater or for patients with recent sun exposure, a bleaching cream such as 4% hydroquinone with or without 0.025% retinoic acid and 2% hydrocortisone may be prescribed as side effects after treatment have been reported to be reduced with the pretreatment use of sunscreens and bleaching creams. Additionally, an oral antiviral medication may be initiated 24 hours before the laser procedure and continued for a total of 7 days in patients with a history of HSV near the laser treatment site (▸ Fig. 8.2).

Patients should be instructed to remove hair by shaving, trimming, or chemical depilation either immediately before or within a short time point prior to the procedure. The hair should be cut to approximately 1 mm in length to minimize plume and prevent subsequent epidermal damage, allowing the energy to be delivered to the desired target. Importantly, all patients should avoid mechanical epilation of hairs in the treatment area for at least 3 to 4 weeks prior to treatment, as these methods remove an intact hair shaft, which contains the target

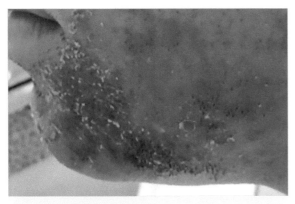

Fig. 8.2 Impetiginized herpetic eruption 4 days after laser treatment of facial hair. Subsequent treatments were without recurrence with the use of oral prophylaxis prior and following treatment.

chromophore for LHR. Thus, plucking, waxing, threading, or other physical methods of hair removal are discouraged as the hair shaft within the dermal portion of the hair follicle is necessary for successful LHR.

Immediately prior to treatment, makeup should be removed to allow for maximum laser energy delivery and to minimize light scatter. A topical anesthetic cream may be applied to the treatment area prior to the procedure in order to minimize patient discomfort. These agents should be applied to the treatment areas 30 minutes to 1 hour prior to treatment. Popular prescribed and over-the-counter topical anesthetics include a eutectic mixture of lidocaine 2.5% and prilocaine 2.5% cream (EMLA cream) or topical 4% lidocaine cream (LMX cream). One study did not find a statistically significant difference in pain control between these two topical anesthetics.[42] Compounded prescriptions containing lidocaine, tetracaine, and/or betacaine may be used as a stronger topical anesthetic. Regardless, topical anesthetics should be used with caution on large skin surface areas, as systemic toxicity has previously been reported.[23] Importantly, any topical anesthetic agent should be removed from the area prior to treatment.

Several other methods can be used to minimize patient discomfort during LHR, such as the use of cold air blowing on the adjacent skin surface, cold compresses to the treated skin surface, the application of prechilled rollers prior to each pulse, and pneumatic skin-flattening (PSF) devices. PSF technology reduces treatment discomfort based on the principles of the gate control therapy, in which activation of the non-nociceptive nerve fibers interferes with signal transmission from pain fibers, thereby inhibiting pain. The PSF suction device generates contact and compression between a transparent sapphire window and the skin, activating the tactile and pressure receptors prior to laser irradiation, thereby blocking the transmission of pain to the brain. This technology has

demonstrated success in decreasing patient discomfort with IPL devices as well as with other laser systems.[43,44, 45,46] It should be noted that the combined use of cooling agents can have a negative outcome in treating darker skin types or tanned skin where proper cooling of the epidermis is essential to avoid complications. The combination of a cold air blowing device and a directed cooling spray that is designed to work with a specific laser system may impact the effectiveness of the primary cooling agent as the blowing cold air will misdirect the coolant emitted from the laser device at the target tissue, thereby creating a zone of epidermis that may not be adequately cooled.

Immediately prior to treatment, the patient should be placed in a comfortable position so as to also permit maximum accessibility to the target surfaces. All staff members and the patient must wear protective glasses or goggles with a minimum optical density specific for the wavelength of the light being used. The use of a vacuum to remove smoke plume from vaporized hair is important to minimize the potentially toxic inhalation of smoke and the malodorous scent of burnt hair. It is advisable for all staff present in the room to wear adequate respiratory protection with an N95 mask due to particulate matter that is released during laser photoepilation.

The laser/light device should be calibrated to ensure proper energy delivery. Laser parameters should be tailored to each patient and device to ensure maximum efficacy with minimal side effects. The highest tolerated fluence and the largest spot size should be used to obtain efficient and optimal results. Mild traction on the skin with slight pressure may help provide uniform treatment and prevent capillary blood flow, which may interfere with light transmission to the hair follicles. Applying gentle skin traction decreases the relative depth of the bulb and bulge relative to the skin surface. The treatment should be systematic so as to avoid missed or skipped areas and prevent excessive overlaps of pulses. In general, individuals performing laser- and light-based hair removal should be properly trained in order to have a clear understanding of the proper use of these devices and a thorough knowledge of undesirable side effects and complications.

The treated skin should be monitored for 5 minutes after the initiation of treatment for desired erythema and perifollicular edema (▶ Fig. 8.3). If any whitening, vesiculation, or forced epidermal separation (positive Nikolsky's sign) are noted, the fluence must be decreased and repeat monitoring observed at the lower energy. In general, the treatment fluence should be at 75% of the Nikolsky sign threshold fluence.

8.7 Postoperative Care

After laser/light treatment, the skin can be gently patted with cool compresses to alleviate discomfort and remove any charred hair stubble from the skin surface. In general,

Fig. 8.3 Immediate posttreatment perifollicular erythema and edema after alexandrite laser in type I skin.

Table 8.5 Complications of laser/light hair removal

Epidermal vesiculation/burning

Dyspigmentation

Hyperpigmentation

Hypopigmentation

Scarring

Leukotrichia

Paradoxical hypertrichosis

Acneiform eruptions

Hyperhidrosis

Urticaria

Reticulate erythema

Ocular injury

patients should be instructed to avoid topical agents that can be irritating for a few days after treatment. Makeup may be applied on the next day unless blistering or crusts develop. Any trauma, such as picking or excoriating the area, should be avoided. Additionally, proper sun protection during the immediate postoperative period is imperative.

Patients should be made aware of the expected posttreatment presence of perifollicular edema, erythema, and acneiform eruptions. The perifollicular edema will have a variable duration, lasting minutes to 1 or 2 days. The use of cool compresses or ice will hasten its regression. When treating body sites with very dense and coarse hairs, the degree of edema tends to be great, lasting up to 1 week in some cases. Application of a low-potency topical corticosteroid may be helpful. In rare and severe cases, oral corticosteroids may be used to minimize perifollicular edema and aid in patient comfort. Purpura is rarely observed after LHR and, if present, tends to resolve over 2 weeks. Analgesics are generally not required unless extensive areas are treated.

Additionally, patients should be informed that the treated hair will continue to "grow" or shed for 1 to 2 weeks after treatment, with the discharge of follicular hair shafts occurring several days after the treatment session. Patients can shave, tweeze, or wax these treated hairs to expedite their removal once all inflammation has resolved. Depending on the treatment site, patients will note hair regrowth of those hairs not in anagen during treatment 2 to 6 weeks afterward. Importantly, treatment intervals are largely patient and site dependent, with the interval based on the presence of some regrowth from previous sessions. In general, treatments should occur every 6 to 8 weeks for the face, axillae, and bikini areas where regrowth is faster, and every 8 to 12 weeks for legs, chests, arms, and back where regrowth is slower.

8.8 Complications and Their Management

LHR is generally considered safe, with rare complications that are often transient in nature. The majority of side effects associated with LHR are due to epidermal injury and include blistering, dyspigmentation, and rarely scarring.[47] When blistering occurs, it may require localized wound care and a mid-potency corticosteroid cream may be recommended. Other less common side effects of LHR include acneiform eruptions, hyperhidrosis, urticaria, and reticulate erythema (▶ Table 8.5).[48] Skin containing a great amount of melanin has a greater risk of side effects. Therefore, selecting the proper wavelength and/or device, as well as patient avoidance of sun tanning prior to treatment, is essential to mitigate the potential for adverse events. In a comparative study of alexandrite laser, diode laser, and IPL, the diode laser was associated with a greater frequency of side effects, with the lowest frequency noted to be with the alexandrite laser. Importantly, all side effects reported in this study were temporary in nature.[49]

8.8.1 Dyspigmentation

Dyspigmentation are pigmentary changes that include either hyperpigmentation or hypopigmentation. This occurs most frequently in patients who do not avoid skin exposure before or after treatment and in patients with Fitzpatrick skin type III or greater (▶ Fig. 8.4).

Hyperpigmentation usually results from inflammatory injury, leading to stimulation of melanin production from epidermal melanocytes, or is due to epidermal disruption, allowing for an increase in melanin within macro-

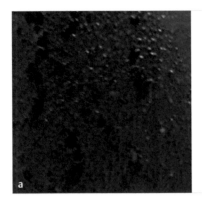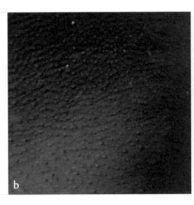

Fig. 8.4 (a) Two days after treatment with 1,064-nm Nd:YAG laser with a mismatch with coolant spray and laser leading to superficial crusting. **(b)** Two months after superficial burn with complete resolution and no residual dyspigmentation.

phages of the dermis. It is usually reversible in nature, but tends to resolve slowly over time, often taking months to years for full resolution. Additionally, the use of bleaching agents, such as hydroquinone, can help reduce the development of hyperpigmentation due to epidermal injury in darker skin phototypes. Importantly, patients should be counseled that topical hydroquinone creams may rarely cause an irritant dermatitis with long-term use.

Hypopigmentation, on the other hand, may be transient or permanent. Transient hypopigmentation often results from the thermal destruction of excess epidermal pigments and occurs if there is significant epidermal melanin present, such as from a tan. If an individual has variations in skin color, very commonly observed in the genital area, caution should be used with wavelength and fluence considerations.

Normal repigmentation usually occurs in areas of hypopigmentation over a variable period of time, ranging from weeks to months. If significant thermal injury to the melanocytes occurs, preventing melanin production, the resulting hypopigmentation may be permanent. The risk of permanent hypopigmentation is highest when there is an inappropriate selection of a shorter-wavelength laser/light device for darker skin phototypes. However, with proper selection of wavelength, fluence, and appropriate epidermal cooling, the risk of hypopigmentation is markedly reduced. When the hypopigmentation is clearly associated with mild epidermal injury of tanned skin and a sparing of untreated skin in between individual pulses of the laser, a pattern of hypopigmented spots is very apparent. Treating the entire area of hypopigmented and normally pigmented skin with a thulium 1,927-nm laser will hasten the return to a uniform pigment in most cases.

Interestingly, hypopigmentation after laser-assisted hair removal in combination with dynamic cryogen spray cooling systems has also been described in the literature. The exact pathophysiology of this entity is controversial, with speculation that it may be due to a cold-induced injury from the cryogen agent or a laser-induced thermal injury. Epidermal protection is only complete when a cooling device is held perpendicular and in contact to the skin surface. If a handpiece is angled 6 degrees or more from perpendicular when using a dynamic cooling device, a crescent-shaped burn may likely result due to incomplete cryogen coverage of the laser spot.[50] The transient dyspigmentation that occurs is likely a result of the thermal injury due to the mismatch of laser beam spot dimension and adequate cryogen. However, a prolonged cryogen spray duration used during dynamic cooling devices may also result in hyperpigmentation due to a cold-induced inflammatory injury. This phenomenon is most notable in darker skin phototypes.

8.8.2 Leukotrichia

Temporary or permanent leukotrichia has been reported after laser- and light-based hair removal therapies. This phenomenon is thought to represent the destruction of the melanocytes within the hair follicles without destruction of the germinative cells. Temporary leukotrichia may represent a transient arrest in melanin synthesis by damaged but viable melanocytes. Hair color restoration often occurs once the melanocytes become functional again and occurs more frequently in younger patients, whose melanocytes may be less susceptible to permanent thermal damage. Permanent melanocyte destruction likely occurs in patients with persistent leukotrichia of treated hair. Permanent leukotrichia was reported in 29 of 770 patients of Fitzpatrick skin types I to IV treated for unwanted facial and submental hair using a noncoherent IPL system with a 650-nm flashlamp filter. The white hairs were found to be as thick as the pretreatment black hairs. The use of sufficient fluences to induce germinative cell death concurrently with melanocyte death is critical in avoiding this side effect.

8.8.3 Paradoxical Hypertrichosis

Paradoxical hypertrichosis, the induction of terminal hair from vellus hair, is a well-known side effect of LHR.[51,52] The incidence of this side effect ranges from 5% to as high as 10% in some studies and has been reported in all skin phototypes. Increased hair growth tends to occur within the treated areas as well as in the adjacent, untreated skin. The most common sites for paradoxical hypertrichosis include the jawline, neck, and cheeks of women with darker skin phototypes. However, these changes have also been reported to occur on the torso. Importantly, anatomic sites at higher risk of paradoxical hypertrichosis tend to contain finer vellus hairs, which are then converted to terminal hairs due to the thermal induction of follicular maturation. Interestingly, the resultant hairs tend to appear coarser and darker than the hairs initially treated.[53,54] It is speculated that sublethal fluences may result in his paradoxically increased hair growth and use of highest tolerated fluence tends to minimize these occurrences. However, significant pain needs to be recognized and may be a warning that fluences are too high, potentially leading to tissue destruction. Treatment of paradoxical hypertrichosis consists of additional LHR of involved areas. Cooling the skin adjacent to the treatment area and confining the laser energy to the target area have demonstrated success in reducing the incidence of this side effect.

8.8.4 Acneiform Eruptions

The occurrence of acneiform eruptions, defined as small pustules in a follicular distribution, has been noted to occur in 6% of those treated with laser- and light-based therapies for hair removal. This transient complication usually occurs on the face in younger women and may be treated with standard acne therapies.

8.8.5 Hyperhidrosis

Hyperhidrosis is an uncommon, transient side effect of LHR and is thought to abate with regrowth of hair in the involved area. When occurring after LHR, it most commonly occurs in the axilla. Hyperhidrosis after treatment with a 1,064-nm Nd:YAG laser was reported in one study and lasted at least 1 year prior to resolving.[56]

8.8.6 Urticaria

Urticaria has been described in patients treated with a variety of lasers for hair removal, often occurring in treatment areas and lasting up to several days after laser therapy.[55,57] Many of these patients were previously treated with lasers without consequences. Patients often note severe pruritus in association with the urticaria, and antihistamines, topical, and systemic corticosteroids may often be used with improvement. At present, the etiology of the urticaria remains unclear.

8.8.7 Reticulate Erythema

Reticular erythema, defined as a nonblanching reddish blue lacelike erythema, is a very rare side effect that has been described after LHR for with the 800-nm diode laser. This rare side effect appeared in individuals treated after an average of 2.7 treatments. Although the etiology remains unclear, it is suspected that this may represent a variant of erythema ab igne.

8.8.8 Ocular Injury

Although ocular injury is the least common complication of LHR, it is considered the most important. Laser injuries to the eye are oftentimes permanent and include destruction of the retina, iris, and ocular epithelium, potentially leading to partial or complete blindness.[58] The mechanism for ocular injury is not clear in all cases, but it is believed that the relatively nonpigmented eyelids may lead to transmission of laser energy through the lids, resulting in absorption by the heavily pigmented iris and ciliary body.[58] The rolled contour of the orbital rim was also thought to allow for improper positioning of the laser handpiece, resulting in a portion of the beam being directed through the eyelid.

The use of longer-wavelength lasers increases the likelihood of ocular injury when treating the ocular area due to the greater depth of penetration. Thus, caution should be exercised if performing LHR in the periorbital region and use of longer-wavelength lasers/light devices within the orbital rim should be avoided. In fact, a number of case reports detail severe eye injuries resulting from LHR of the eyebrows, even in the presence of appropriate eye protection.

8.9 Conclusion

Utilizing the theory of selective photothermolysis, there are several laser and light sources now available for safe and effective hair removal. Although numerous studies have confirmed the long-term efficacy of laser- and light-assisted technology for hair removal, the ability to achieve long-lasting hair removal largely depends on hair color, skin phototype, and treatment fluence. Permanent hair reduction has proven difficult, likely due in part to the broad distribution of pluripotent cells, and no laser-specific parameters provide predictable permanent hair follicle destruction to date.

Although patients with fair skin and dark hair have demonstrated the greatest benefit of laser- and light-assisted technologies for hair removal, studies using devices with longer wavelengths, longer pulse durations, and epidermal cooling have demonstrated safety and efficacy in use of darker-skinned individuals. Whereas further challenges include the need to develop a means to eliminate light and nonpigmented hair, advancing technologies and broadening the understanding of follicular biology will allow for further improved means of hair removal.

At present, dermatologists are seeing an increasing number of complications from laser- and light-assisted hair reduction by nondermatologists and nonphysicians. Although state laws and regulations determine who can perform laser/light hair reduction, patient safety is best maintained when a physician determines the appropriateness of the patient for hair removal. Regardless, it is absolutely paramount that an appropriately trained individual be the one who performs the procedure and the physician should always be present on-site during the procedure should the procedure be delegated to a nonphysician. If complications occur, the physician is best trained to provide treatment due to the thorough understanding of the hair anatomy and laser–tissue interactions.

8.10 Pearls and Pitfalls

- Ensure all cosmetics and sunscreen are removed prior to treatment on the face.
- Ensure all pigment/self tanner is removed prior to treatment.
- Ensure the cryogen is functioning prior to treatment to ensure the skin gets cooled properly.
- Ensure you are using the correct wavelength for the skin type you are treating.
- Try a few pulses and see the laser tissue interaction before proceeding.
- If patient complains of pain, stop and consider lowering the fluence or pulse duration.
- Consider rescheduling the patient should they have a herpetic outbreak on the face and you are planning to treat that area.
- Ensure patients do not wax or pluck for at least 3 to 4 weeks before treatments.
- Remind patients not to be tan prior to their treatment.
- Review the consent with patient and review realistic expectations and number of treatments needed.

References

[1] Benson A. On the treatment of partial trichiasis by electrolysis. BMJ. 1882; 2(1146):1203–1204

[2] Minkis K, Bernstein LJ. Lasers and light devices for hair removal. In: Geronemus RG, Bernstein LJ, Hale EK, et al, eds. Lasers and Related Technologies in Dermatology. 1st ed. Vol. 1. New York, NY: McGraw-Hill; 2013

[3] Stebbins WG, Tsao SS, Hruza GJ, Hanke CW. Laser hair removal. In: Robinson JK, Hanke, CW, Siegel DM, Fratila A, Bhatia A, eds. Surgery of the Skin: Procedural Dermatology. 3rd ed. Elsevier Inc.; New York, NY: 2015:509–523

[4] Anderson RR, Parrish JA. Selective photothermolysis: precise microsurgery by selective absorption of pulsed radiation. Science. 1983; 220(4596):524–527

[5] Grossman MC, Dierickx C, Farinelli W, Flotte T, Anderson RR. Damage to hair follicles by normal-mode ruby laser pulses. J Am Acad Dermatol. 1996; 35(6):889–894

[6] Dierickx CC, Grossman MC, Farinelli WA, Anderson RR. Permanent hair removal by normal-mode ruby laser. Arch Dermatol. 1998; 134 (7):837–842

[7] Finkel B, Eliezri YD, Waldman A, Slatkine M. Pulsed alexandrite laser technology for noninvasive hair removal. J Clin Laser Med Surg. 1997; 15(5):225–229

[8] Lask G, Elman M, Slatkine M, Waldman A, Rozenberg Z. Laser-assisted hair removal by selective photothermolysis. Preliminary results. Dermatol Surg. 1997; 23(9):737–739

[9] Ohyama M. Hair follicle bulge: a fascinating reservoir of epithelial stem cells. J Dermatol Sci. 2007; 46(2):81–89

[10] Festa E, Fretz J, Berry R, et al. Adipocyte lineage cells contribute to the skin stem cell niche to drive hair cycling. Cell. 2011; 146(5):761–771

[11] Natow AJ. Chemical removal of hair. Cutis. 1986; 38(2):91–92

[12] Smith G. The removal of superfluous hairs by electrolysis. BMJ. 1886; 1(1308):151–152

[13] Richards RN, Meharg GE. Electrolysis: observations from 13 years and 140,000 hours of experience. J Am Acad Dermatol. 1995; 33(4): 662–666

[14] Crosby PD, Rittmaster RS. Predictors of clinical response in hirsute women treated with spironolactone. Fertil Steril. 1991; 55(6):1076–1081

[15] Görgü M, Aslan G, Aköz T, Erdoğan B. Comparison of alexandrite laser and electrolysis for hair removal. Dermatol Surg. 2000; 26(1): 37–41

[16] Altshuler GB, Anderson RR, Manstein D, Zenzie HH, Smirnov MZ. Extended theory of selective photothermolysis. Lasers Surg Med. 2001; 29(5):416–432

[17] Trotter MJ, Tron VA, Hollingdale J, Rivers JK. Localized chrysiasis induced by laser therapy. Arch Dermatol. 1995; 131(12):1411–1414

[18] Almoallim H, Klinkhoff AV, Arthur AB, Rivers JK, Chalmers A. Laser induced chrysiasis: disfiguring hyperpigmentation following Q-switched laser therapy in a woman previously treated with gold. J Rheumatol. 2006; 33(3):620–621

[19] Waldman A, Bolotin D, Arndt KA, et al. ASDS Guidelines Task Force: consensus recommendations regarding the safety of lasers, dermabrasion, chemical peels, energy devices, and skin surgery during and after isotretinoin use. Dermatol Surg. 2017; 43(10):1249–1262

[20] Khatri KA. The safety of long-pulsed Nd:YAG laser hair removal in skin types III–V patients during concomitant isotretinoin therapy. J Cosmet Laser Ther. 2009; 11(1):56–60

[21] Khatri KA, Garcia V. Light-assisted hair removal in patients undergoing isotretinoin therapy. Dermatol Surg. 2006; 32(6):875–877

[22] Khatri KA. Diode laser hair removal in patients undergoing isotretinoin therapy. Dermatol Surg. 2004; 30(9):1205–1207, discussion 1207

[23] Elsaie ML. Cardiovascular collapse developing after topical anesthesia. Dermatology. 2007; 214(2):194

[24] Goldberg DJ, Littler CM, Wheeland RG. Topical suspension-assisted Q-switched Nd:YAG laser hair removal. Dermatol Surg. 1997; 23(9): 741–745

[25] Rao K, Sankar TK. Long-pulsed Nd:YAG laser-assisted hair removal in Fitzpatrick skin types IV-VI. Lasers Med Sci. 2011; 26(5):623–626

[26] Davoudi SM, Behnia F, Gorouhi F, et al. Comparison of long-pulsed alexandrite and Nd:YAG lasers, individually and in combination, for leg hair reduction: an assessor-blinded, randomized trial with 18 months of follow-up. Arch Dermatol. 2008; 144(10):1323–1327

[27] Li R, Zhou Z, Gold MH. An efficacy comparison of hair removal utilizing a diode laser and an Nd:YAG laser system in Chinese women. J Cosmet Laser Ther. 2010; 12(5):213–217

[28] Sommer S, Render C, Sheehan-Dare R. Facial hirsutism treated with the normal-mode ruby laser: results of a 12-month follow-up study. J Am Acad Dermatol. 1999; 41(6):974–979

[29] McCoy S, Evans A, James C. Long-pulsed ruby laser for permanent hair reduction: histological analysis after 3, 4 1/2, and 6 months. Lasers Surg Med. 2002; 30(5):401–405

[30] Eremia S, Li CY, Umar SH, Newman N. Laser hair removal: long-term results with a 755 nm alexandrite laser. Dermatol Surg. 2001; 27(11): 920–924

[31] Campos VB, Dierickx CC, Farinelli WA, Lin TY, Manuskiatti W, Anderson RR. Hair removal with an 800-nm pulsed diode laser. J Am Acad Dermatol. 2000; 43(3):442–447

[32] Kopera D. Hair reduction: 48 months of experience with 800 nm diode laser. J Cosmet Laser Ther. 2003; 5(3–4):146–149

[33] Lou WW, Quintana AT, Geronemus RG, Grossman MC. Prospective study of hair reduction by diode laser (800 nm) with long-term follow-up. Dermatol Surg. 2000; 26(5):428–432

[34] Ibrahimi OA, Kilmer SL. Long-term clinical evaluation of a 800-nm long-pulsed diode laser with a large spot size and vacuum-assisted suction for hair removal. Dermatol Surg. 2012;38(6):912–917

[35] Braun M. Comparison of high-fluence, single-pass diode laser to low-fluence, multiple-pass diode laser for laser hair reduction with 18 months of follow up. J Drugs Dermatol. 2011;10(1):62–65

[36] Weiss RA, Weiss MA, Marwaha S, Harrington AC. Hair removal with a non-coherent filtered flashlamp intense pulsed light source. Lasers Surg Med. 1999; 24(2):128–132

[37] Goh CL. Comparative study on a single treatment response to long pulse Nd:YAG lasers and intense pulse light therapy for hair removal on skin type IV to VI: is longer wavelengths lasers preferred over shorter wavelengths lights for assisted hair removal. J Dermatolog Treat. 2003; 14(4):243–247

[38] McGill DJ, Hutchison C, McKenzie E, McSherry E, Mackay IR. A randomised, split-face comparison of facial hair removal with the alexandrite laser and intense pulsed light system. Lasers Surg Med. 2007; 39(10):767–772

[39] Yaghmai D, Garden JM, Bakus AD, Spenceri EA, Hruza GJ, Kilmer SL. Hair removal using a combination radio-frequency and intense pulsed light source. J Cosmet Laser Ther. 2004; 6(4):201–207

[40] Sadick NS, Shaoul J. Hair removal using a combination of conducted radiofrequency and optical energies: an 18-month follow-up. J Cosmet Laser Ther. 2004; 6(1):21–26

[41] Sochor M, Curkova AK, Schwarczova Z, Sochorova R, Simaljakova M, Buchvald J. Comparison of hair reduction with three lasers and light sources: prospective, blinded and controlled study. J Cosmet Laser Ther. 2011; 13(5):210–215

[42] Guardiano RA, Norwood CW. Direct comparison of EMLA versus lidocaine for pain control in Nd:YAG 1,064 nm laser hair removal. Dermatol Surg. 2005; 31(4):396–398

[43] Fournier N. Hair removal on dark-skinned patients with pneumatic skin flattening (PSF) and a high-energy Nd:YAG laser. J Cosmet Laser Ther. 2008; 10(4):210–212

[44] Yeung CK, Shek SY, Chan HH. Hair removal with neodymium-doped yttrium aluminum garnet laser and pneumatic skin flattening in Asians. Dermatol Surg. 2010; 36(11):1664–1670

[45] Lask G, Friedman D, Elman M, Fournier N, Shavit R, Slatkine M. Pneumatic skin flattening (PSF): a novel technology for marked pain reduction in hair removal with high energy density lasers and IPLs. J Cosmet Laser Ther. 2006; 8(2):76–81

[46] Bernstein EF. Pneumatic skin flattening reduces pain during laser hair reduction. Lasers Surg Med. 2008; 40(3):183–187

[47] Lim SP, Lanigan SW. A review of the adverse effects of laser hair removal. Lasers Med Sci. 2006; 21(3):121–125

[48] Radmanesh M, Azar-Beig M, Abtahian A, Naderi AH. Burning, paradoxical hypertrichosis, leukotrichia and folliculitis are four major complications of intense pulsed light hair removal therapy. J Dermatolog Treat. 2008; 19(6):360–363

[49] Toosi S, Ehsani AH, Noormohammadpoor P, Esmaili N, Mirshams-Shahshahani M, Moineddin F. Treatment of trichostasis spinulosa with a 755-nm long-pulsed alexandrite laser. J Eur Acad Dermatol Venereol. 2010; 24(4):470–473

[50] Kelly KM, Svaasand LO, Nelson JS. Further investigation of pigmentary changes after alexandrite laser hair removal in conjunction with cryogen spray cooling. Dermatol Surg. 2004; 30(4, Pt 1):581–582

[51] Desai S, Mahmoud BH, Bhatia AC, Hamzavi IH. Paradoxical hypertrichosis after laser therapy: a review. Dermatol Surg. 2010; 36(3):291–298

[52] Alajlan A, Shapiro J, Rivers JK, MacDonald N, Wiggin J, Lui H. Paradoxical hypertrichosis after laser epilation. J Am Acad Dermatol. 2005; 53(1):85–88

[53] Willey A, Torrontegui J, Azpiazu J, Landa N. Hair stimulation following laser and intense pulsed light photo-epilation: review of 543 cases and ways to manage it. Lasers Surg Med. 2007; 39(4):297–301

[54] Aydin F, Pancar GS, Senturk N, et al. Axillary hair removal with 1064-nm Nd:YAG laser increases sweat production. Clin Exp Dermatol. 2010; 35(6):588–592

[55] Bernstein EF. Severe urticaria after laser treatment for hair reduction. Dermatol Surg. 2010; 36(1):147–151

[56] Aydin F, Pancar GS, Senturk N, Bek Y, Yuksel EP, Canturk T, Turanli AY. Axillary hair removal with 1064-nm Nd:YAG laser increases sweat production. Clin Exp Dermatol. 2010;35(6):588–592

[57] Moteno-Arias GA, Tiffon T, Marti T, Camps-Fresneda A. Urticaria vasculitis induced by diode laser photoepilation. Dermatol Surg. 2000; 26(11):1082–1083

[58] Brilakis HS, Holland EJ. Diode-laser-induced cataract and iris atrophy as a complication of eyelid hair removal. Am J Ophthalmol. 2004; 137(4):762–763

9 Tattoo Removal

Richard L. Lin, Alexa B. Steuer, Andrea Tan, and Jeremy A. Brauer

Summary

The prevalence of tattoos continues to increase, with the rising popularity and shift in cultural attitudes regarding body art and self-expression. Concurrently, tattoo removal procedures have also seen an increase in demand, due to either regret or changes in personal or professional life events. Over the past few decades, laser procedures have become the gold standard for safe and effective tattoo removal. Quality switched, or Q-switched, nanosecond pulse duration lasers have long been considered state of the art; however, more recently, picosecond pulse duration lasers have become the new standard of care. Additionally, adjunctive treatment modalities, such as the perfluorodecalin-infused silicone patch, have been shown to aid in rapidly reducing laser-induced opaque whitening, thus allowing for an increased number of passes in rapid sequence without increasing the risk of adverse events. These advances hold promise for improved treatment experience and enhanced clinical outcomes in laser tattoo removal moving forward.

Keywords: tattoo removal, laser, Q-switched laser, nanosecond, picosecond, perfluorodecalin

9.1 Introduction

Tattoo removal procedures have shifted dramatically over the course of history. The first evidence of attempted tattoo removal was observed in Egyptian mummies dated back to 4,000 BC; the ancient Greeks used salt abrasion or a paste made from white garlic cloves mixed with Alexandrian cantharidin.[1] Tattoo removal later shifted to excisional and destructive procedures such as surgical excision, cryotherapy, dermabrasion, or thermal cautery.[2] However, while still utilized for small or otherwise difficult to treat tattoos, these surgical procedures have the potential to result in poor cosmetic outcomes and significant scarring.[2]

The idea of laser tattoo removal began in 1963 when Leon Goldman first showed that 0.5-millisecond pulses from a ruby (694 nm) laser effectively targeted pigmented structures of the skin.[3] Despite this initial success, laser tattoo removal was performed largely by nonselective, continuous wave source lasers such as the argon and CO_2 into the 1980s.[4] In 1983, Anderson and Parrish introduced the concept of selective photothermolysis that allowed for laser-based destruction of specific components of the skin, such as pigment or melanin, while leaving surrounding tissue intact.[5] This formed the basis of modern tattoo removal.

9.2 Modalities and Treatment Options

Modern tattoo removal techniques and devices are derived from the principle of selective photothermolysis.[5] Different chromophores found in the skin (such as melanin, ink particles, hemoglobin, and water) preferentially absorb different wavelengths of light. As long as a target chromophore has greater optical absorption at some wavelength than surrounding tissue, it can be targeted selectively by a laser. Subsequently, the energy delivered by the photons is converted to thermal energy and dissipated at a rate determined by thermal relaxation time, or the time taken for a chromophore to lose half of its heat via diffusion. Thermal relaxation time is proportional to the size of target chromophore. For example, tattoo particles may have a thermal relaxation time of few nanoseconds, whereas leg venules correspond to a thermal relaxation time on the order of 100 milliseconds.[6] A pulse duration that is shorter than a chromophore's thermal relaxation time will ideally limit heat damage to only the targeted chromophore, whereas a pulse duration that is longer than the thermal relaxation time may result in the transfer of heat energy to the surrounding skin and cause unintended damage.[7] On the basis of selective thermolysis, the development of nanosecond Q-switched lasers, specifically the ruby (694-nm) laser, alexandrite laser (755 nm), and neodymium:yttrium aluminum garnet (Nd:YAG) laser (1,064 or 532 nm [frequency doubled]), made the treatment of tattoos possible.[8]

Although nanosecond lasers can be effective in tattoo removal, success is often achieved only after numerous treatment sessions. This is especially the case where specific colors are more recalcitrant or show pigmentary changes following laser irradiation.[9,10] Therefore, attempts have been, and continue to be, made to improve the process. In 1998, greater efficiency in the clearance of black tattoos was observed with picosecond rather than nanosecond pulse durations.[11] Rather than relying solely on thermal energy to destroy the tattoo particles, it has since been shown that these picosecond duration lasers heat their targets within such a short period of time to cause thermal expansion and vibration. This effect ultimately leads to photomechanical stress and fracture of the tattoo particles.[8] These subsequent fragments are smaller than what is observed after destruction by nanosecond lasers, and therefore likely better removed by circulating macrophages. By relying less upon a photothermal effect to achieve effect, picosecond pulse duration lasers minimize the potential for collateral injury to surrounding tissues. Smaller studies have demonstrated improvement in removal of traditionally more difficult tattoo colors, namely blue, green, and yellow pigments.[12,13]

Although it took more than a decade for the picosecond pulse duration laser to translate from benchtop to bedside, numerous picosecond devices are now commercially available. Commonly utilized wavelengths in these picosecond devices include 532, 694, 755, and 1,064 nm, with a range of 375 to 750 picoseconds; however, some devices also allow for nanosecond pulses.

Beyond selective photothermolysis and photoacoustolysis, fractional photothermolysis with ablative and nonablative fractional lasers has been successfully utilized in tattoo removal.[14,15,16] With laser excitation, tattoo pigments such as white and brown, which generally contain titanium oxide or ferric oxide, can turn black through a reduction reaction.[17] As these resurfacing lasers primarily target water and not pigment contained within exogenous tattoo particles, they offer another option for removal for certain ink colors. The infrared wavelengths are absorbed by water to damage (nonablative) or remove (ablative) microscopic columns of skin, called microscopic treatment zones (MTZs).[14] The areas around the zones of injury are unaffected and create an environment favorable for rapid wound healing.[14] Therefore, fractional lasers remove tattoo pigment physically, as well as by creating microscopic channels through which the pigment can migrate upward. It is then eliminated transepidermally in the form of exfoliated necrotic debris within approximately 1 week of treatment.[14,15,16]

9.3 Indications

The motivations for tattoo removal vary from individual to individual and are often multifactorial and complex. Prominent reasons for removal include unwanted details (such as the name of a prior partner), outdated tattoos, or inappropriateness of the tattoo regarding employment. A study comparing the motivations for tattoo removal in 1996 with those in 2006 found an increase in the prevalence of women getting as well as removing tattoos, compared to their male counterparts.[18] Ultimately, the increase in female patients requesting tattoo removal was linked to an increase in negative societal connotations for women versus men with visible tattoos, particularly for women in the professional job market.[18]

9.4 Procedural Planning and Counseling

9.4.1 Preoperative Evaluation

Prior to laser tattoo removal, it is imperative for the clinician to take a thorough past medical, surgical, and allergy history. Specifically, does the patient report any known medical conditions, or is the patient currently or has recently taken medications that could affect wound healing; similarly, it is important to determine if there is a history of gold therapy, keloid, postinflammatory pigmentary alteration, or current or recent use of isotretinoin. If treating on or around the mouth, determine history of oral herpes simplex virus. In addition to medical and surgical history, the patient should be asked if they have experienced any adverse events to laser treatments previously, including known allergic reactions. Recent or planned sun exposure or application of artificial tanner must also be discussed, as these lasers will target pigment whether endogenous or exogenous, potentially increasing the risk of complications. Therefore, it is advised not to treat tanned skin, and to avoid and protect healing areas from the sun afterward.

It is also important to get a good history of the tattoo of concern. If determined to be an amateur tattoo, this may have different clinical and management implications and expectations than a professionally administered tattoo. The pigment deposition in an amateur tattoo tends to have a much wider distribution throughout the dermis. Pigment density is generally lower and less uniform than that of a professional tattoo. Decreased density and fewer ink components found in an amateur tattoo generally translates to fewer treatment sessions required for removal. One study found a mean difference of 4.5 versus 8.6 visits for the removal of amateur versus professional tattoos, respectively.[19] The age of the tattoo itself is an important factor in pretreatment evaluation. Older tattoos that have started to fade are easier to remove and require fewer treatments. In addition to the age and type of tattoo, the colors of the tattoo are important. Specifically, it is important to determine if "white" ink or other colors that may have incorporated white were used to yield the final color. This is because treatment of these colors with nanosecond and picosecond lasers can result in a graying or darkening of the tattoo, known as "paradoxical darkening." Therefore, the colors will dictate which wavelength, or even type of laser, or lasers are most appropriate for removal (▶ Table 9.1).

Table 9.1 Tattoo ink colors and optimal device

Color	Wavelength (nm)	Pulse duration
Black	694; 755; 1,064	nanosecond; picosecond
Blue	755, 785	picosecond
Green	755, 785	nanosecond; picosecond
Purple	755, 785	picosecond
Red	532	nanosecond; picosecond
Yellow	532	nanosecond; picosecond
Orange	532	nanosecond; picosecond

Fitzpatrick skin type of the patient is another factor to consider in tattoo removal. Epidermal melanin often acts as the primary competing chromophore in laser tattoo removal. Due to differences in melanosome size and distribution, patients of skin of color are at greater risk of pigmentary alterations such as hypopigmentation and hyperpigmentation; they are also at increased risk of hypertrophic scarring and keloid formation.[20,21] In patients with darker skin types, threshold responses will normally occur at lower fluences, and longer wavelength devices such as the 1,064-nm Nd:YAG laser should be used to minimize epidermal damage.[21] Use of a protective barrier, such as hydrogel pads or the perfluorodecalin (PFD) infused silicone patch, may provide additional epidermal protection, minimizing risks. Regardless of skin type, patients with recent skin damage due to sun exposure should be instructed to delay treatment.

The specific location of a tattoo also presents unique challenges when evaluating for laser removal. Tattoos that are located on the distal extremities are subject to less lymphatic drainage, which causes less pigment clearance after laser treatment and requires more treatments to achieve complete removal.[22] The area of skin containing the tattoo itself should also be closely inspected to make sure that there are no signs of any malignant or premalignant lesions that can be hidden by certain tattoo pigments.[23] Another significant, but often overlooked, aspect of treatment that should be discussed with the patient is that of realistic expectations regarding treatment course, possible posttreatment appearance/clearance, and cost and time of treatment. Successful tattoo removal requires multiple treatment sessions, and the cost of, and time commitment to, the process can become considerable.[24]

9.4.2 Treatment Selection

Ultimately, laser selection is largely based on the primary pigments contained within the tattoo of concern. Because of the ever-increasing complexity of the pigments used in modern tattoos, as well as the cultural trend of an increasing number of pigments in each individual piece, it may be necessary for the use of multiple wavelengths, and possibly multiple devices and approaches, for removal of an individual tattoo. This combination approach is the preferred treatment method of the authors, potentially utilizing a PFD patch with nanosecond, picosecond, ablative, and/or nonablative lasers over the course of complete tattoo removal.

Nanosecond Lasers

The Q-switched nanosecond pulse duration lasers regularly utilized in tattoo removal include the ruby, Nd:YAG with and without a potassium titanyl phosphate (KTP) crystal, and the alexandrite lasers.[24,25] The Q-switched ruby laser was one of the first lasers to be employed in tattoo removal and operates at the 694-nm wavelength.[25] This laser has been most successful in removal of black and, less so, blue tattoo pigments. This wavelength is less effective with removal of red or orange pigments from the skin due to the reflection, as opposed to absorption, of light from the ruby source.[25] The targeting of black pigments makes the Q-switched ruby laser ideal for the removal of amateur tattoos, which most commonly utilize India ink pigment.[25,26]

The Q-switched Nd:YAG laser emits light in the infrared range at 1,064 nm.[26,27] This laser is commonly modified by the addition of a KTP crystal, allowing for the doubling of the laser frequency, "frequency doubled," so the same laser can operate at the 532-nm wavelength.[26,27] At the 1,064-nm wavelength, the Q-switched Nd:YAG laser provides excellent removal of black and dark blue pigments. The 1,064-nm wavelength has a deeper penetration and lower absorption by melanin, making it a safer choice for patients of skin of color. When operating at the 532-nm wavelength, the Q-switched Nd:YAG laser provides effective removal of red, orange, and some yellow pigments. The ability to operate in two different wavelengths makes the Q-switched Nd:YAG laser a choice for a tattoo with multiple pigments.[26,27]

The Q-switched alexandrite laser is another laser that can remove blue and black pigments.[28] Its greatest utility, however, may be its ability to remove green pigments, which are often noticeably left behind, particularly after the use of a Q-switched Nd:YAG laser. The removal of green pigments is possible due to the Q-switched alexandrite laser's emission at the 755-nm wavelength.[19,29] Thus, this laser can act as an excellent complement to other Q-switched lasers.

The selection of nanosecond lasers should be based on the primary pigments contained in the tattoo that need to be removed, as well as the patient skin type. Due to the ever-increasing number and complexity of the pigments used in modern tattoos, it may be necessary to use multiple lasers with different wavelengths for complete removal.

Picosecond Lasers

Picosecond lasers became commercially available within the last decade and are now considered by many to be the first choice for laser tattoo removal (▶ Fig. 9.1). As previously mentioned, closer approximation of thermal relaxation times of smaller particles and photomechanical effects allow these lasers to minimize thermal damage to surrounding tissues. Specifically, diameters of most tattoo pigment particles are between 10 and 100 nm, corresponding to a thermal relaxation time shorter than 10 nanoseconds, falling into the "subnanosecond" or picosecond range.[30,31] Early picosecond pulse duration lasers generated these pulses via mode locking, a process involving an oscillator coupled to an amplifier.[30] Picosecond lasers presently in use employ passive Q-switching, thus

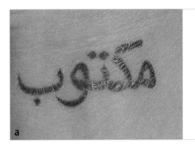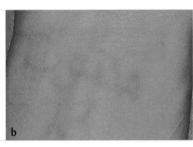

Fig. 9.1 Black tattoo treatment with 1,064-nm picosecond pulse duration laser. (a) Baseline. (b) Clearance after three sessions. (These images are provided courtesy of Dr. E. Victor Ross.)

reducing the need for bulky equipment while operating at multiple wavelengths and being more amenable to clinical practice.[30]

Laboratory studies on picosecond pulse duration lasers demonstrated superior clearance of tattoo pigment when compared to clearance by nanosecond pulse duration lasers.[11] Some pigments that have conventionally been more difficult to remove, such as blue, green, and yellow, have responded well to the picosecond laser.[12,13] As tattoo removal can be time-consuming and costly, the ability to potentially achieve clearance in fewer treatment sessions is of significant importance. Clinical trials, of which there are few, have only been done with small sample sizes. Therefore, although some studies have cited greater clearance with the picosecond laser than the nanosecond laser, any conclusions may lack definitive generalizability. A recent systematic review remarked on the scarcity of high-quality studies available.[31,32,33,34]

Picosecond laser treatment is associated with similar potential risks seen with nanosecond devices including but not limited to pain, dyspigmentation, erythema, edema, pinpoint bleeding, and scarring.[31,34] Studies assessing the safety of picosecond lasers reported comparable safety with regard to clinical scarring and histopathologic fibrosis.[12,31,32,33] Additionally, as with nanosecond lasers, picosecond lasers, when possible, should not be used on tattoos that may have iron oxide in the ink due to risk of paradoxical darkening, instead considering use of ablative lasers. There are occasions, however, where it may behoove the physician to intentionally induce this reaction and then continue to treat the tattoo, a technique that has been successfully demonstrated using a picosecond laser.[35]

The first commercially available picosecond laser was a 755-nm alexandrite laser with a pulse duration of 750 picoseconds. The Nd:YAG-based frequency-doubled 1,064-/532-nm picosecond laser was subsequently developed by two different companies, employing a two-stage system that effectively targets purple, red, yellow, and orange pigments in addition to black.[36] These systems incorporate three wavelengths, including 670 and 785 nm, as well as the option to treat at 2-nanosecond pulse duration. In recent years, more picosecond lasers have become available and operate at two or more wavelengths with multiple pulse durations, giving physicians the ability to target a spectrum of colors.

Ablative and Nonablative Lasers

Through fractional photothermolysis, ablative and nonablative fractionated treatment can offer an alternative method of tattoo removal for colors recalcitrant to selective photothermolysis.[14,15,16] Nonablative lasers utilize wavelengths in the near-infrared spectrum (1,320, 1,440, 1,540, 1,550, and 1,927 nm), whereas ablative lasers use energy in the mid-infrared spectrum (2,940 or 2,790 nm), or far-infrared spectrum (10,600 nm). Successful combination treatment with the carbon dioxide laser and Q-switched ruby laser has been reported and showed improved tattoo removal than with Q-switched ruby laser alone.[16] Similarly, erbium:yttrium aluminum garnet (Er:YAG) fractionated laser alone or in combination with a Q-switched Nd:YAG laser has been successful in patients with allergic tattoo reactions.[15]

An advantage of ablative and nonablative devices for tattoo removal is that the target chromophore is water, not tattoo pigments specifically, which is especially helpful for white, skin-colored, and multicolored tattoos, which as mentioned earlier carry a greater risk of paradoxical darkening. Whereas this can certainly be an advantage, treatment with these devices is not without risk, and multiple treatment sessions are often still necessary given the fractional pattern of injury. Specifically, the risk of excessive thermal damage and/or permanent scarring is greater with these resurfacing devices when compared to nanosecond and picosecond lasers, particularly for individuals of skin of color.

Perfluorodecalin Patch

Although laser tattoo removal is generally regarded as safe and effective, the lengthy treatment period usually required to achieve clearance is a major drawback. Traditional techniques have consisted of a single treatment session administered every 4 to 8 weeks.[37] A recent series demonstrated increased efficacy of removal when four passes are delivered over a single treatment session.[37] Specifically, upon completion of a laser treatment, the patient and treating physician would wait until the epidermal whitening reaction dissipated, at which time another treatment would be performed. The time for this to occur is approximately 20 minutes on average. This method, known as R20, may present practical limitations for both the patient and physician, as the time required for this dissipation of epidermal whitening and subsequent treatment would significantly extend a single office visit.

PFD is a stable, metabolically inert fluorocarbon liquid with several unique properties.[38,39] It has exceptional optical transparency from the ultraviolet (UV) to the far-infrared range.[40] Importantly, it has a well-known property of being able to dissolve gases, which has led to its use in first-generation artificial blood substitutes and liquid ventilation.[38,39] Of particular importance, laser-induced cavitation reaction generates gas bubbles that readily diffuse into the liquid PFD.[39] This critical property affords PFD the unique ability to immediately reduce the whitening reaction caused by this cavitation reaction.

The mechanism by which PFD clears the laser-induced cutaneous immediate whitening reactions in tattoo removal is mainly attributable to this gas transfer through tissues resulting in effective multiple-pass laser tattoo removal.[39] As this layer dissipates, optical clearing may play a role in the mechanism of action, allowing photons to penetrate more deeply with reduced optical scattering.

The safety and efficacy of a PFD-infused silicone patch has also been demonstrated in conjunction with both nanosecond and picosecond lasers.[41,42,43,44] A retrospective review was recently performed, including 45 consecutive patients of Fitzpatrick skin types I to V with black as well as multicolor (black, blue, green, red, and yellow) tattoos. All patients were treated with a 755-nm picosecond laser, with two patients receiving treatment with a 532-nm wavelength in the same treatment session. The mean number of passes per treatment session was 2.6 (range of 1–4 passes) and the mean number of treatment sessions necessary was 2.8 (range of 2–5 treatments). Notably, no dyspigmentation, scarring, textural changes, or unanticipated adverse events were reported.[44]

9.5 Technique

9.5.1 Procedural Preparation

Prior to laser treatment, the surface of the tattoo should be cleaned, and the laser should be calibrated. Providers should review patient's medical, surgical, allergy history; answer any patient questions or concerns; and take measurements and photographs. The informed consent should review risks of (such as pain, unsatisfactory cosmetic outcome, paradoxical darkening, scar, bleeding, and need for further treatments), benefits of, and alternatives to treatment. If necessary, providers should discuss options for anesthesia (topical, infiltrative, nerve block). Providers should also consider performing a test spot as an initial treatment and then bring back for follow-up if there are significant concerns for paradoxical darkening. This allows the physician to observe for the appropriate response and clinical outcome.

9.5.2 Tattoo Removal Procedure

The treatment area is anesthetized as discussed prior to treatment, via a topical ointment or locally injected lidocaine. Eye protection for the patient, physician, and support staff in the room is essential. Protective goggles are wavelength specific; it is important that all staff members involved are familiar with the appropriate safety equipment and protocols. In the case of cosmetic tattoos involving eyelids or eyebrows, utilization of intraocular shields is paramount.

When preferred and appropriate, the PFD is applied to the treatment area immediately followed by the patch. This process is then repeated anywhere from none to three additional passes during one session, depending on factors including but not limited to the anatomic location of the tattoo, Fitzpatrick skin type of the patient, as well as the current state or clearance of the tattoo. Laser treatment should be performed with the use of partially overlapping pulses of the chosen laser. The overlapping of pulses allows the clinician to avoid leaving certain portions of the tattoo untreated and prevent the aesthetically unappealing "honeycomb" appearance that can occur when the pulses are too far apart. The ideal response is tissue whitening in the treated area. An undesired response to the laser presents as epidermal disruption or bleeding that may indicate excessive fluence. In general, the physician should adjust the fluence of the laser accordingly when an undesired response occurs and also note that some pinpoint bleeding can be acceptable. Specifically, with a multiple-pass technique, it is important to take into account the cumulative energy and potential for injury, modifying parameters as necessary over the course of the treatment session.

9.6 Postoperative Management

After the laser procedure is completed, postoperative instructions should be reviewed with the patient, including but not limited to the application of an emollient and bandaging to the area for at least 1 week, or until healed, as well as appropriate sun protection. Expectations of skin whitening of the skin, which generally fades within 20 minutes, as well as the healing process should also be reviewed, including crusting, blistering, or pinpoint bleeding, and anticipatory guidelines should be provided. The treatment interval is determined by several factors, including skin type and anatomic location, but in general laser tattoo removal should not be performed sooner than 4 weeks. Some patients may experience an urticarial eruption following the laser treatment. Should this occur, patients are instructed to notify the physician and appropriate steps taken, including possible administration of an oral antihistamine and documentation of the subsequent reaction.

9.7 Potential Complications and Management

Complications of laser removal are often divided by time course into immediate and delayed reactions.[6] Many of the immediate reactions were those previously mentioned such as an urticarial reaction, pain, crusting, blistering, pinpoint hemorrhage, and paradoxical darkening. The most common long-term complications with laser treatment include hypopigmentation, hyperpigmentation, and scarring; patients should be appropriately counseled regarding sun protection and avoidance after treatment in order to minimize these complications (▶ Fig. 9.2). Rarely, the laser removal of red and yellow inks can cause the patient to develop an anaphylactic reaction or more commonly a systemic allergic reaction that is delayed weeks to months after treatment. This reaction is the result of the body's immune response to the specific chemicals and compounds that are released and carried away. Once identified, these reactions should be treated appropriately with topical, intralesional, or possibly oral corticosteroids and antihistamines.

Furthermore, in order to protect physicians and staff from the smoke emitted during tattoo removal, especially with ablative laser treatment, smoke evacuator, surgical mask, and/or other occlusive barriers should be used to minimize exposure to airborne contaminants.[45,46]

9.8 Pearls, Pitfalls, and Future Directions

The field of tattoo removal has been dynamic in recent years, especially with regard to shifting cultural attitudes toward tattoos, complex motives for seeking tattoo removal, and improving techniques and advancements in technology. Laser treatment continues to be the gold standard for safe and effective tattoo removal. Although the Q-switched nanometer laser is currently the most common treatment modality for these patients, the picosecond laser has rapidly come to be considered the new standard of care by many.

Selection of the appropriate patient, device, and parameters, in addition to following thorough pre-, intra-, and postoperative protocols, can minimize the risk of complications and maximize patient experience and results. Potential pitfalls such as unwanted hypo- or hyperpigmentation may occur with laser tattoo removal, especially in patients of skin of color. The selection of an appropriate laser, as well as counseling of patients regarding diligent sun protection before and after treatment, may also help minimize these complications. In addition, tattoo removal often requires multiple treatment sessions to achieve the desired cosmetic outcome; realistic and practical expectations should be discussed with the patient in each individual case. Given the potential discomfort, burden, cost, and time

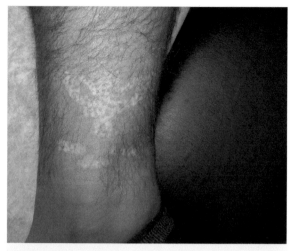

Fig. 9.2 Tattoo complication—dyspigmentation observed after treatment with a 50-nanosecond Q-switched alexandrite laser. (This image is provided courtesy of Dr. Brian Biesman.)

required, implementing a treatment strategy to allow for the largest amount of laser passes per session is becoming ever more essential. More recent advances, such as the PFD patch, can help rapidly reduce laser-induced opaque whitening to facilitate more passes in rapid sequence without additional adverse events. Incorporation of acoustic shock waves has recently been reported in conjunction with picosecond laser treatment for tattoo removal with promising potential.[47] These advances hold promise for improved patient experience and clinical outcomes in laser tattoo removal moving forward.

References

[1] Adatto MA, Halachmi S, Lapidoth M. Tattoo removal. Curr Probl Dermatol. 2011; 42:97–110

[2] de Moll EH. Tattoos: from ancient practice to modern treatment dilemma. Cutis. 2018; 101(5):E14–E16

[3] Goldman L, Blaney DJ, Kindel DJ,et al. Effect of the laser beam on the skin: preliminary report. J Invest Dermatol. 1963;40:121–122

[4] Apfelberg DB, Maser MR, Lash H, White DN, Flores JT. Comparison of argon and carbon dioxide laser treatment of decorative tattoos: a preliminary report. Ann Plast Surg. 1985; 14(1):6–15

[5] Anderson RR, Parrish JA. Selective photothermolysis: precise microsurgery by selective absorption of pulsed radiation. Science. 1983; 220(4596):524–527

[6] Naga LI, Alster TS. Laser tattoo removal: an update. Am J Clin Dermatol. 2017; 18(1):59–65

[7] Barua S. Laser-tissue interaction in tattoo removal by Q-switched lasers. J Cutan Aesthet Surg. 2015; 8(1):5–8

[8] Kasai K. Picosecond laser treatment for tattoos and benign cutaneous pigmented lesions (secondary publication). Laser Ther. 2017; 26(4): 274–281

[9] Ross EV, Yashar S, Michaud N, et al. Tattoo darkening and nonresponse after laser treatment: a possible role for titanium dioxide. Arch Dermatol. 2001; 137(1):33–37

[10] Peach AH, Thomas K, Kenealy J. Colour shift following tattoo removal with Q-switched Nd-YAG laser (1064/532). Br J Plast Surg. 1999; 52 (6):482–487

[11] Ross V, Naseef G, Lin G, et al. Comparison of responses of tattoos to picosecond and nanosecond Q-switched neodymium: YAG lasers. Arch Dermatol. 1998; 134(2):167–171

[12] Brauer JA, Reddy KK, Anolik R, et al. Successful and rapid treatment of blue and green tattoo pigment with a novel picosecond laser. Arch Dermatol. 2012; 148(7):820–823

[13] Alabdulrazzaq H, Brauer JA, Bae YS, Geronemus RG. Clearance of yellow tattoo ink with a novel 532-nm picosecond laser. Lasers Surg Med. 2015; 47(4):285–288

[14] Manstein D, Herron GS, Sink RK, Tanner H, Anderson RR. Fractional photothermolysis: a new concept for cutaneous remodeling using microscopic patterns of thermal injury. Lasers Surg Med. 2004; 34 (5):426–438

[15] Ibrahimi OA, Syed Z, Sakamoto FH, Avram MM, Anderson RR. Treatment of tattoo allergy with ablative fractional resurfacing: a novel paradigm for tattoo removal. J Am Acad Dermatol. 2011; 64(6): 1111–1114

[16] Weiss ET, Geronemus RG. Combining fractional resurfacing and Q-switched ruby laser for tattoo removal. Dermatol Surg. 2011; 37(1): 97–99

[17] McIlwee BE, Alster TS. Treatment of cosmetic tattoos: a review and case analysis. Dermatol Surg. 2018; 44(12):1565–1570

[18] Armstrong ML, Roberts AE, Koch JR, Saunders JC, Owen DC, Anderson RR. Motivation for contemporary tattoo removal: a shift in identity. Arch Dermatol. 2008; 144(7):879–884

[19] Alster TS. Q-switched alexandrite laser treatment (755 nm) of professional and amateur tattoos. J Am Acad Dermatol. 1995; 33(1): 69–73

[20] Alexis AF. Lasers and light-based therapies in ethnic skin: treatment options and recommendations for Fitzpatrick skin types V and VI. Br J Dermatol. 2013; 169 Suppl 3:91–97

[21] Jones A, Roddey P, Orengo I, Rosen T. The Q-switched ND:YAG laser effectively treats tattoos in darkly pigmented skin. Dermatol Surg. 1996; 22(12):999–1001

[22] Sardana K, Ranjan R, Ghunawat S. Optimising laser tattoo removal. J Cutan Aesthet Surg. 2015; 8(1):16–24

[23] Pohl L, Kaiser K, Raulin C. Pitfalls and recommendations in cases of laser removal of decorative tattoos with pigmented lesions: case report and review of the literature. JAMA Dermatol. 2013; 149(9): 1087–1089

[24] Bernstein EF. Laser tattoo removal. Semin Plast Surg. 2007; 21(3): 175–192

[25] Taylor CR, Anderson RR, Gange RW, Michaud NA, Flotte TJ. Light and electron microscopic analysis of tattoos treated by Q-switched ruby laser. J Invest Dermatol. 1991; 97(1):131–136

[26] Kilmer SL, Anderson RR. Clinical use of the Q-switched ruby and the Q-switched Nd:YAG (1064 nm and 532 nm) lasers for treatment of tattoos. J Dermatol Surg Oncol. 1993; 19(4):330–338

[27] Kilmer SL, Lee MS, Grevelink JM, Flotte TJ, Anderson RR. The Q-switched Nd:YAG laser effectively treats tattoos. A controlled, dose-response study. Arch Dermatol. 1993; 129(8):971–978

[28] Fitzpatrick RE, Goldman MP. Tattoo removal using the alexandrite laser. Arch Dermatol. 1994; 130(12):1508–1514

[29] Zelickson BD, Mehregan DA, Zarrin AA, et al. Clinical, histologic, and ultrastructural evaluation of tattoos treated with three laser systems. Lasers Surg Med. 1994; 15(4):364–372

[30] Adatto MA, Amir R, Bhawalkar J, et al. New and advanced picosecond lasers for tattoo removal. Curr Probl Dermatol. 2017; 52:113–123

[31] Reiter O, Atzmony L, Akerman L, et al. Picosecond lasers for tattoo removal: a systematic review. Lasers Med Sci. 2016; 31(7):1397–1405

[32] Lorgeou A, Perrillat Y, Gral N, Lagrange S, Lacour JP, Passeron T. Comparison of two picosecond lasers to a nanosecond laser for treating tattoos: a prospective randomized study on 49 patients. J Eur Acad Dermatol Venereol. 2018; 32(2):265–270

[33] Saedi N, Metelitsa A, Petrell K, Arndt KA, Dover JS. Treatment of tattoos with a picosecond alexandrite laser: a prospective trial. Arch Dermatol. 2012; 148(12):1360–1363

[34] Pinto F, Große-Büning S, Karsai S, et al. Neodymium-doped yttrium aluminium garnet (Nd:YAG) 1064-nm picosecond laser vs. Nd:YAG 1064-nm nanosecond laser in tattoo removal: a randomized controlled single-blind clinical trial. Br J Dermatol. 2017; 176(2): 457–464

[35] Bae YSC, Alabdulrazzaq H, Brauer J, Geronemus R. Successful treatment of paradoxical darkening. Lasers Surg Med. 2016; 48(5): 471–473

[36] Bernstein EF, Schomacker KT, Basilavecchio LD, Plugis JM, Bhawalkar JD. A novel dual-wavelength, Nd:YAG, picosecond-domain laser safely and effectively removes multicolor tattoos. Lasers Surg Med. 2015; 47(7):542–548

[37] Kossida T, Rigopoulos D, Katsambas A, Anderson RR. Optimal tattoo removal in a single laser session based on the method of repeated exposures. J Am Acad Dermatol. 2012; 66(2):271–277

[38] Littlejohn GR, Gouveia JD, Edner C, Smirnoff N, Love J. Perfluorodecalin enhances in vivo confocal microscopy resolution of Arabidopsis thaliana mesophyll. New Phytol. 2010; 186(4):1018–1025

[39] Reddy KK, Brauer JA, Anolik R, et al. Topical perfluorodecalin resolves immediate whitening reactions and allows rapid effective multiple pass treatment of tattoos. Lasers Surg Med. 2013; 45(2): 76–80

[40] Ding H, Lu JQ, Wooden WA, Kragel PJ, Hu XH. Refractive indices of human skin tissues at eight wavelengths and estimated dispersion relations between 300 and 1600 nm. Phys Med Biol. 2006; 51(6): 1479–1489

[41] Biesman BS, O'Neil MP, Costner C. Rapid, high-fluence multi-pass q-switched laser treatment of tattoos with a transparent perfluorodecalin-infused patch: a pilot study. Lasers Surg Med. 2015; 47(8):613–618

[42] Biesman BS, Costner C. Evaluation of a transparent perfluorodecalin-infused patch as an adjunct to laser-assisted tattoo removal: fa pivotal trial. Lasers Surg Med. 2017; 49(4):335–340

[43] Brauer JA, Geronemus R, O'Neil MP. Perfluorodecalin-infused patch in picosecond and Q-switched laser-assisted tattoo removal: assessments of optical transparency, chemical stability, and safety. J Am Acad Dermatol. 2018; 79(3):AB218

[44] Feng H, Geronemus RG, Brauer JA. Safety of a perfluorodecalin-infused silicone patch in picosecond laser-assisted tattoo removal: a retrospective review. Dermatol Surg. 2019; 45(4):618–621

[45] Lewin JM, Brauer JA, Ostad A. Surgical smoke and the dermatologist. J Am Acad Dermatol. 2011; 65(3):636–641

[46] Heppt W, Metelmann HR, Heppt M, Feller G, Vent J. General precautions and safety aspects of facial laser treatment. Facial Plast Surg. 2018; 34(6):588–596

[47] Vangipuram R, Hamill SS, Friedman PM. Accelerated tattoo removal with acoustic shock wave therapy in conjunction with a picosecond laser. Lasers Surg Med. 2018; 50(9):890–892

10 Leg Vein Treatment

Jeffrey F. Scott, Nina Lucia Tamashunas, and Margaret Mann

Summary

Leg veins can be categorized as spider veins, reticular veins, and varicose veins. This chapter reviews all the different approaches to treatment, providing pearls and pitfalls to improve patient outcomes.

Keywords: varicose veins, reticular veins, spider veins, ablation, sclerotherapy, microphlebectomy, venous insufficiency, phlebectomy, telangiectasia, matting, great saphenous vein, small saphenous vein

10.1 Introduction

The clinical spectrum of chronic venous disease of the legs is vast and spans telangiectasias (spider veins), reticular veins, varicose veins, edema, and stasis dermatitis (▶ Fig. 10.1). Nearly 25% of patients progress to advanced disease, including lipodermatosclerosis, atrophie blanche, and ulceration.[1] The prevalence of chronic venous disease is high and increases with age; telangiectasias and reticular veins affect approximately 80% of adults aged 18 to 64 years and varicose veins affect approximately 60% of adults older than 50 years.[2] The economic burden of chronic venous disease is also significant as the estimated cost of treating venous disease of the legs is $3 billion per year in the United States.[3]

Symptoms of chronic venous disease of the legs include, but are not limited to, pain, achiness, heaviness, cramping, itching, tingling, swelling, and restless legs. Patients with chronic venous insufficiency generally have a reduced quality of life and frequently suffer with depression and social isolation, all of which correlate with the severity of venous disease.[4,5,6,7] The clinical, etiology, anatomy, and pathophysiology (CEAP) classification system designates severity of venous disease and is particularly useful for risk stratification (▶ Table 10.1).[8,9,10] For example, the CEAP classification for a patient with primary superficial varicose veins resulting from reflux would be $C_2E_pA_sP_R$.

The majority of symptomatic leg veins result from venous hypertension, which is most commonly caused by reflux through incompetent vein valves, but can also result from venous outflow obstruction (e.g., thrombosis, congenital anomaly) or from failure of the calf muscle pump system (e.g., obesity, immobility).[1] Pregnancy, infection, and phlebitis are also predisposing factors. Reflux most often occurs in the superficial veins, including the great saphenous vein (GSV) and small saphenous vein (SSV), but it can also affect the superficial and deep systems simultaneously (▶ Fig. 10.2).[11] Over time, venous hypertension induces dilation, weakening, and stretching of veins, clinically manifesting as telangiectasias, reticular veins, and varicose veins.

10.1.1 Treatment Options Available

The treatment of leg veins is influenced by the size of the involved veins, the source and location of reflux, and disease severity (▶ Table 10.2). Early identification and treatment of chronic venous disease can reduce the risk of disease progression, including ulcer formation and recurrence.[12,13,14,15,16] The goals of treatment are to prevent disease progression, alleviate symptoms, and improve quality of life. The mainstay of nonoperative treatment is compression therapy, which consists of compression stockings or compression bandages, physical therapy, and manual lymphatic drainage.[1] Compression stockings improve reflux, reduce edema and hyperpigmentation, and improve quality of life.[17,18] Long-term compression therapy also results in a lower rate of ulcer recurrence.[19] Nonsteroidal anti-inflammatory drugs (NSAIDs), frequent leg elevation, weight loss, and exercise also serve as conservative treatment options.

The operative treatments of leg veins can be organized into four main categories: (1) surgical ligation and stripping, (2) thermal ablation, (3) nonthermal ablation, and (4) ambulatory phlebectomy. Historically, treatment of GSV and SSV reflux was performed under general or epidural anesthesia using high surgical ligation at the saphenofemoral junction (SFJ) and/or saphenopopliteal junction, respectively, with or without stripping of the vein.[20] Surgical ligation without stripping of the GSV has a much higher recurrence rate than ligation with stripping.[21] Long stripping was gradually replaced with short stripping to reduce the risk of saphenous nerve damage. Open surgical management results in durable outcomes with success rates of approximately 75% at 5 years, as well as improved quality of life and decreased ulcer recurrence rates.[12,22,23,24] However, surgical high ligation and stripping often results in significant short-term morbidity, including ecchymoses, hematomas, and pain.[23]

More recently, minimally invasive treatment options of GSV and SSV reflux aim to reduce surgical trauma and improve long-term outcomes. These include thermal ablative techniques, such as endovenous laser ablation (EVLA), radiofrequency ablation (RFA), and endovenous steam ablation (EVSA), as well as nonthermal ablative techniques, such as ultrasound-guided foam sclerotherapy (UGFS), Varithena, mechanochemical sclerotherapy (ClariVein), and non-sclerosant-based techniques (VenaSeal). These minimally invasive options can be performed in the outpatient setting without general or epidural anesthesia and are characterized by fewer complications, less postoperative pain, and faster recovery times compared to open surgical management.[21,23,25,26,27,28] Meta-analyses and a Cochrane review suggest similar

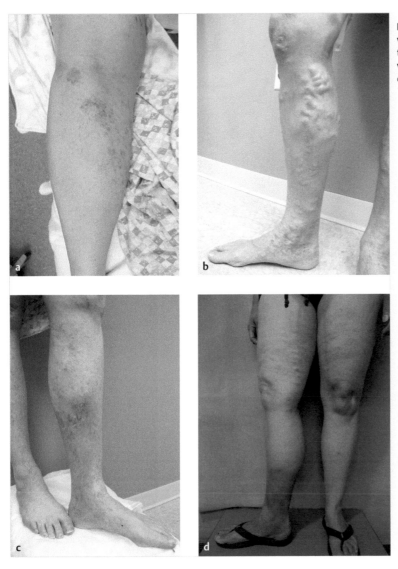

Fig. 10.1 The clinical spectrum of chronic venous disease of the legs, including **(a)** telangiectasias (spider veins), **(b)** reticular veins, **(c)** varicose veins, and **(d)** stasis dermatitis.

Table 10.1 Clinical, etiology, anatomy, and pathophysiology classification

Clinical (C)	Etiology (E)	Anatomy (A)	Pathophysiology (P)
C_0: No visible or palpable signs of venous disease	E_C: congenital	A_S: superficial veins	P_R: reflux
C_1: Telangiectasia	E_P: primary	A_D: deep veins	P_O: obstruction
C_2: Varicose veins	E_S: secondary	A_P: perforating veins	
C_3: Edema			
C_4: Skin changes (stasis dermatitis)			
C_5: Healed venous leg ulcer			
C_6: Active venous leg ulcer			

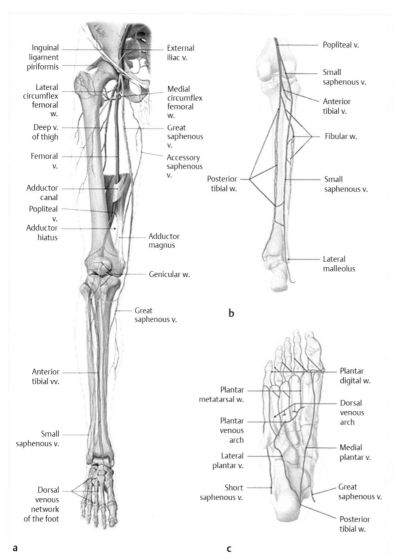

Fig. 10.2 (a–c) Venous anatomy of the leg, including the saphenofemoral junction, femoral vein, great saphenous vein, and small saphenous vein. (From: Schünke M, Schulte E, Schumacher U, Voll M, Wesker K, Johnson N, ed. THIEME Atlas of Anatomy, Volume 1: General Anatomy and Musculoskeletal System. 3rd Edition. Illustration by Karl Wesker and Marcus Voll. © Thieme 2020.)

Table 10.2 Treatment of leg veins based on the source of disease

Source of disease	Treatment options
GSV/SSV reflux	• Surgical ligation ± stripping • Thermal ablation: RF, laser, steam • Nonthermal ablation: UGFS, chemical ablation (Varithena microfoam), MOCA (ClariVein), cyanoacrylate adhesive (VenaSeal)
Varicose veins (tributary disease)	• Ambulatory phlebectomy • UGFS
Reticular veins	• Liquid sclerotherapy • Foam sclerotherapy
Telangiectasias	• Liquid sclerotherapy

Abbreviations: GSV, great saphenous vein; MOCA, mechano-chemical ablation; RF, radiofrequency; SSV, small saphenous vein; UGFS, ultrasound-guided foam sclerotherapy.

efficacies for EVLA, RFA, UGFS, and surgical ligation and stripping.[27,28,29,30]

Thermal ablation involves the production of significant heat within the vein, leading to transmural vein wall injury, desquamation of the endothelium, and exposure to thrombogenic material.[31] Specifically, EVLA induces damage using electromagnetic radiation (808–1,569 nm), targeting either hemoglobin or water depending on the wavelength chosen, and converting it to heat. Steam bubbles develop at the tip of the laser fiber and distribute along the endothelium to provide homogenous thermal injury.[32] The efficacy of EVLA is high, with occlusion rates greater than 95% immediately following treatment and decreasing with time to 93% at 3 years and 88% at 5 years.[25,33,34,35] Moreover, a meta-analysis demonstrated significantly higher efficacy of EVLA for leg varicosities compared to RFA, vein stripping, and UGFS.[24] Most EVLA devices utilizing different wavelengths have similar efficacy, with longer wavelengths resulting in lower energy absorption and possibly fewer complications.[36,37] In contrast, RFA delivers thermal energy of 80 to 120 °C directly to the vein endothelium and, therefore, requires direct contact between the vein wall and catheter.[38] The success rate of RFA is 90% at 2 years, with similar outcomes to surgical ligation and stripping, but lower efficacy and higher recurrence rates than EVLT.[28,39,40,41,42] Finally, EVSA, which is currently not approved by the Food and Drug Administration (FDA), uses steam to thermally damage the vein.[43] Pressurized sterile water is injected into a microtube, heated by an electric current, and emitted at the tip of a handpiece as steam pulses at 150 °C. After traveling through a catheter connected to the handpiece, the steam exits into the vein at a reduced temperature of 120 °C. The success rate of EVSA is 96% at 1 year and is not inferior to EVLA at 6 months.[43,44,45] However, the longer-term efficacy of EVSA has not been well defined.

Nonthermal ablation involves injecting a liquid or foam solution into the lumen of the targeted vein, damaging the endothelium of the vessel wall, inducing an inflammatory response, and, ultimately, leading to localized thrombosis and reabsorption of the target vein.[46] By avoiding the use of thermal energy, tumescent anesthesia is not needed, reducing intraoperative pain and the risk of nerve injury and skin damage. All nonthermal ablative modalities use sclerosants apart from VenaSeal, which uses a proprietary cyanoacrylate-based adhesive.[47,48] Sclerosants are classified according to their mechanism of action as a detergent, hypertonic solution, or chemical irritant.[49,50,51] Detergents, including sodium tetradecyl sulfate (STS) and polidocanol, damage endothelial cells by extracting cell surface proteins. Hypertonic solutions, including hypertonic saline and dextrose/sodium chloride, primarily damage endothelial cells through cellular dehydration. Finally, chemical irritants, including glycerin, damage endothelial cells by disrupting chemical bonds on cell surface proteins. Firm fibrotic indurations form within treated veins, followed by gradual absorption.

UGFS utilizes foamed sclerosants to damage endothelial cells. Compared to liquid sclerosants, foamed sclerosants allow for treatment of larger veins because the foamed solution completely fills the lumen of the vein and is not rapidly diluted by blood. This allows for increased contact time between the sclerosant and the vessel wall, thereby inducing greater amounts of endothelial injury. For example, the efficacy of foamed sclerosants is 76.8% for the treatment of saphenous veins versus 39.5% for liquid sclerotherapy.[52] Occlusion rates for UGFS depend on the diameter of the vein and the concentration of injected foam.[53] Smaller volumes and lower concentrations of foamed solution can be utilized to limit local and systemic side effects.

UGFS for varicose veins improves disease-specific health-related quality of life and patient-reported outcomes 5- to 8 years after treatment, and only 15.3% of legs require re-treatment after 5 years.[54] Although the immediate success rate of UGFS is high and approaches 90% at 6 months, success rates diminish over time.[54,55,56,57,58,59] The 3-year success rate of UGFS for obliteration of the GSV is 81%, which is comparable to the clinical outcomes of surgical stripping with high ligation.[60,61] However, UGFS was inferior to both EVLA and RFA in several randomized clinical trials.[28,55,56,62] UGFS is ideal for tortuous GSV that may not be accessible by catheter-based treatment modalities.

Similar to UGFS, Varithena utilizes 1% polidocanol delivered in a proprietary canister using low nitrogen concentrations to facilitate quick absorption.[63,64] Varithena is FDA approved for the treatment of incompetent GSV, accessory saphenous veins, and visible varicosities of the GSV system above and below the knee. The Varithena canister is capable of generating more consistent bubble size within the microfoam compared to physician-prepared compounds,[46] with no reported cases of pulmonary emboli or clinically important neurologic or visual adverse events reported. In contrast, ClariVein is a mechanochemical technique that uses a high-speed (2,000–3,500 revolutions per minute [rpm]) rotary wire system to mechanically disrupt the endothelium before administration of liquid sclerosants to increase the degree of endothelial cell damage.[65,66] ClariVein is FDA-approved as a proprietary infusion catheter but is not specifically indicated for the treatment of saphenous vein insufficiency. Early occlusion rates with ClariVein are 87 to 99%, with 2-year occlusion rates of 96 to 97%.[65,66,67,68] Finally, a nonsclerosant-based technique for nonthermal ablation is the VenaSeal system, which uses a proprietary cyanoacrylate adhesive and is FDA approved for the treatment of saphenous vein insufficiency.[47,48] VenaSeal is distinct from all other ablative methods in that it does not require endothelial damage or sclerosis, and postoperative compression is not necessary. The efficacy of VenaSeal is comparable to those of other modalities, with an immediate occlusion rate above 90%, a 2-year occlusion rate of 92%, and similar outcomes as RFA for the treatment of GSV reflux at 3 months.[47,48,69] These nonthermal ablative modalities are preferred when access near the lower third of the leg is necessary to treat the entire GSV or SSV. Thermal techniques in this area are associated with higher risks of nerve injury.

Liquid and foam sclerosants are also used for the treatment of varicose veins, reticular veins, and telangiectasias. Physician-prepared foamed sclerosants are considered off-label for the treatment of reticular veins and nontruncal varicose veins but have a long record of success and safety.[70] The two most common sclerosants used in the United States are the detergents STS and polidocanol, both of which are FDA approved for the treatment of reticular veins and telangiectasias. Hypertonic saline and glycerin, which are both off-label treatment options, are used less commonly. Hypertonic saline is rapidly diluted in blood, reducing its efficacy over a short distance. Similarly, glycerin is very viscous and can be challenging to inject.

A Cochrane review of 10 studies for treatment of leg telangiectasias revealed no differences in efficacy or patient satisfaction between any one sclerosing agent but confirmed sclerotherapy's superiority to normal saline placebo.[71] Treatment is successful in 95% of patients at 12 and 16 weeks, and 78 and 84% of patients are satisfied or very satisfied at 12 and 26 weeks, respectively.[71,72] Moreover, another Cochrane review of 17 studies for treatment of leg varicose veins revealed no difference in efficacy for any one sclerosing agent or dose, with an improvement in symptoms and cosmetic appearance observed for all formulations.[73] For reticular veins, prospective studies using up to three treatments with 1% polidocanol or 1% STS reveal high success rates.[72]

Finally, ambulatory phlebectomy (stab avulsion, microextraction) is used to treat relatively superficial varicose veins mainly in outpatient setting under local or tumescent anesthesia.[74] The varicosities must be visible and palpable on the surface of the skin. Similar to surgical ligation and stripping, ambulatory phlebectomy exteriorizes and physically removes segments of varicose veins of any size and location.[75] Ambulatory phlebectomy can be used alone or in combination with surgical ligation or any modality of thermal or nonthermal ablation of the GSV or SSV. Ulcer recurrence after EVLA is less frequent in patients treated with ambulatory phlebectomy for varicose veins at the time of thermal ablation.[76]

10.2 Indications

Leg veins are treated for both cosmetic and therapeutic purposes. Treatment of symptomatic GSV or SSV reflux unresponsive to conservative treatment is indicated to (1) relieve symptoms, (2) improve the severity of underlying reflux and venous hypertension, and (3) reduce the risk of developing complications associated with chronic venous disease.[1,14,15,16] In the absence of GSV or SSV reflux, cosmetically unacceptable telangiectasias, reticular veins, or varicose veins can be treated using sclerotherapy or ambulatory phlebectomy with excellent success. Asymptomatic telangiectasias and reticular veins may be treated with liquid sclerotherapy, and asymptomatic varicose veins may be treated with foam sclerotherapy or ambulatory phlebectomy. Treatment with foam sclerotherapy and ambulatory phlebectomy is also indicated for symptomatic varicose veins unresponsive to conservative treatment with compression stockings, NSAIDs, frequent leg elevation, weight loss, and exercise. However, treating the source of the venous disease is critical. If reflux is present, treatment with sclerotherapy or ambulatory phlebectomy will not yield satisfactory results unless paired with a thermal or nonthermal ablative technique to address the source of the reflux.

10.3 Preoperative Considerations

10.3.1 Patient Selection

Patients presenting with symptomatic veins or skin findings suggestive of chronic venous disease should be evaluated with a thorough history and physical examination, as well as duplex ultrasound (US) to define the venous anatomy and identify areas of significant reflux. Although diagnostic testing is not required for asymptomatic patients with telangiectasias and reticular veins, duplex US should be used to evaluate venous anatomy as significant small vessel disease on the medial aspect of the thigh or calf may be the sign of underlying reflux in the GSV or SSV, respectively.

The clinical history should include the duration of venous disease, prior pregnancies, and history of deep venous thrombosis (DVT). The physical examination should include a visual inspection of the legs and assessment of peripheral pulses. A complete examination involves an evaluation of the entire course of the accessible portions of each vein. Unless the patient clearly describes unilateral symptoms, duplex US should be performed bilaterally. The patient should stand during the duplex US examination, and sources of venous reflux and courses of veins amenable to treatment should be marked out on the legs and documented on a vein map (▶ Fig. 10.3). CEAP classification should be determined. An US technician should be consulted for specific technical considerations for documenting saphenous vein anatomy, size, and reflux.

Patients with significant comorbidities should initially be offered less invasive treatment options, such as nonthermal ablation and compression. Morbidly obese patients are also at higher risk of developing postoperative complications, including DVT, pulmonary embolism (PE), wound infections, fat necrosis, seromas, and hematomas. Contraindications for the treatment of leg veins are provided in ▶ Table 10.3.

10.4 Technical Aspects of Treatment

The goal of this section is to provide a step-by-step overview of the essential technical aspects of leg vein treatments performed under local or tumescent anesthesia (thermal and nonthermal ablation, ambulatory phlebectomy).

10.4.1 Thermal Ablation of the GSV

Patient preparation is similar for all three thermal ablative techniques (EVLA, RFA, and EVSA) and all are performed in the outpatient setting with tumescent anesthesia (▶ Fig. 10.4). An oral benzodiazepine, such as lorazepam or diazepam, may be given as needed for anxiety. Conscious sedation is rarely required. The treatment room is kept warm to prevent vasoconstriction, and heating pad may be useful.

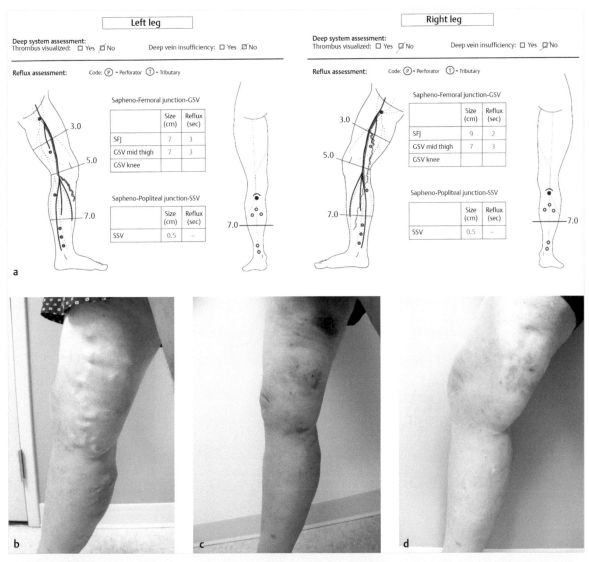

Fig. 10.3 Representative example of a vein map. (**a**) Ultrasound venous reflux study showing reflux in the GSV bilaterally with presence of tributary varicose veins. (**b**) Clinical presentation of the patient's right leg pretreatment. (**c**) 1 week posttreatment with appropriate ecchymosis to the thigh and phlebectomy sites. (**d**) 1 month posttreatment with resolution of varicosities.

Table 10.3 Contraindications to the treatment of leg veins

- Allergies to compounds used for treatment
- Acute superficial or deep venous thrombosis
- Local or systemic infection
- Immobility
- Advanced peripheral vascular disease
- Severe systemic disease
- Pregnancy or breastfeeding
- Hypercoagulable or bleeding disorders
- Known patent foramen ovale (foam sclerotherapy)

First, the source(s) of reflux and venous anatomy are confirmed with duplex US. The probe is placed on the inguinal crease to identify the SFJ. The GSV is visualized arising from the SFJ and can be followed distally along the medial thigh to the medial calf. Refluxes at the SFJ and along the GSV are confirmed by compressing the thigh or calf or having the patient perform the Valsalva maneuver. With the US probe angled slightly oblique toward the heart, a blue color on the color flow Doppler function indicates blood flow toward the heart after distal compression. Upon releasing compression, a red color indicates blood flow toward the feet, or reflux (► Fig. 10.5).

Next, the GSV is carefully mapped from the SFJ to the distal calf using a marking pen. It is helpful to use a pen cap to firmly press the skin and create an indentation immediately prior to wiping off the US gel and marking. Incompetent valves, areas of dilation and tortuosity, and depth of the GSV are noted. Additionally, major

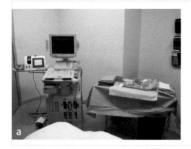
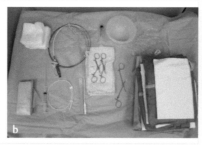

Fig. 10.4 Thermal ablation treatment room setup. (a) Endovenous laser device, ultrasound, and surgical tray. (b) Close-up of surgical tray showing (from *left*, counterclockwise) ultrasound gel packet, spinal needle on 3-mL syringe for access, guidewire, #11 blade, surgical towels and towel clamps, hemostat, sterile surgical gowns, saline basin, 5-mL syringe for flushing, blue laser fiber, gauze.

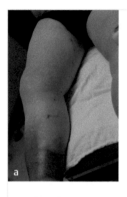
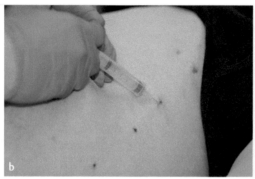
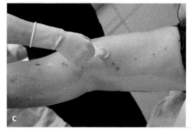
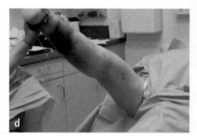

Fig. 10.5 Prepping patient for endovenous laser ablation. (a) The vein is premarked under ultrasound guidance. (b) Local anesthesia with 1% lidocaine without epinephrine is placed subdermally along the course of the vein. (c) The patient is then prepped with a ChloraPrep applicator and (d) draped in a sterile fashion.

tributaries at the SFJ and any perforating veins, communicating veins, or sizable tributaries of the GSV are recorded.

The optimal site for percutaneously accessing the GSV is now chosen. Any segment of the GSV greater than 3 mm in diameter is suitable for obtaining access. It is typically most advantageous to choose a location on the distal thigh or proximal lower leg as the GSV is larger and straighter directly above and below the knee. Of note, the saphenous nerve runs close to the GSV below the knee, increasing the risk of nerve injury in this location. Inject a small amount of 1% lidocaine without epinephrine to produce a dermal wheal at regular intervals (~5 cm) along the marked GSV. To prevent vasoconstriction, epinephrine is omitted and the injection is made as superficial and with as little lidocaine as possible.

Next, the entire leg is prepped with copious amounts of an antiseptic applicator (ChloraPrep) containing chlorhexidine gluconate and isopropyl alcohol from groin to foot. The leg is then draped in a sterile fashion, with extra care taken to drape the groin and foot (▶ Fig. 10.6). As

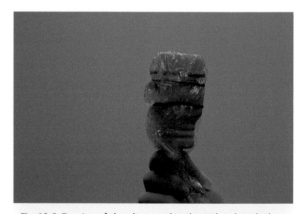

Fig. 10.6 Draping of the ultrasound probe with gel applied on head within sterile sleeve.

thermal ablative techniques are performed under US guidance, the US probe must also be inserted into a sterile sleeve with gel, draped in a sterile fashion, and secured to the patient in a position that is easy to access. The US monitor should be placed within the treatment room in a convenient location to see throughout the procedure (► Fig. 10.7).

Obtaining venous access can begin once the patient is prepped in a sterile fashion. This is the essential step of any thermal or nonthermal ablative technique. Correct patient positioning is critical for successfully accessing the GSV. A number of strategies can be used for GSV vasodilation and to facilitate obtaining venous access, including applying local heat to the leg with a heating pad prior to sterilization, positioning the patient in reverse Trendelenburg position to increase venous pressure, and applying a small amount of 2% nitroglycerin to the access site. Additionally, the hip should be externally

rotated to relax the leg and position the GSV in an optimal orientation. Under US guidance, a venous puncture needle (16–21 gauge) is percutaneously inserted at a shallow angle following the course of the GSV (► Fig. 10.8). The needle is swiftly inserted into the skin, as quick advancement of the needle in one smooth motion is often required to puncture the vein. The needle is carefully advanced toward the GSV at the correct depth. The GSV wall can be palpated with the needle under US guidance and flash back of venous blood return should be noted to confirm correct positioning (► Fig. 10.9).

Once percutaneous venous access is obtained, a guidewire is passed through the puncture needle into the GSV and carefully advanced proximally toward the SFJ under US guidance. If resistance is met and advancement is

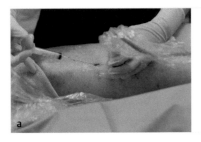
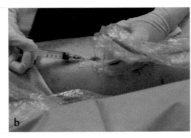

Fig. 10.7 (a) Correct insertion of the needle at a shallow angle under ultrasound guidance. (b) Flashback seen with correct placement into the vein.

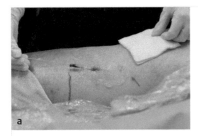
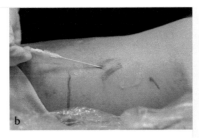
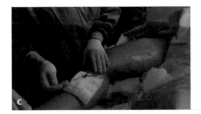
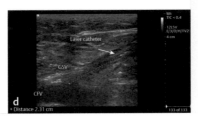

Fig. 10.8 (a) Advancement of guidewire into the vein, (b) followed by the introducer. (c) Withdrawal of the guidewire and advancement of the laser fiber into the GSV toward the saphenofemoral junction. Note the red laser aiming beam. (d) Laser fiber positioned close to the saphenofemoral junction (no closer than 2 cm).

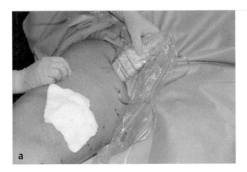
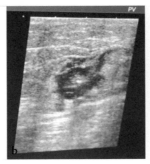

Fig. 10.9 (a) Placement of tumescent anesthesia along the course of the vein under ultrasound guidance. (b) Filling of the para-vessel space between the fascial envelop and the outer vein surface with tumescent anesthesia. Hyperechoic (white) dot is the laser fiber on cross section.

difficult due to vasospasm, GSV tortuosity, small diameter, thrombotic remnants, or side branches, it is often helpful to stretch the skin at various angles to attempt to straighten the course of the GSV. Alternatively, a smaller guidewire can be used. These maneuvers will allow passage of the guidewire in the vast majority of cases. If the guidewire still cannot be safely advanced proximally without meeting resistance, then venous access should be obtained proximal to the troublesome segment.

Once the guidewire is in position, the venous puncture needle can be removed and the sheath catheter is inserted over the guidewire. First, make a small incision over the access site using a no. 11 blade to facilitate advancement of the guiding sheath catheter over the guidewire and into the lumen of the GSV. The sheath catheter gently dilates the GSV and stabilizes percutaneous access. The guidewire can be removed once the sheath catheter is visualized within the GSV as confirmed by US. The laser device should be turned on and placed in standby mode before insertion of the laser fiber. Most laser fibers emit a focused, round, and red aiming beam that confirms correct alignment and setup of the system. Troubleshoot according to the manufacturer's instructions if no aiming beam is visualized. Appropriate laser safety glasses should be worn by the patient and all staff members in the room.

With the sheath catheter in place and the laser device in standby mode, the laser fiber can be safely advanced through the catheter into the lumen of the GSV and toward the SFJ under US guidance. The tip of the laser fiber should be advanced no closer than 2 to 3 cm from the SJF and at least 1 cm distal to the superior epigastric vein or other major tributary veins (► Fig. 10.10). The tip of the laser fiber should be confirmed by US in both the

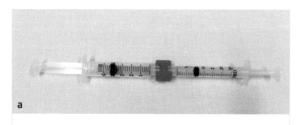

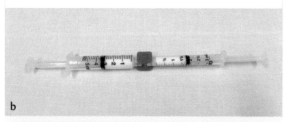

Fig. 10.10 (a, b) Preparation of foamed sclerosants using the Tessari method. 1 mL of liquid sclerosant is placed in one syringe and 4 mL of air is placed in the second syringe. Rapid alternating pushing of the plunger 10 to 15 times creates foam sclerosant.

transverse and longitudinal directions. Once the tip of the laser fiber is in proper position, the sheath catheter can be pulled almost all the way out so that only the laser fiber remains within the GSV.

Next, tumescent anesthesia (0.1% lidocaine with 1,000,000 epinephrine) is infiltrated with a 21- to 25-gauge needle along the entire planned treatment area. Up to 35 mg/kg of dilute lidocaine as a tumescent solution is well tolerated and safe, but in most cases, no more than 500 mL of tumescent anesthesia is necessary for treatment. Infiltration can begin proximally at the SFJ or distally at the access site. An automatic infusion pump on low-flow settings is typically used, but hand injection can also be used for finer control. Tumescent anesthesia should be injected between the fascial envelope and outer GSV surface (► Fig. 10.11). Approximately 5 to 10 mL/cm of vein is injected to provide at least 1 cm of tumescent solution circumferentially around the vein. In thin patients or those with a superficial GSV, additional tumescent anesthesia should be placed to position the GSV at least 1 to 2 cm below the surface of the skin to reduce the risk of skin burn. The patient should now be placed in Trendelenburg position to facilitate collapse of the GSV. Goals of tumescent anesthesia include (1) to provide local anesthesia to the vein during treatment; (2) to provide a cooling area to minimize thermal injury to surrounding tissues, including skin, soft tissue, nerves, and arteries; and (3) to vasoconstrict and compress the GSV so that little to no blood remains in the treated sections.

Once sufficient tumescent anesthesia is infiltrated along the entire planned treatment area, laser parameters, which depend on the size of the GSV, pullback speed of the laser fiber, and the power and wavelength of the laser device, are selected. Just prior to activating the laser, confirmation that the tip of the laser fiber is at least 2 cm distal to the SFJ should be obtained with US in both the transverse and longitudinal directions. The pullback speed of the laser fiber can be controlled by careful hand movements or automated with a pullback device. The total amount of energy delivered per centimeter is a product of the power of the device (W) and the withdrawal velocity of the fiber (cm/s). Approximately 60 to 80 J of energy should be delivered per centimeter of GSV treated. Higher doses of energy result in a higher efficacy but more side effects.[77,78]

Patient preparation for RFA is similar to EVLA and includes mapping the GSV, sterile prepping, obtaining venous access, and infiltrating the leg with tumescent anesthesia. The tip of the RFA catheter should also be positioned at least 2 to 3 cm distal to the SFJ under US guidance. The RFA catheter is then connected to a radiofrequency generator. One key difference between RFA and EVLA is that RFA relies on direct contact between the catheter and vein wall to induce thermal damage. Manual compression of the vein during treatment is recommended by some to enhance contact between the RFA catheter and the vein endothelium. Newer models of RFA devices contain a thermocouple on the RFA catheter that monitors and maintains a constant temperature of the endothelium (85–90 °C) during withdrawal via a feedback system.[79] The catheter is typically withdrawn in 7-cm segments (or 3 cm for shorter veins) in 20-second intervals.

Patient preparation for EVSA is identical to EVLA and RFA. The steam ablative catheter is advanced no closer than 2 to 3 cm to the SFJ. After device activation, two pulses of steam are delivered to dispel condensed water from the catheter, and three pulses are subsequently released at the tip of the catheter. The steam ablative catheter is pulled back in stepwise increments of 1 cm, with two to four pulses (one pulse = 60 J) of steam released per centimeter, to induce thermal damage to the vein wall. The exact number of required pulses depends on the GSV diameter.

10.4.2 Nonthermal Ablation of the GSV

UGFS uses either 1 to 2% foamed STS or 1 to 3% foamed polidocanol. The optimal concentration of foamed sclerosant for a given vein size is not established, but, in general, higher concentrations of sclerosant are used for larger veins. Foamed sclerosants are best administered into larger veins under US guidance because they are easily visualized as echogenic solutions and can be accurately monitored during injection. UGFS can be performed with local anesthesia to the access site, but use of tumescent anesthesia does not improve the efficacy or patient satisfaction of UGFS.[80] The most widely used method for preparing foamed sclerosants is the Tessari method, which utilizes two Luer lock syringes with low silicone content connected by a three-way stopcock (▶ Fig. 10.12).[81] One syringe contains 1 mL of sclerosant and the other syringe contains 4 mL of room air or CO_2/ O_2 gas mixture. With the third port closed, the syringes are pressed back and forth 10 to 20 times through the three-way stopcock to produce a foamed solution, which is only stable for approximately 2 minutes.[82,83] The foamed solution is then slowly injected percutaneously into the GSV under US guidance. Treatment of the GSV usually requires 6 to 8 mL of total solution, whereas the SSV usually requires 4 to 6 mL of solution. The volume of foam injected should not exceed 10 mL, as higher volumes are associated with more side effects. The patient typically remains lying down on the table for 5 minutes after injection to optimize contact between the foam and the vein endothelium.

One limitation of UGFS is variability in preparation of the physician-prepared foam sclerosant due to differences in mixing techniques and/or ratio of sclerosant to air. To address this limitation, Varithena contains 1% polidocanol foam prepared and delivered in a proprietary canister containing low nitrogen concentrations that facilitate quick absorption. Similar to UGFS, Varithena is injected percutaneously into the GSV under US guidance with the leg elevated to 45 degrees. Importantly, any perforator veins must be identified and precisely mapped so that they can be manually compressed before and during

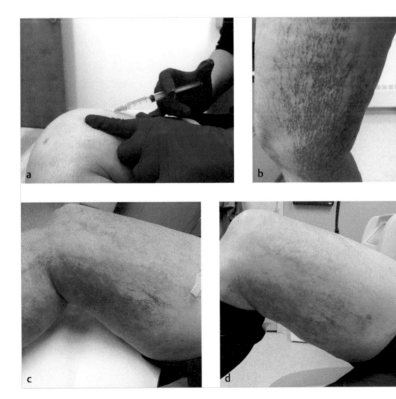

Fig. 10.11 Injection of telangiectasias and reticular veins with liquid sclerotherapy. (a) Bend the needle 45 degree to facilitate a parallel approach to the very superficial spider veins. (b) Before sclerotherapy. (c) One month posttreatment with residual hyperpigmentation. (d) Improvement in pigmentation at 3 months.

injection. Similar to UGFS, Varithena can be injected using only local anesthesia to the access site and does not require tumescent anesthesia. The volume of Varithena should be limited to 5 mL per injection and 15 mL per treatment session. Treatment sessions should be separated by at least 5 days.

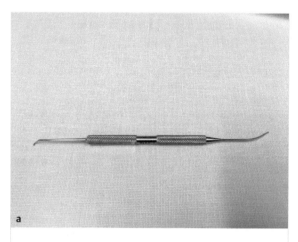

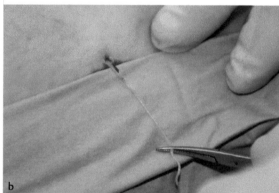

Fig. 10.12 Microphlebectomy. (a) Representative example of a skin hook used for ambulatory phlebectomy. (b) Vein removal assisted with hemostat.

ClariVein utilizes a proprietary mechanochemical technique with any liquid sclerosant. Similar to UGFS, local anesthesia is only required at the venous access site. After percutaneous access is obtained, US guidance is used to advance the catheter within a sheath into the GSV until the wire is positioned 2 cm distal to the SFJ. Next, the motor drive unit is connected and activated at 3,500 rpm for 2 to 3 seconds to promote vasospasm. The liquid sclerosant of choice is infused through the distal catheter port near the rotary wire, and the catheter is withdrawn at a rate of 1 to 2 mm/s.

Finally, VenaSeal utilizes a proprietary non-sclerosant-based technique using cyanoacrylate, which acts as a glue to directly seal the vein shut. After percutaneous access is obtained with local anesthesia to the access site, the catheter is advanced under US guidance and positioned 5 cm distal to the SFJ. After triggering the device, 0.1 mL of VenaSeal adhesive is delivered. The catheter is then withdrawn 1 cm, and another 0.1 mL of adhesive is delivered. The catheter is withdrawn another 3 cm, and the vein is manually compressed for 3 minutes. After compression, 0.1 mL of adhesive is delivered every 3 cm of GSV to be treated, and 30 seconds of compression is delivered after every administration of adhesive.

Treatment of varicose veins, reticular veins, and telangiectasias for therapeutic or cosmetic purposes is best accomplished with sclerotherapy (liquid or foam) and ambulatory phlebectomy. Both STS and polidocanol can be used on almost all sizes of telangiectasias, reticular veins, and varicose veins. Although there is little consensus on when to use liquid versus foam sclerosants, it is generally accepted that telangiectasias are best treated with liquid sclerosants and reticular veins and varicose veins greater than 4 mm are best treated with foam sclerosants.[84,85,86] Similar to UGFS, the lowest concentration of sclerosant in the smallest volume that will be effective for a given vein diameter should be used (▶ Table 10.4).[86,87] For telangiectasias and reticular veins, less than 1 mL is usually needed at any single injection site. Additionally, a European Consensus Meeting on foam sclerotherapy

Table 10.4 Choice of sclerosant based on vein size

Vein size (mm)	Recommended effective concentration (%)					
	Liquid sclerosant				Foam sclerosant	
	Sodium tetradecyl sulfate	Polidocanol	Hypertonic saline	Glycerin	Sodium tetradecyl sulfate	Polidocanol
Matting	0.1	0.25	–	40–50	–	–
Telangiectasia (< 1 mm)	0.1–0.2	0.25–0.5	11.7	50–72	–	–
Venulectasia (1–2 mm)	0.2–0.5	0.5–1.0	11.7–23.4	–	–	–
Reticular vein (2–4 mm)	0.33–0.5	1.0–2.0	23.4	–	0.2–0.5	0.5–1.0
Varicose veins (> 4 mm)	0.5–1.0	2.0–5.0	–	–	0.5–1.0	0.75–2.5

in 2006 recommended that the maximum dose should be limited to less than 10 mL per session.[88] As described earlier, foam sclerosants are prepared by a physician immediately before injection using the Tessari method.[81]

Sclerotherapy should be performed in a warm and comfortable environment with the patient supine or prone, depending on the areas to be injected. Adequate lighting is essential, and specialized vein lights can be used for magnification and better visualization of deeper veins. Sclerosants are typically injected with 30- or 32-gauge needles attached to 3-mL syringes, but butterfly needles may also be used. The treatment area is first cleansed with copious amounts of isopropyl alcohol using cotton balls. The needle should be bent at 45 degrees to facilitate a parallel approach to the skin and effective percutaneous cannulation of the target vein. A relatively linear segment of vein should be chosen as the access site to facilitate successful cannulation. The sclerosant should be injected slowly under low pressure to prevent rupture. Immediate disappearance of the target vein beginning proximally and extending distally is visualized with successful injection. After a few seconds, blood flows back into the veins, and the successfully treated veins will develop erythematous wheals. The injection should immediately be stopped if a bleb develops or disappearance of the target vein is not observed as the sclerosant is likely infiltrating the dermis. Foam sclerotherapy and liquid sclerotherapy typically require one to two treatments and two to three treatments, respectively.

STS is available in 1 and 3% concentrations, and polidocanol is available in 0.5 and 1% concentrations. STS is typically diluted to 0.25% for treating telangiectasias and 0.5% for treating reticular veins. Similarly, polidocanol is typically diluted to 0.5% for treating telangiectasias and 1% for treating reticular veins. Hypertonic saline is available at a concentration of 23.4%, which can be diluted to 11.7% for the off-label treatment of fine telangiectasias and other small veins. Finally, glycerin is available as a 72% solution that is compounded 2:1 with 1% lidocaine and epinephrine for the off-label treatment of telangiectasias and reticular veins.

10.4.3 Ambulatory Phlebectomy

Ambulatory phlebectomy, or Muller's phlebectomy, is used alone or in conjunction with thermal and nonthermal ablation to treat superficial varicose veins under local anesthesia. A critical step in successful ambulatory phlebectomy is precise preoperative mapping of varicosities with the patient in a standing position, as many varicosities will resolve with the patient lying down. Transillumination mapping with specialized vein lights can also be used to allow better visualization. The main advantage of ambulatory phlebectomy is its excellent cosmetic outcome due to the small size of the microincisions. First, the skin overlying the varicose veins is anesthetized with

superficial injections of 1% lidocaine without epinephrine or with very dilute concentrations of epinephrine (1:25,000). Tumescent anesthesia is commonly used for large treatment areas because it increases patient comfort and safety, particularly when combining ambulatory phlebectomy with thermal ablation modalities such as EVLA. Tumescent anesthesia is also advantageous because it facilitates vein extraction by hydrodissection of the vein from fibrous adhesions as it infiltrates the fat under pressure.

Microincisions 1 to 3 mm in length over the varicose veins should be made with a no. 11 blade (or 18-gauge needle) parallel to the long axis of the leg (vertical), except around the knee where they should be made parallel to the relaxed skin tension lines (horizontal). The microincisions should be spaced approximately 3 to 5 cm apart, but the exact distance will depend on the size and orientation of the vein. Microincisions should not be widened with a hemostat because the trauma can increase the risk of postinflammatory hyperpigmentation (PIH). Hooks are the primary instruments used in ambulatory phlebectomy, and, although many shapes and sizes exist, the majority are simple modifications of the original hook designed by Muller. The hook is carefully insertion through the microincision, avoiding inadvertent trauma to the wound margin. The target vein is exteriorized by slowly and gently pulling it through the microincision. The hook rarely needs to be inserted more than 2 to 3 mm below the skin. Once exteriorized, the vein is secured with a mosquito clamp and traction is applied to lift the vein through the skin. The vein is then secured with a second mosquito clamp and divided with scissors. The two ends are independently extracted from the microincision using a combination of slow and deliberate circular motions and traction to release adhesions and free up the longest segment of the varicose vein as possible. When pulling a vein, the skin adjacent to the microincision may become depressed. This is a fibrous attachment of the varicose vein and indicates the location for the next microincision. If the varicose vein breaks, it is often easier and safer to make additional microincisions rather than trying to retrieve the broken vein through the original microincision. If significant bleeding occurs, the patient should be placed in Trendelenburg position with firm pressure applied to each microincision using a gloved finger. The majority of microincisions do not need closure and heal without a perceptible scar. Microincisions can be closed for hemostasis with 5–0/6–0 absorbable or nonabsorbable suture or Steri-Strips.

10.5 Postoperative Instructions

A critical element of postoperative care for the majority of leg vein treatments is compression therapy. After thermal ablation (EVLA, RFA, EVSA) of the GSV, thigh-high compression stockings are worn continuously for 2 to

Table 10.5 Characteristics of compression stockings

Compression stockings	Treatment	Indications
Class III (30–40 mm Hg)	• Thermal ablation (EVLA, RFA, EVSA) • Nonthermal ablation (UGFS, Varithena, ClariVein, VenaSeal)	• GSV/SSV reflux • Severe varicose vein • Venous leg ulcers • Severe edema • Lymphedema
Class II (20–30 mm Hg)	• Sclerotherapy (liquid, foam)	• Mild/moderate varicose veins • Reticular veins • Telangiectasias
Class I (15–20 mm Hg)	• Sclerotherapy (liquid)	• Telangiectasias

Abbreviations: EVLA, endovenous laser ablation; EVSA, endovenous steam ablation; GSV, great saphenous vein; RFA, radiofrequency ablation; SSV, small saphenous vein; UGFS, ultrasound-guided foam sclerotherapy.

3 days and then daily for 3 weeks. Although evidence supporting the efficacy of compression stocking to improve clinical outcomes after thermal ablation is lacking, it may reduce pain and improve physical function during the first week after treatment.[89,90,91] Class III compression stockings (30–40 mm Hg) are most often prescribed. patients are instructed to ambulate in the office for 20 to 30 minutes before putting on the compression stockings (▶ Table 10.5). Patients are encouraged to pursue normal activities for the first 24 hours after the procedure, including ambulation as tolerated, to reduce the risk of thrombotic complications. Hot baths, jogging, and heavy lifting should be avoided for 1 to 2 weeks. Patients should be assessed for flow within the GSV and for extension of a junctional thrombus into the femoral vein with duplex US a week after treatment. Follow-up typically occurs 1 week and 2 to 6 months after the procedure to assess its short-term efficacy.

Postoperative care for patients undergoing UGFS, Varithena, ClariVein, and VenaSeal is similar. Although thigh-high compression stockings (30–40 mm Hg) are commonly prescribed after UGFS, evidence supporting the efficacy of this intervention is lacking.[59] Similarly, thigh-high compression stockings are also commonly prescribed after Varithena and ClariVein treatment. Notably, no compression is required after VenaSeal treatment given its unique mechanism of action with the cyanoacrylate adhesive.

In contrast to thermal and nonthermal ablation of the GSV, compression therapy after sclerotherapy of varicose veins, reticular veins, and telangiectasias is essential because it allows the vein walls to remain in proximity, maximizing endothelial damage. Compression therapy after sclerotherapy improves the clinical clearance of

vessels and reduces the risk of bruising and PIH.[92,93] Cotton balls with adhesive tape are applied along the course of varicose veins treated with foam sclerotherapy for 24 hours. Class II compression stockings (20–30 mm Hg) are typically prescribed after treatment of reticular and varicose veins. Over-the-counter class I compression stockings (15–20 mm Hg) are recommended if only telangiectasias are treated. Compression stockings are worn continuously for the first 1 to 2 days, and then daily for 2 to 3 weeks, with the most critical time for compression stockings appearing to be within the first 3 days.[94] Importantly, compression stockings should cover the entire treated area, and thigh-high compression stockings are typically recommended because sources of reflux contributing to telangiectasias can include reticular and perforator veins that extend above the knee even for treatments confined to the lower leg.

Cotton balls and nonadhesive tape are applied directly to the microincisions after ambulatory phlebectomy. The treated leg is then wrapped circumferentially from the ankle to the groin for 48 hours. Patients ambulate in the office for 10 to 15 minutes to ensure that there is no postoperative bleeding and that the wrappings are well tolerated.

10.6 Potential Complications and How to Manage

Types of complications are fairly uniform across treatment modalities. Nearly all patients have pain and bruising after thermal ablation, which resolves by 2 weeks. EVSA and RFA appear to be associated with less pain than EVLA.[41,45] Tylenol 1 g alternating with ibuprofen 800 mg every 4 hours is sufficient for pain control in the majority of patients. Almost all patients also report a transient burning taste and smell during the procedure.[95] Uncommon complications include mild leg numbness, paresthesias, PIH, burns, scars, localized hematomas, and superficial thrombophlebitis, all of which are self-limiting. Superficial thrombophlebitis has an incidence of 5% after RFA, and can be treated with warm compresses and pain control.[96] The majority of self-limiting complications from thermal ablation can be mitigated through proper use of tumescent anesthesia. The incidence of paresthesia and skin burns during RFA drops from 14.5 to 1.8%, and from 9.1 to 0.5%, respectively, with the use of tumescent anesthesia.[42] The incidence of paresthesia after EVSA is also very low (2%).[45]

DVT occurs in up to 5.7% of EVLA cases, most often from direct extension of the thrombus from the GSV into the common femoral vein.[97,98] PE following EVLA has been reported, but a direct correlation with a DVT from the procedure has not been established.[99] Of note, the steam bubbles produced during EVSA collapse locally and do not confer risk of air embolisms. Anticoagulation should be prescribed for DVT diagnosed on postoperative duplex US.

The complications of UGFS, Varithena, ClariVein, and VenaSeal are similar to those described for thermal ablation techniques. UGFS carries an increased risk of small vein ruptures, leading to PIH and telangiectatic matting.[52] Venous perforation is also possible with the ClariVein system given the mechanical nature of the device, but this complication has not yet been reported. No DVT, PE, significant paresthesias, or skin necrosis have been associated with the ClariVein system.[66] There was no difference in complications rates between treatment with VenaSeal and RFA, but the rates of superficial phlebitis and device-related complications were higher with VenaSeal compared to RFA.[48]

Complications of sclerotherapy depend on the type, formulation, and concentration of sclerosant. The most common complications of sclerotherapy are telangiectatic matting and PIH. Telangiectatic matting, which occurs after sclerotherapy in 15 to 24% of cases, refers to the development of fine capillary networks within the treated area resulting from neoangiogenesis.[100,101] PIH occurs in approximately 33% of cases, which can be significantly reduced with compression therapy.[100,101,102] The risk of telangiectatic matting and PIH can be minimized by injecting the leg while elevated, under minimal pressure, and with the minimal concentration and volume of sclerosant necessary and by prescribing compression stockings postoperatively. Fitzpatrick skin types IV to VI should be treated with lower concentrations and volumes of sclerosants as these patients have the highest risk of developing PIH after sclerotherapy. A test area can also be considered. Additionally, postsclerotherapy coagulum present within reticular and varicose veins should be extracted with a no. 11 blade to minimize the risk of PIH by preventing deposition of hemosiderin from erythrocyte extravasation. Although PIH resolves within 6 months in 70% of cases with sun protection and avoidance of ultraviolet radiation, Q-switched laser, hydroquinone, and topical retinoids may be prescribed, particularly when an inflammatory component is present.[94,101,102,103]

Uncommon and self-limited complications include sclerosant extravasation leading to cutaneous necrosis, superficial thrombophlebitis, cough, and transient visual disturbances including scotomas.[101] Cutaneous necrosis and ulcerations may heal well with optimal wound care involving petrolatum and occlusive dressings. Extravasation can be prevented by using proper injection technique, injecting slowly, visualizing the flow of sclerosant into the treated veins, and immediately stopping if a bleb forms. Nitroglycerin 2% paste can be applied if blanching is observed, and massage may be helpful to resolve blebs. Moreover, tight compression should be avoided over bony sites at high risk of ulceration, including the ankle. Superficial thrombophlebitis occurs in less than 1% of cases within a few weeks, and responds well to coagulum extraction, continued use of compression stockings, and NSAIDs. Transient visual disturbances are reported in less

than 2% of cases and are postulated to represent a form of migraine aura resulting from the release of endothelin-1 from the treated veins.[104]

Rare and serious complications of sclerotherapy include arterial injections, nerve damage (saphenous and sural nerve), DVT/PE, myocardial infarction, and anaphylaxis.[105,106,107] Although all sclerosants pose some risk, polidocanol is associated with very rare allergic reactions, a very low risk of cutaneous necrosis, and very little pain with injection. Skin necrosis and PIH can occur with extravasation of STS, but the risk of telangiectatic matting appears to be lower.[71,73] Hypertonic saline is associated with the most injection pain, likely due to irritation of free nerve endings.[108] Finally, glycerin rarely causes extravasation necrosis and PIH and has a low risk of anaphylaxis.

Foam sclerotherapy poses unique challenges given the injection of gas bubbles.[109] Severe complications, including transient ischemic attacks, as well as chest tightness and cough are quite rare, and the majority are associated with UGFS involving large quantities of foam solution.[106,110,111] However, most neurological events are thought to be physiologically related to migraine headaches related to endothelin released locally from the treated vein, rather than gas bubbles migrating to the brain.[88,112,113] Moreover, the presence of gas bubble does not necessarily correlate with neurological symptoms. Of note, Varithena may have a lower risk for cerebrovascular complications from gas emboli in high-risk patients with right-to-left shunts.[114] If neurologic symptoms are present, administration of oxygen and prompt referral to a stroke center are recommended.

10.6.1 Ambulatory Phlebectomy

Reported advantages of ambulatory phlebectomy over sclerotherapy include a lower risk of scarring and PIH. Scarring can be further reduced by ensuring the microincisions are as small as possible and minimizing skin trauma from the use of dissectors and forceps. In a multicenter analysis of 36,000 ambulatory phlebectomies performed in France, complications were rare and included telangiectatic matting (1.5%), blister formation (1%), superficial thrombophlebitis (0.05%), PIH (0.03%), postoperative bleeding (0.03%), temporary nerve damage (0.05%), and permanent nerve damage (0.02%).[115] Telangiectatic matting will typically fade after several months and may be prevented with a longer duration of compression therapy. Superficial thrombophlebitis can occur a few days after treatment and is best managed with compression therapy and NSAIDs. Moreover, intraoperative extraction of sensory nerves leads to an immediate burning and sharp pain, which, if occurring in the ankle or foot, are most likely to result in temporary postoperative paresthesias.[116]

Certain areas of the leg, including the feet, pretibial, and popliteal regions, are associated with higher complication rates. Pretibial microincisions commonly injure ascending lymphatic vessels, resulting in seromas and lymphoceles.[117] Prolonged edema can occur after treatment of the dorsal foot, and lymphatic pseudocysts can complicate treatment of the popliteal region. For quicker resolution, these lymphatic collections can be drained, followed by compression therapy. Finally, careful application of postoperative dressings is essential in preventing additional complications, including hematoma, blistering, nerve injury, ischemia, and bleeding. For example, the lateral fibular head is a common area for pressure-induced injury to the deep and superficial peroneal nerves.

10.7 Pearls and Pitfalls

10.7.1 Thermal Ablation

- There is significant heterogeneity in the definitions of efficacy reported in the literature, which highlights the need for standardizing outcomes to enable comparisons of future trials.[118] Important clinical outcomes to patients include symptomatic relief, improvement in quality of life, prevention of venous ulceration, and aesthetic improvement.
- The majority of studies on thermal ablation modalities only report short-term outcomes, and only a few studies report outcomes past 5 years. Additional long-term follow-up is needed to establish the durability of these treatments.
- The laser fiber or catheter tip should be visualized by US throughout the procedure.
- It is often easier to infiltrate tumescent anesthesia proximal to distal, rather than distal to proximal, along the course of the GSV.
- During treatment, one hand holds the US probe and the other hand pulls the laser fiber or catheter. A footswitch controls firing of the device. The laser fiber or catheter tip must be visualized throughout the entire treatment until it exits the vein.
- Firing of the laser fiber or catheter must be stopped before the tip is pulled out of the vein in order to avoid a skin burn. The sheath catheter must also be removed prior to device firing as the heat will cause the plastic of the catheter to melt and break into pieces.
- Use lower-energy settings below the knee due to an increased risk of injuring the common peroneal nerve as it courses superficially around the lateral aspect of the knee.
- After treatment, hold pressure at the venous access site for hemostasis.
- For symptomatic venous disease with reflux, up to 3 months of conservative therapy may be required for insurance coverage of thermal ablation of the GSV or SSV.
- Be especially careful with thermal ablation of the distal segments of the GSV and SSV due to the high risk of

nerve injury resulting in paresthesia. One should avoid thermal ablation of the GSV below the mid to distal calf, as the saphenous nerve runs in close proximity to the GSV in this location. Similarly, thermal ablation of the SSV should be performed no lower than mid-calf level due to the proximity of the sural nerve.

10.7.2 Nonthermal Ablation

- UGFS may require additional treatments to achieve the same efficacy as EVLA, RFA, or EVSA.
- Ensure that the venous access site is planned before preparing foamed sclerosants using the Tessari method. It is helpful for an assistant to prepare the foam while the GSV or SSV is visualized with US at the planned access site.
- When performing liquid sclerotherapy, be sure the needle is bent and approaches the target vein as parallel to the skin as possible to facilitate percutaneous access. A linear segment of vein is easier to cannulate than a tortuous segment.
- Inject sclerosants slowly and under low pressure.
- The first 3 days after nonthermal ablation is the most critical time period for wearing compression stockings.
- VenaSeal is the only thermal or nonthermal ablative modality that does not require compression stockings after treatment.

10.7.3 Ambulatory Phlebectomy

- Avoid making microincisions directly over the skin markings to prevent tattooing.
- Varicose veins are sometimes connected to perforating veins. When exteriorizing these varicose veins, the patient may experience pain as traction is applied to the perforator.
- Ambulatory phlebectomy can be challenging to perform on the pretibial leg and dorsal foot due to a paucity of subcutaneous fat in these locations. The anterior knee can also be difficult because of its thicker skin and underlying fibrotic tissue.
- Never pull the vein forcefully out from the microincision because varicose veins are typically fragile, particularly in older patients.
- Be especially careful with phlebectomy at the lateral knee. The common peroneal nerve runs along the lateral fibular head and divides in the deep and superficial peroneal nerve. Injury to the deep peroneal nerve can result in foot drop.

References

[1] Bergan JJ, Schmid-Schönbein GW, Smith PD, Nicolaides AN, Boisseau MR, Eklof B. Chronic venous disease. N Engl J Med. 2006; 355(5): 488–498

[2] Evans CJ, Fowkes FG, Ruckley CV, Lee AJ. Prevalence of varicose veins and chronic venous insufficiency in men and women in the general

population: Edinburgh Vein Study. J Epidemiol Community Health. 1999; 53(3):149–153

[3] McGuckin M, Waterman R, Brooks J, et al. Validation of venous leg ulcer guidelines in the United States and United Kingdom. Am J Surg. 2002; 183(2):132–137

[4] Kahn SR, M'lan CE, Lamping DL, Kurz X, Bérard A, Abenhaim LA, VEINES Study Group. Relationship between clinical classification of chronic venous disease and patient-reported quality of life: results from an international cohort study. J Vasc Surg. 2004; 39 (4):823–828

[5] Franks PJ, Moffatt CJ. Health related quality of life in patients with venous ulceration: use of the Nottingham health profile. Qual Life Res. 2001; 10(8):693–700

[6] van Korlaar I, Vossen C, Rosendaal F, Cameron L, Bovill E, Kaptein A. Quality of life in venous disease. Thromb Haemost. 2003; 90(1):27–35

[7] Kaplan RM, Criqui MH, Denenberg JO, Bergan J, Fronek A. Quality of life in patients with chronic venous disease: San Diego population study. J Vasc Surg. 2003; 37(5):1047–1053

[8] Carpentier PH, Cornu-Thénard A, Uhl JF, Partsch H, Antignani PL, Société Française de Médecine Vasculaire, European Working Group on the Clinical Characterization of Venous Disorders. Appraisal of the information content of the C classes of CEAP clinical classification of chronic venous disorders: a multicenter evaluation of 872 patients. J Vasc Surg. 2003; 37(4):827–833

[9] Eklöf B, Rutherford RB, Bergan JJ, et al. American Venous Forum International Ad Hoc Committee for Revision of the CEAP Classification. Revision of the CEAP classification for chronic venous disorders: consensus statement. J Vasc Surg. 2004; 40(6):1248–1252

[10] Porter JM, Moneta GL, International Consensus Committee on Chronic Venous Disease. Reporting standards in venous disease: an update. J Vasc Surg. 1995; 21(4):635–645

[11] Maurins U, Hoffmann BH, Lösch C, Jöckel KH, Rabe E, Pannier F. Distribution and prevalence of reflux in the superficial and deep venous system in the general population: results from the Bonn Vein Study, Germany. J Vasc Surg. 2008; 48(3):680–687

[12] Barwell JR, Davies CE, Deacon J, et al. Comparison of surgery and compression with compression alone in chronic venous ulceration (ESCHAR study): randomised controlled trial. Lancet. 2004; 363 (9424):1854–1859

[13] Tenbrook JA, Jr, Iafrati MD, O'donnell TF, Jr, et al. Systematic review of outcomes after surgical management of venous disease incorporating subfascial endoscopic perforator surgery. J Vasc Surg. 2004; 39(3):583–589

[14] Samuel N, Carradice D, Wallace T, Smith GE, Chetter IC. Endovenous thermal ablation for healing venous ulcers and preventing recurrence. Cochrane Database Syst Rev. 2013(10):CD009494

[15] Gohel MS, Heatley F, Liu X, et al. EVRA Trial Investigators. A randomized trial of early endovenous ablation in venous ulceration. N Engl J Med. 2018; 378(22):2105–2114

[16] Abdul-Haqq R, Almaroof B, Chen BL, Panneton JM, Parent FN. Endovenous laser ablation of great saphenous vein and perforator veins improves venous stasis ulcer healing. Ann Vasc Surg. 2013; 27 (7):932–939

[17] Motykie GD, Caprini JA, Arcelus JI, Reyna JJ, Overom E, Mokhtee D. Evaluation of therapeutic compression stockings in the treatment of chronic venous insufficiency. Dermatol Surg. 1999; 25(2):116–120

[18] Andreozzi GM, Cordova R, Scomparin MA, Martini R, D'Eri A, Andreozzi F, Quality of Life Working Group on Vascular Medicine of SIAPAV. Effects of elastic stocking on quality of life of patients with chronic venous insufficiency. An Italian pilot study on Triveneto Region. Int Angiol. 2005; 24(4):325–329

[19] Gohel MS, Barwell JR, Taylor M, et al. Long term results of compression therapy alone versus compression plus surgery in chronic venous ulceration (ESCHAR): randomised controlled trial. BMJ. 2007; 335(7610):83

[20] Wolf B, Brittenden J. Surgical treatment of varicose veins. J R Coll Surg Edinb. 2001; 46(3):154–158

[21] Rutgers PH, Kitslaar PJ. Randomized trial of stripping versus high ligation combined with sclerotherapy in the treatment of the incompetent greater saphenous vein. Am J Surg. 1994; 168(4):311–315

[22] Michaels JA, Campbell WB, Brazier JE, et al. Randomised clinical trial, observational study and assessment of cost-effectiveness of the treatment of varicose veins (REACTIV trial). Health Technol Assess. 2006; 10(13):1–196, iii–iv

[23] Lurie F, Creton D, Eklof B, et al. Prospective randomized study of endovenous radiofrequency obliteration (closure procedure) versus ligation and stripping in a selected patient population (EVOLVeS Study). J Vasc Surg. 2003; 38(2):207–214

[24] van den Bos R, Arends L, Kockaert M, Neumann M, Nijsten T. Endovenous therapies of lower extremity varicosities: a meta-analysis. J Vasc Surg. 2009; 49(1):230–239

[25] Min RJ, Khilnani N, Zimmet SE. Endovenous laser treatment of saphenous vein reflux: long-term results. J Vasc Interv Radiol. 2003; 14(8):991–996

[26] Ostler AE, Holdstock JM, Harrison CC, Price BA, Whiteley MS. Strip-tract revascularization as a source of recurrent venous reflux following high saphenous tie and stripping: results at 5–8 years after surgery. Phlebology. 2015; 30(8):569–572

[27] Pan Y, Zhao J, Mei J, Shao M, Zhang J. Comparison of endovenous laser ablation and high ligation and stripping for varicose vein treatment: a meta-analysis. Phlebology. 2014; 29(2):109–119

[28] Rasmussen LH, Lawaetz M, Bjoern L, Vennits B, Blemings A, Eklof B. Randomized clinical trial comparing endovenous laser ablation, radiofrequency ablation, foam sclerotherapy and surgical stripping for great saphenous varicose veins. Br J Surg. 2011; 98(8):1079–1087

[29] Siribumrungwong B, Noorit P, Wilasrusmee C, Attia J, Thakkinstian A. A systematic review and meta-analysis of randomised controlled trials comparing endovenous ablation and surgical intervention in patients with varicose vein. Eur J Vasc Endovasc Surg. 2012; 44(2):214–223

[30] Nesbitt C, Bedenis R, Bhattacharya V, Stansby G. Endovenous ablation (radiofrequency and laser) and foam sclerotherapy versus open surgery for great saphenous vein varices. Cochrane Database Syst Rev. 2014(7):CD005624

[31] Fan CM, Rox-Anderson R. Endovenous laser ablation: mechanism of action. Phlebology. 2008; 23(5):206–213

[32] Proebstle TM, Lehr HA, Kargl A, et al. Endovenous treatment of the greater saphenous vein with a 940-nm diode laser: thrombotic occlusion after endoluminal thermal damage by laser-generated steam bubbles. J Vasc Surg. 2002; 35(4):729–736

[33] Navarro L, Min RJ, Boné C. Endovenous laser: a new minimally invasive method of treatment for varicose veins: preliminary observations using an 810 nm diode laser. Dermatol Surg. 2001; 27 (2):117–122

[34] Min RJ, Zimmet SE, Isaacs MN, Forrestal MD. Endovenous laser treatment of the incompetent greater saphenous vein. J Vasc Interv Radiol. 2001; 12(10):1167–1171

[35] Disselhoff BC, der Kinderen DJ, Kelder JC, Moll FL. Five-year results of a randomised clinical trial of endovenous laser ablation of the great saphenous vein with and without ligation of the saphenofemoral junction. Eur J Vasc Endovasc Surg. 2011; 41(5):685–690

[36] Kabnick LS. Outcome of different endovenous laser wavelengths for great saphenous vein ablation. J Vasc Surg. 2006; 43(1):88–93

[37] Proebstle TM, Moehler T, Gül D, Herdemann S. Endovenous treatment of the great saphenous vein using a 1,320 nm Nd:YAG laser causes fewer side effects than using a 940 nm diode laser. Dermatol Surg. 2005; 31(12):1678–1683, discussion 1683–1684

[38] Goodyear SJ, Nyamekye IK. Radiofrequency ablation of varicose veins: best practice techniques and evidence. Phlebology. 2015; 30(2) Suppl:9–17

[39] Weiss RA, Weiss MA. Controlled radiofrequency endovenous occlusion using a unique radiofrequency catheter under duplex guidance to eliminate saphenous varicose vein reflux: a 2-year follow-up. Dermatol Surg. 2002; 28(1):38–42

[40] Helmy ElKaffas K, ElKashef O, ElBaz W. Great saphenous vein radiofrequency ablation versus standard stripping in the management of primary varicose veins-a randomized clinical trial. Angiology. 2011; 62(1):49–54

[41] Ahadiat O, Higgins S, Ly A, Nazemi A, Wysong A. Review of endovenous thermal ablation of the great saphenous vein: endovenous laser therapy versus radiofrequency ablation. Dermatol Surg. 2018; 44(5):679–688

[42] Merchant RF, Pichot O, Myers KA. Four-year follow-up on endovascular radiofrequency obliteration of great saphenous reflux. Dermatol Surg. 2005; 31(2):129–134

[43] van den Bos RR, Milleret R, Neumann M, Nijsten T. Proof-of-principle study of steam ablation as novel thermal therapy for saphenous varicose veins. J Vasc Surg. 2011; 53(1):181–186

[44] Milleret R, Huot L, Nicolini P, et al. Great saphenous vein ablation with steam injection: results of a multicentre study. Eur J Vasc Endovasc Surg. 2013; 45(4):391–396

[45] van den Bos RR, Malskat WS, De Maeseneer MG, et al. Randomized clinical trial of endovenous laser ablation versus steam ablation (LAST trial) for great saphenous varicose veins. Br J Surg. 2014; 101 (9):1077–1083

[46] Kugler NW, Brown KR. An update on the currently available nonthermal ablative options in the management of superficial venous disease. J Vasc Surg Venous Lymphat Disord. 2017; 5(3):422–429

[47] Proebstle TM, Alm J, Dimitri S, et al. The European multicenter cohort study on cyanoacrylate embolization of refluxing great saphenous veins. J Vasc Surg Venous Lymphat Disord. 2015; 3(1):2–7

[48] Morrison N, Gibson K, McEnroe S, et al. Randomized trial comparing cyanoacrylate embolization and radiofrequency ablation for incompetent great saphenous veins (VeClose). J Vasc Surg. 2015; 61 (4):985–994

[49] Duffy DM. Sclerosants: a comparative review. Dermatol Surg. 2010; 36 Suppl 2:1010–1025

[50] American Academy of Dermatology. Guidelines of care for sclerotherapy treatment of varicose and telangiectatic leg veins. J Am Acad Dermatol. 1996; 34(3):523–528

[51] Rabe E, Breu FX, Cavezzi A, et al. Guideline Group. European guidelines for sclerotherapy in chronic venous disorders. Phlebology. 2014; 29(6):338–354

[52] Hamel-Desnos C, Allaert FA. Liquid versus foam sclerotherapy. Phlebology. 2009; 24(6):240–246

[53] Myers KA, Jolley D, Clough A, Kirwan J. Outcome of ultrasound-guided sclerotherapy for varicose veins: medium-term results assessed by ultrasound surveillance. Eur J Vasc Endovasc Surg. 2007; 33(1):116–121

[54] Darvall KA, Bate GR, Bradbury AW. Patient-reported outcomes 5–8 years after ultrasound-guided foam sclerotherapy for varicose veins. Br J Surg. 2014; 101(9):1098–1104

[55] Belcaro G, Nicolaides AN, Ricci A, et al. Endovascular sclerotherapy, surgery, and surgery plus sclerotherapy in superficial venous incompetence: a randomized, 10-year follow-up trial—final results. Angiology. 2000; 51(7):529–534

[56] Biemans AA, Kockaert M, Akkersdijk GP, et al. Comparing endovenous laser ablation, foam sclerotherapy, and conventional surgery for great saphenous varicose veins. J Vasc Surg. 2013; 58(3):727–34.e1

[57] Chapman-Smith P, Browne A. Prospective five-year study of ultrasound-guided foam sclerotherapy in the treatment of great saphenous vein reflux. Phlebology. 2009; 24(4):183–188

[58] Blaise S, Bosson JL, Diamand JM. Ultrasound-guided sclerotherapy of the great saphenous vein with 1% vs. 3% polidocanol foam: a multicentre double-blind randomised trial with 3-year follow-up. Eur J Vasc Endovasc Surg. 2010; 39(6):779–786

[59] Hamel-Desnos CM, Guias BJ, Desnos PR, Mesgard A. Foam sclerotherapy of the saphenous veins: randomised controlled trial with or without compression. Eur J Vasc Endovasc Surg. 2010; 39(4):500–507

[60] Shadid N, Ceulen R, Nelemans P, et al. Randomized clinical trial of ultrasound-guided foam sclerotherapy versus surgery for the incompetent great saphenous vein. Br J Surg. 2012; 99(8):1062–1070

[61] Pang KH, Bate GR, Darvall KA, Adam DJ, Bradbury AW. Healing and recurrence rates following ultrasound-guided foam sclerotherapy of superficial venous reflux in patients with chronic venous ulceration. Eur J Vasc Endovasc Surg. 2010; 40(6):790–795

[62] Gonzalez-Zeh R, Armisen R, Barahona S. Endovenous laser and echo-guided foam ablation in great saphenous vein reflux: one-year follow-up results. J Vasc Surg. 2008; 48(4):940–946

[63] Todd KL, III, Wright DI, VANISH-2 Investigator Group. The VANISH-2 study: a randomized, blinded, multicenter study to evaluate the efficacy and safety of polidocanol endovenous microfoam 0.5% and 1.0% compared with placebo for the treatment of saphenofemoral junction incompetence. Phlebology. 2014; 29(9):608–618

[64] King JT, O'Byrne M, Vasquez M, Wright D, VANISH-1 Investigator Group. Treatment of truncal incompetence and varicose veins with a single administration of a new polidocanol endovenous microfoam preparation improves symptoms and appearance. Eur J Vasc Endovasc Surg. 2015; 50(6):784–793

[65] van Eekeren RR, Boersma D, Holewijn S, Werson DA, de Vries JP, Reijnen MM. Mechanochemical endovenous ablation for the treatment of great saphenous vein insufficiency. J Vasc Surg Venous Lymphat Disord. 2014; 2(3):282–288

[66] Witte ME, Reijnen MM, de Vries JP, Zeebregts CJ. Mechanochemical endovenous occlusion of varicose veins using the ClariVein® device. Surg Technol Int. 2015; 26:219–225

[67] Elias S, Raines JK. Mechanochemical tumescentless endovenous ablation: final results of the initial clinical trial. Phlebology. 2012; 27 (2):67–72

[68] Bishawi M, Bernstein R, Boter M, et al. Mechanochemical ablation in patients with chronic venous disease: a prospective multicenter report. Phlebology. 2014; 29(6):397–400

[69] Almeida JI, Javier JJ, Mackay E, Bautista C, Proebstle TM. First human use of cyanoacrylate adhesive for treatment of saphenous vein incompetence. J Vasc Surg Venous Lymphat Disord. 2013; 1(2):174–180

[70] Palm MD, Guiha IC, Goldman MP. Foam sclerotherapy for reticular veins and nontruncal varicose veins of the legs: a retrospective review of outcomes and adverse effects. Dermatol Surg. 2010; 36 Suppl 2:1026–1033

[71] Schwartz L, Maxwell H. Sclerotherapy for lower limb telangiectasias. Cochrane Database Syst Rev. 2011(12):CD008826

[72] Rabe E, Schliephake D, Otto J, Breu FX, Pannier F. Sclerotherapy of telangiectases and reticular veins: a double-blind, randomized, comparative clinical trial of polidocanol, sodium tetradecyl sulphate and isotonic saline (EASI study). Phlebology. 2010; 25(3):124–131

[73] Tisi PV, Beverley C, Rees A. Injection sclerotherapy for varicose veins. Cochrane Database Syst Rev. 2006(4):CD001732

[74] Kabnick LS, Ombrellino M. Ambulatory phlebectomy. Semin Intervent Radiol. 2005; 22(3):218–224

[75] Ramelet AA. Phlebectomy. Technique, indications and complications. Int Angiol. 2002; 21(2) Suppl 1:46–51

[76] Marston WA, Crowner J, Kouri A, Kalbaugh CA. Incidence of venous leg ulcer healing and recurrence after treatment with endovenous laser ablation. J Vasc Surg Venous Lymphat Disord. 2017; 5(4):525–532

[77] Timperman PE. Prospective evaluation of higher energy great saphenous vein endovenous laser treatment. J Vasc Interv Radiol. 2005; 16(6):791–794

[78] Proebstle TM, Moehler T, Herdemann S. Reduced recanalization rates of the great saphenous vein after endovenous laser treatment with increased energy dosing: definition of a threshold for the endovenous fluence equivalent. J Vasc Surg. 2006; 44(4):834–839

[79] Zikorus AW, Mirizzi MS. Evaluation of setpoint temperature and pullback speed on vein adventitial temperature during endovenous radiofrequency energy delivery in an in-vitro model. Vasc Endovascular Surg. 2004; 38(2):167–174

[80] Devereux N, Recke AL, Westermann L, Recke A, Kahle B. Catheter-directed foam sclerotherapy of great saphenous veins in combination with pre-treatment reduction of the diameter employing the principals of perivenous tumescent local anesthesia. Eur J Vasc Endovasc Surg. 2014; 47(2):187–195

[81] Tessari L, Cavezzi A, Frullini A. Preliminary experience with a new sclerosing foam in the treatment of varicose veins. Dermatol Surg. 2001; 27(1):58–60

[82] McAree B, Ikponmwosa A, Brockbank K, Abbott C, Homer-Vanniasinkam S, Gough MJ. Comparative stability of sodium tetradecyl sulphate (STD) and polidocanol foam: impact on vein damage in an in-vitro model. Eur J Vasc Endovasc Surg. 2012; 43(6):721–725

[83] Rabe E, Pannier F, for the Guideline Group. Indications, contraindications and performance: European Guidelines for Sclerotherapy in Chronic Venous Disorders. Phlebology. 2014; 29 (1) s uppl:26–33

[84] Kahle B, Leng K. Efficacy of sclerotherapy in varicose veins: prospective, blinded, placebo-controlled study. Dermatol Surg. 2004; 30(5):723–728, discussion 728

[85] Palm MD. Commentary: choosing the appropriate sclerosing concentration for vessel diameter. Dermatol Surg. 2010; 36 Suppl 2: 982

[86] Sadick NS. Choosing the appropriate sclerosing concentration for vessel diameter. Dermatol Surg. 2010; 36 Suppl 2:976–981

[87] Erkin A, Kosemehmetoglu K, Diler MS, Koksal C. Evaluation of the minimum effective concentration of foam sclerosant in an ex-vivo study. Eur J Vasc Endovasc Surg. 2012; 44(6):593–597

[88] Breu FX, Guggenbichler S, Wollmann JC. 2nd European Consensus Meeting on Foam Sclerotherapy 2006, Tegernsee, Germany. Vasa. 2008; 37 Suppl 71:1–29

[89] Bakker NA, Schieven LW, Bruins RM, van den Berg M, Hissink RJ. Compression stockings after endovenous laser ablation of the great saphenous vein: a prospective randomized controlled trial. Eur J Vasc Endovasc Surg. 2013; 46(5):588–592

[90] Ayo D, Blumberg SN, Rockman CR, et al. Compression versus no compression after endovenous ablation of the great saphenous vein: a randomized controlled trial. Ann Vasc Surg. 2017; 38:72–77

[91] Ye K, Wang R, Qin J, et al. Post-operative benefit of compression therapy after endovenous laser ablation for uncomplicated varicose veins: a randomised clinical trial. Eur J Vasc Endovasc Surg. 2016; 52 (6):847–853

[92] Nootheti PK, Cadag KM, Magpantay A, Goldman MP. Efficacy of graduated compression stockings for an additional 3 weeks after sclerotherapy treatment of reticular and telangiectatic leg veins. Dermatol Surg. 2009; 35(1):53–57, discussion 57–58

[93] Kern P, Ramelet AA, Wütschert R, Hayoz D. Compression after sclerotherapy for telangiectasias and reticular leg veins: a randomized controlled study. J Vasc Surg. 2007; 45(6):1212–1216

[94] Weiss RA, Sadick NS, Goldman MP, Weiss MA. Post-sclerotherapy compression: controlled comparative study of duration of compression and its effects on clinical outcome. Dermatol Surg. 1999; 25(2):105–108

[95] Klem TM, Stok M, Grotenhuis BA, et al. Benzopyrene serum concentration after endovenous laser ablation of the great saphenous vein. Vasc Endovascular Surg. 2013; 47(3):213–215

[96] Almeida JI, Raines JK. Radiofrequency ablation and laser ablation in the treatment of varicose veins. Ann Vasc Surg. 2006; 20(4):547–552

[97] Krnic A, Sucic Z. Bipolar radiofrequency induced thermotherapy and 1064 nm Nd:Yag laser in endovenous occlusion of insufficient veins: short term follow up results. Vasa. 2011; 40(3):235–240

[98] Puggioni A, Kalra M, Carmo M, Mozes G, Gloviczki P. Endovenous laser therapy and radiofrequency ablation of the great saphenous vein: analysis of early efficacy and complications. J Vasc Surg. 2005; 42(3):488–493

[99] Ravi R, Rodriguez-Lopez JA, Trayler EA, Barrett DA, Ramaiah V, Diethrich EB. Endovenous ablation of incompetent saphenous veins: a large single-center experience. J Endovasc Ther. 2006; 13(2):244–248

[100] Guex JJ, Schliephake DE, Otto J, Mako S, Allaert FA. The French polidocanol study on long-term side effects: a survey covering 3,357 patient years. Dermatol Surg. 2010; 36 Suppl 2:993–1003

[101] Goldman MP, Sadick NS, Weiss RA. Cutaneous necrosis, telangiectatic matting, and hyperpigmentation following sclerotherapy. Etiology, prevention, and treatment. Dermatol Surg. 1995; 21(1):19–29, quiz 31–32

[102] Georgiev M. Postsclerotherapy hyperpigmentations: a one-year follow-up. J Dermatol Surg Oncol. 1990; 16(7):608–610

[103] Tafazzoli A, Rostan EF, Goldman MP. Q-switched ruby laser treatment for postsclerotherapy hyperpigmentation. Dermatol Surg. 2000; 26 (7):653–656

[104] Frullini A, Da Pozzo E, Felice F, Burchielli S, Martini C, Di Stefano R. Prevention of excessive endothelin-1 release in sclerotherapy: in vitro and in vivo studies. Dermatol Surg. 2014; 40(7):769–775

[105] Marrocco-Trischitta MM, Guerrini P, Abeni D, Stillo F. Reversible cardiac arrest after polidocanol sclerotherapy of peripheral venous malformation. Dermatol Surg. 2002; 28(2):153–155

[106] Ceulen RP, Sommer A, Vernooy K. Microembolism during foam sclerotherapy of varicose veins. N Engl J Med. 2008; 358(14):1525–1526

[107] Engelberger RP, Ney B, Clair M, et al. Myocardial infarction after ultrasoundguided foam sclerotherapy for varicose veins: a case report and review of the literature of a rare but serious adverse event. Vasa. 2016; 45(3):255–258

[108] Peterson JD, Goldman MP, Weiss RA, et al. Treatment of reticular and telangiectatic leg veins: double-blind, prospective comparative trial of polidocanol and hypertonic saline. Dermatol Surg. 2012; 38(8): 1322–1330

[109] Morrison N, Neuhardt DL. Foam sclerotherapy: cardiac and cerebral monitoring. Phlebology. 2009; 24(6):252–259

[110] Bush RG, Derrick M, Manjoney D. Major neurological events following foam sclerotherapy. Phlebology. 2008; 23(4):189–192

[111] Forlee MV, Grouden M, Moore DJ, Shanik G. Stroke after varicose vein foam injection sclerotherapy. J Vasc Surg. 2006; 43(1):162–164

[112] Frullini A, Barsotti MC, Santoni T, Duranti E, Burchielli S, Di Stefano R. Significant endothelin release in patients treated with foam sclerotherapy. Dermatol Surg. 2012; 38(5):741–747

[113] Frullini A, Felice F, Burchielli S, Di Stefano R. High production of endothelin after foam sclerotherapy: a new pathogenetic hypothesis for neurological and visual disturbances after sclerotherapy. Phlebology. 2011; 26(5):203–208

[114] Regan JD, Gibson KD, Rush JE, Shortell CK, Hirsch SA, Wright DD. Clinical significance of cerebrovascular gas emboli during polidocanol endovenous ultra-low nitrogen microfoam ablation and correlation with magnetic resonance imaging in patients with right-to-left shunt. J Vasc Surg. 2011; 53(1):131–137

[115] Almeida JI, Raines JK. Ambulatory phlebectomy in the office. Perspect Vasc Surg Endovasc Ther. 2008; 20(4):348–355

[116] Ramelet AA. Complications of ambulatory phlebectomy. Dermatol Surg. 1997; 23(10):947–954

[117] Olivencia JA. Complications of ambulatory phlebectomy. Review of 1000 consecutive cases. Dermatol Surg. 1997; 23(1):51–54

[118] Kundu S, Lurie F, Millward SF, et al. American Venous Forum, Society of Interventional Radiology. Recommended reporting standards for endovenous ablation for the treatment of venous insufficiency: joint statement of the American Venous Forum and the Society of Interventional Radiology. J Vasc Surg. 2007; 46(3): 582–589

11 Lasers and Lights in Acne

Samantha Gordon, Jordan Borash, and Emmy M. Graber

Summary

Acne is traditionally treated by prescribing topical and oral medications. However, there are patients who do not want to use such medications, have contraindications to these medications, or see suboptimal results with these medications. Such patients may be good candidates for acne treatment with laser and light devices. A multitude of laser and light devices has been explored for their use in acne and herein we report on the dermatology literature of such devices as well as practical advice for employing this technology to treat acne patients.

Keywords: acne, acne vulgaris, lasers, lights, devices, potassium titanyl phosphate laser, pulsed dye laser, infrared lasers, fractional CO_2 laser, intense pulsed light, blue light, red light, photodynamic therapy, photopneumatic therapy, handheld at home devices, radiofrequency devices, fractional microneedling radiofrequency

11.1 Introduction

Acne is a multifactorial disease of the pilosebaceous glands, resulting from abnormal keratinization, increased sebum production, inflammation, and *Propionibacterium acnes* (recently reclassified as *Cutibacterium acnes* and thus subsequently referred to herein as *C. acnes*).[1,2,3,4] It affects up to 70 to 87% of the population and has severe psychosocial consequences with profound effects on quality of life.[1,5] Treatment in a timely manner is important to minimize its negative impact and the potential for permanent scarring.[1]

Conventional treatments for acne vulgaris have traditionally included topical and oral retinoids, topical and oral antibiotics, and hormonally based treatments.[6,7] However, topical agents are often not adequate in the treatment of scarring acne, and oral medications have issues with safety, teratogenicity, resistance, and compliance.[1] *C. acnes* is now reported to have greater than 60% resistance to the most common antibiotics used in the treatment of acne, limiting the utility of this standard treatment.[7] Lasers and lights provide minimally invasive alternatives for the treatment of acne, with improved safety, efficacy, and convenience as compared to many of the conventional treatments.[1,8]

Lasers and lights treat acne through two main mechanisms, which target *C. acnes* and/or the sebaceous glands.[1,3] The first mechanism works through photoactivation of porphyrins produced by *C. acnes*.[1,3,9] This results in a photodynamic reaction with production of highly reactive free radicals that in turn destroy the *C. acnes*.[3,9] Porphyrin absorption and excitation is most efficient near the Soret band, that is between 400 and 430 nm.[9] Therefore, lasers and light devices operating within these wavelengths will theoretically be the most effective lasers to combat *C. acnes*. However, given the relatively low wavelength of light, depth of penetration into the skin is limited and may therefore prevent the light from even reaching the *C. acnes*.

The second mechanism of action in which lasers and light devices work to improve acne is by damaging sebaceous glands. Energy from lasers that target water, and thus secondarily collagen, is converted to heat in the dermis, which collaterally damages the sebaceous glands.[1] This secondarily decreases *C. acnes* by reducing available sebum as *C. acnes* survives by the presence of sebum.[3,9]

There are many different lasers and light sources that work based on the above principles, and these will each be discussed in the following sections.

11.2 Modalities

11.2.1 Lasers

Potassium Titanyl Phosphate Laser

The 532-nm potassium titanyl phosphate (KTP) laser provides an ideal wavelength for photoactivation of bacterial porphyrins, resulting in production of free radicals and bacterial cell death.[3] However, its low depth of penetration limits its ability to reach *C. acnes*, and thus its utility as an effective treatment for acne.

Several small studies have assessed the efficacy of KTP in the treatment of acne. Lee demonstrated 60 to 70% clearance of acne lesions, which increased to 80 to 95% if used in conjunction with a 1,064-nm neodymium:yttrium aluminum garnet (Nd:Yag) laser.[10] Sadick showed that the use of KTP following photodynamic therapy (PDT) improved treatment efficacy from 32 to 52%.[7] Yilmaz et al demonstrated 26.4 and 39.7% reduction in Michaelson acne severity score (MASS) at 1 and 4 weeks, respectively, in patients treated twice weekly with KTP, and 21.2 and 31.4% improvement at 1 and 4 weeks, respectively, in those treated once weekly.[3]

Despite the above reports demonstrating some efficacy, there seems to be no consensus on frequency of treatments, ranging from every 3 days up to every 4 weeks.[3,7,10] Total number of treatments in the above studies ranged from three to six.[3,7,10] Settings varied as well, including spot sizes of 2 to 4 mm, pulse durations of 7 to 50 milliseconds, and fluences of 5 to 15 J/cm^2.[3,10] Follow-up time was minimal in all studies, thus limiting our knowledge of the duration of effectiveness.

KTP lasers are relatively well tolerated, with most patients experiencing minimal erythema.[3,7] Other potential side effects include edema, transient crusting, and pigmentary changes in dark-skinned patients.[3]

Pulsed Dye Laser

The 585- or 595-nm pulsed dye laser (PDL) works by targeting oxygenated hemoglobin, resulting in endothelial disruption and decreased inflammation.[5,11] Furthermore, it reduces comedone formation and promotes collagen production through heating of the perivascular dermis, which stimulates fibroblast proliferation and procollagen messenger ribonucleic acid (mRNA) expression.[5,11]

Despite its common use for the treatment of vascular lesions, studies regarding its utility in acne are limited. Several reports have shown only minimal, if any, improvement in inflammatory lesions after multiple treatments, with results that were short-lived.[1,5,12,13] Of note, Leheta demonstrated that 46.2% of patients treated with PDL showed marked improvement of their acne, with results that were more sustained than in patients whose acne was treated with topical benzoyl peroxide and tretinoin or trichloracetic acid chemical peels.[5]

Treatments in reported studies ranged from only once or twice to up to six sessions, spaced every 2 weeks. The 585-nm laser was used with a pulse duration of 350 microseconds, spot size of 7 mm, and fluence of 3 J/cm^2, and the 595-nm laser was used with a pulse duration of 10 milliseconds, spot size of 7 mm, and fluence of 8 J/cm^2.[5,12,13]

The treatments are overall well tolerated, with the majority of patients only experiencing mild transient erythema and mild pain.[1,5,11,13]

Infrared Lasers

650 microsecond 1,064-nm Laser

The 650 microsecond 1,064-nm laser has been FDA cleared to treat mild to moderate inflammatory acne. It reduces the inflammation of acne by damaging the sebaceous glands via bulk heating of the dermis. Additionally, it coagulates the vessels in the dermis, resulting in reduced blood supply surrounding the pilosebaceous unit. A recent double-blind randomized control study using this laser demonstrated its efficacy. Consisting of 20 subjects with either moderate or severe acne, half of the patients in the study received laser treatments, while the other half received sham laser treatments. The subjects were treated at weeks 0, 2, 4, and 8, with a final follow up visit at week 12. Treatments were done without anesthesia. The treatment group showed a decrease of inflammatory lesions by 42% at week 12 compared with a 26% decrease in inflammatory lesions in the sham treatment group. Only minutes of transient erythema was noted after each treatment.[14] While the 650 microsecond 1,064-nm laser shows promise, further studies are needed in a larger population and with longer follow-up periods to determine the efficacy in treating acne.

Nd:Yag 1,060-nm laser with gold microparticles

A more recent approach to treat acne with lasers is with the preapplication of gold microparticles. These gold microparticles comprise a gold outer coating wrapped around a silica core. After massage of these particles into the skin, and thus penetration into the pilosebaceous unit, a 1,064-nm laser is employed. The gold preferentially absorbs light at the 1,064-nm wavelength, facilitating a photothermal reaction and consequently damaging the sebaceous gland.[15] Early studies suggest that weekly treatment for three consecutive treatments result in significant improvement of several months' duration. More recent studies show that these results may be magnified with pretreatment and concomitant treatment with a topical retinoid/benzoyl peroxide product (▸ Fig. 11.1, ▸ Fig. 11.2, ▸ Fig. 11.3).

1,450- and 1,320-nm Lasers

The 1,450- and 1,320-nm infrared lasers target water in dermal collagen, resulting in production of heat, which diffuses to collaterally damage sebaceous glands and reduce sebum production.[1,8,16]

Jih et al showed a 63.8 and 48.4% reduction after two treatments in patients treated with 14 and 16 J/cm^2, respectively, which increased to a 75.1 and 70.6% reduction after three treatments.[8] These improvements were maintained at 3-, 6-, and 12-month follow-up visits.[8] Bernstein demonstrated a 78% improvement in patients treated with a high-energy (13–14 J/cm^2) single pass, and a 68% improvement in those treated with a low-fluence (8–11 J/cm^2) double pass.[17] Reported treatment regimens were spaced from weekly to every 4 weeks, with a total of 3 to 10 treatments.[8,16,17]

Although these studies demonstrated improvement in acne, pain limits utility of this laser, with many patients

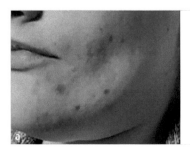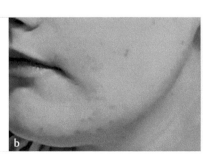

Fig. 11.1 (a) Before Sebacia treatment. (b) Six months after Sebacia treatment.

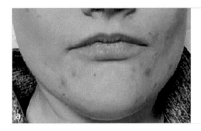

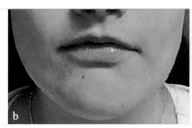

Fig. 11.2 (a) Before Sebacia treatment.
(b) Six months after Sebacia treatment.

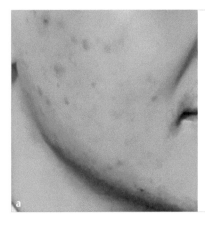

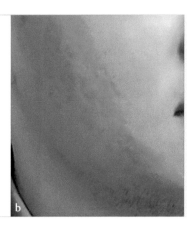

Fig. 11.3 (a) Before Sebacia treatment.
(b) Six months after Sebacia treatment.

requiring local topical anesthetic.[17] Decreasing the energy to 8 to 12 J/cm^2, coupled with a double-pass treatment, can help reduce associated pain while maintaining efficacy.[8,17] Other reported, but less common side effects include edema, hypo- or hyperpigmentation, acneiform eruptions, blistering, and crusting.[1,16]

1,726-nm Laser

1,726 nm is a new wavelength utilized to selectively target the sebaceous gland, thereby preventing and treating acne. The unique 1,726-nm wavelength selectively targets sebum and at 1,726 nm, sebum preferentially absorbs more light than water.[18] This allows the sebaceous glands to be selectively targeted with minimal damage to the surrounding structures and without damage to the epidermis.[19] Currently in the United States, there are two 1,726-nm lasers with FDA clearance for treating acne. The first 1,726-nm laser with FDA clearance for treating acne in the United States is manufactured by Cutera. It has FDA clearance for treating mild, moderate, and severe acne and also has clearance by Health Canada for treating both acne and acne scars. In the pivotal study to achieve FDA clearance, 104 subjects, all 16 years of age and older, were evaluated with acne ranging from mild to severe. Each patient received three full face laser treatments (excluding the nose), spaced 1 month apart. The laser was used as monotherapy, as no other oral or topical acne agents were employed. Patients were followed 1, 3, 6, and 12 months after the final treatment. Eighty percent of subjects who completed the 3-month follow-up achieved at least a 50% reduction in their inflammatory acne lesion count. Forty-seven percent of subjects achieved at least a

2-point improvement in their IGA score compared to baseline. The most common side effects of the treatment were postinflammatory erythema and edema, which were transient and for most patients resolved within minutes after procedure completion. There were no reports of hypo- or hyperpigmentation. Anesthesia was not needed for the treatments and most patients reported a pain score of 3 to 4 out of 10[20] (▶ Fig. 11.4, ▶ Fig. 11.5).

The other 1,726-nm laser that has FDA clearance in the United States to treat acne is manufactured by Acurre. It has FDA clearance for treating mild to severe inflammatory acne vulgaris and also has European clearance for treating moderate acne vulgaris. Like the other 1,726-nm laser, it selectively damages the sebaceous glands while the epidermis remains intact. It utilizes highly controlled air cooling and a real-time temperature monitoring feedback safety feature. In the pilot study, 16 patients had select areas of the face and back treated. The contralateral area was not treated. Topical and injectable local anesthetics were used for the treatments. Each patient received four treatments, spaced 1 month apart. Patients were followed 1 and 3 months after the final treatment. There were significant reductions in papules and pustules on the treated side compared to the untreated contralateral side. At the 3 month post treatment completion follow-up, there was an 80% inflammatory lesion count reduction. The laser results showed statistically significant improvements in inflammatory lesions on the treatment side. The most common side effect of the treatment was papules appearing within 24 hours of treatment and resolving within a week without scarring.[21]

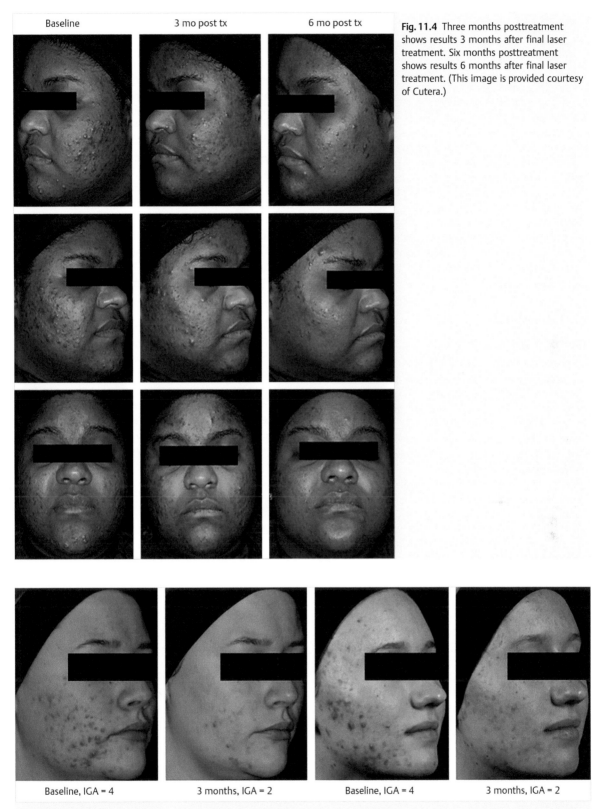

| Baseline | 3 mo post tx | 6 mo post tx |

Fig. 11.4 Three months posttreatment shows results 3 months after final laser treatment. Six months posttreatment shows results 6 months after final laser treatment. (This image is provided courtesy of Cutera.)

| Baseline, IGA = 4 | 3 months, IGA = 2 | Baseline, IGA = 4 | 3 months, IGA = 2 |

Fig. 11.5 Patient A's Baseline IGA=4 and 3 months after final treatment, IGA=2. Patient B's baseline IGA=4 and 3 months after final treatment, IGA=2. (This image is provided courtesy of Cutera.)

Fractional CO_2 Laser

Unlike all of the above-mentioned lasers, the CO_2 laser is an ablative laser treatment, causing obliteration of the epidermis and part of the dermis. Newer CO_2 lasers operate in a fractional manner such that the laser produces a pixelated ablation of the skin, leaving interspersed normal tissue. Through this ablation, the CO_2 laser causes destruction of sebaceous glands, reducing sebum production and follicular plugging.[22]

Shin et al showed a 54% reduction of papule counts and a 41% reduction of pustule counts in patients treated with one to two sessions of fractional CO_2.[22] However, patients had notable side effects, including pain, erythema, edema, hyperpigmentation, and crusting, with an average downtime of 11.8 days.[22] Despite its efficacy in reduction of acneiform lesions, it is not recommended for the treatment of acne given its marked potential side effects without long-lasting benefit.

11.2.2 Lights

Intense Pulsed Light

Intense pulsed light (IPL) treats acne through several mechanisms of action, which are related to its delivery of light over a broad spectrum (500–1,200 nm).[2] The lower wavelengths in this spectrum, given their proximity to the Soret band, act primarily to reduce *C. acnes* by activating porphyrins. The higher wavelengths, given their preference to be absorbed by water, improve acne by causing sebaceous gland coagulation.

IPL is difficult to study, given the plethora of IPL machines and their inherent differences in fluence and emitted light spectrum. For instance, Deshpande demonstrated reduction in acne lesion count in 80% of patients treated with IPL, as well as improvements in erythema in the majority of patients.[23] However, Mei et al only demonstrated 51% reduction in global lesion counts; this was increased to 75.2% when combined with PDT.[2] Choi et al compared IPL with PDL in a split-faced trial.[24] They showed that while IPL was associated with an earlier and more profound improvement in inflammatory lesions, this was followed by a rebound aggravation within several weeks, as opposed to PDL, which was associated with a gradual and sustained improvement.[24]

Total number of treatments in the above studies varied from one to four; these were spaced weekly to twice weekly.[2,23]

Side effects included erythema, edema, blistering, and crusting.[1,23,24]

Blue and Red Light (without Photosensitizers)

Blue light (407–420 nm) is bactericidal, whereas red light (620–700 nm) is anti-inflammatory.[1] Bacterial protoporphyrin IX and coproporphyrin III have peak absorption at 415 nm, which lies within the blue light spectrum (407–420 nm).[1,25,26] This results in photoactivation of *C. acnes* with development of free oxygen radicals and subsequent bacterial cell damage and death.[1,16,25,27] A limitation of blue light is its poor penetration into the skin; however, when combined with longer wavelengths, deeper penetration can be promoted.[1]

Red light influences the release of cytokines from macrophages, which has anti-inflammatory effects and stimulates fibroblast proliferation.[1,27] The production of growth factors results in healing and wound repair.[1,27] Additionally, the deeper penetration of red light results in photothermolysis of sebaceous glands; the exact mechanism of action is unknown, however.[1]

Papageorgiou et al showed a 76% improvement in inflammatory acneiform lesions in patients treated with combined blue-red light therapy; this improvement was superior to blue light monotherapy.[27] Other studies have demonstrated that improvement with blue and red light is more effective than topical clindamycin, but less effective than PDL, IPL, or PDT.[1] Additionally, treatment with blue and red light is associated with high rates of relapse following discontinuation.[1]

Treatment is relatively well tolerated, with minimal reported side effects. Some patients report mild dryness, erythema, and pigmentary changes, but the irritation and pruritus are less than that reported with topical benzoyl peroxide.[1,25,26,27] Treatments are applied two to four times per week, for a total of 4 to 8 weeks.[25,27]

11.2.3 Photodynamic Therapy

PDT employs topical photosensitizers combined with a light source in order to treat acne.[1] The exogenous photosensitizers are absorbed by the pilosebaceous units, where they are metabolized by the heme biosynthesis pathway.[2] The porphyrins that are produced, including protoporphyrin IX (which is produced in excess by *C. acnes*), are photoactivating, resulting in singlet oxygen and free radical production.[1] This subsequently destroys cell nuclei and membranes, ultimately resulting in cell death of *C. acnes*.[2,6] The sebaceous glands also undergo phototoxic injury, resulting in decreased sebum output.[2,6] In combination, this results in reduction of keratinocyte shedding and follicular obstruction.[1,2] Antimicrobial PDT (aPDT) combines topical antibiotics with PDT, allowing for a lower photosensitizer concentration and lower light fluence to be used.[28]

Photosensitizers include aminolevulinic acid (ALA), liposomal ALA, methyl aminolevulinate (MAL), indole-3-acetic acid (IAA), and indocyanine green (ICG).[1] However, the ideal incubator is unclear, along with the time of incubation (30 min–5 h). Light sources include IPL, red light, blue light, ultraviolet (UV) light, PDL, and KTP.[1]

Several studies compare different incubators, and have shown red light to be more effective than IPL for inflammatory lesions; however, IPL was better tolerated, with less pain and erythema.[29]

PDT is difficult to study given the variety of different incubators, incubator times, and light sources, many of which show improvement in the treatment of acne. However, all studies show selective improvement of inflammatory lesions over noninflammatory comedones. Alexiades-Armenakas showed a 77% clearance rate of inflammatory lesions when used with long-pulsed PDL.[1,30]

Despite its effectiveness, PDT is associated with more side effects than other light treatments. Patients commonly report pain, erythema, and edema.[2,6] Less commonly seen side effects include hyperpigmentation, perifollicular pustular eruptions, exudate, and crusting, which are more pronounced with longer incubation times.[1,2]

11.2.4 Photopneumatic Therapy

Photopneumatic therapy uses negative suction pressure to draw target skin into a machine tip, while simultaneously delivering broadband pulsed light.[31,32,33] The suction allows for sebaceous glands to be brought closer to the surface of the skin, with the goal of more efficient energy transmission.[32,33] This vacuum effect results in opening of pores and sebaceous glands, allowing for mechanical removal of sebum, bacteria, and other impurities, opening closed comedones and clogged hair follicles.[31,32,33] The device then delivers broadband light (400–1,200 or 500–1,200 nm) to the treatment area, which works through the mechanisms described earlier, resulting in both anti-inflammatory and bactericidal effects.[31,32] Ultrastructural studies of treated skin demonstrate thermal injury to both *C. acnes* and the pilosebaceous units.[33]

Various studies have demonstrated a 64 to 69% reduction in inflammatory acne lesions, and a 41 to 44% reduction in noninflammatory lesions. Percent improvement increased in patients with more severe baseline disease.[31] Other studies evaluating patient satisfaction revealed some degree of perceived improvement in 82 to 94% of patients.[31,32]

Treatment wavelengths vary depending on the exact device used. The original photopneumatic device, Isolaz, delivered broadband light from 400 to 1,200 nm.[31] The newer photopneumatic device, TheraClearX, delivers broadband light from 500 to 1,200 nm.[34] Treatment intervals range from every 1 to 4 weeks, with one to two passes per treatment, for a total of three to five sessions.[31,32,33] Lower fluences and longer wavelengths are recommended in darker skin types to prevent unwanted thermal damage.[31]

Side effects include slight pain, transient erythema, edema, rare purpura, hyper- or hypopigmentation, and/

or exacerbation of preexisting acne.[31,32] In one study, edema and erythema were noted to improve in severity as the treatment series progressed.[33]

11.2.5 Handheld at Home Devices

Most at-home devices for the treatment of acne employ light in the visible spectrum (red and/or blue light) or heat.[35] The blue and red light devices work through bactericidal and anti-inflammatory mechanisms, as discussed earlier. Combined light and heat devices (LHE) use broad-spectrum light combined with direct heating. The light activates a photochemical reaction in *C. acnes*, like that seen with red and blue light, while the heat accelerates the photochemical reaction and thermally alters sebaceous glands.[36,37] The bacteria respond to heat via "heat shock responses," which result in transcription of genes producing heat shock proteins.[35] This causes bacteria to self-destruct and undergo apoptosis.[36]

Studies evaluating the efficacy of these treatments are difficult to assess, given that they are often small studies without control groups, are unblended, and often industry sponsored (thus introducing potential bias). Although some studies show reduction of up to 76.8% of inflammatory acne lesions, others show limited efficacy, with reduction of lesion duration by 1 day on average.[37]

These treatments are self-applied anywhere from twice weekly to up to twice daily by consumers at home.[36] They are relatively safe, with patients reporting transient warmth and dryness; however, they are quite time intensive.[35,37]

11.2.6 Radiofrequency

There are few studies that look at the use of radiofrequency devices in the treatment of acne. They work by heating dermal tissues and increasing metabolism of sebaceous glands, which results in gland shrinkage and decreased sebum output.[38,39] The simultaneous cooling of the epidermis prevents any superficial damage.[39] Furthermore, the pilosebaceous unit has higher electrical resistance as compared to surrounding tissues, which allows for selective follicular heating.[38] This minimizes side effects, which are limited to mild pain.

Yu and Huang demonstrated a 42% reduction in active acne lesions for patients who received six weekly treatments, and this response was sustained at follow-up visits at 4 weeks.[38]

11.2.7 Fractional Microneedling Radiofrequency

Fractional microneedling radiofrequency (FMR) uses an array of microneedles to deliver current to the dermis, resulting in heat production and thermal injury, as described earlier.[39,40] However, traditional radiofrequency is limited by its depth of penetration, and microneedles help overcome this, allowing for dermal delivery.[40,41] Insulation ensures that the radiofrequency is only delivered at the tip of each needle, ensuring targeted delivery to the dermis and preventing epidermal damage.[41] Microneedles further affect acne pathogenesis through their own mechanism of action, by promoting secretion of growth factors which recruit keratinocytes and fibroblasts.[41] This ultimately results in collagen synthesis and remodeling.[40,41]

Min et al demonstrated an 80% reduction in inflammatory acne lesions, and a 65% reduction in noninflammatory lesions after two treatments of FMR, spaced 4 weeks apart.[40] Molecular studies from these patients revealed a decrease in inflammatory markers, specifically nuclear factor-kappa B (NF-κB) and interleukin 8 (IL-8), the latter of which has been shown to correlate with acne grade.[40] Additionally, patients demonstrated a statistically significant decrease in sebum excretion, which was sustained at follow-up at 2 months. This desirable effect is thought to be secondary to the deeper penetration provided by the microneedles, which allows for greater heating of sebaceous glands.[40]

Kim et al similarly revealed a 90.11% reduction in inflammatory lesions 3 months after three total treatments, each spaced 4 weeks apart.[41] Noninflammatory lesions showed a 76.64% reduction at this 3-month follow-up. Mean decrease in sebum excretion at 3 months was 36.99%.

These studies used an applicator tip compromised of 49 insulated microneedles. Treatments were delivered every 4 weeks at a radiofrequency level of 2 to 3 for 50 to 80 milliseconds, with a depth of 1.5 mm. Passes were delivered with slight overlap, and totaled between two and three per treatment.[40,41]

Treatment was well tolerated aside from pain and transient erythema, swelling, pinpoint bleeding, scaling, and crusting. These all subsided within 1 week.[40,41]

11.3 Patient Selection

Acne patients desiring to undergo laser treatment for their acne must primarily understand that there is no laser or light device that offers a permanent cure for their acne. They must also realize that results are variable and that there is a downtime or healing time associated with most modalities. Therefore, the practitioner must set up realistic expectations when counseling the patient and forgo treatment on those with unrealistic expectations.

Many of the lasers and devices, especially those in the visible wavelength, are safest when performed on patients when their skin is at their fairest (not suntanned). A preexisting suntan may increase the risk of side effects such as dyspigmentation and scarring. Those with active skin infections, such as impetigo or herpes simplex virus, should not undergo treatment. Patients with a history of herpes simplex virus may need prophylactic treatment with oral antiviral medications.

It was previously dogma that acne patients having undergone treatment with oral isotretinoin had to wait 6 to 12 months before undergoing a laser or light procedure due to a potential increased risk of scarring. However, more research is now suggesting that treatment immediately after isotretinoin treatment or even during isotretinoin treatment may be safe.

11.4 Technique/Postoperative Instructions

The practitioner should be experienced with each laser and light device prior to using it on acne patients as acne is not commonly treated with lasers and lasers are often reserved for other cutaneous conditions. Technique is dependent upon the device used and the previously mentioned settings for each device are not necessarily the ideal settings. Additionally, settings may vary based upon skin phototype. Postoperative instructions vary among the lasers and devices. The physician should provide both verbal and written instructions to the patient regarding postoperative care.

11.5 Potential Complications and Management of Complications

Complications of laser treatments are mentioned earlier for each specific laser and include the following: prolonged erythema, edema, crusting, blistering, dyspigmentation, scarring, and infection. Erythema will resolve with time and edema can be minimized with ice and/or oral corticosteroids. Sun avoidance should be strictly adhered to after any laser treatment to prevent dyspigmentation especially in those who experience crusting or blistering. Any infections that result from a treatment should be swiftly treated with the appropriate antimicrobial and should be followed carefully to minimize the risk of scarring. It has been reported that some laser treatments result in a temporary acne flare. Whether this is due to the device itself or the postoperative care (i.e., topicals that are applied) remains to be determined. As with any complication, close communication and follow-up with the patient remains critical for ensuring patient safety and satisfaction.

11.6 Pearls and Pitfalls

As mentioned earlier, the practitioner offering laser or light treatment should be experienced with device use and should set up realistic expectations for the patient. A deficiency in either device experience or patient communication will result in subpar outcomes and low satisfaction. The practitioner must understand and convey to the patient that although they may be helpful, lasers and lights are not the gold standard for treating acne and that other topical and oral therapeutic modalities may be preferred.

References

[1] Tong LX, Brauer JA. Lasers, light, and the treatment of acne: a comprehensive review of the literature. J Drugs Dermatol. 2017; 16 (11):1095–1102

[2] Mei X, Shi W, Piao Y. Effectiveness of photodynamic therapy with topical 5-aminolevulinic acid and intense pulsed light in Chinese acne vulgaris patients. Photodermatol Photoimmunol Photomed. 2013; 29(2):90–96

[3] Yilmaz O, Senturk N, Yuksel EP, et al. Evaluation of 532-nm KTP laser treatment efficacy on acne vulgaris with once and twice weekly applications. J Cosmet Laser Ther. 2011; 13(6):303–307

[4] Dréno B, Pécastaings S, Corvec S, Veraldi S, Khammari A, Roques C. Cutibacterium acnes (Propionibacterium acnes) and acne vulgaris: a brief look at the latest updates. J Eur Acad Dermatol Venereol. 2018; 32(2) Suppl 2:5–14

[5] Leheta TM. Role of the 585-nm pulsed dye laser in the treatment of acne in comparison with other topical therapeutic modalities. J Cosmet Laser Ther. 2009; 11(2):118–124

[6] Orringer JS, Sachs DL, Bailey E, Kang S, Hamilton T, Voorhees JJ. Photodynamic therapy for acne vulgaris: a randomized, controlled, split-face clinical trial of topical aminolevulinic acid and pulsed dye laser therapy. J Cosmet Dermatol. 2010; 9(1):28–34

[7] Sadick N. An open-label, split-face study comparing the safety and efficacy of Levulan kerastick (aminolevulonic acid) plus a 532 nm KTP laser to a 532 nm KTP laser alone for the treatment of moderate facial acne. J Drugs Dermatol. 2010; 9(3):229–233

[8] Jih MH, Friedman PM, Goldberg LH, Robles M, Glaich AS, Kimyai-Asadi A. The 1450-nm diode laser for facial inflammatory acne vulgaris: dose-response and 12-month follow-up study. J Am Acad Dermatol. 2006; 55(1):80–87

[9] Rai R, Natarajan K. Laser and light based treatments of acne. Indian J Dermatol Venereol Leprol. 2013; 79(3):300–309

[10] Lee MW. Combination 532-nm and 1064-nm lasers for noninvasive skin rejuvenation and toning. Arch Dermatol. 2003; 139(10):1265–1276

[11] Yoon HJ, Lee DH, Kim SO, Park KC, Youn SW. Acne erythema improvement by long-pulsed 595-nm pulsed-dye laser treatment: a pilot study. J Dermatolog Treat. 2008; 19(1):38–44

[12] Orringer JS, Kang S, Hamilton T, et al. Treatment of acne vulgaris with a pulsed dye laser: a randomized controlled trial. JAMA. 2004; 291 (23):2834–2839

[13] Lekwuttikarn R, Tempark T, Chatproedprai S, Wananukul S. Randomized, controlled trial split-faced study of 595-nm pulsed dye laser in the treatment of acne vulgaris and acne erythema in adolescents and early adulthood. Int J Dermatol. 2017; 56(8):884–888

[14] Kesty K, Goldberg DJ. 650 µsec 1064nm Nd:YAG laser treatment of acne: a double-blind randomized control study. J Cosmet Dermatol. 2020; 19(9):2295–2300

[15] Painthankar DY, Sakamoto FH, Farinelli WA, et al. Acne treatment based on selective photothermolysis of sebaceous follicles with topically delivered light-absorbing gold microparticles. J Invest Dermatol. 2015; 135(7):1727–1734

[16] Noborio R, Nishida E, Morita A. Clinical effect of low-energy double-pass 1450nm laser treatment for acne in Asians. Photodermatol Photoimmunol Photomed. 2009; 25(1):3–7

[17] Bernstein EF. A pilot investigation comparing low-energy, double pass 1,450nm laser treatment of acne to conventional single-pass, high-energy treatment. Lasers Surg Med. 2007; 39(2):193–198

[18] Sakamoto FH, Doukas AG, Farinelli WA, Tannous Z, Shinn M, Benson S, et al. Selective photothermolysis to target sebaceous glands: theoretical estimation of parameters and preliminary results using a free electron laser. Lasers Surg Med. 2012; 44(2):175–183

[19] Tanghetti Emil A, et al. Safety and efficacy data in a pilot study of the treatment of acne with a 1726 nm fibre laser. In: Lasers in Surgery and Medicine. Vol. 52. Wiley: USA, 2020

[20] Data on file. FDA clearance study. Cutera Inc

[21] Tanghetti E, Geronemus R, Bloom B, Anderson RR, Ross EV, Sakamoto, FW. Safety and efficacy data in a pilot study of the treatment of acne with a fiber laser. Poster accepted for presentation at 40th ASLMS Annual Conference. 2020 April 29 - May 3. Phoenix, AZ, USA

[22] Shin JU, Lee SH, Jung JY, Lee JH. A split-face comparison of a fractional microneedle radiofrequency device and fractional carbon dioxide laser therapy in acne patients. J Cosmet Laser Ther. 2012; 14(5):212–217

[23] Deshpande AJ. Efficacy and safety evaluation of high-density intense pulsed light in the treatment of grades II and IV acne vulgaris as monotherapy in dark-skinned women of child bearing age. J Clin Aesthet Dermatol. 2018; 11(4):43–48

[24] Choi YS, Suh HS, Yoon MY, Min SU, Lee DH, Suh DH. Intense pulsed light vs. pulsed-dye laser in the treatment of facial acne: a randomized split-face trial. J Eur Acad Dermatol Venereol. 2010; 24 (7):773–780

[25] Tremblay JF, Sire DJ, Lowe NJ, Moy RL. Light-emitting diode 415 nm in the treatment of inflammatory acne: an open-label, multicentric, pilot investigation. J Cosmet Laser Ther. 2006; 8(1):31–33

[26] Ammad S, Gonzales M, Edwards C, Finlay AY, Mills C. An assessment of the efficacy of blue light phototherapy in the treatment of acne vulgaris. J Cosmet Dermatol. 2008; 7(3):180–188

[27] Papageorgiou P, Katsambas A, Chu A. Phototherapy with blue (415 nm) and red (660 nm) light in the treatment of acne vulgaris. Br J Dermatol. 2000; 142(5):973–978

[28] Pérez-Laguna V, Pérez-Artiaga L, Lampaya-Pérez V, et al. Bactericidal effect of photodynamic therapy, alone or in combination with mupirocin or linezolid, on Staphylococcus aureus. Front Microbiol. 2017; 8:1002

[29] Zhang L, Wu Y, Zhang Y, et al. Topical 5-aminolevulinic photodynamic therapy with red light vs intense pulsed light for the treatment of acne vulgaris: a spilt face, randomized, prospective study. Dermatoendocrinol. 2017; 9(1):e1375634

[30] Alexiades-Armenakas M. Long-pulsed dye laser-mediated photodynamic therapy combined with topical therapy for mild to severe comedonal, inflammatory, or cystic acne. J Drugs Dermatol. 2006; 5(1):45–55

[31] Rajabi-Estarabadi A, Choragudi S, Camacho I, Moore KJ, Keri JE, Nouri K. Effectiveness of photopneumatic technology: a descriptive review of the literature. Lasers Med Sci. 2018; 33(8):1631–1637

[32] Lee EJ, Lim HK, Shin MK, Suh DH, Lee SJ, Kim NI. An open-label, split-face trial evaluating efficacy and safty of photopneumatic therapy for the treatment of acne. Ann Dermatol. 2012; 24(3):280–286

[33] Narurkar VA, Gold M, Shamban AT. Photopneumatic technology used in combination with profusion therapy for the treatment of acne. J Clin Aesthet Dermatol. 2013; 6(9):36–40

[34] http://www.theraclearx.com/

[35] Hession MT, Markova A, Graber EM. A review of hand-held, home-use cosmetic laser and light devices. Dermatol Surg. 2015; 41(3):307–320

[36] Sadick NS, Laver Z, Laver L. Treatment of mild-to-moderate acne vulgaris using a combined light and heat energy device: home-use clinical study. J Cosmet Laser Ther. 2010; 12(6):276–283

[37] Gold MH, Sensing W, Biron JA. Clinical efficacy of home-use blue-light therapy for mild-to moderate acne. J Cosmet Laser Ther. 2011; 13(6):308–314

[38] Yu JN, Huang P. Use of a TriPollar radio-frequency device for the treatment of acne vulgaris. J Cosmet Laser Ther. 2011; 13(2):50–53

[39] Lee KR, Lee EG, Lee HJ, Yoon MS. Assessment of treatment efficacy and sebosuppressive effect of fractional radiofrequency microneedle on acne vulgaris. Lasers Surg Med. 2013; 45(10):639–647

[40] Min S, Park SY, Yoon JY, Suh DH. Comparison of fractional microneedling radiofrequency and bipolar radiofrequency on acne and acne scar and investigation of mechanism: comparative randomized controlled clinical trial. Arch Dermatol Res. 2015; 307 (10):897–904

[41] Kim ST, Lee KH, Sim HJ, Suh KS, Jang MS. Treatment of acne vulgaris with fractional radiofrequency microneedling. J Dermatol. 2014; 41 (7):586–591

12 Chemical Peels

Ezra Hazan, Seaver L. Soon, and Hooman Khorasani

Summary

Chemical peels are a safe and cost-effective treatment for a variety of cosmetic and medical conditions. They work by inducing epidermal and dermal ablation at varying levels, depending on the chemical and concentration, among other factors. Superficial peels penetrate to the level of the epidermis and can treat acne, melasma, skin texture, and fine lines with little to no downtime. Medium-depth peels penetrate to the level of the papillary dermis and can be used to treat scarring, fine lines, and signs of photoaging, such as actinic keratoses and lentigines. Deep peels ablate to the level of the reticular dermis and can be used to treat focal scars or for facial resurfacing of deep wrinkles. Proper patient selection, peel and concentration selection, pre- and postpeel regimen, technique, and postprocedure care are all essential in performing an effective peel. When used in the appropriate skin type, peels are well tolerated and considered safe.

Keywords: chemical peels, resurfacing, melasma, wrinkles, photoaging, TCA, Jessner's solution

12.1 Introduction

Chemical peeling, or chemexfoliation, is the application of caustic acidic or basic compounds, which leads to cutaneous destruction at different depths. As the ablated skin layers exfoliate, or "peel," normal wound healing takes place, which brings with it rejuvenation and desired clinical results. Chemical peels were introduced in the literature over a century ago for resurfacing. They have since evolved into a cornerstone of cosmetic rejuvenation but maintain noncosmetic applications. Chemical peels carry a long history of safety and efficacy with relatively low cost and straightforward technical application. They can be employed alone or in combination with other invasive and noninvasive procedures and cosmeceuticals for overall facial rejuvenation.

12.2 Modalities/Treatment Option Available

12.2.1 Peel Categorizations

Chemical peels are categorized by the depth of their penetration, as superficial, medium, and deep. The depth in turn depends on the chemical and its concentration, number of coats applied and contact time, peel technique, treatment location, and prepeel preparation.

Peels can be applied to a focal area (like a scar), a single cosmetic subunit, or the entire face. Segmental peeling refers to the differential peeling of various cosmetic subunits since different levels of ablation may be required in various cosmetic subunits.

12.2.2 Mechanism of Action

The clinical endpoint of most chemical peels is defined by erythema or the level of frosting, which correlates with keratocoagulation and penetration into the dermis.[1] This has been best described in the context of trichloroacetic acid (TCA) peeling. Level I frosting is described as scant patchy frosting with a background of erythema (▶ Fig. 12.1). This is seen in superficial peels, if any frosting is seen at all. Level II frosting is uniform white coating with visible underlying erythema (▶ Fig. 12.2). Level III frosting is a white enamel coating without background erythema (▶ Fig. 12.3); this indicates penetration into the papillary or upper reticular dermis, as seen in medium-depth peels.[1]

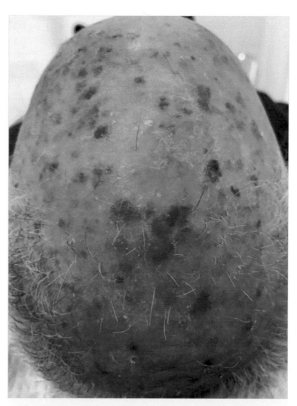

Fig. 12.1 Male scalp treated with Jessner's solution demonstrating level I frost: patchy, reticulate "frost" with diffuse background erythema. Notably, the so-called frost of Jessner's solution represents salicylic acid crystal precipitation, rather than keratin coagulation, which occurs with the frost that develops with trichloroacetic acid. (This image is provided courtesy of Dr. Seaver L. Soon.)

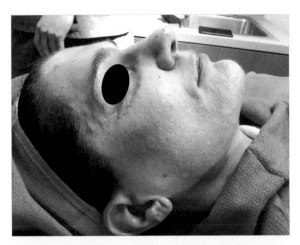

Fig. 12.3 Patient at the completion of the Brody medium-depth peel using solid CO_2 and trichloroacetic acid 35% demonstrating level III frost: solid white frost without visible background erythema. (This image is provided courtesy of Dr. Seaver L. Soon.)

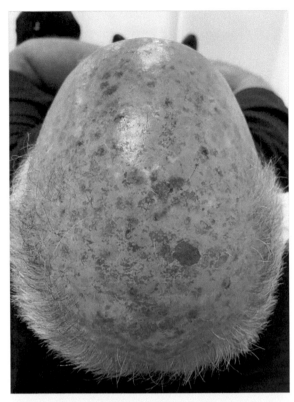

Fig. 12.2 Male scalp after application of multiple coats of trichloroacetic acid 35% demonstrating level II frost: diffuse white frosting with some background erythema. The circular erosive patch on the right vertex represents a thin seborrheic keratosis that was inadvertently removed during the peeling procedure. (This image is provided courtesy of Dr. Seaver L. Soon.)

Some superficial peels, for example, glycolic acid (GA), may be time dependent and require neutralization, whereas other peels such as salicylic acid (SA) or TCA are self-limited in their action and thus do not require neutralization.

12.2.3 Peel Categories

Superficial Peels

Superficial peels cause injury limited to the epidermis and may extend to, but not through, the dermoepidermal junction. They are usually well tolerated with some stinging and burning, and may produce level I frosting. Postprocedure erythema and exfoliation may last up to a few days with superficial peels. These peels are best applied every 2 to 4 weeks for a total of four to six treatments, with progressively increasing strength, as needed and tolerated. Regular, maintenance peels should also be incorporated to sustain the clinical improvement, which can wane to prepeel levels within a few months as a result of normal epidermal turnover.[2] It should be noted that multiple superficial peels do not equate to a medium-depth or deep peel. Pre- and postpeel topical

regimens are essential for optimal outcome and results. Common superficial peels include 10 to 25% TCA, tretinoin, 20 to 30% SA, GA, Jessner's solution (JS), lactic acid, and pyruvic acid.

Salicylic Acid

SA is a beta-hydroxy acid with anti-inflammatory, antimicrobial, keratolytic, comedolytic, and depigmenting properties.[3] SA carries inherent anesthetic properties, making it potentially less painful than other superficial peels. It is present in JS or can be used alone in higher concentrations. SA produces less inflammation than other peels, making it a preferred agent for those susceptible to postinflammatory hyperpigmentation (PIH), and even for treating PIH and melasma.[4] Its comedolytic and anti-inflammatory properties make it a great choice for both comedonal and inflammatory acne. A lipophilic derivative of SA, lipohydroxy acid (LHA), has less skin penetration than SA, enhancing tolerability.[5]

Tretinoin

Tretinoin or, all-trans retinoic acid, peels can be used as superficial peels. Aside from retinoids being used as a mainstay topical treatment for acne and photoaging, they can be applied as peels using 0.5 to 1.0% concentrations. These peels can be used to treat acne, melasma, and PIH. They are self-limited peels that do not require neutralization.

Trichloroacetic Acid

TCA can be used as a superficial, medium-depth, or deep peel, depending on the concentration. The concentration of TCA should be defined using the weight to volume method because other methods can significantly change the relative strength.[6] TCA is a keratolytic and denatures epidermal and dermal proteins. After it has coagulated a certain amount of protein, it self-neutralizes. Further coats or another peel solution may be used at that time to deepen the peel for the desired outcome. Stinging and burning begins almost immediately, and progressively worsens over the first 2 to 3 minutes, then subsides as white frosting appears. TCA 10 to 20% can produce level I frosting and are effective in treating acne.[7] TCA can be effective in treating dyspigmentation, but PIH is a concern, especially with darker Fitzpatrick skin phototype (FSP). Lower concentrations of TCA allow for more controlled reactions, which may lengthen the overall procedure time but provide a safe way to treat darker FSP patients.[8]

Jessner's Solution

JS consists of 14% resorcinol, 14% SA, and 14% lactic acid in 95% ethanol. Modified JS (MJS) contains 17% lactic acid, 17% SA, and 8% citric acid in 95% ethanol. MJS removed resorcinol, which can cause thyroid toxicity, allergic contact dermatitis, and PIH as a contact irritant. These ingredients are keratolytics. Depending on the number of coats applied, they may cause exfoliation from the level of the stratum corneum to the upper layers of the epidermis. These peels can be used alone as a superficial peeling agent and may be repeated every 2 to 3 months, or can be combined with other peels. The clinical endpoint is blotchy erythema or uniform frosting, depending on the desired depth.[4] Commonly, they are combined with another peel, like TCA, for a moderate-depth penetration. Jessner's peels are used to treat acne, PIH, lentigines, skin dullness, freckles, and photodamage[9] (▶ Fig. 12.4).

Alpha Hydroxy Acids

Alpha hydroxy acids (AHAs) include glycolic, pyruvic, and lactic acids, among others. They are naturally formed in foods and induce exfoliation and even epidermolysis at higher concentrations. Over time, they can lead to epidermal thickening, increased dermal collagen, and improved pigmentation.[10] Glycolic and pyruvic acid peels require neutralization with a basic compound, like 5% sodium bicarbonate, or to be rinsed off with water after an appropriate duration of a few minutes. GA is the most commonly used AHA and is available over the counter or for physician purchase. Depending on the concentration, monthly or once to twice weekly applications can be used to treat acne, photoaging, and melasma. Lactic acid and pyruvic acid are less commonly used AHAs. AHAs are widely available in cosmeceuticals for peripeel use as well as part of daily maintenance regimen.

Medium-Depth Peels

Medium-depth peels cause full-thickness epidermal injury, which extends into the papillary or upper reticular dermis. With ablation past the basement membrane,

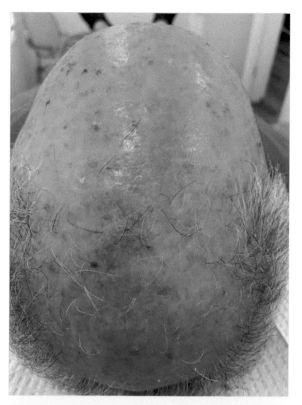

Fig. 12.4 Improvement in lentigines and photodamage of the male scalp using a combination of Jessner's solution followed by trichloroacetic acid 35% (Monheit variation). Result at 2 weeks post-peel. See ▶ Fig. 12.1 for pretreatment comparison. (This image is provided courtesy of Dr. Seaver L. Soon.)

extending down to the level of the papillary dermis, inflammation and collagen remodeling occurs with progressive improvement over the following months. TCA 50% is a medium-depth peel, but has fallen out of favor, given the significant risk of scarring.[7] More commonly, safer concentrations of TCA, usually 35%, are preceded by another superficial peeling agent (such as JS or GA 70%) or a physical agent, such as solid CO_2 (dry ice; ▶ Fig. 12.5). In these cases, a superficial peel acts as a primer to allow for a more even and controlled penetration of TCA, thereby minimizing "hot spots," which are prone to scarring. Medium-depth peels result in epidermal necrosis at day 3 with re-epithelialization occurring at days 7 to 10. They address Glogau level II photoaging, lentigines, actinic keratosis, dyschromias, and mild acne scarring and may serve to blend demarcation lines of other resurfacing procedures[4] (▶ Fig. 12.4). Analgesia may or may not be necessary for medium-depth peeling, but may be achieved by nonsteroidal anti-inflammatory drugs (NSAIDs), anxiolytics, or trigeminal nerve blocks. Common medium-depth peels include Jessner's peel combined with TCA 35% (Monheit's method), GA 70% + TCA 35%

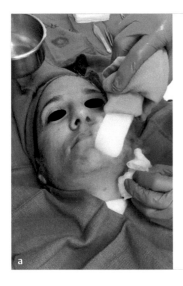
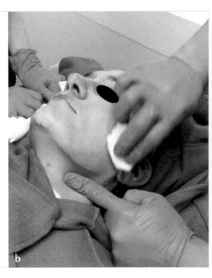

Fig. 12.5 (a) In the Brody variation of medium-depth peeling, a solid block of dry ice is dipped in a solution of 3:1 acetone and alcohol and applied to the skin in gliding movement for cold-induced epidermolysis. **(b)** This skin preparation allows for even papillary dermal penetration of trichloro-acetic acid (TCA) 35%, as evident in the uniform level II frost. (These images are provided courtesy of Dr. Seaver L. Soon.)

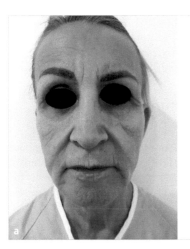
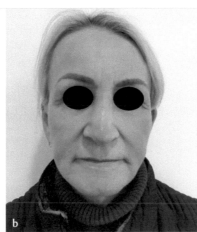

Fig. 12.6 (a,b) This patient underwent a full-face peeling with 33% phenol and 1.1% croton oil (Hetter formula) with significant improvement in static rhytids and overall skin quality. Notably she has had no injectable filler or neurotoxin, demonstrating the lifting and wrinkle softening effects of phenol–croton oil induced tissue remodeling. Result at 6 months post-peel. (These images are provided courtesy of Dr. Seaver L. Soon.)

(Coleman's method), or solid CO_2 + TCA 35% (Brody's method). These combination peels produce a safer and more uniform medium-depth peel. When using combination peels, the second peel may commence once the clinical endpoint of the first peel is met.

Deep Chemical Peels

Deep chemical peels penetrate to the mid-reticular dermis and cause collagen and elastic fiber remodeling. They are composed principally of phenol and croton oil at different concentrations, in combination with a surfactant and water. The formula created by Baker and Gordon had been the standard for decades and consisted of 2.1% croton oil and 49.3% phenol. In 1999, Dr Hetter showed that croton oil, a powerful cytotoxic resin, is the active ingredient.[11] Different concentrations of croton oil may be used to cater to different desired depths. Deep peels are indicated for patients with Glogau type III and IV photoaging and severe

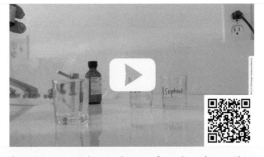

Video 12.1 A properly mixed Hetter formula is shown. This particular peel uses 2 mL of 88% phenol, 2 drops of croton oil, 8 drops of septisol, and 3 mL of water.

acne scarring (▶ Fig. 12.6, ▶ Video 12.1). Additionally, TCA 80 to 100% can be used focally to treat ice pick or boxcar scars, earlobe tears, and xanthelasma.[3]

Phenol–Croton Oil

Phenol–croton oil peels, although they can have dramatic results, also carry significantly more risk. Phenol is known to be cardiotoxic and can precipitate an arrhythmia. Preoperative medical history, electrocardiogram, and laboratory tests including complete blood count (CBC) and comprehensive metabolic panel (CMP) are important prerequisites to patient selection. Cardiac monitoring is required for full-face phenol–croton oil peels, although this is not required for segmental deep chemical peels, where 1 to 2% body surface area is treated with a deep peel (where 1% body surface area is defined as the size of the patient's palm, without fingers) and the remainder of the face is blended with a medium-depth peel.[12] For full-face phenol–croton oil peels, a 10- to 15-minute safety pause should be allowed between cosmetic subunits to allow for phenol and croton oil metabolism and excretion.

12.3 Indications

Applications for chemical peels include both cosmetic and medical conditions. Medical conditions range from epidermal lesions, including actinic keratoses, to acne and pigmentary alterations, including melasma. Cosmetic indications include photoaging, rhytids, blending of demarcation lines from other procedures, and scarring.

12.3.1 Acne

Chemical peels are best utilized as an adjunct to continued medical therapy in acne. They work synergistically; peels produce more rapid results and allow for better penetration of topical therapies. Superficial peels are best utilized to treat acne. These include 30% SA, 30 to 70% GA, and JS. These are safe and effective in mild-to-moderate comedonal and inflammatory acne. Most clinical trials repeated peels every 2 weeks.[10,13] In a split-face, randomized, double-blind trial with 20 patients, SA 30% and GA 30% were similarly effective.[14]

12.3.2 Photoaging

Photoaging describes the summation of skin changes related to chronic sun exposure, namely, irregular pigmentation, atrophy, and wrinkling. Superficial peels can be used to treat fine superficial lines but would require a series of multiple treatments. A split-face study showed that 5 to 10% LHA was equally effective and tolerated as 20 to 50% GA in reducing facial fine lines/wrinkles and hyperpigmentation.[15] Medium-depth and deep peels may be used to treat deeper wrinkles as they result in neocollagenesis, and can be combined with other surgical and nonsurgical cosmetic procedures (▸ Fig. 12.7). Compared to CO_2 laser resurfacing to Baker's phenol peel for upper lip rhytids, Chew et al showed superior improvement with the peel than the laser[16] (▸ Fig. 12.8).

12.3.3 Postinflammatory Hyperpigmentation

GA and SA are most commonly used to treat PIH. One study showed that serial GA peels, in addition to a topical regimen consisting of 0.05% tretinoin cream nightly and hydroquinone 2%/GA 10% gel twice daily, resulted in improved hyperpigmentation compared to the topical regimen alone.[17] Another study, using colorimetric analysis, found that serial biweekly SA 30% peels successfully lightened dark-complected, Asian skin.[18]

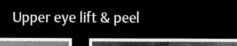

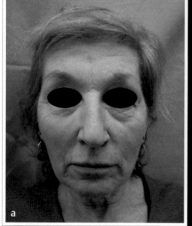
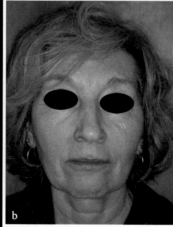

Fig. 12.7 (a, b) Example of a patient who had a trichloroacetic acid (TCA) 35% and upper blepharoplasty. (These images are provided courtesy of Dr. Hooman Khorasani.)

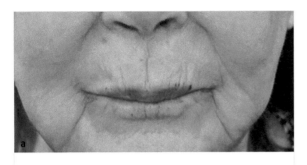

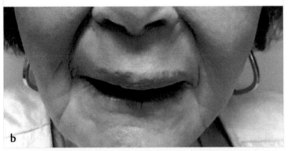

Fig. 12.8 (a, b) Example of a patient with segmental perioral phenol peel not requiring cardiac monitoring. (These images are provided courtesy of Dr. Hooman Khorasani.)

12.3.4 Melasma

Chemical peels can be effective in treating the epidermal variant of melasma using superficial peels and adhering to pre- and postpeel regimens. SA, LA, GA, and JS are the most common peels used for melasma. A split-face study showed similar efficacy between JS and 92% LA in treating melasma; treatment sessions ranged from two to five sessions.[19] A study of dark-skinned patients showed that weekly applications of 1% tretinoin was as effective as, and better tolerated than, weekly 70% GA, in treating melasma.[20]

12.3.5 Scarring

Medium and deep chemical peels may be used to treat acne scarring. Deep phenol peels may also be used for moderate-to-severe acne scarring.[13] JS-TCA 35% peel was performed on 15 Iraqi patients with ice pick and atrophic acne scars. Most received three sessions, with the majority experiencing moderate improvement based on evaluation of serial photographs. PIH was seen in darker FSP but resolved by the 3-month follow-up.[21] In 2002, Lee et al introduced the CROSS (chemical reconstruction of skin scars) technique by applying high TCA concentrations directly and focally into ice pick scars. This leads to focal ablation with rapid healing given the intact adjacent adnexal structures.[22] Lee et al studied 33 patients using 65% TCA and 32 patients using 100% TCA. Two blinded independent clinicians rated good clinical responses in 82 and 94% of patients. Higher treatment courses (five to six sessions) yielded better

results.[22] A 100% TCA CROSS was shown to be safe and effective even in darker FSP.[23]

12.3.6 Actinic Keratosis

A single peel of JS with TCA 35% has also been shown to be as effective as twice daily topical 5-fluorouracil cream for 3 weeks in treatment of actinic keratosis.[24] A study by Tse et al showed that GA-TCA was effective in treating photodamaged skin and slightly more effective than JS-TCA in treating actinic keratosis, with similar healing and downtime.[25] Curettage of hyperkeratosis overlying the actinic keratosis may be performed to hypertrophic actinic keratosis to enable peel penetration and optimize outcomes.

12.4 Patient Selection

12.4.1 History and Physical Examination

A comprehensive history and physical examination are essential in selecting appropriate patients for chemical peels. Special attention should be paid to FSP, prior scarring, and hyperpigmentation. Other pertinent history includes prior peels, resurfacing procedures, invasive and noninvasive lifting procedures, smoking history, and radiation therapy in the area.

Medication history is also important. Topical bleaching agents, such as hydroquinone, may be used pre- and postprocedurally to minimize PIH, especially in darker skin types. Isotretinoin is used frequently for recalcitrant acne. For patients on isotretinoin, a recent American Society for Dermatologic Surgery (ASDS) task force concluded that superficial peels can be safely used in this patient subset. However, insufficient evidence was available to support the use of medium or deep peels in patients who have used isotretinoin within the last 6 months due to a theoretical risk of delayed healing and potential increased risk of scar.[26]

The Glogau photoaging classification system categorizes degrees of sun damage and indicates appropriate level of peeling. Type I is seen in younger patients with mild photodamage and is best managed with superficial peels. Type II, moderate photoaging with dynamic rhytides and some lentigines, may be treated with medium-depth peels. Type III, advanced photoaging patients, with significant dyschromia, actinic keratosis, and static rhytids, may be best served with medium-depth or deep peels. Type IV, severe photoaging, requires deep peeling with surgical rhytidectomy.[27]

12.4.2 Contraindications

Some relative contraindications to chemical peels include active inflammatory skin disease or infection on the face. Patients with poor wound healing, related to undermining surgery within 12 months, or from prior radiation therapy, a history of hypertrophic, or keloidal scarring should be aware that chemical peels may increase the risk of scar formation, especially with medium and deep peels. There are insufficient data on peels in pregnancy and lactation; therefore, they are typically deferred.

It is essential for patients to have realistic expectations in terms of results and downtime, as well as risks. Proper patient selection and education is essential for good outcomes.

12.4.3 Preoperative and Consideration in Darker Skin Types

Tretinoin, or another topical retinoid, applied nightly for 2 to 4 weeks prior to the peel enables even penetration and reduces healing time.[3] FSP IV to VI should stop 1 week prior to the procedure to minimize the risk of PIH. Applying the retinoid on top of a moisturizer can minimize irritation. If retinoid dermatitis develops, peeling should be postponed given the risk of overpenetration and resultant prolonged erythema.[4]

As mentioned earlier, it is common to treat peel patients with bleaching agents periprocedurally. This may minimize the risk of PIH, especially in patients with FSP III or higher. Hydroquinone 2 to 8% twice daily may be used. One of the authors of this chapter (HK) uses Triluma compounded with 8% hydroquinone from a local compounding pharmacy.

Photoprotection should be practiced for 2 to 4 weeks before and after chemical peel, and includes broad-spectrum sunscreen (sun protection factor [SPF] 30 or higher) as well as physical protection from the sun (hats, shade, etc.).

Antiviral prophylaxis is recommended for all patients undergoing medium and deep peels, and may be considered for superficial peels in those with a sensitive history of herpes virus outbreaks. Recommended dosing is valacyclovir 500 mg or 1 g twice daily for 5 to 7 days, beginning the day of the procedure, and may be extended until full re-epithelialization (may need a 14-day course for deep peels).

Test spots may be helpful in darker FSP patients to better predict those who may develop PIH. Pre- and posttreatment with bleaching agents is essential in this population. Clinical endpoints of erythema and frosting may be more difficult to interpret in dark-skinned individuals, and may consequently lead to overtreatment. It is prudent to start with lower concentrations and fewer passes in darker skin types. Combinations of lower concentration peels may be safer than a single peel solution.[28] One of the authors of this chapter (HK) does not perform any medium or deep chemical peels in any individual with FSP III or above.

12.5 Technique

12.5.1 Preprocedure

The skin must be cleaned of any surface impurities prior to peel application. Any makeup and debris are removed

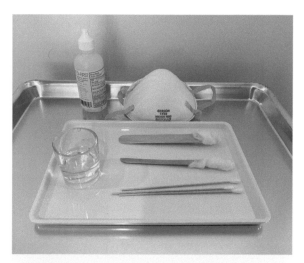

Fig. 12.9 Phenol tray, which includes (*back, left to right*) saline eye wash and N95 mask and (*front, left to right*) glass vessel with mixed phenol–croton oil solution and peel applicators. (This image is provided courtesy of Dr. Seaver L. Soon.)

by the patient washing their own face. Degreasing is an important step to create a smooth surface for an even application, penetration, and clinical response. A study showed no difference using one of four degreasing agents: acetone, alcohol, Hibiclens, or Freon skin degreaser.[29]

A procedure tray should be prepared prior to commencing the peel (▶ Fig. 12.9). The peeling solution should be poured into a basin. The applicators, which may include gauze, cotton balls, brushes, or cotton-tip applicators, should be prepared and opened. Specialized brushes, which minimize waste and speed application time, may be used for superficial peels. Extra gauze should be available on the tray to use to dab any dripping peeling solution. Saline flushes must be readily available in order to rinse the eye in case of inadvertent contact. Anesthesia for superficial peels is not typically necessary. Patients will experience a stinging and burning sensation, which is overall tolerated well. A fan or cool forced air can aid in comfort, in addition to background music and gentle conversation. Music is an excellent distraction and one of the authors of this chapter (HK) prefers to have the Svonos speaker system in each room connected to a desired music service such as Spotify where patients may choose the music. Medium-depth peels usually require nerve blocks, oral NSAIDs, and/or oral or intramuscular anxiolytic or sedative in addition to cool forced air. Full-face deep phenol peels may require intravenous (IV) sedation, although one of the authors of this chapter (SS) performs full-face and segmental phenol–croton oil peeling with oral hydration and anxiolytics. Topical anesthetics may alter the penetration of the peel and therefore their application should be used with caution.

12.5.2 Clinical Endpoints

Chemical peels have clinical endpoints that signal adequate dosing. Understanding when these endpoints are met allows one to properly execute an effective peel, for example, whether another pass is required or if gauze should be applied to remove excess solution. Some peels only produce erythema, whereas others are time-based peels without a reliable clinical endpoint. Peels that penetrate into the dermis produce frosting, which is the clinical sign of dermal protein coagulation. There are three levels of frosting correlating with different depths of dermal penetration. Level I is light reticular frost with erythema (▶ Fig. 12.1); level II has a confluence of light white frost with erythema (▶ Fig. 12.2); and level III is solid white frost (▶ Fig. 12.3).

Epidermal slide is a sign of extension to the papillary dermis in medium-depth peels. It is due to edema, which creates an exaggerated wrinkling upon pinching the skin. This sign is transient; as epidermal and dermal proteins coagulate together, the epidermis re-adheres to the dermis.[30]

12.5.3 Procedure

Peels should be performed quickly and efficiently to minimize discomfort. Most providers position themselves at the head of the bed and with the patient supine. The peel applicators are dipped into the peeling solution; they should be saturated but not dripping with fluid. Different amounts of saturation are used for different areas. Higher saturations may be used for thicker, more sebaceous skin, like the glabella, nose, and medial cheeks and forehead. The peel is started from the forehead and systematically worked downward on the face. On the cheeks, one should apply the peel from the medial cheeks laterally, which will deposit more solution medially, where there is more resistance to scarring.

Feathering peel application into the hairline and below the mandibular shadow will hide demarcation lines. In treating rhytids, stretching the skin will allow an even application into the skin folds. Smaller, deeper rhytids may be treated focally with the wooden end of a cotton-tip applicator.

Before applying another coat of peeling solution, one must wait to observe the clinical endpoint to evolve to avoid overapplication of solution. For most solutions, this is achieved in 3 to 5 minutes, with the exception of AHAs such as GA, which are time-dependent.

The periorbital region is usually saved for last and is done cautiously. Cotton-tip applicators are dipped but not fully saturated and are "rolled" into the lower eyelid skin from the infraorbital crease. Additionally, two dry cotton-tip applicators can be held at the medial and lateral canthi to prevent inadvertent acid leaking into the eye and tears from trickling down the cheek, which may theoretically carry the peeling solution onto thinner neck skin, which may be more prone to scar. A dry gauze may be held in the nondominant hand to catch inadvertent leaks onto the neck.

Hyperkeratotic lesions, such as seborrheic keratosis, actinic keratosis, or dermal lesions such as sebaceous hyperplasia may be gently and safely treated with hyfrecation and curettage prior to chemical peeling directly over the wound.

To treat ice pick scars using the TCA CROSS technique, sharpened wooden applicators are dipped into 65 to 100% TCA. The TCA is focally applied by pressing the tip into the atrophic scar. Frosting should be expected within 10 seconds of application. Multiple treatment sessions spaced 1 to 3 months apart are typically required.

When combining with other surgical procedures, the chemical peel is performed first. When done in conjunction with a blepharoplasty, plastic eye shields are inserted prior to placing a 5-mm rim of Aquaphor along the tarsal plate. The chemical peel is then performed to its desired clinical endpoint.

12.5.4 Specific Peels

Glycolic Acid

GA peels are time dependent, and range from 15 seconds to 2 minutes. Mild erythema, microvesiculation and pinpoint frosting around acne lesions may be clinical endpoints in addition to patient comfort level. After adequate time and/or clinical endpoints, GA peels must be neutralized with 5% sodium bicarbonate or rinsed off with water. In addition to higher concentration, longer application times may be warranted in subsequent treatments.[7]

Salicylic Acid

Peels are self-limited and do not require neutralization. Typically, they are left on the skin for 5 to 6 minutes before wiping off the SA crystals with a wet washcloth. Clinically, there is immediate white precipitation, which can inform the applicator of any potential skip areas that can then be spot-treated. SA has inherent anesthetic properties, making it less painful. SA peels can come in two different vehicles. The hydroalcoholic vehicle evaporates leaving a pseudofrost and mild desquamation after 2 days. A polyethylene glycol vehicle increases follicular penetration without pseudofrost or desquamation. In a study by Dainichi et al, the polyethylene glycol SA peels were effective and very well tolerated—less stinging, less burning, and no peeling or PIH.[4,31]

Tretinoin

Tretinoin peels are not time dependent and do not require neutralization. They leave a yellowish hue to the skin, which can indicate the treated areas. Fine white desquamation is expected 2 to 3 days after the peel.

Jessner's Solution

JS is also self-limited and does not require neutralization. This peel is typically left on the skin for 5 to 6 minutes and then wiped off with a wet washcloth. JS will lead to erythema and speckled whitening. Patients will experience mild stinging and burning. Repeat layered may be used after a few minutes' delay, which can lead to more confluent whitening. If JS is used as a priming peel, the second peeling agent, commonly TCA, is applied on top of the JS after about 6 minutes. In this setting, the priming peel is applied further down, below the jaw, so as to stagger the demarcation of treated and untreated skin.

Trichloroacetic Acid

TCA peels cause whitening as it coagulates protein and penetrates the epidermis and dermis. This process takes approximately 30 seconds, after which it cannot be diluted or removed. Burning and discomfort begin within a few seconds of application and reach their peak after about 30 to 90 seconds.[7] The onset of whitening signals the onset of pain relief as well as protein coagulation.

Phenol–Croton Oil

Phenol peels penetrate the skin rapidly to the level of the reticular dermis, producing level III frosting. While performing these peels, one should wait 10 to 15 minutes between each cosmetic unit to minimize toxicity.[32]

12.5.5 Neutralization

GA and pyruvic acid peels require neutralization after a time endpoint (typically 2 minutes) or a clinical endpoint (either pain, focal erythema, or frost) is achieved using 5% sodium bicarbonate or water to dilute the peeling solution.

12.6 Postpeel Instructions

12.6.1 In-Office

After the peel is complete, a thin layer of petrolatum ointment or emollient is applied. Forced cool air, cold, wet gauze, or ice packs may be used after medium-depth peels for pain relief. This is followed by bland petrolatum ointment application.

For superficial peels, erythema may last for a few hours or up to 2 days and resolve with fine desquamation on days 3 to 4, depending on the peel used. Deeper peels can expect swelling onset for the first 2 days and darkening of the skin, especially lentigines and keratosis after 24 hours. Medium-depth and deep peels will desquamate and re-epithelialize at around days 7 to 10. Residual erythema will fade over 1 month or 2 to 3 months for medium-depth and deep peels, respectively. All patients should be instructed not to pick at or peel off the desquamating skin.

12.6.2 At Home

For home care, superficial peels require only using gentle cleaner and bland moisturizer two to three times per day. For deeper peels, dilute acetic acid may be used as an antiseptic wash to cleanse the area followed by repeated application of bland petrolatum ointment three to five times per day until re-epithelization is complete (7–12 days). One of the authors of this chapter (HK) prefers to switch patients from Aquaphor to coconut oil by day 3 as Aquaphor can be extremely comedogenic with prolonged use.

Continued photoprotection and sunscreen should be maintained throughout. Routine and maintenance skin regimen can be restarted once the skin has fully re-epithelialized.

12.7 Complications and Their Management

12.7.1 Scarring

When treating off the face, there is a higher risk of scarring given the fewer adnexal structures that aid in healing. Thus, only superficial peels should be used off the face. Recent isotretinoin use, facial surgery, or smoking may increase risk of scarring.[33] Focal erythema and induration may portend incipient scarring and should be treated using intralesional or high-potency topical corticosteroids. Pulsed dye lasers may also be used to treat incipient hypertrophic or keloid scars. Bony prominences, such as the zygoma or mandible, are at higher risk of scarring. Other areas of the face prone to scarring include the lateral and inferior cheek, particularly in non-hair-bearing female skin.

12.7.2 Infection

Infection after peeling can be of bacterial, viral, or fungal origins. Patients with concern for infection should be seen in the office for evaluation, culture, and potassium hydroxide preparation, if needed. Clinical signs for bacterial infection include pain and honey-crusting; clinical signs for herpetic infection include pain and scalloped, punched-out erosions or vesicles; and clinical sings for candidal infection include itch and satellite pustulosis. Candidal infection is the diagnosis that is often overlooked as it typically presents much later during the postoperative phase. Prophylactic broad-spectrum antibiotics, treatment dosing of valacyclovir (1 g thrice a day) and oral antifungals should be instituted promptly based on clinical suspicion to prevent scarring.

12.7.3 Postinflammatory Pigment Alteration

Whenever performing a procedure that injures skin, there is a risk of causing hyper- or hypopigmentation, particularly in FSP III or higher patients and with deeper peels. Strict adherence to pre- and postpeel regimens may guard against this potential complication and test spots may be useful for, but not entirely predictive of, response prior to proceeding with full-face peeling. One of the authors of the chapter (HK) does not recommend any type of medium or deep chemical peels in patients with FSP III or higher.

12.7.4 Acne and Folliculitis

Acne and folliculitis may flare postpeel, possibly from occlusive postpeel emollients. These are best managed with oral tetracycline class oral antibiotics since topical therapy may be irritating.

12.7.5 Pruritus

Patients may experience itching during the healing period. Cool compresses, emollients, and oral antihistamines may provide relief. Low- to mid-potency topical corticosteroids may also be used cautiously, with deference to the risk of steroid atrophy.

12.7.6 Prolonged Erythema

Prolonged erythema is defined as erythema beyond 3 months for medium-depth peels and 6 months for deep peels. Postpeel erythema typically self-resolves, but for prolonged erythema, topical steroids or a pulsed dye laser can be employed.

12.8 Pearls and Pitfalls

Choose a few peels to offer in your practice. These peels will be available to your patients as treatments for the various cosmetic and/or medical indications that commonly present to your office. You will become an expert in these peels—from the pre- and postprocedure requirements to effective counseling and ideal patient selection. You will form efficiencies with your entire medical team and staff to safely and effectively perform these peels in a cost-effective manner.

Become familiar with specific applicators and stick to those since they may vary in the amount of solution they transfer to the skin, leading to unpredictable results.

Perform your first peels on family and friends. Ask for feedback during the procedure and during their recovery. Ask them permission to take photographs, which you can then use to counsel patients.

Whenever using peels to blend demarcation lines from other resurfacing procedures, the peel should be performed first. This will prevent the peel solution from penetrating deeper into adjacent resurfaced skin. Avoid medium or deep peels in darker skin individuals.

References

[1] Soleymani T, Lanoue J, Rahman Z. A practical approach to chemical peels: a review of fundamentals and step-by-step algorithmic protocol for treatment. J Clin Aesthet Dermatol. 2018; 11(8):21–28

[2] Butler PE, Gonzalez S, Randolph MA, Kim J, Kollias N, Yaremchuk MJ. Quantitative and qualitative effects of chemical peeling on photo-aged skin: an experimental study. Plast Reconstr Surg. 2001; 107(1): 222–228

[3] Lee KC, Wambier CG, Soon SL, et al. International Peeling Society. Basic chemical peeling: Superficial and medium-depth peels. J Am Acad Dermatol. 2019; 81(2):313–324

[4] Monheit GD, Chastain MA. Chemical and mechanical skin resurfacing. In: Bolognia JL, Schaffer JV, Lorenzo C, eds. Dermatology. 4th ed. Beijing, China: Elsevier; 2018:2593–2609

[5] Zeichner JA. The use of lipohydroxy acid in skin care and acne treatment. J Clin Aesthet Dermatol. 2016; 9(11):40–43

[6] Bridenstine JB, Dolezal JF. Standardizing chemical peel solution formulations to avoid mishaps. Great fluctuations in actual concentrations of trichloroacetic acid. J Dermatol Surg Oncol. 1994; 20(12):813–816

[7] Cox SE, Butterwick KJ. Chemical peels. In: Robinson JK, eds. Surgery of the Skin: Procedural Dermatology. Philadelphia, PA: Elsevier; 2005:463–482

[8] Safoury OS, Zaki NM, El Nabarawy EA, Farag EA. A study comparing chemical peeling using modified Jessner's solution and 15% trichloroacetic acid versus 15% trichloroacetic acid in the treatment of melasma. Indian J Dermatol. 2009; 54(1):41–45

[9] Puri N. Efficacy of modified Jessner's peel and 20% TCA versus 20% TCA peel alone for the treatment of acne scars. J Cutan Aesthet Surg. 2015; 8(1):42–45

[10] Castillo DE, Keri JE. Chemical peels in the treatment of acne: patient selection and perspectives. Clin Cosmet Investig Dermatol. 2018; 11: 365–372

[11] Hetter GP. An examination of the phenol-croton oil peel: part IV. Face peel results with different concentrations of phenol and croton oil. Plast Reconstr Surg. 2000; 105(3):1061–1083, discussion 1084–1087

[12] Lee KC, Sterling JB, Wambier CG, et al. International Peeling Society. Segmental phenol-Croton oil chemical peels for treatment of periorbital or perioral rhytides. J Am Acad Dermatol. 2019; 81(6): e165–e166

[13] Rendon MI, Berson DS, Cohen JL, Roberts WE, Starker I, Wang B. Evidence and considerations in the application of chemical peels in skin disorders and aesthetic resurfacing. J Clin Aesthet Dermatol. 2010; 3(7):32–43

[14] Kessler E, Flanagan K, Chia C, Rogers C, Glaser DA. Comparison of alpha- and beta-hydroxy acid chemical peels in the treatment of mild to moderately severe facial acne vulgaris. Dermatol Surg. 2008; 34 (1):45–50, discussion 51

[15] Oresajo C, Yatskayer M, Hansenne I. Clinical tolerance and efficacy of capryloyl salicylic acid peel compared to a glycolic acid peel in subjects with fine lines/wrinkles and hyperpigmented skin. J Cosmet Dermatol. 2008; 7(4):259–262

[16] Chew J, Gin I, Rau KA, Amos DB, Bridenstine JB. Treatment of upper lip wrinkles: a comparison of 950 microsec dwell time carbon dioxide laser with unoccluded Baker's phenol chemical peel. Dermatol Surg. 1999; 25(4):262–266

[17] Burns RL, Prevost-Blank PL, Lawry MA, Lawry TB, Faria DT, Fivenson DP. Glycolic acid peels for postinflammatory hyperpigmentation in

black patients. A comparative study. Dermatol Surg. 1997; 23(3): 171–174, discussion 175

[18] Ahn HH, Kim IH. Whitening effect of salicylic acid peels in Asian patients. Dermatol Surg. 2006; 32(3):372–375, discussion 375

[19] Sharquie KE, Al-Tikreety MM, Al-Mashhadani SA. Lactic acid chemical peels as a new therapeutic modality in melasma in comparison to Jessner's solution chemical peels. Dermatol Surg. 2006; 32(12):1429–1436

[20] Khunger N, Sarkar R, Jain RK. Tretinoin peels versus glycolic acid peels in the treatment of Melasma in dark-skinned patients. Dermatol Surg. 2004; 30(5):756–760, discussion 760

[21] Al-Waiz MM, Al-Sharqi AI. Medium-depth chemical peels in the treatment of acne scars in dark-skinned individuals. Dermatol Surg. 2002; 28(5):383–387

[22] Lee JB, Chung WG, Kwahck H, Lee KH. Focal treatment of acne scars with trichloroacetic acid: chemical reconstruction of skin scars method. Dermatol Surg. 2002; 28(11):1017–1021, discussion 1021

[23] Bhardwaj D, Khunger N. An assessment of the efficacy and safety of CROSS technique with 100% TCA in the management of ice pick acne scars. J Cutan Aesthet Surg. 2010; 3(2):93–96

[24] Witheiler DD, Lawrence N, Cox SE, Cruz C, Cockerell CJ, Freemen RG. Long-term efficacy and safety of Jessner's solution and 35% trichloroacetic acid vs 5% fluorouracil in the treatment of widespread facial actinic keratoses. Dermatol Surg. 1997; 23(3):191–196

[25] Tse Y, Ostad A, Lee HS, et al. A clinical and histologic evaluation of two medium-depth peels. Glycolic acid versus Jessner's trichloroacetic acid. Dermatol Surg. 1996; 22(9):781–786

[26] Waldman A, Bolotin D, Arndt KA, et al. ASDS guidelines task force: consensus recommendations regarding the safety of lasers, dermabrasion, chemical peels, energy devices, and skin surgery during and after isotretinoin use. Dermatol Surg. 2017; 43(10): 1249–1262

[27] Glogau RG, Matarasso SL. Chemical face peeling: patient and peeling agent selection. Facial Plast Surg. 1995; 11(1):1–8

[28] Abdel-Meguid AM, Taha EA, Ismail SA. Combined Jessner solution and trichloroacetic acid versus trichloroacetic acid alone in the treatment of melasma in dark-skinned patients. Dermatol Surg. 2017; 43(5):651–656

[29] Peikert JM, Krywonis NA, Rest EB, Zachary CB. The efficacy of various degreasing agents used in trichloroacetic acid peels. J Dermatol Surg Oncol. 1994; 20(11):724–728

[30] Obagi ZE, Obagi S, Alaiti S, Stevens MB. TCA-based blue peel: a standardized procedure with depth control. Dermatol Surg. 1999; 25 (10):773–780

[31] Dainichi TD, Ueda S, Imayama S, Furue M. Excellent clinical results with a new preparation for chemical peeling in acne: 30% salicylic acid in polyethylene glycol vehicle. Dermatol Surg. 2008;34:891–899

[32] Wambier CG, Lee KC, Soon SL, et al. International Peeling Society. Advanced chemical peels: phenol-croton oil peel. J Am Acad Dermatol. 2019; 81(2):327–336

[33] Costa IMC, Damasceno PS, Costa MC, Gomes KGP. Review in peeling complications. J Cosmet Dermatol. 2017; 16(3):319–326

13 Light-Emitting Diode Photomodulation

Robert Weiss and Robert D. Murgia

Summary

Light-emitting diode (LED) arrays for photomodulation are useful for collagen stimulation, textural smoothing, and overall photorejuvenation. Additional modalities include photodynamic therapy, wound healing, and reduction of inflammation from a variety of sources. Cellular rescue from ultraviolet damage and other toxic insults has been shown in small studies. Thermal nonablative photorejuvenation and nonthermal LED photomodulation have a synergistic effect, whereas LED photomodulation delivered immediately post thermal-based treatment can reduce both inflammation and the thermally induced erythema and edema of ablative and nonablative treatments. Delivery of LED light immediately before and after thermal injury appears to increase both anti-inflammatory and protective effects. The first written report discussing the use of photomodulation to improve facial wrinkles was published in 2002. In regard to the investigation of LED light for skin modulating properties, clinical tests and fibroblasts cultures demonstrated that specific packets of energy of precise wavelengths combined with a very explicit proprietary pulse sequencing "code" lead to upregulation of collagen type I synthesis and a reduction of matrix metalloproteinases with exposure to 590-/870-nm low-energy light. Because LEDs employ a nonthermal, light-based mechanism, few pretreatment precautions are required prior to exposure, and therapy is safe for all skin types. Exposure time may vary from 35 seconds to 20 minutes depending on the clinical indication and LED device, and minimal to no aftercare is required following treatment.

Keywords: light-emitting diode, photomodulation, photorejuvenation, fibroblasts, collagen, photodynamic therapy, wound healing

13.1 Introduction

Photorejuvenation, a process whereby light energy sources are used to reverse or repair the process of photoaging or environmental damage to the skin, encompasses many procedures using light- or laser-based technology to reverse the effects of dermal collagen degeneration. Photorejuvenation typically delivers a selective thermal injury confined to the papillary and upper reticular dermis leading to activation of fibroblasts and synthesis of new collagen and extracellular matrix material.[1] However, nonablative photorejuvenation refers to the controlled use of thermal energy to accomplish this goal without disturbance of the overlying epidermis and with minimal to no downtime.[2] Additional objectives include improvement of pigmented and vascular signs of sun-induced aging, a lessening of superficial dyspigmentation (both dermal and epidermal), a reduction in dermal telangiectasias, and the appearance of an overall smoother texture.[3] Nonablative modalities include intense pulsed light (IPL), pulsed dye laser (PDL), 532-nm green light (potassium titanyl phosphate [KTP] laser), and various infrared wavelengths, including 1,064, 1,320, 1,450, and 1,540 nm.[2]

A photorejuvenation effect using a nonthermal stimulation of cells requiring low-energy, narrow-band light with specific pulse sequences and durations has been termed photomodulation.[4] Light-emitting diode (LED) photomodulation is a novel category of nonthermal, light-based treatment designed to regulate activity of cells rather than relying on thermal wound-healing mechanisms.[5] Initially, photomodulation was recognized from the use of LED and low-level laser therapy (LLLT) for stimulation of plant growth and wound healing for oral mucositis.[6,7] The concept of regulation of cell activity, either up or down, by low-energy light has been discussed in the past, yet remarkable or consistent results have been lacking.[7,8] Wavelengths previously examined included a 670-nm LED array,[7] a 660-nm array,[9] and higher infrared wavelengths.[10] Durations of exposure and fluence were variable in these studies with energy as high as 4 J/cm² required for results.[7]

The first written report discussing the use of photomodulation to improve facial wrinkles was published in 2002. Clinical tests and fibroblast cultures were used while investigating LED light for skin modulating properties. It was demonstrated that specific packets of energy of precise wavelengths combined with a very explicit proprietary pulse sequencing "code" lead to upregulation of collagen type I synthesis in fibroblast culture using reverse transcription–polymerase chain reaction (RT-PCR) to measure collagen type I. In both the fibroblast and clinical models, collagen synthesis was accompanied by reduction of matrix metalloproteinases (MMP), in particular MMP-1 or collagenase, with exposure to 590-/870-nm low-energy light.[4]

More specifically, photomodulation occurs via stimulation of mitochondrial cell organelles using the proper "packets" of photons as well as the linked up- or downregulation of mitochondrial gene activities. This leads to upregulation of the mitochondrial cytochrome oxidase electron transport pathway and associated mitochondrial deoxyribonucleic acid (DNA) gene modulation. As a result, several factors have been observed in LED-exposed fibroblasts including an increase in adenosine triphosphate (ATP) production, a modulation of reactive oxygen species, a reduction and prevention of apoptosis, a stimulation of

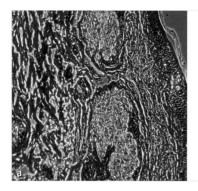
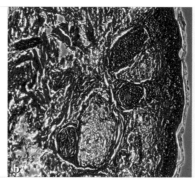

Fig. 13.1 (a,b) Masson staining of human periorbital biopsy 6 months post 4 weeks of thrice a week exposure to 590-/870-nm light-emitting diode (LED) photomodulation (250 milliseconds on time/100 milliseconds off time/100 repetitions at 4.0 mW/cm²). (These images are provided courtesy of David McDaniel.)

angiogenesis, an increase of blood flow, and the induction of transcription. This upregulation of fibroblast collagen synthesis has also been found to correlate with the clinical and histological observation of increased dermal collagen on treated human skin[3,11,12] (▶ Fig. 13.1, ▶ Fig. 13.2).

LEDs employ high-efficiency semiconductors to produce completely noncoherent, noncollimated light at wavelengths ranging from 247 to 1,300 nm.[12,13] LEDs have a typical lamp life of up to 100,000 hours and thus are extremely versatile and durable. Additionally, maintenance and alignment issues tend to be negligible since LEDs do not require expensive or dangerous high-voltage power supplies or complex optics. Therapy is entirely painless, and the availability of large LED panel arrays allows the entire face to be treated in a few minutes or less.[2]

13.2 Modalities

There are several manufacturers of LED arrays producing various wavelengths. Wavelengths are often referred to by their associated colors including blue (400–470 nm), yellow (565–590 nm), red (630–700 nm), and near infrared (700–1,200 nm). Each wavelength has unique photomodulatory properties and longer wavelengths produce deeper tissue penetration.[12,13] Blue light has demonstrated efficacy in acne vulgaris by exhibiting a phototoxic effect on heme metabolism of *Propionibacterium acnes* and reducing inflammatory cytokines.[14]

Photomodulated yellow light has the ability to alter gene expression and increase conversion of adenosine diphosphate (ADP) to ATP in cultured fibroblasts via absorption of photons by mitochondrial protoporphyrin IX.[15] Red LEDs are known to upregulate collagen synthesis and reduce MMPs, whereas infrared light has the ability to enhance wound remodeling by increasing circulation via nitric oxide formation.[12,16] Several of the available devices are mentioned below.

The GentleWaves photomodulation unit, manufactured by LightBioscience of Virginia Beach, Virginia, United States, uses a full-face panel to produce yellow light (590/ 870 nm) for photorejuvenation. Additionally, GlobalMed Technologies of Glen Allen, California, United States,

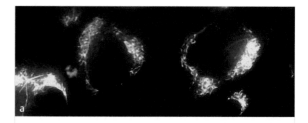
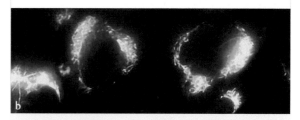

Fig. 13.2 (a,b) Pre- and immediate post-single 590-/870-nm light-emitting diode (LED) photomodulation treatment (250 milliseconds on time/100 milliseconds off time/100 repetitions at 4.0 mW/cm²) of cultured human skin fibroblasts grown on glass coverslips and incubated with the mitochondrial membrane potential probe JC-1. A shift from red fluorescence to green indicates membrane depolarization occurred during exposure. (These images are provided courtesy of David McDaniel.)

produces several LED devices under the Omnilux brand. Omnilux blue transmits blue light (415 nm) for treating acne vulgaris and photodamage. The red light of the Omnilux revive2 (633 nm) is used for photodynamic therapy (PDT) and may also be used to address acne vulgaris, dyschromia, and photoaging. The Omnilux plus transmits infrared light (830 nm) for treatment of photoaging and to accelerate wound healing.[17] Due to issues unrelated to efficacy, some devices are no longer being manufactured at this time (▶ Fig. 13.3).

13.3 Clinical Indications

LED arrays for photomodulation have been found to be beneficial for collagen stimulation, textural smoothing, PDT, alopecia, and reduction of inflammation associated with acne vulgaris, herpes simplex and zoster, acute and chronic wounds, oral mucositis, atopic dermatitis, and even retinal injury. LED photomodulation may be used either alone or in combination with a variety of standard, nonablative rejuvenation procedures in the office setting (▶ Table 13.1).

13.3.1 Photorejuvenation

Treatments may be performed using the GentleWaves yellow light (590/870 nm) LED photomodulation unit equipped with a full-face panel. One hundred pulses are delivered with a pulse duration of 250 milliseconds and an off-interval of 100 milliseconds. An energy density is set at 0.15 J/cm^2 and treatment lasts for approximately 35 seconds. Specific pulsing sequence parameters, the foundation for the "code" of LED photomodulation, were used in a multicenter clinical trial examining 90 patients, who received a series of 8 LED treatments over a 4-week

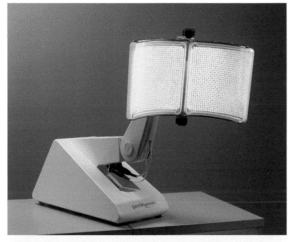

Fig. 13.3 GentleWaves light-emitting diode (LED) photomodulation device. (These images are provided courtesy of David McDaniel.)

period.[11] Digital imaging data provided quite favorable results with over 90% of patients improving by at least one Fitzpatrick photoaging category and 65% of patients demonstrating global improvement in facial texture, fine lines, background erythema, and pigmentation. Results peaked at 4 to 6 months following completion of a series of eight treatments[18] (▶ Fig. 13.4).

Others have confirmed that additional wavelengths of LED light, using both red and infrared, may be effective for improvement in skin texture. In a report of 136 patients, who received 30 treatments over a 15-week period, there was an improvement in skin complexion and skin feeling. Four treatment groups were treated twice a week with either 611- to 650-nm or 570- to 850-nm polychromatic light and compared with controls. Although irradiances and treatment durations varied in all treatment groups, blinded clinical evaluation of photographs confirmed significant improvement in the intervention groups compared with the control.[19]

When LED photomodulation is given independently with the 590-/870-nm pulsing array, patients who present with mild-to-moderate or severe photoaging receive eight treatments over 4 weeks. Alternatively, patients may instead receive LED photomodulation immediately following a nonablative treatment such as IPL, PDL, KTP, or infrared lasers, including 1,064, 1,320, or 1,450 nm. We have found that combining LED photomodulation with other modalities results in more effective clinical results along with faster resolution of erythema, which is believed to be due to the anti-inflammatory effects of LED photomodulation.

13.3.2 Anti-Inflammatory Effects

After treating thousands of patients with photomodulation over the course of several years, we have observed the reduction of erythema from a variety of origins. Reduction of erythema may be induced from a wide range of skin injuries, including, but not limited to, radiation therapy,

Table 13.1 LED wavelengths and associated clinical applications

Wavelength (nm)	400–470	570–590	630–700	800–1,200
Deepest layer targeted	Epidermis	Papillary dermis	Adnexa	Adnexa and reticular dermis
Depth of LED penetration	<1 mm	0.5–2 mm	2–3 mm	5–10 mm
Clinical treatment applications	• Acne • Psoriasis • Atopic dermatitis	• Photorejuvenation • Wound healing • Psoriasis • Atopic dermatitis • Post-laser and IPL treatment • Retinopathy	• Photodynamic therapy • Photorejuvenation • Mucositis • Post-laser treatment • Retinopathy/macular edema • Alopecia	• Wound healing • Photorejuvenation • Combination therapy • Herpes simplex and zoster • Alopecia

Abbreviations: IPL, intense pulsed light; LED, light-emitting diode.

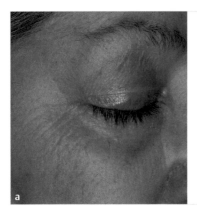
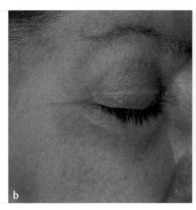

Fig. 13.4 (a,b) Clinical images of progressive improvement in the appearance of periorbital wrinkles, and other skin quality at 6 months post exposure to 4 weeks of thrice a week treatments of 590/870-nm light-emitting diode (LED) photomodulation (250 milliseconds on time/100 milliseconds off time/100 repetitions at 4.0 mW/cm²). (These images are provided courtesy of David McDaniel.)

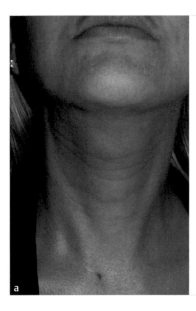
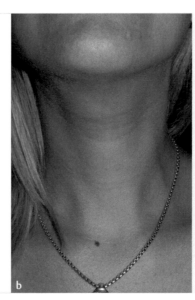

Fig. 13.5 (a,b) Clinical images of improvement of atopic dermatitis post exposure to four treatments over 2 weeks of 590-/870-nm light-emitting diode (LED) photomodulation (250 milliseconds on time/100 milliseconds off time/100 repetitions at 4.0 mW/cm²) after 2 weeks. All topicals withdrawn 2 weeks prior to GentleWaves LED treatment.

thermal laser treatments, ultraviolet (UV) burns, and blunt trauma. Furthermore, patient feedback following a series of GentleWaves LED photomodulation treatments for atopic dermatitis, to diminish bruising, and to aid second degree burns is quite encouraging. Treatment of atopic eczema patients withdrawn from all topical medications has led to rapid clearance within three to four treatments over 1 to 2 weeks (▶ Fig. 13.5).

We believe that the anti-inflammatory effects of LED photomodulation result in a faster resolution of erythema from any multitude of sources. Although the mechanism is still not completely understood, downregulation by photomodulation of a number of inflammatory mediators, such as lymphocytes or macrophages, is suspected. Studies examining human skin fibroblasts and clinical biopsies have shown a reduction in interleukin-1β1 (IL-1β1) and IL-6.[11]

A landmark study examined radiation dermatitis and whether LED photomodulation can alter and improve outcomes of intensity-modulated radiation treatments (IMRT) on cutaneous breast tissue. Nineteen patients with malignancy of the breast were treated with GentleWaves LED photomodulation immediately following all sessions of radiation therapy. Treatments were for post-lumpectomy patients, who received a full course of IMRT. Skin reactions were monitored at weekly intervals using the National Cancer Institute (NCI) grading criteria. Age-matched controls ($n = 28$) received IMRT without post-treatment LED photomodulation. Results of this study revealed that LED treatment had a significantly positive effect. Of LED-treated patients, 18 (94.7%) had grade 0 or 1 reaction and only 1 patient (5.3%) demonstrated a grade 2 or 3 reaction. Among controls, 4 (14.3%) had a grade 1 reaction and 24 (85.7%) had a grade 2 or 3 reaction. Of the non-LED-treated patients, 67.9% had skin reactions with itching or moist desquamation requiring interruption of treatment. Only 5% of the LED-treated group had to interrupt treatment, however. It was concluded that not only did GentleWaves LED photomodulation treatments delivered immediately post each IMRT reduce the incidence of adverse NCI criteria skin reactions, but they also allowed the full course of treatment, resulting in a final smooth skin texture with improvement of skin elasticity following radiation treatment.[20]

Studies have also shown that LED photomodulation can accelerate resolution of post-IPL erythema. Khoury and Goldman examined 15 subjects randomized to receive LED treatment to one side of the face immediately post-IPL treatment for photodamage. Erythema scores on the first visit were found to be statistically significantly lower on the LED-treated side. This finding led to a conclusion that LED photomodulation treatment can shorten time to resolution of erythema and reduce posttreatment discomfort following IPL treatment.[21] This study confirms our observations.

Additional data support an anti-inflammatory effect for LED photomodulation following UV-induced erythema. Results from a solar simulator indicate a photoprotective effect when delivered after UV radiation. This concept demonstrates a rescue from UV-induced damage even after unintended UV radiation has occurred. We have observed a noticeable reduction in UV erythema when LED photomodulation is delivered within hours after UV exposure. The use of 590-/870-nm GentleWaves LED photomodulation produced significant downregulation of dermal matrix degrading enzymes initially stimulated by UV exposure.[11] Additionally, a pilot study found that treatment using a 635-nm wavelength LED array decreases the intensity and duration of postfractional CO_2 laser treatment.[22]

Similar to wound healing, photomodulation has been examined following several types of toxic injury for its preventative and protective effects. Testing requiring exposure to LED light for protection against the toxic actions of methanol-derived formic acid in a rodent model of methanol toxicity has proved successful. Eells et al demonstrated that LED arrays protected the retina from the histopathologic changes induced by methanol on mitochondrial oxidative metabolism in vitro as well as retinal protection in vivo. Photomodulation is thought to enhance recovery from retinal injury and other ocular diseases in which mitochondrial dysfunction is thought to play a role.[23]

Photomodulation has also been successful in treating other retinal diseases, such as diabetic retinopathy. Recently, twice daily treatment for 80 seconds with a 670-nm LED array was reported to demonstrate a statistically significant reduction of macular thickness by 20%, whereas controls demonstrated an increase in thickness of 3% on average.[24] Other in vitro tests on retinal pigment epithelial cells with acute injury from blue light wavelengths showed a sevenfold reduction in vascular endothelial growth factor (VEGF) expression at 24 hours post-LED exposure using LED photomodulation at 590/870 nm delivered at 0.1 J/cm².[25]

Several randomized control trials have used LED arrays for the treatment of acne vulgaris. One group reported a 52% reduction in lesion count compared to no treatment controls after a 414-nm LED delivered at 17.6 J/cm² was used every other day for a period of 8 weeks.[26] A similar study conducted on mild-to-moderate inflammatory acne treated 45 patients with high-intensity pure blue light, 415 nm and 48 J/cm², twice weekly for 4 to 8 weeks. Ninety percent of the patients were satisfied with the results after 8 weeks and, objectively, lesion counts were reduced by 50%.[27] More recently, UV-free blue light has shown great potential in the treatment of hyperkeratotic lesions, such as in psoriasis. A prospective, randomized long-term study consisting of 47 patients showed statistically significant improvement of treated plaques after 4 weeks of use with a 453-nm at-home UV-free blue light device.[28]

Wavelengths of 830 and 1,072 nm have proved beneficial for treatment of recurrent facial herpes simplex virus (HSV) and herpes zoster virus (HZV). Four treatments with 830-nm LED phototherapy, each lasting 10 minutes, given over 10 days along with oral famciclovir resulted in faster healing time, less atrophic scarring, and less postinflammatory hyperpigmentation compared to famciclovir treatment alone.[29] Other trials using 1,072-nm LED arrays resulted in a reduction in re-epithelialization time of 2 to 3 days.[30,31]

13.3.3 Photodynamic Therapy

LED red light (630 nm) has been used for years in combination with a sensitizer (5-aminolevulinic acid) for the treatment of actinic keratoses with PDT.[32] When exposed to light of the correct wavelength, the photosensitizer produces cytotoxic reactive oxygen species that oxidizes the plasma membrane of targeted cells leading to cell and tissue destruction. Due to a lower metabolic rate, there is less sensitizer absorbed by adjacent normal tissue leading to decreased reactivity. One of the absorption peaks of the metabolic product of levulinic acid, protoporphyrin IX, is known to absorb strongly at 630-nm red light. A red LED panel emitting at 633 ± 6 nm (Omnilux revive², GlobalMed Technologies) is currently used for this purpose.[17] We have also used the full-face panel 590-/870-nm LED array for facilitating PDT. This therapy is delivered by application of aminolevulinic acid (Levulan DUSA, Wilmington, Massachusetts, United States) for 45 minutes followed by exposure to continuous (nonpulsed) 590-/870-nm LED for 15 minutes for a cumulative dose of over 70 J/cm². Results have shown reduction of actinic damage, including improvement of skin texture and a reduction of actinic keratoses.[3]

13.3.4 Alopecia

The efficacy of LED photomodulation and LLLT for hair loss has been reported in several published studies. This novel treatment has been found to promote hair growth in both men and women with androgenetic alopecia

(AGA) and female pattern hair loss, respectively.[33] Regarding the mechanism of action, the most widely accepted theory states that photomodulation activates epidermal stem cells in the hair follicle bulge leading to a shift toward the anagen phase.[34] Wavelengths employed to stimulate hair regrowth must be able to penetrate superficial tissue and typically range from 600 to 700 nm, as well as infrared.[35]

In 2007, the first 655-nm LLLT device (HairMax Lasercomb, Lexington Intl., LLC) containing a single-laser module with nine emulated beams was approved for the treatment of hair loss. Of the 110 male subjects suffering from AGA, those treated with the device three times weekly for 15 minutes had a mean increase in terminal hair density of + 19.8 hairs/cm², whereas subjects in the sham device group had a mean decrease of –7.6 hairs/cm² after 26 weeks.[36] More recently, multiple studies have reported that 655-nm red light was found to significantly improve hair counts in both men and women with AGA.[37,38]

13.4 Patient Selection/ Contraindications/Preoperative Care

Because LEDs employ a nonthermal, light-based mechanism, few pretreatment precautions are required prior to exposure, and therapy is safe for all skin types. Eye protection may be worn for patient comfort. However, LEDs are tuned to operate at a lower maximum permissible exposure compared to laser sources, making it safe for the direct view of the light source. Treatments are reduced to a low-energy density, whereas power does not reach more than 50 mW.[39] Since many of our patients receive treatment following various nonablative procedures, patients may be encouraged to use a gentle cleanser or to apply a mild potency topical steroid prior to therapy. Although LED treatment is considered safe, any history of underlying photosensitive disorders or recent use of photosensitizing medications is considered a contraindication to treatment.

13.5 Procedure

Patients are positioned close to the light source. The irradiance level on the surface of the skin is critical to achieving the required photomodulation effect. Part of the specifications in an LED array requires minimum and maximum working distances from the skin. If the subject is too close to the LED array, the treatment may produce minimal or no response. We suggest placing the panel at a distance of 4 cm from the patient's skin.[40] Exposure time may vary from 35 seconds to 20 minutes depending on the clinical indication as well as LED device.

13.6 Postoperative Instructions

Minimal-to-no aftercare is required following treatment. Patients treated with PDT should apply sunscreen before leaving the office and avoid exposure to the sun for approximately 24 to 72 hours, as the topically applied photosensitizer may continue to cause skin sensitivity on treatment areas. All patients should be educated on proper sun protection practices, such as the daily use of sunscreens along with sun protective clothing.

13.7 Potential Complications

To date, no serious complications regarding LED photomodulation have been reported in the literature. Although rare, few incidences of adverse events exist, and complaints of a mild burning sensation, minimal erythema, and postinflammatory hyperpigmentation have been noted in a minority of randomized controlled trials.

13.8 Pearls

Photomodulation employs nonthermal light treatments to regulate cells rather than invoking thermal wound-healing mechanisms. Research suggests that along with the ability to stimulate cells to perform certain functions using low-energy light packets and to enhance cell metabolism, LED photomodulation is a very safe, fast, effective, and affordable treatment for collagen stimulation, textural smoothing, PDT, and the reduction of inflammation.

References

[1] Nelson JS, Majaron B, Kelly KM. What is nonablative photorejuvenation of human skin? Semin Cutan Med Surg. 2002; 21 (4):238–250

[2] Weiss RA, McDaniel DH, Geronemus RG. Review of nonablative photorejuvenation: reversal of the aging effects of the sun and environmental damage using laser and light sources. Semin Cutan Med Surg. 2003; 22(2):93–106

[3] Weiss RA, McDaniel DH, Geronemus RG, et al. Clinical experience with light-emitting diode (LED) photomodulation. Dermatol Surg. 2005; 31(9, Pt 2):1199–1205

[4] McDaniel D, Weiss RA, Geronemus RG, Ginn L, Newman J. Light-tissue interaction II: photothermolysis vs photomodulation clinical applications. Lasers Surg Med. 2002; 14:25

[5] McDaniel DH, Weiss RA, Geronemus RG, Ginn L, Newman J. Light-tissue interactions I: photothermolysis vs photomodulation laboratory findings. Lasers Surg Med. 2002:25

[6] Whelan HT, Smits RL, Jr, Buchman EV, et al. Effect of NASA light-emitting diode irradiation on wound healing. J Clin Laser Med Surg. 2001; 19(6):305–314

[7] Whelan HT, Connelly JF, Hodgson BD, et al. NASA light-emitting diodes for the prevention of oral mucositis in pediatric bone marrow transplant patients. J Clin Laser Med Surg. 2002; 20(6):319–324

[8] Whelan HT, Buchmann EV, Dhokalia A, et al. Effect of NASA light-emitting diode irradiation on molecular changes for wound healing in diabetic mice. J Clin Laser Med Surg. 2003; 21(2):67–74

[9] Walker MD, Rumpf S, Baxter GD, Hirst DG, Lowe AS. Effect of low-intensity laser irradiation (660 nm) on a radiation-impaired wound-healing model in murine skin. Lasers Surg Med. 2000; 26(1):41–47

[10] Lowe AS, Walker MD, O'Byrne M, Baxter GD, Hirst DG. Effect of low intensity monochromatic light therapy (890 nm) on a radiation-impaired, wound-healing model in murine skin. Lasers Surg Med. 1998; 23(5):291–298

[11] Weiss RA, McDaniel DH, Geronemus RG, Weiss MA. Clinical trial of a novel non-thermal LED array for reversal of photoaging: clinical, histologic, and surface profilometric results. Lasers Surg Med. 2005; 36(2):85–91

[12] Barolet D. Light-emitting diodes (LEDs) in dermatology. Semin Cutan Med Surg. 2008; 27(4):227–238

[13] Calderhead RG, Vasily DB. Low Level Light Therapy with Light-Emitting Diodes for the Aging Face. Clin Plast Surg. 2016; 43(3):541–550

[14] Shnitkind E, Yaping E, Geen S, Shalita AR, Lee WL. Anti-inflammatory properties of narrow-band blue light. J Drugs Dermatol. 2006; 5(7):605–610

[15] Weiss RA, Weiss MA, Geronemus RG, McDaniel DH. A novel non-thermal non-ablative full panel LED photomodulation device for reversal of photoaging: digital microscopic and clinical results in various skin types. J Drugs Dermatol. 2004; 3(6):605–610

[16] Barolet D, Roberge CJ, Auger FA, Boucher A, Germain L. Regulation of skin collagen metabolism in vitro using a pulsed 660 nm LED light source: clinical correlation with a single-blinded study. J Invest Dermatol. 2009; 129(12):2751–2759

[17] Omnilux. Omnilux LED. 2019. Available at: https://omniluxled.com/

[18] Weiss RA, McDaniel D, Geronemus RG, Weiss MA, Newman J. Non-ablative, non-thermal light emitting diode (LED) phototherapy of photoaged skin. Lasers Surg Med. 2004; 16:31

[19] Wunsch A, Matuschka K. A controlled trial to determine the efficacy of red and near-infrared light treatment in patient satisfaction, reduction of fine lines, wrinkles, skin roughness, and intradermal collagen density increase. Photomed Laser Surg. 2014; 32(2):93–100

[20] DeLand MM, Weiss RA, McDaniel DH, Geronemus RG. Treatment of radiation-induced dermatitis with light-emitting diode (LED) photomodulation. Lasers Surg Med. 2007; 39(2):164–168

[21] Khoury JG, Goldman MP. Use of light-emitting diode photomodulation to reduce erythema and discomfort after intense pulsed light treatment of photodamage. J Cosmet Dermatol. 2008; 7(1):30–34

[22] Oh IY, Kim BJ, Kim MN, Kim CW, Kim SE. Efficacy of light-emitting diode photomodulation in reducing erythema after fractional carbon dioxide laser resurfacing: a pilot study. Dermatol Surg. 2013; 39(8):1171–1176

[23] Eells JT, Henry MM, Summerfelt P, et al. Therapeutic photobiomodulation for methanol-induced retinal toxicity. Proc Natl Acad Sci U S A. 2003; 100(6):3439–3444

[24] Tang J, Herda AA, Kern TS. Photobiomodulation in the treatment of patients with non-center-involving diabetic macular oedema. Br J Ophthalmol. 2014; 98(8):1013–1015

[25] McDaniel DH, Weiss RA, Geronemus R, Weiss MA. LED Photomodulation "Reverses" Acute Retinal Injury. Annual meeting of

the American Society for Laser Medicine and Surgery, Boston, MA, April 5–9, 2006

[26] Ash C, Harrison A, Drew S, Whittall R. A randomized controlled study for the treatment of acne vulgaris using high-intensity 414 nm solid state diode arrays. J Cosmet Laser Ther. 2015; 17(4):170–176

[27] Tremblay JF, Sire DJ, Lowe NJ, Moy RL. Light-emitting diode 415 nm in the treatment of inflammatory acne: an open-label, multicentric, pilot investigation. J Cosmet Laser Ther. 2006; 8(1):31–33

[28] Pfaff S, Liebmann J, Born M, Merk HF, von Felbert V. Prospective randomized long-term study on the efficacy and safety of UV-free blue light for treating mild psoriasis vulgaris. Dermatology. 2015; 231(1):24–34

[29] Park KY, Han TY, Kim IS, Yeo IK, Kim BJ, Kim MN. The effects of 830 nm light-emitting diode therapy on acute herpes zoster ophthalmicus: a pilot study. Ann Dermatol. 2013; 25(2):163–167

[30] Dougal G, Lee SY. Evaluation of the efficacy of low-level light therapy using 1072 nm infrared light for the treatment of herpes simplex labialis. Clin Exp Dermatol. 2013; 38(7):713–718

[31] Hargate G. A randomised double-blind study comparing the effect of 1072-nm light against placebo for the treatment of herpes labialis. Clin Exp Dermatol. 2006; 31(5):638–641

[32] Tarstedt M, Rosdahl I, Berne B, Svanberg K, Wennberg AM. A randomized multicenter study to compare two treatment regimens of topical methyl aminolevulinate (Metvix)-PDT in actinic keratosis of the face and scalp. Acta Derm Venereol. 2005; 85(5):424–428

[33] Gupta AK, Daigle D. The use of low-level light therapy in the treatment of androgenetic alopecia and female pattern hair loss. J Dermatolog Treat. 2014; 25(2):162–163

[34] Avci P, Gupta GK, Clark J, Wikonkal N, Hamblin MR. Low-level laser (light) therapy (LLLT) for treatment of hair loss. Lasers Surg Med. 2014; 46(2):144–151

[35] Chung H, Dai T, Sharma SK, Huang YY, Carroll JD, Hamblin MR. The nuts and bolts of low-level laser (light) therapy. Ann Biomed Eng. 2012; 40(2):516–533

[36] Leavitt M, Charles G, Heyman E, Michaels D. HairMax LaserComb laser phototherapy device in the treatment of male androgenetic alopecia: a randomized, double-blind, sham device-controlled, multicentre trial. Clin Drug Investig. 2009; 29(5):283–292

[37] Lanzafame RJ, Blanche RR, Bodian AB, Chiacchierini RP, Fernandez-Obregon A, Kazmirek ER. The growth of human scalp hair mediated by visible red light laser and LED sources in males. Lasers Surg Med. 2013; 45(8):487–495

[38] Lanzafame RJ, Blanche RR, Chiacchierini RP, Kazmirek ER, Sklar JA. The growth of human scalp hair in females using visible red light laser and LED sources. Lasers Surg Med. 2014; 46(8):601–607

[39] Alster TS, Wanitphakdeedecha R. Improvement of postfractional laser erythema with light-emitting diode photomodulation. Dermatol Surg. 2009; 35(5):813–815

[40] Weiss RA, Deland MM, Geronemus RG, McDaniel DH. Letter: light-emitting diode photomodulation and radiation dermatitis. Dermatol Surg. 2011; 37(6):885–886

14 Combining Treatments

Rhett A. Kent and Sabrina Guillen Fabi

Summary

There are many noninvasive and minimally invasive therapeutic modalities available for use in cosmetic dermatology, each having its own place in the aesthetic armamentarium. Initial treatments were developed slowly over decades. More recently, an influx of resources into the field has caused the pace of product development to surge. The goals of aesthetically inclined patients, historically out of reach without surgical intervention, may now be achievable through the use of multiple modalities in the dermatologist's office. This has led to the practice of combining treatments for delivery in sequence or on the same day in an attempt to efficiently maximize outcomes. Furthermore, as downtime is a significant concern to patients, by performing therapies during a single visit, their recovery may be carried out in unison, shortening the overall recovery time. Although combination therapy is common in aesthetic practices, many of these regimens have been derived from clinical experience. Regardless, publications are accumulating to support many of these clinically established combination approaches. This chapter will discuss both published and experience-based recommendations on delivering combination noninvasive and minimally invasive aesthetic treatments. Although some background will be given, in-depth explanations of the mechanisms of action behind individual treatment modalities, as well as expanded discussions of their individual uses and techniques, will be better found in other chapters.

Keywords: combination, cosmetic, aesthetic, noninvasive, treatment, therapy, intervention

14.1 A General Approach

As with all aesthetic consultations, an individualized approach to combination aesthetic therapy begins with understanding the patient's needs. Although a patient may present with a specific request, the clinician must rely on their expertise to fully evaluate the anatomy and prioritize interventions based on the anatomical changes that account for the patient's complaint. By educating and empowering the patient to refocus on potentially overlooked therapeutic targets, the clinician can proceed with an appropriate plan to achieve the optimal result. Through formulating a long-term plan, the clinician can offer a schedule that takes into account those interventions that can be performed together or are better delivered in sequential order. It is important to note that although not discussed in detail here, it is vital to know the limits of these therapies and when to recommend

surgical options to patients with more advanced aging changes and/or higher expectations of outcomes. Still when surgical options are pursued, these too can be combined with less invasive modalities to maximize results. Additionally, as clinicians find new uses of approved interventions, they may become accepted without companies seeking U.S. Food and Drug Administration (FDA) clearances. Thus, many of these recommendations include off-label uses of interventions.

14.1.1 The Ideals of Beautification

A more mature patient who is seeking a return to a youthful appearance or blunting of age-related changes is by definition seeking rejuvenation. Alternatively, a patient who presents without these age-related changes but looking to enhance or alter their natural features is approached with a lens of beautification. The latter can be achieved by altering angles or proportions to achieve more desirable features. In most patients, both rejuvenation and beautification techniques are used simultaneously.

To understand the approach to beautification, an understanding of ideal proportions and features is vital. At the basic level, the face is comprised of a set of features whose shapes, sizes, and orientation to each other come together to create their unique appearance. By altering the characteristics of these features in ways that approximate, or even exaggerate, the ideal, one can increase a person's subjective attractiveness.[1] Of course, one should not attempt to drastically change every face to fit a uniform model. Instead, our approach is to make subtle changes with these ideals in mind, having the goal of enhancing their unique appearance. Keep this in mind when considering intervening on any distinctive feature such as a dimple. Although changing such distinctive features may make them subjectively more attractive to a blinded evaluator, it carries the risk of losing identifying features that provide individuality to themselves and distinctness to the world around them.

Ideals are dependent on gender and, of course, gender preferences.[2] The ideal female facial shape is an oval, formed by curves.[3] A man's face is wider, formed by sharper angles, with more prominent lower facial features of the jawline and chin.[3,4] That being said, in Asians, who tend to seek cosmetic interventions for beautification more regularly than Caucasian populations, the ideal facial shape is an oval or heart shaped regardless of gender.[5] The focal point of the midface in women is prominent and lateral, whereas the midface is relatively flat in men.[4,6]

Horizontally, the ideal face can be split into three segments (► Fig. 14.1a): (1) the hairline to the glabella,

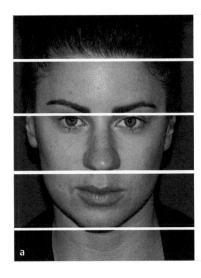
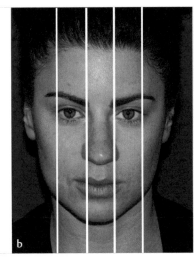

Fig. 14.1 (a) Horizontally, the ideal face can be split into three segments: (1) the hairline to the glabella, (2) the glabella to the bottom of the nose, and (3) below the nose to the menton.[2] (b) Vertically, the ideal face can be split into five segments, with each fifth being the width of the intercanthal distance.[2] As depicted, the lines that form the central segment traverse the nasal ala, the medial canthus, and the medial brow.[8]

(2) the glabella to the bottom of the nose, and (3) below the nose to the menton.[2] The ideal proportions of these horizontally split segments are variable, somewhat dependent on ethnicity.[7] Even without considering these ethnic variations, analyzing the face by splitting it into proportions can reveal asymmetries and disproportions. These may serve as targets of beautification interventions or cautionary guidance to avoid interventions that would exaggerate already disproportionate features.

Ideal vertical facial proportions can be defined using the following framework. Divide the face into vertical fifths (▶ Fig. 14.1b), with each fifth being the width of the intercanthal distance.[2] As depicted, the lines that form the central segment traverse the nasal ala, the medial canthus, and the medial brow.[8] The lateral brow should sit at a similar height as the medial counterpart, at a point on a line drawn from the lateral point of the nasal ala, and traversing the lateral canthus (▶ Fig. 14.2).[8] Having a distinct peak of the brow arch is important in women, with this point lifting above the orbital ridge.[9] The peak of the brow arch should sit above an area ranging from the lateral limbus to the lateral canthus.[8,9,10] Conversely, men should have a less prominent arch and peak,[9] sitting lower, along their more prominent orbital ridge.[4] These ideals were based on classical measurements recorded in ancient Greece and, within the United States, are most applicable to Caucasian women.[7,11] However, many of these ideals are conserved across ethnicities, with higher ethnic variability regarding the width of lips, width of the distal nose, and the distance between the eyes.[7,11]

14.1.2 The Processes of Aging

The forces of aging come from both within (intrinsic aging) and our environment (extrinsic aging). Intrinsic aging is expressed with increasing chronological age as result of the ongoing effects of genetically driven physiological and/or pathological processes. Extrinsic forces most notably include ultraviolet (UV) radiation, to which lighter skin types are particularly susceptible. Oxidative damage is a common pathway that translates the forces of aging into molecular effects.[12] Oxidative damage leads to an inflammatory milieu of cytokines, eosinophils, mast cells, and mononuclear cells.[13] Stress on fibroblasts lead to decreased collagen production, as well as increased matrix metalloproteinase activity, which degrades collagen and elastin.[13] Oxidative damage also leads to progressive telomere shortening linked to cellular senescence and death.[14]

Intrinsic skin aging is primarily manifested by atrophic tissue changes to skin, soft tissue, and bone. The decline of bone mass begins after reaching a peak in the second to third decade of life, becoming significantly less in the fourth decade and continues perpetually at variable speeds leading to loss of our strongest structural framework.[15,16] With receding bony support of the face comes the shifting of soft-tissue compartments, which also variably display atrophic changes. These compartments, vulnerable to gravity, will slowly begin their downward migration. Ultimately this leads to increased skin laxity and the inversion of the youthful facial shape, referred to as an inverted triangle. Loss of bony support precipitates increases in the resting tone of mimetic muscles, which contributes to rhytide formation. Histologically, epidermal and dermal atrophy are the predominant skin changes.[17] Extrinsic aging forces exaggerate these signs of chronological aging, effects best demonstrated by individuals whose daily UV exposure was unequally exerted on one side of their face. The side with heavier exposure shows asymmetrically advanced photoaging, in particular increased laxity, and progressed rhytides of the cheek and periorbitally infraorbital lines and crow's feet.[18]

Extrinsic aging is also responsible for pigmentary, vascular, and textural abnormalities, all more common in lighter, more susceptible skin types. Specifically, UV-induced melanogenesis and melanocytosis lead to solar

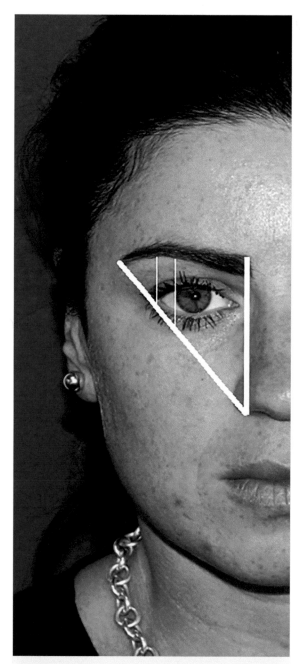

Fig. 14.2 The lateral brow should sit at a similar height as the medial counterpart, at a point on a line drawn from the lateral point of the nasal ala, and traversing the lateral canthus.[8] In women, a distinct peak of the brow arch should lift above the orbital ridge at a point ranging from the lateral limbus to the lateral canthus (depicted as the area between the *thin white lines*).[8,9,10]

manifestations of photoaging include telangiectasia and erythema, which tend to position on the lateral face, a useful clinical clue to differentiate these from centrally located rosacea.[22] Solar purpura, classically evident in the sun-exposed areas of the upper extremities, is due to progressive dermatoporosis, resolving with dyspigmentation from hemosiderin deposition.[23] Textural abnormalities range from coarse skin texture, a cobblestone effect from elastosis to epidermal growths of benign, premalignant, and malignant varieties.[17]

Histologically, extrinsically aged skin is marked by irregular epidermal growth with variably atrophic and hyperplastic changes.[24] The epidermis loses its support with flattening of the previously undulating dermoepidermal junction.[25] In the dermis, collagen, supportive elastic fibers, and extracellular matrix materials atrophy accompanied by thickening of fibrous septa and accumulation of solar elastosis.[24,25]

Teeth are vulnerable to intrinsic aging as well as to a unique set of extrinsic forces specific to their function. The latter defined as attrition, abrasion, and erosion, together lead to tooth wear, which manifests as a loss of structural support, quality, and alignment. Clinically, facial aesthetics are impacted at rest and more directly when smiling. Although not discussed further, cosmetic dentistry is a growing field that can offer a multitude of interventions to address these issues and maximize outcomes of your patients.

14.1.3 Principles of Combination Aesthetic Therapy

As described, aging is complex, affecting tissues from the epidermal surface to the supportive bony framework. Therefore, there is no single intervention that can optimally address each of the components of the aging individual. Furthermore, even when restricting attention to addressing one of these facets, combination approaches may achieve superior outcomes.

▶ Table 14.1 lists the tissue types that serve as targets for rejuvenation and/or beautification and the predominant noninvasive or minimally invasive modalities that have utility for their intervention. Through careful examination, a prioritized list of tissues contributing to the patient's concerns can be made. Once these priorities are defined, the practitioner can choose from the modalities based on availability, cost, downtime, and other patient factors.

14.2 Combining Injections, Implants, and Energy-Based Devices

Soft-tissue augmentation and neurotoxins are the most popular nonsurgical cosmetic treatments.[26] Thus, their utilities should at least be considered during any patient's evaluation for cosmetic enhancement. Furthermore, these

lentigines and dyspigmentation.[19,20] Solar lentigines start developing in the second decade of life, affecting not only the vast majority of Caucasians by age 70 years but also commonly other ethnicities.[19,21] Notable vascular

Table 14.1 List of therapeutic targets and their corresponding available modalities for intervention

Therapeutic target	Modalities for intervention
Epidermal targets	
• Pigment (melanin)	• Devices that directly target melanin: IPL, 585- to 595-nm PDL with compression handpiece, Q-switched and picosecond lasers including the 532-nm KTP, 694-nm ruby, 755-nm alexandrite, and 1,064-nm Nd:YAG • Indirectly improve pigmentation via resurfacing: Ablative and nonablative, continuous wave, and fractionated lasers in the infrared spectrum including 1,320-nm Nd:YAG, 1,440- to 1,450-nm diode, 1,540-nm erbium glass, 1,550-nm diode, 1,927-nm diode, 1,927-nm thulium, 2,940-nm Er:YAG, and 10,600-nm CO_2
• Texture (resurfacing)	Ablative and nonablative, continuous wave, and fractionated lasers in the infrared spectrum (options detailed above)
Dermal targets	
• Vascularity (hemoglobin)	585- to 595-nm PDL, 532-nm KTP, 755-nm alexandrite, 1,064-nm Nd:YAG, IPL
• Collagen/elastin	IPL (with light emission up to 1,200 nm); ablative and nonablative, fractionated > continuous wave lasers in the infrared spectrum (options detailed above)
• Pigment (melanin)	Q-switched and picosecond lasers as referenced above
Subcutaneous tissue	
• Excess fat	Deoxycholic acid, cryolipolysis, monopolar RF, ultrasound, 1,060-nm diode hyperthermic laser, low-level laser therapy (LLLT), High-Intensity Focused Electromagnetic (HIFEM) technology
• Fat atrophy or structural migration	Soft-tissue fillers
• SMAS, retaining ligaments	MFU
• Laxity	Thread/suture lifts, MFU, RF; ablative and nonablative, fractionated, and continuous wave lasers in the infrared spectrum

Abbreviations: CO_2, carbon dioxide laser; Er:YAG, erbium-doped yttrium aluminum garnet laser; IPL, intense pulsed light; KTP, potassium titanyl phosphate laser; MFU, microfocused ultrasound; Nd:YAG, neodymium-doped yttrium aluminum garnet laser; PDL, pulsed dye laser; RF, radiofrequency.

injections are commonly performed during the same session. Although either order is acceptable, we prefer injecting soft-tissue fillers prior to neurotoxin, regardless of whether injections are performed on the same day or in intervals. Filler may necessitate massage after placement, which, if performed after toxin placement, risks unintentional redistribution of the toxin.

Advanced techniques with combination injectable medications maximize outcomes of rejuvenation and beautification. In addition to filling atrophic regions and diminishing rhytides, contouring should be performed with principles of sexual dimorphism in mind (▶ Fig. 14.3). For example, for women with square faces, softening the angles of the lower face can be performed with neurotoxin by chemodenervation of the masseter muscles, and/or parotid glands. When concomitant with a flattened chin, filler into the pogonion can restore three dimensionality to the face and a curved, feminine, seemingly smaller chin. Alternatively, for men with less prominent jawlines, soft-tissue augmentation can be used to build the mandibular angle and jawline. When accompanied by facial and submental fullness, the addition of injection lipolysis, as well as other fat targeting modalities, may be safely coadministered.[27]

In general, we are comfortable performing these injectable interventions during the same session as energy-based devices. In this context, we typically perform injections as the last step of the regimen primarily to avoid contamination of the device heads or the airborne spread of blood. Although some have cited concerns that performing energy-based interventions after injections may denature the deposited products, or cause their diffusion, overall the evidence does not support this. Furthermore, detrimental interactions to soft-tissue fillers or biostimulatory agents have not been shown when followed by intense pulsed light (IPL), infrared lasers, microfocused ultrasound (MFU), or monopolar radiofrequency (RF) treatments.[28,29,30,31,32,33,34]

Although, synergistic effects are not always apparent,[35] the benefits of performing injectable and energy-based interventions during the same session is convenient and

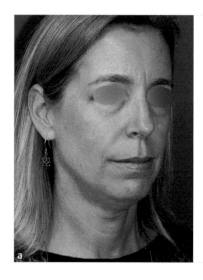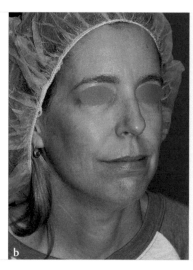

Fig. 14.3 A 44-year-old woman pictured **(a)** before and **(b)** 1 month after injection of three syringes of a VYCROSS hyaluronic acid filler 20 mg/mL (Juvéderm Voluma, Allergan, Irvine, California, United States) to the cheeks, chin, and gonial angle, followed by same day onabotulinumtoxin A (Botox, Allergan) to the glabella, forehead, crow's feet, depressor anguli oris, and mentalis muscles.

shortens total recovery time relative to performing them on sequential visits. Additionally, if using devices that target different tissue planes, combining therapies does not confer an increased risk.[36] However, with multiple interventions comes increased pain associated with the delivering of the chosen therapies. Comfort has a strong correlation with patient satisfaction, and the practitioner should consider offering a combination of analgesia and anesthesia to meet the projected pain level. Depending on the procedures and the individual's pain tolerance, a combination of topical anesthetics, nerve blocks, oral analgesics, oral anxiolytics, and/or nitrous oxide sedation can usually provide adequate analgesia.

When performing absorbable thread lifts in combination with injectables, we recommend performing the lift procedure first as the repositioning may change filler targets and minimize toxin spread from manipulation of threads. When combining lasers or other device treatments with thread lifts, we reserve those known to cause moderate-to-severe diffuse erythema and/or swelling for separate sessions to avoid distortion of the tissue being repositioned. One author (SGF) will perform an IPL treatment or spot treatments, such as with pulsed dye laser (PDL) for discreet vessels, Q-switched or picosecond laser for individual lentigines, on the same day prior to the absorbable thread lift.

14.3 Combination Laser and Light Therapies for Specific Targets

14.3.1 Dyspigmentation

Every face tells a story, and when approaching facial dyschromia, one must carefully assess the diversity of causative pathologies having accumulated over time. When a person displays multiple pigmentary pathologies, this is referred to as complex dyspigmentation.[37] In addition to ill-defined mottled pigmentation and discrete lesions

(solar lentigines, ephelides) that may result from UV exposure, frequently patients have other contributing lesions such as melasma and/or postinflammatory hyper- or hypopigmentation that has resulted from a number of causes, such as acne or mechanical trauma. Looking at ▶ Table 14.1, we see a number of lasers that can improve both epidermal and dermal pigmentation. Each of these listed modalities has been validated for use in treating dyspigmentation as stand-alone therapies. Furthermore, investigations have revealed each of their unique strengths, and by layering treatments with complementary modalities, additive or synergistic effects may be achieved.

When the focus is dyspigmentation alone, it is particularly beneficial to combine therapies that have different mechanisms of action, or penetrate to different tissue levels. For example, IPL can treat both discrete pigmented lesions and ill-defined background dyspigmentation; however, many choose to combine IPL with Q-switched or picosecond laser treatments to more efficiently treat discrete pigmented lesions.[37,38] Additionally, layering a third device with a separate mechanism of action, such as the 1,927-nm thulium nonablative laser, can further provide improvement in complex dyspigmentation.

A combination approach is also useful when treating lesions with a component of deep dermal pigmentation, such as is classically seen with nevus of Ota or Hori's nevus.[39,40,41] With these lesions, combining Q-switched lasers of various wavelengths to treat both superficial and deep melanin can improve outcomes.[41] Alternatively, resurfacing immediately prior to Q-switched laser treatment may work synergistically by improving penetration of the latter.[39,40] Multiple resurfacing modalities have been helpful for this purpose including ablative lasers,[40] nonablative lasers,[39] or both. Extrapolating from this evidence, these approaches may also be useful when treating postinflammatory hyperpigmentation or other diagnoses where both superficial and deep pigmentations are clinically evident.

More commonly, however, dyspigmentation is accompanied by other pathologies, and together, combination therapies can target each of the contributing components. For example, IPL tends to have a greater effect on concomitant vascular abnormalities, whereas ablative and nonablative fractional lasers are slightly better at improving texture.[42] Thus, by combining these in a single session (▶ Fig. 14.4), an efficient intervention can achieve greater overall improvement by impacting all metrics including dyspigmentation, vascularity, and texture.[43,44] One study on such a strategy treating lentigines in Asian skin had good results with Q-switched Nd:YAG (neodymium-doped yttrium aluminum garnet laser) for discrete lesions followed by fractional erbium resurfacing for the entire face, which offered improvements in lentigines as well as other parameters.[21]

Melasma is a unique pigmentary disorder, and we have learned more recently that in some patients, there is a significant contribution from the underlying vasculature.[45,46] This appears to be true particularly for melasma patients who have grossly visible underlying erythema or widened capillaries on dermoscopy.[47,48] For such patients, studies have shown that combining a modality to target vasculature, such as PDL,[48] IPL,[49] or long-pulsed Nd:YAG,[45] with standard Q-switched lasers leads to superior results.[48,49] One author (SGF) prefers an IPL to address both pigment and redness in Fitzpatrick skin types I to III, or PDL followed by either a 1,927-nm thulium laser or 1,927-nm diode laser in Fitzpatrick skin types IV and V.[46,50] There are high risks of postinflammatory hyperpigmentation or melasma rebounding when treating with energy-based devices in this population. Yet again, using a combination of light or lasers may achieve efficacy while permitting the use of less aggressive energy settings, which when combined with adequate cooling decreases the risk of these complications.[49]

14.3.2 Vascular Abnormalities

Combining energy-based therapies can be useful when treating a variety of cosmetically concerning vascular lesions. In particular, combining modalities that have different mechanisms of action, penetrate to different tissue levels, and/or have complementary strengths can improve outcomes.

Facial erythema, telangiectasias, angiomas, and periorbital veins are among the most common vascular lesions presenting to the aesthetic dermatologist. Discrete lesions (telangiectasia, angiomas, and periorbital veins) are best treated until reaching indicators of vessel damage, either with an endpoint of purpura indicating coagulation or blanching indicating vascular contraction.[51,52] This can be performed with a number of devices whose energy is absorbed preferentially by oxyhemoglobin when treating redness and deoxyhemoglobin when treating blue reticular veins (▶ Table 14.1). Although carrying a higher burden of cosmetic downtime, purpuric PDL treatments are possibly the most effective.[52,53,54] However, evidence also indicates that by combining 1,064-nm Nd:YAG with PDL treatments, highly effective clearance rates are achieved while permitting subpurpuric PDL parameters.[55] This can be particularly useful in darker skin types as purpuric PDL settings carry a higher risk of pigmentary complications.

Conversely, facial erythema is best treated with subpurpuric PDL parameters, as purpuric treatments may exacerbate erythema.[52] Thus, in erythematotelangiectatic rosacea where erythema and telangiectasia are seen concurrently, combination therapies, such as 1,064-nm Nd:YAG with subpurpuric PDL, may achieve successful treatment of both components.[56] In addition, RF is an emerging therapy for both erythematotelangiectatic rosacea and papulopustular rosacea, leaving the possibility of

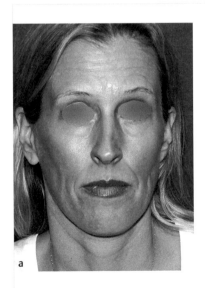
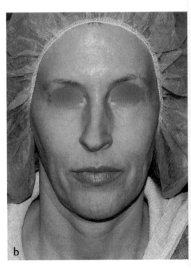

Fig. 14.4 A 44-year-old woman pictured (a) before and (b) after 5 years of twice a year combination treatments with intense pulsed light (IPL), followed with same-day poly-L-lactic acid (Sculptra, Galderma Laboratories, L.P., Fort Worth, Texas, United States) to the medial and lateral cheeks, chin, pyriform fossa, and temples, immediately followed by the 1,440-nm diode laser (Clear and Brilliant, Solta Medical Inc., Pleasanton, California, United States). Then on consecutive visits, the patient had a Cohesive Polydensified Matrix hyaluronic acid (Belotero, Merz North America, Inc., Raleigh, North Carolina, United States) injected into the nasolabial folds, and three times a year treatments with abobotulinumtoxin A (Dysport, Ipsen Biopharmaceuticals, Inc., Basking Ridge, New Jersey, United States) toxin to the glabella, crow's feet, and frontalis muscles.

further improvement by combining RF with laser or light modalities.[57]

14.3.3 Resurfacing

Resurfacing options include a range of technologies from chemical peels, dermabrasion, and laser modalities, detailed in ▶ Table 14.1.

Traditionally, energy-based resurfacing options primarily encompassed nonablative and ablative laser systems and their fractional counterparts. Lasers in these classes target tissue water, variably heating epidermal and/or dermal tissues to incite a wound-healing response that has been refined over recent decades. Traditional fully ablative erbium-doped yttrium aluminum garnet (Er:YAG) and carbon dioxide (CO_2) laser systems are the most aggressive resurfacing options, whose energy vaporizes tissue water, resulting in the ablation of the epidermis and/or superficial dermis.[58,59] More conservative, nonablative laser systems offer a significantly dampened version of this, heating tissue in a controlled manner without ablation.[60]

Fractionating lasers, both ablative and nonablative, work to decrease the surface area of heated tissue by limiting laser energy to uniform columnar subunits named the microthermal zone (MTZ).[61] When applied fractionally, laser energy penetrates far deeper into dermal tissue relative to nonfractionated therapies. Primarily with ablative fractional lasers, various handpieces have been developed that adjust the shape of the MTZ. Here, larger MTZs lead to superficial treatments that work to improve texture. Conversely, deep penetration is achieved with smaller MTZs, leading to advantageous dermal remodeling that spreads to interwoven areas of nontreated tissue. Considering the differences in their patterns of induced tissue damage, it is easy to see how combining resurfacing therapies may offer a more comprehensive approach to resurfacing.

Beginning with the combination approach to traditional fully ablative laser treatment, evidence suggests there may be certain advantages relative to single-modality treatment. Although both Er:YAG and CO_2 are fully ablative therapies, Er:YAG is more efficiently absorbed by tissue water, leading to superficial ablation, whereas CO_2 reaches the upper dermis, leading to tissue contraction, which correlates with more dramatic improvement of deep rhytides. Although results are less dramatic, the benefits of Er:YAG compared to CO_2 is primarily associated with a significantly hastened recovery and decreased adverse effects.

A combination of CO_2 and Er:YAG can achieve both intermediate results and an intermediate recovery compared to these treatments alone.[62] Furthermore, in multiple investigations, CO_2 followed by Er:YAG worked primarily to speed recovery time and decrease the adverse events associated with CO_2 resurfacing.[62,63,64] Laser settings may be kept the same regardless of whether it is used in combination or alone; however, some evidence supports a lower number of

CO_2 laser passes when followed with Er:YAG laser.[62,63,64] Later a device with the capabilities of delivering dual CO_2 and Er:YAG treatments simultaneously was developed. This device achieves improved operative homeostasis, outcomes in rhytides, texture, and patient satisfaction when compared to Er:YAG alone.[65] Furthermore, these results were reproducible on both the neck[65] and face, with the highest improvement produced periorally.[66] Notably, switching the order of CO_2 and Er:YAG therapies when used in combination may alter results. A histological study using the sequential combination of Er:YAG followed by CO_2 led to an increase in collagen production and a remodeled elastic network.[67] Although clinical studies are yet to be published, using the Er:YAG to ablate the entire epidermis prior to the deeper penetrating CO_2 laser appeared to further accentuate CO_2-led tissue contraction.[67]

With the arrival of fractionated lasers, a number of combination regimens employing fractional and traditional ablative lasers have shown utility. These regimens take advantage of the improved recovery of fractionated lasers while reserving the more aggressive fully ablative lasers for resistant regions. Such resistance is frequently encountered in the periorbital and perioral regions where rhytides are more pronounced compared to other facial zones. Thus, one option is to provide full-face rejuvenation with the less aggressive, fractional ablative laser, while reserving traditional fully ablative lasers for smaller cosmetic units that are more problematic regions.[68]

Fractionated lasers also penetrate deeper, the depth of penetration increasing with increasing fluency. Accordingly, a full-facial combination treatment of fractional CO_2 followed by fully ablative Er:YAG has shown benefit. This combination harnesses the superficial results of a fully ablative Er:YAG treatment while gaining the deeper impact of fractional CO_2 on deep rhytides.[69]

Alternatively, a combination of fractional ablative treatments can also provide dual depth resurfacing with a further decrease in adverse effects and recovery time. To accomplish this, fractionated laser parameters can be adjusted to superficial or deeper treatment levels between passes. Another option is to use a combination of the various handpieces for fractional ablative lasers developed for this purpose.[70]

Nonablative lasers can also be combined to yield well-suited combination regimens. Although there are less published works on combination nonablative lasers, these treatments likely far outnumber ablative combinations given their increasing proportion of total resurfacing procedures.[26]

14.4 Combining Other Modalities

14.4.1 Photodynamic Therapy

Photodynamic therapy (PDT) was first developed as a field therapy for neoplasia that harnesses a tumor-specific, photochemical reaction used commonly to treat nonmelanoma skin cancers and their precursors. However, incidentally, PDT was shown to impart a superior cosmetic result when compared to other modalities for treating keratinocyte neoplasms. This has been confirmed by multiple systematic reviews and meta-analyses that have shown PDT outcomes to have better overall cosmesis when compared to cryotherapy, topical imiquimod, and 5-fluorouracil.[71,72] This correlated clinically with improved rhytides, skin texture, and firmness, and histologically with increased dermal collagen and a reduction in epidermal thickness, solar elastosis, and dermal inflammatory infiltrate.[73,74] As such, PDT has developed as a stand-alone cosmetic therapy for skin rejuvenation of photodamaged skin, as well as a treatment for acne vulgaris, sebaceous hyperplasia, and rosacea.[75,76,77]

Although off-label, there are a wide variety of modifications that can be utilized to optimize results and the practicality of therapy. In addition to modifications of altering incubation times, significant improvement has been shown with alterations of the illuminator. Both FDA-approved regimens utilize polychromatic sources of light, one a blue fluorescent lamp emitting a 417-nm wavelength near the Soret band and the other a red light-emitting diode (LED) emitting wavelengths peaking at the 630-nm Q-band. However, with time, other light sources and laser devices have been utilized to photoexcite the protoporphyrin IX molecule including green light, artificial white light, daylight, the 532-nm KTP laser (potassium titanyl phosphate), the 585- to 595-nm PDL, and 500- to 1,200-nm IPL.[78,79,80]

The benefits of utilizing lasers or IPL systems for PDT include the quick application compared to the time required for red and blue light regimens. Additionally, a combination of light or laser sources may be utilized sequentially in a single PDT session in order to maximize photobleaching of the photosensitizer and amplify the benefits. A retrospective study looked at patients treated with aminolevulinic acid (ALA) PDT utilizing either blue light alone, blue light + PDL, blue light + IPL, blue light + PDL + IPL, and blue light + red light + IPL + PDL.[81] They found that with the additive combinations of blue light + PDL + IPL, maximal benefit was achieved.[81] The addition of red light to this regimen further led to significantly less erythema, peeling, acne flares, and pain.[81] In the context of scar treatment, PDT has also shown efficacy and safety when combined with resurfacing lasers.[82]

14.4.2 Radiofrequency

RF technologies have accumulated evidence over recent decades, establishing a multitude of applications in cosmetic dermatology. The mechanism is based on the creation of an electrical current within the target tissue. Dependent on the tissue impedance, the current is converted to heat, ultimately leading to controlled thermal damage and a wound-healing response. RF devices can be noninvasive, using a specific number of electrodes to exert energy without skin penetration, or minimally

invasive, using extenders to reach deeper tissue layers.[83] Devices can be monopolar, bipolar, or multipolar, depending on the number of electrodes.

RF devices of all types have traditionally been used to improve skin laxity and for contouring. Tightening can occur when energy is directed to the dermis at 60 °C to denature collagen bonds and stimulate new collagen production while keeping epidermal temperatures below 45 °C to avoid epidermal compromise.[84] Whereas RF energy within the subcutaneous fat induces lipolysis when adequately heated at 50 °C for a minimum of 1 minute, it can also have a tissue-tightening effect here via effects on the fibrous septa.[84] Temperature-controlled RF is a minimally invasive option where a probe is inserted directly within the tissues under tumescent anesthesia, completely avoiding the epidermis and exerting the greatest effect on laxity and contouring of all the RF devices. Minimally invasive RF options also include microneedling RF devices. Although it also has an effect on skin tightening, microneedling RF devices are also used for treatment of dyspigmentation, texture, and general photorejuvenation.[83]

Combination RF regimens can be safely combined with laser and/or light therapies sequentially or on the same day to achieve additive or even synergistic results.[85,86] When components of a multimodal regimen are delivered at standard treatment parameters, adverse effects and recovery are typically similar to the most aggressive delivered modality when used alone. However, various combinations have evidence of providing for lower levels of adverse effects compared to solo treatments.[87]

With the arrival of RF technologies, a multitude of combination approaches have been explored. In particular, adding an RF modality that focuses on improving laxity and rhytides can supplement laser and light regimens, which have limited ability to impact these outcomes, especially on deeper tissues. Many regimens utilizing laser, light, and RF employ multimodal devices that are aimed at providing a comprehensive therapy, whether delivered sequentially or simultaneously.[88,89] One such device delivers IPL and bipolar RF simultaneously, producing IPL-associated improvement in dyspigmentation, and vascularity, whereas RF provides for enhanced treatment of rhytides.[90] A combination of bipolar RF with minimally invasive RF devices, including microneedle RF, can provide a similar comprehensive photorejuvenation treatment. Another device delivers fractional ablative CO_2 laser and bipolar RF which is intended to resurface and tighten.[87]

Combination RF, laser, and/or light devices have also been developed for a focused, multimodal approach to skin tightening. These devices combine technologies in which both modalities are aimed at maximizing improvement of laxity and rhytides, working together to create a dynamic wound-healing stimulus. These include those harnessing bipolar RF followed immediately by diode laser treatment, another combining bipolar RF with infrared light.[88,89] A series of either treatment can significantly improve laxity and facial rhytides.[89] Furthermore, despite differences between their technologies, both devices deliver similar results.[89] Another study evaluated the combination of these devices, having patients undergo RF and 900-nm diode laser followed immediately by bipolar RF and IPL, which showed incremental improvement in rhytides, laxity, and other signs of photodamage.[91]

14.4.3 Microneedling

Microneedling is a relatively safe, minimally invasive procedure that has gained popularity in recent years. Microneedling devices are outfitted with regularly spaced needles that are applied to the skin to induce numerous micro-wound channels in order to stimulate a wound-healing response.[92,93,94] The controlled tissue damage stimulates dermal remodeling, collagenesis, and elastic fiber production.[95] Furthermore, the damage to the epidermis is thought to be negligible, decreasing the risk of dyspigmentation and providing a safe option for skin of color.[96]

Relatively little has been published regarding the use of microneedling combined with other procedures. Furthermore, a large proportion of the publications on combination treatments involving microneedling focus on its use to assist in dermal drug delivery of another compound such as chemical peels or platelet-rich plasma (PRP).[97] That being said, based on the experiences of colleagues who regularly perform microneedling, it has been safely incorporated into combination regimens involving soft-tissue fillers, neurotoxins, and nonablative lasers. Due to the pinpoint bleeding and edema that follows this procedure, microneedling is typically performed at the end of the sequence of same-day combination treatments.

14.4.4 Chemical Peels

Chemical peels are a well-established, relatively cheap therapy. In the world of rejuvenation, chemical peels are primarily used for resurfacing and dyspigmentation. In addition to their use with microneedling as mentioned earlier, studies have reported on their combination with lasers. Specifically, combinations of 15 to 25% trichloroacetic acid with or without Jessner's solution have been combined with pigment targeting lasers, including the 510-nm pigmented lesion dye laser and Q-switched 755-nm alexandrite laser.[98] These treatments led to improvement in the majority of patients, without increased complications reported.[98]

14.4.5 Microfocused Ultrasound

MFU was introduced onto the aesthetic market as an innovative technology for skin tightening and noninvasive lifting. MFU generates acoustic waves that converge at predetermined depths to create thermal energy within the tissue.[99] The thermal energy is delivered in regularly spaced intervals, leading to a precise array of microscopic necrotic zones known as thermal coagulation points (TCPs), stimulating a wound-healing response.[99,100] In addition to targeting the dermis, and subcutaneous fibrous septa, MFU can penetrate far deeper to target musculature and fascia. Using MFU to target each of these tissue levels can produce skin tightening and lifting superior to other noninvasive therapies, and therefore is the only device with a lifting indication. To maximize efficacy, dual-plane treatments should be used.[101] For facial treatments, a key target for MFU is the superficial musculoaponeurotic system (SMAS), a fibrous layer that integrates the dermis, facial musculature, and fascia for the purpose of facial expression.[102] Initially establishing utility on the face, results with MFU were later replicated on the neck, chest, and beyond.[103]

The addition of MFU's ability to lift and tighten greatly improves results and patient satisfaction from combination regimens. Furthermore, as MFU is primarily used to treat deeper structures than those targeted by other interventions, MFU can be safely combined with other interventions including injectables and other energy-based modalities. A case series of over 100 patients reported the same-day combination of PDL or IPL for vasculature, followed by MFU, immediately followed by Q-switched 755-nm alexandrite for macular seborrheic keratoses (SK), followed by ablative fractional laser to the full face and neck.[104] Results from this combined treatment were said to offer patients greater satisfaction than is typically seen from any single laser alone, without any greater risk or increased downtime than seen when resurfacing is performed alone.[104] We find that MFU is particularly useful for contouring of the jawline and upper neck when combined with lower face soft-tissue augmentation, with or without lipolysis (see section on Site-Specific Combination Therapies).

14.5 Considerations for Treatments in Skin of Color

We have learned that even in darker skin types, same-day combination treatments can be performed safely, leading to additive or even synergistic results, shortened overall downtime, and, thus, higher patient satisfaction.[105] That being said, higher Fitzpatrick skin phototypes and certain ethnic origins predispose individuals to a higher rate of pigmentary complications following aesthetic therapies. In general, choosing treatments that cause less disruption of the basal layer is safer. When using energy-based therapies that invariably damage the epidermis, conservative settings are recommended. As many have found, combination therapies can provide improvements while allowing for less aggressive settings. As such, although combination regimens are less reported in darker skin types, they may prove particularly useful in these patients.[21,106]

14.6 Megacombinations

For those patients displaying the whole host of age-related changes, many will present desiring an entire "makeover." In these cases, using a plethora of treatments in concert can provide maximal results in the least amount of time. Many so-called megacombinations have been investigated for their safety and effectiveness. Still, their use in clinical practice appears to be far more common than suggested by published literature.

One study reported on the use of an extensive same-day laser combination used to treat a population with the gamut of complex, advanced aging symptoms. They used the following sequence: 595-nm PDL for telangiectasia and erythema, followed by Q-switched 755-nm alexandrite laser for discrete pigmentary lesions, followed by fractionated CO_2 to regions of resistant rhytides, including 100% coverage of perioral tissues, followed by sculpting of remaining lines with an Er:YAG pulsed device, and finally treated with fractionated CO_2 over the entire face and neck. With this regimen, benefits were sustained at the last evaluation, 1.5 years after treatment.[107] The treatment was tolerated quite well, with the majority of healing taking place in approximately 9 days with no need for specialized wound care.[107] Furthermore, by ensuring adequate anesthesia with a combination of topical anesthesia, nerve blocks, and, in some cases, conscious sedation, treatment-associated pain scores were minimal.[107]

One of the authors (SGF) frequently combines a vascular laser, such as PDL or IPL, followed by a Q-switched device for pigmented SK and/or lighter lentigines, followed by full-face fractionated CO_2 laser treatment, and then treats perioral and periorbital units with fully ablative CO_2 laser followed by a fully ablative erbium laser without coagulation on the same day to get optimal results (▶ Fig. 14.5, ▶ Fig. 14.6).

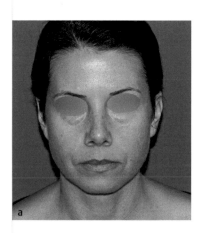
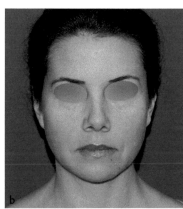

Fig. 14.5 A 36-year-old woman pictured (a) before and (b) 2 years after treatment with onabotulinumtoxin A (Botox, Allergan) to the glabella, crow's feet, frontalis, masseter, mentalis, and depressor anguli oris. After 2 weeks, she was treated with full-face intense pulsed light (IPL), immediately followed by fully ablative 10,600-nm CO_2 (UltraPulse laser, Lumenis, Yokneam, Israel), followed by the fully ablative 2,940-nm Er:YAG laser (Contour TRL, Sciton, Palo Alto, California, United States) periocularly. After 3 months, she was treated with two syringes of VYCROSS hyaluronic acid filler 20 mg/mL (Juvéderm Voluma, Allergan) to the cheeks, chin, and gonial angle and same-day onabotulinumtoxin A (Botox, Allergan) to the glabella, frontalis, crow's feet, masseter, depressor anguli oris, and mentalis.

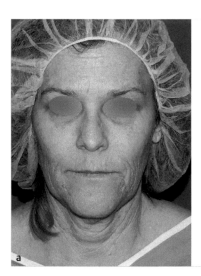
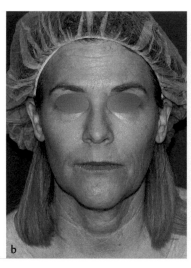

Fig. 14.6 A 50-year-old woman pictured (a) before and (b) after treatment with onabotulinumtoxin A (Botox, Allergan) to the glabella, frontalis, and crow's feet, followed 2 weeks by the same treatment with intense pulsed light (IPL), followed by Q-switched 755-nm alexandrite laser, followed by fully ablative 10,600-nm CO_2 laser (UltraPulse laser, Lumenis), followed by fully ablative 2,940-nm Er:YAG laser (Contour TRL, Sciton) periocularly and periorally, followed by fractionated 10,600-nm CO_2 laser (Fraxel Repair, Solta Medical Inc.).

14.7 Site-Specific Combination Therapy

14.7.1 Periorbital Rejuvenation

The periorbital tissues show early aging changes with contributions from brow descent, dermatochalasis, and orbital fat pseudoherniation.[2] Bone resorption in the periorbital region leads to a widening of the orbital aperture.[108] With this, the eyes appear more sunken, and there is less bone to support surrounding tissue allowing lid ptosis to progress.[108] Furthermore, with concomitant maxillary resorption and inward rotation, both superficial and deep midface fat pads separate from the infraorbital fat pad contributing to the appearance of a tear trough.[2,109]

In order to combat the aging appearance of periorbital tissues, a combination of treatments is particularly effective.[101,102,103,104,105,106,107,108,109,110] Neurotoxins to smooth resting and dynamic rhytides of the glabella, forehead, crow's feet, and/or lower lid can be a great starting point for periorbital intervention. Both properly placed neurotoxins and MFU can provide for a brow lift with completely different mechanisms of action. Combining these for further lifting can be useful, as can RF and ablative lasers for more superficial tightening of periorbital skin. Volumization with midfacial and temporal injection of biostimulating or soft-tissue fillers also helps restore the periorbital region. Moreover, filler treatment of temporal hollows can have a lifting effect on the brow.[111] However, small adjustments in brow position and shape can lead to substantial changes. In Korean women, MFU alone is the treatment of choice for brow lifting as a further exaggerated arch may appear particularly aggressive.[5] Monopolar RF is the treatment of choice for skin tightening of the eyelid itself.[101,102,103,104,105,106,107,108,109,110]

Treatment options for periorbital dark circles include soft-tissue fillers, lasers, light modalities, or combinations thereof to address hollowing, excessive pigmentation, and prominent vasculature.[112] One study investigating a same-day megacombination for periorbital dark circles found a combination of PDL for telangiectasia, followed by fully ablative CO_2 resurfacing, followed by Er:YAG for combination resurfacing over deep rhytides, facial scars, and/or feathering, followed by Q-switched alexandrite lasers for dyspigmentation was highly effective and without additional risk[113] (▶ Fig. 14.7). The use of a Q-switched alexandrite laser was determined necessary if pigmentation was still evident after resurfacing lasers.[113] Pigmentation persistence indicates a significant dermal component of pigmentation, which is known to take longer to respond to laser treatments.[113] Furthermore, after treatment, dyspigmentation was the last component to respond, typically improving 6 to 8 weeks after treatment.[113]

14.7.2 Midfacial Rejuvenation

With the bony resorption of aging, the loss of maxillary support begets the descent of superficial and deep fat pad

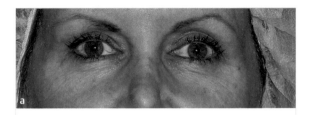
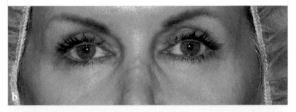

Fig. 14.7 A 54-year-old woman (a) before and (b) 4 years after treatment with the 585-nm pulsed dye laser (Vbeam, Syneron Inc., Irvine, California, United States) immediately followed by fully ablative 10,600-nm CO_2 (UltraPulse laser, Lumenis), followed by the fully ablative 2,940-nm Er:YAG (Contour TRL, Sciton) periocularly.

compartments.[6,108] Although equally prone to photodamage compared to other facial units, rejuvenation of the midface is particularly dependent on the use of soft-tissue fillers to combat these structural changes[114] (▶ Fig. 14.8). When combining soft-tissue fillers with neuromodulators, RF, MFU, lasers, and light modalities in the midface, a number of same-day sequences have been proposed, with significant differences based on provider preference.[114]

14.7.3 Perioral Rejuvenation

The lips and perioral region are a center point of visual attention, and an area where patients seek specific treatment for both enhancement and rejuvenation. Unfortunately, aging is particularly harsh to this region. Maxillary inward rotation causes a lack of support to the levators of the lip and diminishing projection of the lip. This coupled with fat pad atrophy of the vermillion body leads to thinning of the body of the lip, and a flattening of philtral columns. Definition of the vermillion border and cupid's bow is lost. Mandibular resorption causes a lack of support to the depressors of the lip, contributing to a downturning of the oral commissures, and marionette lines. Proper placement of tissue fillers is key to addressing each of the aforementioned issues, redefining structures, combating deep lines, malposition, and restoring fullness of the lips themselves.[115]

When present, deep, radial perioral rhytides can present a therapeutic challenge. Even with the availability of less aggressive options, fully ablative lasers continue to be heavily used for perioral rejuvenation due to their distinct superiority here. Still, at times the deepest of rhytides will survive these fully ablative lasers. In these instances, a low-viscosity hyaluronic acid (HA) filler can

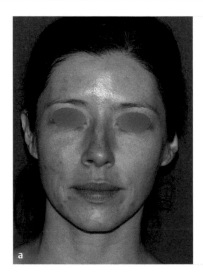
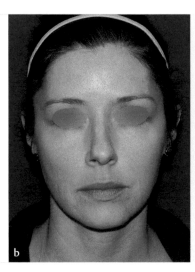

Fig. 14.8 A 32-year-old woman pictured (a) before and (b) 6 years after yearly combination treatments of intense pulsed light, followed immediately by poly-L-lactic acid (Sculptra, Galderma Laboratories, L.P.) to the medial and lateral cheeks, chin, pyriform fossa, and temples, immediately followed by a Cohesive Polydensified Matrix hyaluronic acid (Belotero, Merz North America, Inc.) to the nasolabial folds, followed by onabotulinumtoxin A (Botox, Allergan) to the glabella, crow's feet, frontalis, and depressor anguli oris.

be placed linearly within these refractory rhytides.[115] Neuromodulators can also add to combination therapy of less prominent perioral rhytides. When studied, the combination of fillers and neurotoxins for perioral rejuvenation proved superior to either treatment alone.[116] Additionally, neuromodulators improve the positioning of the lips during animation for a more aesthetically pleasing smile by targeting the levator labii superioris alaeque nasi muscle, and improving the appearance of a "gummy smile."

14.7.4 The Lower Face and Neck

Several intrinsic and extrinsic changes accumulate in the neck with age, making the area a prime focus of patient concern and a potential canvas for the entire spectrum of rejuvenation interventions. The skin of the neck is thin, having a skin thickness that resembles the eyelid more closely than that of the other facial areas.[117] Additionally, skin in the neck lacks the support of pilosebaceous units. Thus, the neck tends to more readily show signs of skin quality loss and aging. As the skin is thin here and the adnexal units drop precipitously relative to the face, the neck is prone to scarring. Due to these variables, traditional fully ablative lasers should be used cautiously or even avoided for resurfacing of the neck. Fractional ablative lasers also carry significant risk and should be used judiciously. Thus, some choose to only use nonablative lasers when choosing among laser resurfacing options for this region.

Neoplasms that harbor attention should be the first priority, removing any SK, acrochordons, etc., that have accumulated over time. Although rare in experienced hands, each of the available methods to accomplish their removal has potential for pigmentary, textural, or scarring complications. Thus, removing these neoplasms first will allow other planned treatments to erase any imperfections induced by earlier treatments. Next, as

the area is open to UV radiation, pigmentation abnormalities are common. With the neck prone to cutaneous atrophy, vascular signs of photodamage are more readily revealed, particularly telangiectasia. When present in combination in this region, telangiectasia, atrophy, hyper- and/or hypopigmentation produce poikiloderma of Civatte. With this range of targets, IPL is the first choice in lighter phototypes, but energy levels should be decreased, and pulse delays increased to account for the lower reservoir of pilosebaceous units. Otherwise, dyspigmentation and vascularity can be treated similar to other areas using more conservative settings.

With bony resorption, the mandible resorbs three dimensionally with age.[108] Changes include decreased vertical height of the mandibular rami and body, as well as decreased mandibular length.[108] Most notably, these changes lead to decreased chin projection, loss of jawline definition and increased soft-tissue laxity of the lower face and neck.[108] This loss of support also accentuates the laxity produced by reductions in skin quality. Furthermore, for those individuals with a history of significant adipose loss, prior stretching of this area may further add to neck skin laxity. Soft-tissue fillers to support and reshape the jawline and chin can be combined with MFU to further contour the neck and decrease skin laxity.

Thread lifts can be applied to redrape soft tissue along the jawline, combating laxity and bringing back youthful definition to these structures.[118] Furthermore, thread lifting has high patient satisfaction in multiple other areas including the midface and eyebrows.[118] Thread lifts are low risk, with minimal adverse effects or safety issues, especially when considering more invasive options.[119] In individuals with particularly thin, atrophic neck skin, we use MFU to improve skin quality prior to performing thread lifts. Of note, in individuals with severe laxity, the tightening effects of MFU and/or thread lifts is usually insufficient. Patients who fit this level of severe laxity should be counseled appropriately in the beginning to avoid disappointment when surgical neck lifts are more appropriate.

In those that accumulate fat in the submental neck, interventions to target the adiposity can also be added or even the sentinel intervention. The "double-chin appearance," which is more common in those who are overweight, is a common focus of patients. Liposuction remains the gold standard, and following the procedure, depending on the baseline laxity of the skin, more redundancy may be noted, although a fair amount of skin contraction typically occurs from liposuction alone. As such, liposuction can be combined with skin-tightening devices, and it has been found to be safe and effective when performed in the same treatment session.[120] The author (SGF) typically performs liposuction immediately followed by a subsurface 1,320-nm laser procedure (CoolLipo, CoolTouch Inc., Roseville, California, United States) at 10 W for typically 6 minutes to the entire area. Subsurface monopolar RF can also be used, with an internal temperature of 60 °C to start and increased as epidermal temperatures tolerate, for a minimum of 25 minutes to the entire area. When paired, results from liposuction will be evident immediately, whereas appreciable skin tightening takes months.[120]

The development of noninvasive lipolysis treatments has widely expanded options to address such unwanted adiposity. Whether it be with injectable deoxycholic acid, cryolipolysis, laser, or RF-assisted lipolysis, we can now offer these treatments for the head and neck, as well as for nonfacial locations. Additionally, neck fullness laterally may be due to submandibular gland enlargement, which can be targeted by neurotoxins similar to the parotid glands.[121,122]

There are two populations of lines on the neck, vertical platysmal banding and horizontal rhytides. Typically developing later in life, increased muscular tone of the platysma may form unsightly vertical bands along the anterior neck. Neurotoxins work well to diminish or even completely soften such platysmal bands. When combined with small-volume neurotoxin injections along the jawline, a so-called Nefertiti lift can help create a sharper jawline.[123] Significant neck laxity can accentuate platysmal bands, and thus combining with MFU can further result in

patients with prominent banding.[124] Notably these can be delivered on the same day, again waiting to perform injections as the last step of combination therapies.[34] On the other hand, although horizontal rhytides can improve with skin-tightening devices and neurotoxins, a low-viscosity HA soft-tissue filler may be needed to adequately soften their appearance.[124]

14.7.5 Chest Rejuvenation

The chest is a prominently photoexposed region prone to displaying the spectrum of skin aging. Like the neck, conservative treatments should be undertaken as skin of the chest is thin and devoid of support from the pilosebaceous unit. As with other photodamaged areas, laser and light therapies to treat vascularity, dyspigmentation, and for resurfacing can be safely applied here with this in mind. MFU has also proven useful for lifting, tightening, and reducing rhytides on the chest.[125] Additionally, biostimulatory fillers and low-viscosity HA soft-tissue fillers are frequently used on the chest to further dampen rhytides and restore volume to this area[126,127] (▶ Fig. 14.9). If to be combined on the same day, MFU is performed first, followed by laser and/or light devices, followed by the filler.

14.7.6 Hand Rejuvenation

For individuals who have undergone rejuvenation efforts on other visible areas, attention is often drawn to the hands, equally conspicuous, and where photodamage remains prominent. To provide a natural, even appearance, the hands should be made to match the face, neck, and chest. A frequent area to develop actinic keratoses (AK) and macular pigmented SK, we prefer treatment of AK with PDT, using sequential PDL, IPL, blue and red light, and SK with IPL layered with Q-switched alexandrite laser. Otherwise similar to other photoexposed areas, the spectrum of laser and light therapies can be utilized for hand dyspigmentation, and vascularity, whereas resurfacing is used to improve skin tone and quality.[28]

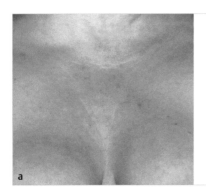 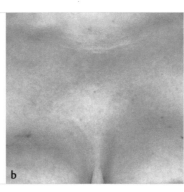

Fig. 14.9 The pictured décolletage **(a)** before and **(b)** 6 months after treatment with MFU-V (Ultherapy, Merz North America, Inc.), immediately followed by one syringe of calcium hydroxylapatite filler (diluted 1:2 with normal saline; Radiesse, Merz North America, Inc.), with filler repeated every 6 weeks for two more treatments.

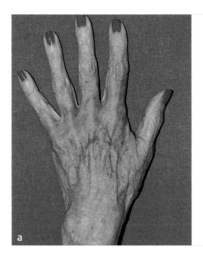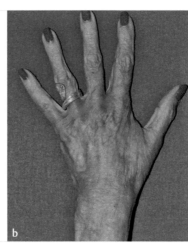

Fig. 14.10 Photoaged left hand pictured **(a)** before and **(b)** 1 month after treatment with intense pulsed light (IPL) immediately followed by 1.5-mL injection of calcium hydroxylapatite (CaHA; Radiesse, Merz North America, Inc.) blended with 0.5 mL of 1% lidocaine (per hand) to address dyschromia and volume loss.

Prominent fat atrophy also occurs in the dorsal hands, defining underlying bony and tendinous structures, as well as making veins more prominent. Soft-tissue fillers are the primary modality for volume restoration in the hand, although biostimulatory fillers and fat transfer are other options.[28,124]

When dyspigmentation and volume loss are addressed on the same day, an IPL or a 1,927-nm diode laser is used first immediately followed by either calcium hydroxylapatite (CaHA; Radiesse, Merz North America, Inc., Raleigh, North Carolina, United States) or a particulate HA gel (Resytlane Lyft, Galderma Laboratories, L.P., Fort Worth, Texas, United States), both of which are FDA cleared for dorsal hand augmentation (▶ Fig. 14.10). With the presence of reticular blue veins in the hands, addressing any concomitant atrophy should be performed first, as these interventions are frequently satisfactory. If this remains a concern, sclerotherapy is a useful, less invasive option; phlebectomy can also be used.[28]

The authors personally utilize foam sclerotherapy using either 0.5% sodium tetradecyl sulfate or 1% polidocanol. Although up to 20 mL of foam can be used on the same day, one author (SGF) finds that 1 mL of sclerosant and 5 mL of total foam are typically adequate per hand. Some experts recommend avoiding sclerotherapy at the same time as other local interventions due to concerns of exacerbating the significant swelling that may occur following sclerotherapy and the need for compression during the weeks following sclerotherapy.[128] The authors do not have experience combining sclerotherapy with other local interventions, and further studies are needed.

14.7.7 Rejuvenation of Other Body Sites

Surgical interventions have pioneered the way in body contouring, an arena that developed in large part to address issues after massive weight loss.[129] That being said, body contouring is also commonly performed for patients seeking improvement from age-related changes. Surgical options commonly include liposuction, excisional procedures, surgical lifts, autologous fat grafting, and implants. Although traditionally performed by plastic surgeons, cosmetic dermatologists variably offer many of these therapies as well. However, newer noninvasive and minimally invasive therapies for lipolysis, collagen stimulation, and skin tightening have made nonsurgical body contouring possible. The emerging use of these less invasive options has shifted expertise in body contouring further in the realm of the cosmetic dermatologist. Additionally, a relationship between surgeons and dermatologists has been created by motivated patients looking to finely tune surgical outcomes with nonsurgical options.

Liposuction is at the top of the most commonly performed surgical procedures, remaining the gold standard intervention to address adiposity and/or adipose-related deformity.[130] However, the advent of noninvasive lipolysis has created many more options for treatment. The buttocks and thighs may preferentially accumulate adiposity over time. When liposuction is foregone, noninvasive lipolysis treatments can be offered as another option. Among lipolysis options are cryolipolysis, RF-assisted devices, laser-assisted devices, high-frequency focused ultrasound, and nonthermal ultrasound. The latter is distinctly less painful, but results are similar.[36]

Additionally, performing skin-tightening treatments in areas that tend to accumulate adiposity such as the buttocks, thighs, and arms can improve cosmesis without addressing the problem directly. When using energy-based device therapies on nonfacial sites, treatments should be initiated with conservative parameters, especially in areas with less support from adnexal structures.[36] Although most commonly used on the head and neck regions, MFU can be applied in nearly any region where skin tightening is desired. When used for body contouring, MFU has shown efficacy on the buttocks, arm, thighs, and above large joints of the extremities.[101,131,132,133] Regional differences in responses have been noted. The upper arms and knees showed superior responses to MFU, compared to the responses of the buttocks and thighs.[101,131] The benefits realized above the knees and elbows are particularly impressive due to the counteracting force associated with the constant repetitive motion at these joints.[101,133] Resurfacing lasers have also been used safely on the extremities for more superficial skin tightening.[134]

Dermal fillers, specifically biostimulatory injectables such as CaHA and poly-L-lactic acid (PLLA; Sculptra, Galderma Laboratories, L.P.), can be added to areas where skin quality is diminished to improve laxity, elasticity, stratum corneum hydration, skin thickness, and density.[124] Based on consensus recommendations, soft-tissue fillers are first-line early interventions and second-line restoration procedures for the chest and hands; they are also efficacious on the upper arm, thighs, buttocks, and abdomen.[135,136,137,138] When using PLLA for biostimulation, larger dilutions (12 mL or more per vial) are recommended for off-facial sites.[138] The author (SGF) uses 16-mL dilutions off the face (▶ Fig. 14.11).

Frequently, the buttocks and thighs exhibit unique signs of aging, including striae and cellulite, requiring a combination approach for optimal rejuvenation. When present, striae rubra's vascular component can be reliably treated with vascular laser and light therapies. Conversely, the textural component is often refractory. In order to diminish the intensity of these atrophic linear plaques, a combination approach may provide more substantial improvements. For example, one study found that microneedle RF and fractionated CO_2 laser provided better improvements of striae than either modality alone.[139] To address both components in striae rubra, vascular lasers can be combined with resurfacing lasers and/or microneedling on the same day as long as the vascular laser is used first.[140]

For fully developed cellulite, we favor subcutaneous subcision, whereas RF devices can be used on more mild or superficial lesions.[36] Suction-assisted subcision is particularly useful, being careful not to treat areas of laxity as this can exacerbate this component.[141] When both superficial and deep cellulite components are present, the procedures can be combined with RF performed prior to subcision.[140] Pairing these interventions with injections of biostimulatory fillers can be particularly useful, as can the addition of MFU when concomitant laxity is present.

The consequences of lifelong venous dependence of the lower extremities create a zone prone to vascular abnormalities. These include venous varicosities of all sizes, as well as matted telangiectasia. Sclerotherapy is the treatment of choice for smaller varicosities and telangiectasias, whereas more invasive options are required for larger lesions.

14.7.8 Patient Selection, Patient Preparation, and Recovery

As those that offer any of the discussed individual therapies will know from experience, proper patient selection is vital to successful treatment outcomes. With combination treatments, patient selection is no different. A long-term regimen of sun protection and topical therapies (antioxidants, retinoids, hydroxy acids, etc.) is best established before pursuing therapies targeting superficial targets (pigment, erythema, rhytides). The regimen will be used to maximize skin quality and maintain improvement reached synergistically with the aforementioned therapies. Additionally, establishing maintenance regimens prior to pursuing device therapies allows the patient to demonstrate compliance with intensive skin care regimens.

Setting expectations is important with any cosmetic therapy. Although the patient may not always know what they want when they enter a consultation, treatment targets should be agreed upon prior to proceeding with therapy. Discussions of recommended options should include a detailed discussion of their associated recoveries. The authors recommend utilizing photographs of prior patients undergoing the proposed therapies to help set expectations and prepare for the recovery process. The authors typically show the patients the before, immediately after, daily, and then weekly photographs during the recovery process and then follow-up months after completing treatment. These photographs prepare the patients far more effectively than words can.

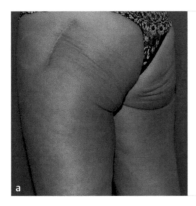 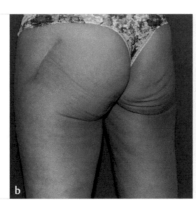

Fig. 14.11 A 60-year-old woman **(a)** before and **(b)** 2 months after treatment with microfocused ultrasound with visualization (MFU-V; Ultherapy, Merz North America, Inc.) to the posterior legs and buttocks, immediately followed by three vials of poly-L-lactic acid (Sculptra, Galderma Laboratories, L.P.) to each buttock (16-mL dilution per vial).

14.7.9 Postoperative Care

Postoperative care is no different than that prescribed during recovery of the individual treatments the patients are receiving.

References

[1] Perrett DI, May KA, Yoshikawa S. Facial shape and judgements of female attractiveness. Nature. 1994; 368(6468):239–242

[2] Bueller H. Ideal facial relationships and goals. Facial Plast Surg. 2018; 34(5):458–465

[3] Goodman GJ. The oval female facial shape: a study in beauty. Dermatol Surg. 2015; 41(12):1375–1383

[4] Keaney TC, Anolik R, Braz A, et al. The male aesthetic patient: facial anatomy, concepts of attractiveness, and treatment patterns. J Drugs Dermatol. 2018; 17(1):19–28

[5] Chao YYY, Chhabra C, Corduff N, et al. PAN-ASIAN CONSENSUS-Key Recommendations for Adapting the World Congress of Dermatology Consensus on Combination Treatment with Injectable Fillers, Toxins, and Ultrasound Devices in Asian Patients. J Clin Aesthet Dermatol. 2017; 10(8):16–27

[6] Paskhover B, Durand D, Kamen E, Gordon NA. Patterns of change in facial skeletal aging. JAMA Facial Plast Surg. 2017; 19(5):413–417

[7] Farkas LG, Katic MJ, Forrest CR, et al. International anthropometric study of facial morphology in various ethnic groups/races. J Craniofac Surg. 2005; 16(4):615–646

[8] Westmore MG. Facial Cosmetics in Conjunction with Surgery. Course presented at the Aesthetic Plastic Surgery Society Meeting, May 1975, Vancouver, British Columbia

[9] Cook TA, Brownrigg PJ, Wang TD, Quatela VC. The versatile midforehead browlift. Arch Otolaryngol Head Neck Surg. 1989; 115 (2):163–168

[10] Griffin GR, Kim JC. Ideal female brow aesthetics. Clin Plast Surg. 2013; 40(1):147–155

[11] Fang F, Clapham PJ, Chung KC. A systematic review of interethnic variability in facial dimensions. Plast Reconstr Surg. 2011; 127(2): 874–881

[12] Saluja SS, Fabi SG. A holistic approach to antiaging as an adjunct to antiaging procedures: a review of the literature. Dermatol Surg. 2017; 43(4):475–484

[13] Poon F, Kang S, Chien AL. Mechanisms and treatments of photoaging. Photodermatol Photoimmunol Photomed. 2015; 31(2):65–74

[14] Kosmadaki MG, Gilchrest BA. The role of telomeres in skin aging/photoaging. Micron. 2004; 35(3):155–159

[15] Demontiero O, Vidal C, Duque G. Aging and bone loss: new insights for the clinician. Ther Adv Musculoskelet Dis. 2012; 4(2): 61–76

[16] Bonati LM, Fabi SG. Treating the young aesthetic patient: evidence-based recommendations. J Drugs Dermatol. 2017; 16(6):s81–s83

[17] Han A, Chien AL, Kang S. Photoaging. Dermatol Clin. 2014; 32(3): 291–299, vii

[18] Mac-Mary S, Sainthillier JM, Jeudy A, et al. Assessment of cumulative exposure to UVA through the study of asymmetrical facial skin aging. Clin Interv Aging. 2010; 5:277–284

[19] Ber RS, Bhawan J. Lentigo. Int J Dermatol. 1996; 35(4):229–239

[20] Eller MS, Yaar M, Gilchrest BA. DNA damage and melanogenesis. Nature. 1994; 372(6505):413–414

[21] Tian BW. Novel low fluence combination laser treatment of solar lentigines in type III Asian skin. J Cutan Aesthet Surg. 2015; 8(4): 230–232

[22] Helfrich YR, Maier LE, Cui Y, et al. Clinical, histologic, and molecular analysis of differences between erythematotelangiectatic rosacea and telangiectatic photoaging. JAMA Dermatol. 2015; 151(8):825–836

[23] Hafsi W, Badri T. Actinic Purpura. Treasure Island, FL: StatPearls Publishing; 2019

[24] El-Domyati M, Attia S, Saleh F, et al. Intrinsic aging vs. photoaging: a comparative histopathological, immunohistochemical, and ultrastructural study of skin. Exp Dermatol. 2002; 11(5):398–405

[25] Contet-Audonneau JL, Jeanmaire C, Pauly G. A histological study of human wrinkle structures: comparison between sun-exposed areas of the face, with or without wrinkles, and sun-protected areas. Br J Dermatol. 1999; 140(6):1038–1047

[26] American Society for Aesthetic Plastic Surgery. Cosmetic Surgery National Data Bank Statistics. 2017. Available at: https://www.surgery.org/sites/default/files/ASAPS-Stats2017.pdf. Accessed October 20, 2018

[27] Anand C. Facial contouring with fillers, neuromodulators, and lipolysis to achieve a natural look in patients with facial fullness. J Drugs Dermatol. 2016; 15(12):1536–1542

[28] Fabi SG, Goldman MP. The safety and efficacy of combining poly-L-lactic acid with intense pulsed light in facial rejuvenation: a retrospective study of 90 patients. Dermatol Surg. 2012; 38(7, Pt 2): 1208–1216

[29] Casabona G. Combined use of microfocused ultrasound and a calcium hydroxylapatite dermal filler for treating atrophic acne scars: a pilot study. J Cosmet Laser Ther. 2018; 20(5):301–306

[30] Goldman MP, Alster TS, Weiss R. A randomized trial to determine the influence of laser therapy, monopolar radiofrequency treatment, and intense pulsed light therapy administered immediately after hyaluronic acid gel implantation. Dermatol Surg. 2007; 33(5):535–542

[31] England LJ, Tan MH, Shumaker PR, et al. Effects of monopolar radiofrequency treatment over soft-tissue fillers in an animal model. Lasers Surg Med. 2005; 37(5):356–365

[32] Shumaker PR, England LJ, Dover JS, et al. Effect of monopolar radiofrequency treatment over soft-tissue fillers in an animal model: part 2. Lasers Surg Med. 2006; 38(3):211–217

[33] Alam M, Levy R, Pajvani U, et al. Safety of radiofrequency treatment over human skin previously injected with medium-term injectable soft-tissue augmentation materials: a controlled pilot trial. Lasers Surg Med. 2006; 38(3):205–210

[34] Cuerda-Galindo E, Palomar-Gallego MA, Linares-Garcíavaldecasas R. Are combined same-day treatments the future for photorejuvenation? Review of the literature on combined treatments with lasers, intense pulsed light, radiofrequency, botulinum toxin, and fillers for rejuvenation. J Cosmet Laser Ther. 2015; 17(1):49–54

[35] Park KY, Park MK, Li K, Seo SJ, Hong CK. Combined treatment with a nonablative infrared device and hyaluronic acid filler does not have enhanced efficacy in treating nasolabial fold wrinkles. Dermatol Surg. 2011; 37(12):1770–1775

[36] Coleman KM, Pozner J. Combination therapy for rejuvenation of the outer thigh and buttock: a review and our experience. Dermatol Surg. 2016; 42 Suppl 2:S124–S130

[37] Park JM, Tsao H, Tsao S. Combined use of intense pulsed light and Q-switched ruby laser for complex dyspigmentation among Asian patients. Lasers Surg Med. 2008; 40(2):128–133

[38] Wang CC, Sue YM, Yang CH, Chen CK. A comparison of Q-switched alexandrite laser and intense pulsed light for the treatment of freckles and lentigines in Asian persons: a randomized, physician-blinded, split-face comparative trial. J Am Acad Dermatol. 2006; 54 (5):804–810

[39] Tian BW. Novel treatment of Hori's nevus: a combination of fractional nonablative 2,940-nm Er:YAG and low-fluence 1,064-nm Q-switched Nd:YAG laser. J Cutan Aesthet Surg. 2015; 8(4):227–229

[40] Manuskiatti W, Sivayathorn A, Leelaudomlipi P, Fitzpatrick RE. Treatment of acquired bilateral nevus of Ota-like macules (Hori's nevus) using a combination of scanned carbon dioxide laser followed by Q-switched ruby laser. J Am Acad Dermatol. 2003; 48(4):584–591

[41] Ee HL, Goh CL, Khoo LS, Chan ES, Ang P. Treatment of acquired bilateral nevus of ota-like macules (Hori's nevus) with a combination of the 532 nm Q-switched Nd:YAG laser followed by the 1,064 nm Q-switched Nd:YAG is more effective: prospective study. Dermatol Surg. 2006; 32(1):34–40

[42] Wu DC, Friedmann DP, Fabi SG, Goldman MP, Fitzpatrick RE. Comparison of intense pulsed light with 1,927-nm fractionated thulium fiber laser for the rejuvenation of the chest. Dermatol Surg. 2014; 40(2):129–133

[43] Kearney C, Brew D. Single-session combination treatment with intense pulsed light and nonablative fractional photothermolysis: a split-face study. Dermatol Surg. 2012; 38(7, Pt 1):1002–1009

[44] Tao L, Wu J, Qian H, et al. Intense pulsed light, near infrared pulsed light, and fractional laser combination therapy for skin rejuvenation in Asian subjects: a prospective multi-center study in China. Lasers Med Sci. 2015; 30(7):1977–1983

[45] Choi YJ, Nam JH, Kim JY, et al. Efficacy and safety of a novel picosecond laser using combination of 1 064 and 595 nm on patients with melasma: a prospective, randomized, multicenter, split-face, 2% hydroquinone cream-controlled clinical trial. Lasers Surg Med. 2017; 49(10):899–907

[46] Zaleski L, Fabi S, Goldman MP. Treatment of melasma and the use of intense pulsed light: a review. J Drugs Dermatol. 2012; 11(11):1316–1320

[47] Park GH, Lee JH, Choi JR, Chang SE. The degree of erythema in melasma lesion is associated with the severity of disease and the response to the low-fluence Q-switched 1064-nm Nd:YAG laser treatment. J Dermatolog Treat. 2013; 24(4):297–299

[48] Kong SH, Suh HS, Choi YS. Treatment of melasma with pulsed-dye laser and 1,064-nm Q-switched Nd:YAG laser: a split-face study. Ann Dermatol. 2018; 30(1):1–7

[49] Yun WJ, Moon HR, Lee MW, Choi JH, Chang SE. Combination treatment of low-fluence 1,064-nm Q-switched Nd: YAG laser with novel intense pulse light in Korean melasma patients: a prospective, randomized, controlled trial. Dermatol Surg. 2014; 40(8):842–850

[50] Vanaman Wilson MJ, Jones IT, Bolton J, Larsen L, Fabi SG. The safety and efficacy of treatment with a 1,927-nm diode laser with and without topical hydroquinone for facial hyperpigmentation and melasma in darker skin types. Dermatol Surg. 2018; 44(10):1304–1310

[51] Chen DL, Cohen JL. Treatment of periorbital veins with long-pulse Nd:YAG laser. J Drugs Dermatol. 2015; 14(11):1360–1362

[52] Iyer S, Fitzpatrick RE. Long-pulsed dye laser treatment for facial telangiectasias and erythema: evaluation of a single purpuric pass versus multiple subpurpuric passes. Dermatol Surg. 2005; 31(8, Pt 1):898–903

[53] Gao L, Gao N, Song W, et al. A retrospective study on efficacy of pulsed dye laser and intense pulsed light for the treatment of facial telangiectasia. J Drugs Dermatol. 2017; 16(11):1112–1116

[54] Alam M, Dover JS, Arndt KA. Treatment of facial telangiectasia with variable-pulse high-fluence pulsed-dye laser: comparison of efficacy with fluences immediately above and below the purpura threshold. Dermatol Surg. 2003; 29(7):681–684, discussion 685

[55] Karsai S, Roos S, Raulin C. Treatment of facial telangiectasia using a dual-wavelength laser system (595 and 1,064 nm): a randomized controlled trial with blinded response evaluation. Dermatol Surg. 2008; 34(5):702–708

[56] Alam M, Voravutinon N, Warycha M, et al. Comparative effectiveness of nonpurpuragenic 595-nm pulsed dye laser and microsecond 1064-nm neodymium:yttrium-aluminum-garnet laser for treatment of diffuse facial erythema: a double-blind randomized controlled trial. J Am Acad Dermatol. 2013; 69(3):438–443

[57] Kim SJ, Lee Y, Seo YJ, Lee JH, Im M. Comparative efficacy of radiofrequency and pulsed dye laser in the treatment of rosacea. Dermatol Surg. 2017; 43(2):204–209

[58] Ratner D, Viron A, Puvion-Dutilleul F, Puvion E. Pilot ultrastructural evaluation of human preauricular skin before and after high-energy pulsed carbon dioxide laser treatment. Arch Dermatol. 1998; 134(5):582–587

[59] Laubach HJ, Tannous Z, Anderson RR, Manstein D. Skin responses to fractional photothermolysis. Lasers Surg Med. 2006; 38(2):142–149

[60] Lupton JR, Williams CM, Alster TS. Nonablative laser skin resurfacing using a 1540 nm erbium glass laser: a clinical and histologic analysis. Dermatol Surg. 2002; 28(9):833–835

[61] Manstein D, Herron GS, Sink RK, Tanner H, Anderson RR. Fractional photothermolysis: a new concept for cutaneous remodeling using microscopic patterns of thermal injury. Lasers Surg Med. 2004; 34(5):426–438

[62] Greene D, Egbert BM, Utley DS, Koch RJ. In vivo model of histologic changes after treatment with the superpulsed CO_2 laser, erbium:YAG laser, and blended lasers: a 4- to 6-month prospective histologic and clinical study. Lasers Surg Med. 2000; 27(4):362–372

[63] Goldman MP, Manuskiatti W. Combined laser resurfacing with the 950-microsec pulsed CO_2 + Er:YAG lasers. Dermatol Surg. 1999; 25(3):160–163

[64] McDaniel DH, Lord J, Ash K, Newman J. Combined CO_2/erbium:YAG laser resurfacing of peri-oral rhytides and side-by-side comparison with carbon dioxide laser alone. Dermatol Surg. 1999; 25(4):285–293

[65] Goldman MP, Marchell NL. Laser resurfacing of the neck with the combined CO_2/Er:YAG laser. Dermatol Surg. 1999; 25(12):923–925

[66] Goldman MP, Marchell N, Fitzpatrick RE. Laser skin resurfacing of the face with a combined CO_2/Er:YAG laser. Dermatol Surg. 2000; 26(2):102–104

[67] Anayb Baleg SM, Bidin N, Suan LP, et al. Combination of Er:YAG laser and CO_2 laser treatment on skin tissue. Photochem Photobiol. 2015; 91(1):134–138

[68] Worley B, Cohen JL. Combination ablative approach to laser therapy in advanced aging of the face. J Drugs Dermatol. 2018; 17(7):796–799

[69] Mittelman H, Furr M, Lay PC. Combined fractionated CO_2 and low-power erbium:YAG laser treatments. Facial Plast Surg Clin North Am. 2012; 20(2):135–143, v

[70] Kotlus BS. Dual-depth fractional carbon dioxide laser resurfacing for periocular rhytidosis. Dermatol Surg. 2010; 36(5):623–628

[71] Patel G, Armstrong AW, Eisen DB. Efficacy of photodynamic therapy vs other interventions in randomized clinical trials for the treatment of actinic keratoses: a systematic review and meta-analysis. JAMA Dermatol. 2014; 150(12):1281–1288

[72] Gupta AK, Paquet M, Villanueva E, Brintnell W. Interventions for actinic keratoses. Cochrane Database Syst Rev. 2012; 12:CD004415

[73] Park MY, Sohn S, Lee ES, Kim YC. Photorejuvenation induced by 5-aminolevulinic acid photodynamic therapy in patients with actinic keratosis: a histologic analysis. J Am Acad Dermatol. 2010; 62(1):85–95

[74] Issa MC, Piñeiro-Maceira J, Vieira MT, et al. Photorejuvenation with topical methyl aminolevulinate and red light: a randomized, prospective, clinical, histopathologic, and morphometric study. Dermatol Surg. 2010; 36(1):39–48

[75] Sun Y, Chen L, Zhang Y, Gao X, Wu Y, Chen H. Topical photodynamic therapy with 5-aminolevulinic acid in Chinese patients with Rosacea. J Cosmet Laser Ther. 2019; 21(4):196–200

[76] Gold MH, Bradshaw VL, Boring MM, Bridges TM, Biron JA, Lewis TL. Treatment of sebaceous gland hyperplasia by photodynamic therapy with 5-aminolevulinic acid and a blue light source or intense pulsed light source. J Drugs Dermatol. 2004; 3(6) Suppl:S6–S9

[77] Itoh Y, Ninomiya Y, Tajima S, Ishibashi A. Photodynamic therapy of acne vulgaris with topical delta-aminolaevulinic acid and incoherent light in Japanese patients. Br J Dermatol. 2001; 144(3):575–579

[78] Osiecka BJ, Nockowski P, Szepietowski JC. Treatment of actinic keratosis with photodynamic therapy using red or green light: a comparative study. Acta Derm Venereol. 2018; 98(7):689–693

[79] O'Gorman SM, Clowry J, Manley M, et al. Artificial white light vs daylight photodynamic therapy for actinic keratoses: a randomized clinical trial. JAMA Dermatol. 2016; 152(6):638–644

[80] Rubel DM, Spelman L, Murrell DF, et al. Daylight photodynamic therapy with methyl aminolevulinate cream as a convenient, similarly effective, nearly painless alternative to conventional photodynamic therapy in actinic keratosis treatment: a randomized controlled trial. Br J Dermatol. 2014; 171(5):1164–1171

[81] Friedmann DP, Goldman MP, Fabi SG, Guiha I. The effect of multiple sequential light sources to activate aminolevulinic Acid in the treatment of actinic keratoses: a retrospective study. J Clin Aesthet Dermatol. 2014; 7(9):20–25

[82] Yin R, Lin L, Xiao Y, Hao F, Hamblin MR. Combination ALA-PDT and ablative fractional Er:YAG laser (2,940 nm) on the treatment of severe acne. Lasers Surg Med. 2014; 46(3):165–172

[83] Sadick N, Rothaus KO. Minimally invasive radiofrequency devices. Clin Plast Surg. 2016; 43(3):567–575

[84] Gentile RD, Kinney BM, Sadick NS. Radiofrequency technology in face and neck rejuvenation. Facial Plast Surg Clin North Am. 2018; 26(2):123–134

[85] Gold MH, Biron JA, Sensing W. Facial skin rejuvenation by combination treatment of IPL followed by continuous and fractional radiofrequency. J Cosmet Laser Ther. 2016; 18(1):2–6

[86] Gold AH, Pozner J, Weiss R. A fractional bipolar radiofrequency device combined with a bipolar radiofrequency and infrared light treatment for improvement in facial wrinkles and overall skin tone and texture. Aesthet Surg J. 2016; 36(9):1058–1067

[87] Cameli N, Mariano M, Serio M, Ardigò M. Preliminary comparison of fractional laser with fractional laser plus radiofrequency for the treatment of acne scars and photoaging. Dermatol Surg. 2014; 40(5):553–561

[88] Doshi SN, Alster TS. Combination radiofrequency and diode laser for treatment of facial rhytides and skin laxity. J Cosmet Laser Ther. 2005; 7(1):11–15

[89] Choi YJ, Lee JY, Ahn JY, Kim MN, Park MY. The safety and efficacy of a combined diode laser and bipolar radiofrequency compared with combined infrared light and bipolar radiofrequency for skin rejuvenation. Indian J Dermatol Venereol Leprol. 2012; 78(2):146–152

[90] Bitter P, Jr, Stephen Mulholland R. Report of a new technique for enhanced non-invasive skin rejuvenation using a dual mode pulsed light and radio-frequency energy source: selective radio-thermolysis. J Cosmet Dermatol. 2002; 1(3):142–143

[91] Alexiades-Armenakas M. Rhytides, laxity, and photoaging treated with a combination of radiofrequency, diode laser, and pulsed light and assessed with a comprehensive grading scale. J Drugs Dermatol. 2006; 5(8):731–738

[92] Camirand A, Doucet J. Needle dermabrasion. Aesthetic Plast Surg. 1997; 21(1):48–51

[93] Fernandes D. Percutaneous collagen induction: an alternative to laser resurfacing. Aesthet Surg J. 2002; 22(3):307–309

[94] Fernandes D. Minimally invasive percutaneous collagen induction. Oral Maxillofac Surg Clin North Am. 2005; 17(1):51–63, vi

[95] Aust MC, Fernandes D, Kolokythas P, Kaplan HM, Vogt PM. Percutaneous collagen induction therapy: an alternative treatment for scars, wrinkles, and skin laxity. Plast Reconstr Surg. 2008; 121(4):1421–1429

[96] Aust MC, Reimers K, Repenning C, et al. Percutaneous collagen induction: minimally invasive skin rejuvenation without risk of hyperpigmentation-fact or fiction? Plast Reconstr Surg. 2008; 122(5):1553–1563

[97] El-Domyati M, Abdel-Wahab H, Hossam A. Combining microneedling with other minimally invasive procedures for facial rejuvenation: a split-face comparative study. Int J Dermatol. 2018; 57(11):1324–1334

[98] Lee GY, Kim HJ, Whang KK. The effect of combination treatment of the recalcitrant pigmentary disorders with pigmented laser and chemical peeling. Dermatol Surg. 2002; 28(12):1120–1123, discussion 1123

[99] White WM, Makin IR, Barthe PG, Slayton MH, Gliklich RE. Selective creation of thermal injury zones in the superficial musculoaponeurotic system using intense ultrasound therapy: a new target for noninvasive facial rejuvenation. Arch Facial Plast Surg. 2007; 9(1):22–29

[100] Laubach HJ, Makin IR, Barthe PG, Slayton MH, Manstein D. Intense focused ultrasound: evaluation of a new treatment modality for precise microcoagulation within the skin. Dermatol Surg. 2008; 34(5):727–734

[101] Alster TS, Tanzi EL. Noninvasive lifting of arm, thigh, and knee skin with transcutaneous intense focused ultrasound. Dermatol Surg. 2012; 38(5):754–759

[102] Whitney ZB, Zito PM. Anatomy, Skin, Superficial Musculoaponeurotic System (SMAS) Fascia. Treasure Island, FL: StatPearls Publishing; 2018

[103] Fabi SG. Microfocused ultrasound with visualization for skin tightening and lifting: my experience and a review of the literature. Dermatol Surg. 2014; 40 Suppl 12:S164–S167

[104] Woodward JA, Fabi SG, Alster T, Colón-Acevedo B. Safety and efficacy of combining microfocused ultrasound with fractional CO_2 laser resurfacing for lifting and tightening the face and neck. Dermatol Surg. 2014; 40 Suppl 12:S190–S193

[105] Gregory A, Chunharas C, Ogilvie P, Humphrey S, Fabi SG. Single Treatment versus Combination Treatment in Patient Retention. Annual Meeting of the American Society for Dermatologic Surgery, October, 2018, Chicago, IL

[106] Guss L, Bolton JG, Fabi SG. Combination therapy in skin of color including injectables, laser, and light devices. Semin Cutan Med Surg. 2016; 35(4):211–217

[107] Wu DC, Fitzpatrick RE. Facial rejuvenation via the sequential combined use of multiple laser modalities: safety and efficacy. Lasers Surg Med. 2016; 48(6):577–583

[108] Shaw RB, Jr, Katzel EB, Koltz PF, et al. Aging of the facial skeleton: aesthetic implications and rejuvenation strategies. Plast Reconstr Surg. 2011; 127(1):374–383

[109] Fezza JP, Massry G. Lower eyelid length. Plast Reconstr Surg. 2015; 136(2):152e–159e

[110] Carruthers J, Burgess C, Day D, et al. Consensus recommendations for combined aesthetic interventions in the face using botulinum toxin, fillers, and energy-based devices. Dermatol Surg. 2016; 42(5):586–597

[111] Langelier N, Beleznay K, Woodward J. Rejuvenation of the upper face and periocular region: combining neuromodulator, facial filler, laser, light, and energy-based therapies for optimal results. Dermatol Surg. 2016; 42 Suppl 2:S77–S82

[112] Friedmann DP, Goldman MP. Dark circles: etiology and management options. Clin Plast Surg. 2015; 42(1):33–50

[113] Manuskiatti W, Fitzpatrick RE, Goldman MP. Treatment of facial skin using combinations of CO_2, Q-switched alexandrite, flashlamp-pumped pulsed dye, and Er:YAG lasers in the same treatment session. Dermatol Surg. 2000; 26(2):114–120

[114] Humphrey S, Beleznay K, Fitzgerald R. Combination therapy in midfacial rejuvenation. Dermatol Surg. 2016; 42 Suppl 2:S83–S88

[115] Ponsky D, Guyuron B. Comprehensive surgical aesthetic enhancement and rejuvenation of the perioral region. Aesthet Surg J. 2011; 31(4):382–391

[116] Carruthers A, Carruthers J, Monheit GD, Davis PG, Tardie G. Multicenter, randomized, parallel-group study of the safety and effectiveness of onabotulinumtoxinA and hyaluronic acid dermal fillers (24-mg/ml smooth, cohesive gel) alone and in combination for lower facial rejuvenation. Dermatol Surg. 2010; 36 Suppl 4:2121–2134

[117] Ha RY, Nojima K, Adams WP, Jr, Brown SA. Analysis of facial skin thickness: defining the relative thickness index. Plast Reconstr Surg. 2005; 115(6):1769–1773

[118] Rezaee Khiabanloo S, Jebreili R, Aalipour E, Saljoughi N, Shahidi A. Outcomes in thread lift for face and neck: a study performed with silhouette soft and promo happy lift double needle, innovative and classic techniques. J Cosmet Dermatol. 2019; 18(1):84–93

[119] Sarigul Guduk S, Karaca N. Safety and complications of absorbable threads made of poly-L-lactic acid and poly lactide/glycolide: experience with 148 consecutive patients. J Cosmet Dermatol. 2018; 17(6):1189–1193

[120] Alexiades-Armenakas M. Combination laser-assisted liposuction and minimally invasive skin tightening with temperature feedback for treatment of the submentum and neck. Dermatol Surg. 2012; 38(6):871–881

[121] Wu WT. Botox facial slimming/facial sculpting: the role of botulinum toxin-A in the treatment of hypertrophic masseteric muscle and parotid enlargement to narrow the lower facial width. Facial Plast Surg Clin North Am. 2010; 18(1):133–140

[122] Cardona I, Saint-Martin C, Daniel SJ. Effect of recurrent onabotulinum toxin A injection into the salivary glands: an ultrasound measurement. Laryngoscope. 2015; 125(10):E328–E332

[123] Levy PM. The "Nefertiti lift": a new technique for specific re-contouring of the jawline. J Cosmet Laser Ther. 2007; 9(4):249–252

[124] Fabi SG, Burgess C, Carruthers A, et al. Consensus recommendations for combined aesthetic interventions using botulinum toxin, fillers, and microfocused ultrasound in the neck, décolletage, hands, and other areas of the body. Dermatol Surg. 2016; 42(10):1199–1208

[125] Fabi SG, Massaki A, Eimpunth S, Pogoda J, Goldman MP. Evaluation of microfocused ultrasound with visualization for lifting, tightening, and wrinkle reduction of the décolletage. J Am Acad Dermatol. 2013; 69(6):965–971

[126] Fabi SG. Noninvasive skin tightening: focus on new ultrasound techniques. Clin Cosmet Investig Dermatol. 2015; 8:47–52

[127] Fabi SG. A Prospective, Randomized, Single-Center, Evaluator-Blinded Clinical Trial Evaluating the Safety, Efficacy, and Patient Satisfaction of Injectable Calcium Hydroxylapatite (Radiesse®) in Combination with Micro-Focused Ultrasound for Rejuvenation of the Aging Chest. Vegas Cosmetic Surgery meeting, June, 2018, Las Vegas, NV

[128] Butterwick K, Sadick N. Hand rejuvenation using a combination approach. Dermatol Surg. 2016; 42 Suppl 2:S108–S118

[129] Almutairi K, Gusenoff JA, Rubin JP. Body contouring. Plast Reconstr Surg. 2016; 137(3):586e–602e

[130] American Society of Plastic Surgeons. 2017. Complete Plastic Surgery Statistics Report. Available at: https://www.plasticsurgery.org/documents/News/Statistics/2017/plastic-surgery-statistics-full-report-2017.pdf. Accessed November 25, 2018

[131] Goldberg DJ, Hornfeldt CS. Safety and efficacy of microfocused ultrasound to lift, tighten, and smooth the buttocks. Dermatol Surg. 2014; 40(10):1113–1117

[132] Gold MH, Sensing W, Biron J. Use of micro-focused ultrasound with visualization to lift and tighten lax knee skin (1). J Cosmet Laser Ther. 2014; 16(5):225–229

[133] Rokhsar C, Schnebelen W, West A, Hornfeldt C. Safety and efficacy of microfocused ultrasound in tightening of lax elbow skin. Dermatol Surg. 2015; 41(7):821–826

[134] Torres O, Kirkland C, Rogachefsky A. Fractionated CO_2 laser treatment for photoaging treatment of the arms and legs. Dermatologist. 2013; 21 (7)

[135] Distante F, Pagani V, Bonfigli A. Stabilized hyaluronic acid of non-animal origin for rejuvenating the skin of the upper arm. Dermatol Surg. 2009; 35 Suppl 1:389–393, discussion 394

[136] Amselem M. Radiesse(®): a novel rejuvenation treatment for the upper arms. Clin Cosmet Investig Dermatol. 2015; 9:9–14

[137] Cogorno Wasylkowski V. Body vectoring technique with Radiesse(®) for tightening of the abdomen, thighs, and brachial zone. Clin Cosmet Investig Dermatol. 2015; 8:267–273

[138] Mazzuco R, Sadick NS. The use of poly-L-lactic acid in the gluteal area. Dermatol Surg. 2016; 42(3):441–443

[139] Ryu HW, Kim SA, Jung HR, Ryoo YW, Lee KS, Cho JW. Clinical improvement of striae distensae in Korean patients using a combination of fractionated microneedle radiofrequency and fractional carbon dioxide laser. Dermatol Surg. 2013; 39(10):1452–1458

[140] Coleman KM, Coleman WP, III, Benchetrit A. Non-invasive, external ultrasonic lipolysis. Semin Cutan Med Surg. 2009; 28(4):263–267

[141] Green JB, Cohen JL. Cellfina observations: pearls and pitfalls. Semin Cutan Med Surg. 2015; 34(3):144–146

15 Neuromodulators and Injection Technique

Gee Young Bae

Summary

Cosmetic use of botulinum neurotoxins (BoNTs) in the field of dermatology has grown beyond the treatment of wrinkles to include facial and body contouring. BoNT treatment has gained popularity owing to factors such as little injury and privacy, dramatic effects, relatively low cost, and negligible downtime. Paradigm shifts such as low-dose modulation rather than high-dose paralysis, frequent combination with fillers, and superficial injection in selective cases presently occur in BoNT treatment. A need, however, exists for a patient-tailored treatment that will produce a more satisfying result without complications. This requires an in-depth knowledge of the products used, a thorough understanding of individual anatomy, both static and functional, and consideration of ethnicity, gender, and age. Herein, we present up-to-date knowledge and techniques regarding BoNT treatment. We have also presented the toxicity and immunogenicity of BoNT, and an in-depth discussion of BoNT treatment for glabellar frown lines, horizontal forehead lines, crow's feet, bunny lines, plunging nose tip, nasal flare, gummy smile, asymmetric lip or smile, nasolabial folds, melomental folds (Marionette folds), perioral wrinkles, cobblestone chin, mouth corners, platysmal bands, horizontal neck lines, facial contouring treating benign masseteric hypertrophy and salivary gland enlargement, body contouring, hyperhidrosis, pain and pruritus, and wound healing.

Keywords: botulinum toxin, wrinkle treatment, smile deformity, facial contouring, masseteric hypertrophy, salivary gland enlargement, body contouring, new use of botulinum toxin

15.1 Introduction

15.1.1 Basic Science of Botulinum Toxin

Botulinum neurotoxins (BoNTs), produced by anaerobic spore-forming bacteria of the genus *Clostridium*, are the most potent toxins known to mankind; however, they have been used as therapeutic agents for a wide range of indications. Although initially thought to inhibit acetylcholine (ACh) release only at neuromuscular junctions, BoNTs are now recognized to act on parasympathetic cholinergic nerve and nociceptive neurons.[1] There are eight serotypes of botulinum toxin (A, B, C1, D, E, F, G, and X) with each possessing different pharmacological properties, and only serotypes A and B are currently available for clinical use.[2] BoNT-A is generally used in clinical practice owing to its higher efficacy and longer duration compared to BoNT-B. BoNT-B exhibits a faster onset of action and higher autonomic efficacy than BoNT-A. However, owing to injection pain associated with its acidic pH (pH 5.6) and the higher rate of neutralizing antibodies, BoNT-B is usually used to treat patients who fail to respond to BoNT-A.[3,4,5]

BoNTs are large protein complexes comprised of a neurotoxin subunit and several nontoxic proteins. The core neurotoxin has a molecular weight of 150 kDa and consists of a heavy chain (HC; 100 kDa) and a light chain (LC; 50 kDa) polypeptide linked via a disulfide bond (▶ Fig. 15.1a). This core neurotoxin is surrounded and protected by complexing proteins or nontoxic accessory proteins (NAPs). The composition of the complexing proteins varies among products with either hemagglutinin (HA) or nontoxic nonhemagglutinin (NTNH).[6] After reconstitution, the neurotoxin rapidly dissociates from the complexing proteins. In the presence of the neurotoxin, the complexing proteins seem to induce immunologic responses and promote antibody formation.

BoNTs inhibit ACh release at the neuromuscular junction via a four-stage process: (1) HC-mediated neurospecific binding of the toxin, (2) endocytosis of BoNT receptor complex, (3) acidification of the endocytic vesicle to allow LC translocation through the membrane, and (4) catalysis of the disulfide bond by thioredoxin (Trx) for the release of LC into the cytoplasm where it is activated as a zinc-dependent endoprotease, cleaving the soluble N-ethylmaleimide-sensitive factor attachment receptor (SNARE) complex, which is essential for neurotransmitter release. The SNARE complex consists of vesicle-associated membrane protein (VAMP), and two target proteins: plasma membrane synaptosomal associated protein 25 (SNAP-25) and syntaxin. BoNT-A removes amino acids from SNAP-25, whereas BoNT-B works by cleaving VAMP. Cleavage of any SNARE proteins from the SNARE complex inhibits membrane fusion and ACh release, terminating muscle contraction[7] (▶ Fig. 15.1b). Muscle paresis occurs 1 to 5 days after injection and reaches its maximal point at 2 weeks. This effect lasts 2 to 3 months before gradually stopping; however, this can last 4 to 6 months based on the treatment area, dose, and formulation used. After repeated injection, reduced muscle contractility and resting tone provide wrinkle prevention effect, which extends the duration of the effect. In addition, muscle atrophy and reduced number of targets with changes in muscle habit can produce a prolonged effect.[8] An initial functional recovery is mediated by new axonal sprouts, which is followed and completed by reestablishment of original terminals.

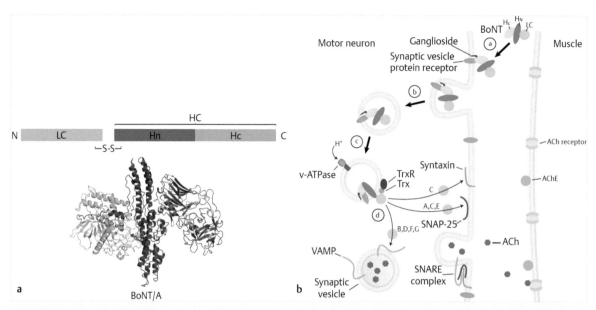

Fig. 15.1 (a) Schematic of the botulinum neurotoxins (BoNT) domain and the structure of BoNT/A. (HC, heavy chain; Hn: translocation domain; Hc: receptor-binding domain; LC, light chain.) **(b)** Mechanism of BoNT intoxication. ⓐ BoNT binds to the neuronal cell membrane via a dual-receptor complex. ⓑ Endocytosis of BoNT-receptor complex. ⓒ Acidification of the endocytic vesicle allows translocation of LC through the membrane. ⓓ Thioredoxin (Trx) catalyzes the disulfide bond, releasing LC into the cytoplasm where it can cleave its soluble N-ethylmaleimide-sensitive factor attachment protein receptor (SNARE) substrate. Cleavage of any SNARE proteins from the SNARE complex inhibits membrane fusion and acetylcholine (ACh) release, terminating muscle contraction. (ACh, acetylcholine; AChE, acetylcholine esterase; TrxR,: thioredoxin reductase.)

15.1.2 Comparison of Products

▶ Table 15.1 contains key information regarding the BoNT products available worldwide. Different neurotoxin formulations are chemically and pharmacologically unique. Their doses cannot be interchanged, and their dose-response curves are not parallel.[9] Various commercially available products differ in formulation, purification process, molecular weight, toxin size, neurotoxin content, complex proteins, stabilizer, biologic activity, and pH.[10,11]

Currently, the following six BoNT preparations have been approved by the U.S. Food and Drug Administration (FDA): one BoNT-B product, rimabotulinumtoxinB (RIMA; Myobloc) and five BoNT-A products, onabotulinumtoxinA (ONA; Botox), abobotulinumtoxinA (ABO; Dysport), incobotulinumtoxinA (INCO; Xeomin), prabotulinumtoxinA-xvfs (PRA; Jeuveau, and daxibotulinumtoxinA (Daxxify, Revance). ONA, the first BoNT product, is the most extensively studied BoNT product, with the other products weighing on the interchangeability based on potency and efficacy. In many clinical studies, INCO was shown to be as effective as ONA when a clinical conversion ratio of 1:1 was used, though some experts concluded that the estimated conversion ratio of INCO and ONA was between 1:0.75 and 1:0.5.[9,12] INCO demonstrated a more rapid onset of action than ONA and ABO.[13] The ONA-to-ABO conversion ratio is approximately 1:2.5 in aesthetic indications.[14] ONA and INCO have comparable spread, whereas ABO has a greater spread than ONA/INCO with respect to anhidrosis.[15]

One of the trends in the cosmetic use of BoNT is the administration of high doses to multiple areas (e.g., treating the whole face or body contouring). This has increased the need for products with lower antigenicity. INCO and Coretox are only composed of neurotoxin proteins and are free of complexing proteins, which may increase the risk of sensitization and antibody formation. New products such as Innotox, Coretox, and Daxxify do not contain albumin or any proteins of animal origin. Currently, the liquid-type BoNT-A, Innotox, is available in addition to the BoNT-B, Myobloc. A ready-to-use liquid formulation has increased safety, with reduced risk of contamination and accurate dosing (Innotox, 4 U/0.1 mL; Myobloc 500 U/0.1 mL).[16] Furthermore, the newest addition, Daxxify, has demonstrated in clinical trials to have a 6-month mean duration. A topical BoNT product using nanoparticle delivery system is under evaluation as a potential treatment for hyperhidrosis, acne, and crow's feet lines.[17,18]

15.1.3 Preparation for Use

Reconstitution with a diluent is necessary for powder-type BoNT products. Saline is most commonly used and diluents such as Ringer's acetate, distilled water, albumin, epinephrine, and hyaluronic acid do not interfere with toxin activity. The use of local anesthetics for reconstitution does not affect toxin potency; however, the risk of an anaphylactic reaction increases. Although BoNT does not appear as fragile as we expected, aggressive reconstitution

Table 15.1 Comparison of BoNT products

Product name	Company	Country	First approval	Formulation	Unit	Serotype/strain	Complex size	Excipient	Storage/shelf life	Approved cosmetic indications
Botox/Vistabel (onabotulinumtoxinA)	Allergan	United States	1989	Vacuum-dried powder	50, 100	Hall A1-hyper	900 kDa	HSA, NaCl	2–8 °C/36 mo	Glabellar line (FDA, EU), primary axillary hyperhidrosis (FDA, EU), lateral canthal line (FDA, EU)
Dysport/Azzalure (abobotulinumtoxinA)	Ipsen	United Kingdom	1990	Lyophilized-powder	300, 500	A1 ATCC3502	500–600 and 900 kDa	HSA, lactose	2–8 °C/24 mo	Glabellar line (FDA, EU)
BTXA	Lanzhou	China	1996	Lyophilized-powder	50, 100	Hall A1-hyper	900 kDa	Bovine gelatine-dextran-sucrose	−20 to approximately −5 °C/36 mo	None
Myobloc (rimabotulinumtoxinB)	Solstice Neuroscience	United States	2000	Liquid	2,500, 5,000, 10,000	B Bean	700 kDa	HSA, sodium succinate,	2–8 °C/36–48 mo	None
Xeomin/Bocouture (incobotulinumtoxinA)	Merz	Germany	2005	Lyophilized-powder	50, 100	A1 ATCC3502	150 kDa	HSA, sucrose	2–8 °C or room temperature up to 25 °C/36 mo	Glabellar line (FDA, EU), combined treatment of upper facial lines[a] (EU)
Meditoxin/Neuronox/Botulift/Siax/Cunox	Medytox	Korea	2006	Lyophilized-powder	50, 100, 150, 200	Hall A1-hyper	900 kDa	HSA, NaCl	2–8 °C or < −5 °C/36 mo	Glabellar frown line (KFDA)
Botulax	Hugel	Korea	2010	Lyophilized-powder	50, 100, 150, 200	A1 CBFC26	900 kDa	HSA, NaCl	2–8 °C/36 mo	Glabellar frown line (KFDA)
Nabota (prabotulinumtoxinA)	Daewoong	Korea	2013	Vacuum-dried powder	50, 100, 150, 200	A	900 kDa	HSA, NaCl	2–8 °C/36 mo	Glabellar frown line, lateral canthal line (KFDA)
Innotox	Medytox	Korea	2013	Liquid	25, 50	Hall A1-hyper	900 kDa	Methionine, polysorbate	2–8 °C/36 mo	Glabellar frown line (KFDA)
Relatox	NPO microgen	Russia	2014	Lyophilized-powder	50, 100	A	900 kDa	Gelatine, maltose	2–8 °C/36 mo	Expression wrinkle (FDA-Russia)
Coretox	Medytox	Korea	2016	Lyophilized-powder	100	Hall A1-hyper	150 kDa	Methionine, polysorbate, sucrose, NaCl	2–8 °C/36 mo	Glabellar frown line (KFDA)
Jeuveau (prabotulinumtoxinA-xvfs)	Evolus	United States	2019	Vacuum-dried powder	100	A	900 kDa	HSA, NaCl	2–8 °C/36 mo	Glabellar frown line (FDA)
Daxxify (daxibotulinumtoxinA-lanm)	Revance	United States	2022	Lypophilized powder	50, 100	A	150 kDa	RTP004	2–8 °C	Glabellar lines (FDA)

Abbreviations: BoNT, botulinum neurotoxin; EU, European Union; FDA, Food and Drug Administration; HSA, human serum albumin; KFDA, Korean Food and Drug Administration.
[a]Glabellar frown lines, lateral periorbital lines, and horizontal forehead lines.

Table 15.2 Botulinum toxin reconstitution

Product	Unit vial	Volume of diluent (mL)	Concentration (U/0.1 mL)	Remarks
Botox	100	5	2	Large area, body treatment
Botox	100	2.5	4	Most commonly used concentration
Botox	100	1.25	8	Small area, precise treatment
Botox	100	1	10	Small area, precise treatment
Xeomin	100	2.5	4	Thorough reconstitution required to dissolve products underneath a cap
Dysport	300	1.5	20	Conversion ratio of 1:2.5 with ONA
Dysport	300	2.5	12	Conversion ratio of 1:2.5 with ONA
Dysport	300	3	10	Conversion ratio of 1:2.5 with ONA

Abbreviation: ONA, onabotulinumtoxinA.

with violent shaking can decrease toxin potency.[19] Reconstitution volumes and their concentrations of Botox, Dysport, and Xeomin are detailed in ▶ Table 15.2. In clinical practice, reconstitution volumes can vary based on location and indication. Lower volumes are often used in areas where minimized diffusion is required for detailed treatment (such as perioral areas), whereas higher volumes are used to facilitate the spread of BoNT in large target areas (for axillary hyperhidrosis or body contouring).[20] Despite the manufacturer's recommendation that a vial be used only once, some studies suggest that a reconstituted and refrigerated vial can be used up to 6 weeks without loss of efficacy.[21] Some reports propose that BoNT may be frozen, thawed, and injected without loss of potency for up to 6 months.[22] Prior to injection, topical anesthesia and/or ice can be applied for pain relief. Treatment areas should be thoroughly cleansed using topical antiseptics such as 4% chlorhexidine.

15.1.4 Patient Selection and Consultation

At the first consultation, doctors should evaluate the extent of photodamage and distinguish wrinkle caused by photoaging from dynamic wrinkle owing to muscle contraction. This helps predict the extent of improvement expected from BoNT treatment and plan for future cosmetic treatment. It is best to propose the need for other combination treatment modality before treatment, if any. Off-label treatment should be clearly disclosed and should be included on the consent form. Doctors should also evaluate the subjective beauty concept of patients and objective characteristics such as age, gender, ethnicity, facial shape, aging pattern, wrinkle types, sociocultural aspects, and the previous history of BoNT treatment or cosmetic surgery, as they can affect the treatment dose and injection technique. It is crucial to observe the face at rest and in motion and record habitual muscle movement

or asymmetry. Before and after photographs (sometimes videos) are also important for precise assessment and treatment planning.

Contraindications for BoNT include the following:
- Hypersensitivity to any of the ingredients in the botulinum product.
- Current infection at injection sites.
- Preexisting neuromuscular junction disorders (myasthenia gravis, amyotrophic lateral sclerosis, and Lambert–Eaton syndrome).

Special precautions should be taken when treating the following patients:
- Those with preexisting swallowing or breathing difficulties.
- Those taking high doses of aminoglycosides, tetracyclines, or other medications that interfere with neuromuscular acetylcholine release and potentiate the effect of BoNT (cyclosporine, benzodiazepine, anticholinergics, etc.).
- Pregnant and breastfeeding women.

BoNT products are pregnancy category C, and thus are not recommended for use during pregnancy. It is reported that, to date, 24 pregnant women have received up to 250 U BoNT-A injections purposely or accidentally. The babies were born without complications, but two miscarriages occurred; it is unclear whether BoNT played a role in the miscarriages. Risks of maternal–infant transmission of botulinum toxin in lactating women are unknown and, thus, treatment is not recommended during lactation. However, experts believe that BoNT can be used during pregnancy and breastfeeding in selective cases.[23]

15.1.5 Ethnic and Gender Consideration

BoNT treatment should be modified based on ethnicity, gender, and age. Generally, Asians tend to have a smaller muscle mass and lower dynamic activity than Caucasians. The upper facial expression muscle is used by Caucasians up to 30% more than Asians.[24] Notably, Asians have a thicker dermis as well as thicker and denser fat compared to Caucasians. These factors therefore lead to fewer wrinkles and lower dose requirements for Asians than Caucasians. Asians favor a slim, V-shaped face than a square face; therefore, lower facial contouring using BoNT has been gaining popularity. It is noteworthy that infraorbital eye-opening treatment (tarsal muscle injection) is not performed on Asians owing to their esthetic preference. Thus, although the use of BoNT for eyebrow lifting to create a high arched eyebrow is popular in the West, this is not performed as frequently on Asians because Asian females do not prefer a high lateral arched-shape; instead, a flat shape is preferred, and this is also the choice of men (straighter eyebrows).

In most areas, men can be treated by the same techniques as women; however, due to increased muscle mass, higher doses are required. As some male patients have a broader corrugator muscle, which requires more lateral injection points, techniques should be adjusted according to individual anatomy.[25]

When a patient receives repeated treatment for a long time, BoNT dose should be readjusted according to the status of muscle atrophy from either aging or BoNT-induced muscle atrophy.[26] Generally, a higher concentration is safe for older patients owing to the laxity of the surrounding soft tissue.

15.1.6 Toxicity and Immunogenicity

Extrapolating from animal experiments, the estimated lethal dose (LD50) in a 70-kg adult would be at least 3,000 U, that is, 30 vials of 100-U BoNT-A products. In most cases, injecting 200 U in one session for cosmetic purposes is not harmful; however, cases of iatrogenic botulism are rarely reported due to systemic spread of BoNT. Symptoms include asthenia, generalized muscle weakness, diplopia, blurred vision, ptosis, dysphagia, dysphonia, dysarthria, urinary incontinence, and breathing difficulties; these symptoms have been reported hours to weeks after injection. In the event of accidental overdose, systemic muscular weakness, paralysis of oropharyngeal, esophageal, or respiratory muscles should be carefully monitored. If iatrogenic botulism is suspected, an antitoxin should be used immediately.[27] For severe botulism, mechanical ventilation, tube feeding, and other general supportive care is necessary until the patient makes a full recovery. Patients with the neuromuscular junction disorders such as myasthenia gravis are particularly susceptible to toxicity.

As BoNT therapy is often continued over many years, some patients may develop detectable antibodies that may or may not affect their biological activity. Only neutralizing antibodies can inhibit the biological activity of the toxin and potentially lead to treatment failure.

Frequency of the development of neutralizing antibodies to different formulations is 0 to 3% and 10 to 44% for BoNT-A and BoNT-B products, respectively. Most immunoresistance cases have been observed when high-dose therapeutic treatments are administered, but this is rarely observed in cosmetic treatments. Several clinical tests including the frontalis antibody test and unilateral brow injection may be used to evaluate a patient's sensitivity to BoNT. A reduced response may suggest the presence of neutralizing antibodies. If immunoresistance is clinically suspected, patient serum is sent to a lab for confirmation. Clinical strategies to reduce potential risk factors include the administration of the lowest effective doses at the longest inter-injection interval.[28] For cases of antibody-induced treatment failure, retreatment with a low antigenicity BoNT product after a drop in antibody titers did not induce antibody-induced treatment failure, thus offering a new treatment opportunity.[29] It is important to distinguish between immunoresistance and treatment nonresponse. Lack of a clinical benefit can be caused by technical issues such as inadequate dosing, failure to accurately identify and inject muscles, or difficulty targeting the intended muscle. Changes in patient state over time and unrealistic patient expectations may impact the perceived success of repeated treatments.

15.1.7 Adverse Reactions

Headache

Headache is the most commonly encountered complication after injection. Although BoNT is used to treat and prevent migraines and tension headaches, it may paradoxically trigger headaches. Headaches usually last 1 to 3 days and require attention and workup if persistent for more than 1 week.

Allergic Reaction

Hypersensitivity reactions, such as anaphylaxis, urticaria, papular eruption, and dyspnea, to the active neurotoxin or any excipients (human albumin, sucrose, lactose) have been reported.[30,31]

Bruise

"If you bruise them, you lose them." This is a famous rhyme among injectors. Although bruise is temporary, it nullifies the advantage of having no downtime with BoNT treatment. Tips to prevent bruise during wrinkle treatment include subdermal or intradermal injections instead of subcutaneous or intramuscular injection, using good lighting to avoid injecting into large vessels, gentle pressure on needle marks for enough time, and discontinuation of aspirin or other anticoagulants for 2 weeks before the procedure. Topical anesthesia cream has vasoconstrictive effects and pain relief itself prevents high blood pressure, which can also increase bruising.

Edema

Patients can experience eyelid edema after forehead or glabella treatment, and malar edema after crow's feet treatment, and whole facial edema after whole face treatment. Severity of edema is dose dependent and is accompanied by a wide range of personal differences. The underlying mechanism of edema may be insufficient lymphatic circulation in the paralyzed muscle. Mild lymphatic edema brings positive cosmetic effect such as a shiny, smooth skin texture.

Masklike Face

Excessive paralysis of facial expression muscles can cause a masklike face, which is unnatural and may cause depression. When treating whole face wrinkles, dose reduction is recommended.

Diffusion to Unwanted Muscle

In 2014, a systematic review of clinical studies was performed to evaluate the safety of botulinum toxin A in aesthetic treatments between 2000 and 2012 using 35 papers with a total of 8,787 subjects.[32] Treatment-related adverse events included blepharoptosis (2.5%), brow ptosis (3.1%), eye sensory disorders (3%) in the upper face and lip asymmetries, and imbalance in the lower face (6.9%); these events resolved spontaneously and were attributed to local diffusion of BoNT into adjacent areas. Diffusion or size of the denervation field of BoNT is determined by the dose and volume of the solution.[33] A massage immediately after injection should be avoided to prevent unwanted diffusion, whereas contraction of the injected muscles for approximately 2 hours after injection is thought to increase product uptake. A slow, gentle injection with the smallest effective volume and the isolation of the target muscle from the surrounding tissue with the noninjecting hand are important to avoid this embarrassing complication.

15.1.8 Pretreatment Assessment

The patient-tailored approach is becoming increasingly important. As a pretreatment assessment, the extent, bulk, action, and counteraction of muscles are carefully examined by asking the patient to contract the target group of muscles; the muscle is, however, relaxed during injection. For example, patients are asked to close their eyes and squeeze tightly to activate the frontalis, corrugator, procerus, nasalis, and orbicularis muscles. Points of injection are then determined based on the extent and activity of the muscle, and the depth and dose determined depending on the bulk of the muscle.[34] Wrinkles develop in the skin where muscle tension acts on most or at the cutaneous insertion of a muscle; a wrinkle itself is, therefore, a very good point

of injection. However, as large vessels can run underneath deep static wrinkles, injection depth is important. In addition, for deep static wrinkles, the need for a filler injection or other combination treatment should be addressed before treatment. Experienced injectors suggest an option of concomitant treatment of counteracting muscles as they can be strengthened or activated through compensatory muscle hyperactivity. The amount of units discussed below refers to ONA and may be carefully extrapolated to other formulations (▶ Table 15.3, ▶ Table 15.4).

15.2 Upper Face

15.2.1 Glabellar Frown Lines

Treatment of glabellar frown lines with botulinum toxin injection is one of the most popular procedures in esthetic medicine. Furthermore, improvement in depressive symptoms after glabellar toxin treatment suggests the new paradigm of using BoNT to target facial muscles that affect negative emotions and mood[35]; BoNT is currently in phase III clinical trials for depression.[36]

Glabellar frown lines are produced by the corrugator supercilii muscle (CSM) and procerus muscle. Superomedial fibers of the orbicularis oculi that interconnect with the frontalis or procerus, termed depressor supercilii muscle, also contribute to frown lines. The CSM originates as three or four thin, rectangular, panel-like muscle groups from a broad osseous origin along the medial supraciliary arch. The CSM travels laterally, with most of the muscle passing through fibers of the orbicularis oculi and the frontalis. A dermal insertion or corrugator dimple is located around the central portion of the eyebrow.[37,38] A total of 20 U (8–40 U) at three to seven points is injected in the glabella; 4 U is injected into the horizontal lines in the radix to target the procerus muscle; 4 U is injected into the belly of the corrugator near its origin (this is usually a bony plateau on the medial supraciliary arch); and a 0.5- to 2-U intradermal injection is added to the corrugator dimple and tail (▶ Fig. 15.2a).

Common adverse effects include headache and a change in facial expression. Decreased visual acuity can occur especially in elderly patients who must use their frowning muscles for visual acuity. The most serious complication, eyelid ptosis, can be caused by paralysis of the levator palpebrae superioris muscle due to BoNT diffusion through the orbital septum. To prevent this occurrence, slow and gentle injection of the lowest possible volume (higher concentration) is necessary, with the needle directed away from the orbit, and blocking of the orbit performed with the noninjecting hand. If ptosis occurs, this may last for 2 to 3 months, and alpha-adrenergic agonist eyedrops such as 0.5% apraclonidine eyedrops (Iopidine, Alcon Labs) should be used three to

Table 15.3 Recommended BoNT dose for face and neck

Indications	Target muscles	Total dose	Injection level
Glabellar frown line	CSM, DSC, procerus	8–40 U	IM
Eyebrow lifting	CSM, DSC, lateral orbicularis oculi	8–16 U	IM and IC
Forehead line	Frontalis	4–20 U	IM or IC
Lateral canthal line	Orbicularis oculi	6–10 U per side	IC
Bunny line	Nasalis transverse part, LLSAN	4 U per side	IC
Nasal flare	Dilator naris	4–8 U per side	IM
	LLSAN	0.5–1 U per side	IM
Nasal tip elevation, plunged nose	DSN	4–8 U	IM
Gummy smile	DSN	2–4 U	IM
	LLSAN, LLS, ZMi	0.5–2 U per side	IM
Nasolabial fold	Lip levators	0.5–2 U per side	IM and IC
Marionette fold	DAO	3–4 U per side	IC
Perioral wrinkle	Orbicularis oris	4–8 U	IC
Cobble stone chin	Mentalis	8–10 U	IM
Mouth frown (mouth corner elevation)	DAO	3–4 U per side	IC
	Mentalis	8–10 U	IM
Nefertiti lift	Platysma	20 U per side	IM or IC
Platysmal bands	Platysma	10 U per band	IC
Horizontal neck line	Platysma	10 U per line	IC

Abbreviations: BoNT, botulinum neurotoxin; CSM, corrugator supercilii muscle; DAO, depressor angularis oris; DSC, depressor supercilli; DSN, depressor septi nasi; IC, intracutaneous; IM, intramuscular; LLSAN, levator labii superioris alaeque nasi; ZMi, zygomaticus minor.

Table 15.4 Recommended BoNT dose for face and body contouring

Indications	Target muscles	Initial dose per side
Benign masseteric hypertrophy	Masseter	20–40 U
Salivary gland enlargement	Parotid gland	20–60 U
	Submandibular gland	20–40 U
Calf contouring	Gastrocnemius and soleus	50–100 U
Thigh contouring	Quadriceps	100–150 U
Shoulder contouring	Trapezius	20–40 U
Upper arm contouring	Deltoid	30–50 U

Abbreviation: BoNT, botulinum neurotoxin.

four times per day. The eyedrops cause contraction of the Müller muscle and 1- to 2-mm elevation of the upper lid. Brow ptosis or blepharochalasis should be distinguished from eyelid ptosis. Brow ptosis usually affects both sides and is recovered by manual lifting of the eyebrows; this does not apply to eyelid ptosis. Medial brow ptosis can occur when glabellar toxin relaxes the inferomedial portion of the frontalis more than the glabellar complex through upward diffusion. This can be alleviated by adopting a careful eyebrow lifting technique; BoNT injection into the brow depressors including the lateral orbicularis oculi leads to 1 to 3 mm of brow lifting[39] (▶ Fig. 15.2b). Aggressive look from altered brow shapes such as "Mephisto eyebrow" or "Samurai eyebrow" can also develop by compensatory hypercontraction of the lateral portion of the frontalis induced by relaxation of the inferomedial frontalis during glabella treatment. A 0.5-U BoNT injection into the most hyperactive point in the lateral forehead can treat Mephisto eyebrow[40] (▶ Fig. 15.2c).

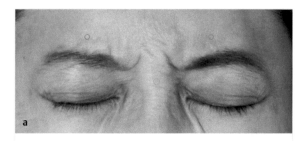

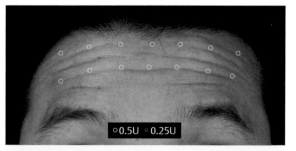

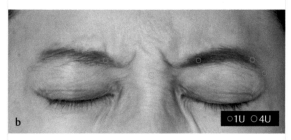

Fig. 15.3 Forehead line injection of 8 U in men. Intradermal small-dose injection near eyebrows.

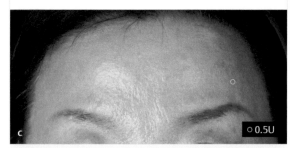

Fig. 15.2 **(a)** Glabellar injection point. **(b)** Eyebrow lifting technique. **(c)** Correcting Mephisto eyebrow.

15.2.2 Horizontal Forehead Lines

Horizontal forehead lines are caused by contraction of the frontalis, which raises the eyebrows and upper eyelid, wrinkling the forehead in the process. The frontalis muscle, the only eyebrow elevator, originates from the galea aponeurotica near the coronal suture. It is inserted into the superciliary ridge of the frontal bone and interconnects with the muscle fibers of brow depressors such as the procerus, corrugator supercilii, and orbicularis oculi muscles. Men typically have greater muscle mass and a larger forehead surface area than women; therefore, they require higher doses. Eyebrows are naturally positioned lower in men, and excessive relaxation of the lower frontalis can result in brow ptosis.[41] The following are groups at high risk of brow ptosis during forehead BoNT treatment: individuals in their late 40 s and above, individuals with blepharochalasis or lateral hooding, individuals with thick and edematous eyelids, and individuals who use their frontalis during eye opening. The total dose administered is 4 to 20 U, and injection protocols for the forehead differ between patients based on muscular anatomy, size, and tone[42]; one to three lines of injection are designed based on forehead size (▶ Fig. 15.3). The initial

injection dose usually starts from 8 U, but in the high-risk group, 4 U is initially injected with an additional injection considered at the 2-week follow-up. For low-dose injection, a large dilution and intradermal injection is helpful for even injections. In addition, a lower-dose injection achieves a more natural result with shorter duration. The antiwrinkle effect of BoNT does not significantly differ between intramuscular and intradermal injections. However, side effects such as eyebrow ptosis and heaviness are more prominent after intramuscular injection and can be prevented by intradermal injections in the lower forehead near the eyebrows.[43]

As previously mentioned, BoNT treatment of the glabella and frontalis muscle impacts the position and configuration of the eyebrow. Brow shapes such as "Mephisto eyebrow" or "Samurai eyebrow" can develop if the injection is performed overly central. Preexisting amount of frontalis weakening is important for this brow expression change.

15.2.3 Lateral Canthal Lines (Crow's Feet)

Lateral canthal lines or crow's feet are caused by the contraction of the orbicularis oculi muscle. The orbicularis oculi muscle is composed of three portions: orbital, preseptal, and pretarsal. Orbital fibers originate from the superior and inferior orbital edges that insert into the medial and lateral canthal ligaments and interconnect with the frontalis, corrugator, and procerus muscles. As this is a circular muscle, and facial expression wrinkles develop vertically to the muscular contraction vector, wrinkles appear radially from the orbit, and are not only found in lateral areas. A snap test is useful to determine whether eyelid skin is sufficiently elastic for the performance of BoNT injections. When the skin retraction time is greater than 3 seconds, there is an increased risk of eyelid edema and scleral exposure.

The average injection dose is 6 to 10 U per side, and dose is inserted into each wrinkle based on severity (▶ Fig. 15.4). Typically, injections are given 1.5 cm from the lateral canthus and 1 cm lateral to the bony orbital rim.

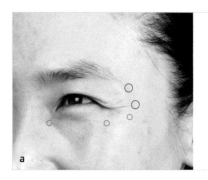
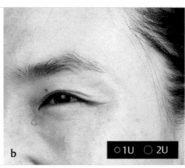

Fig. 15.4 Crow's feet intracutaneous injection divided according to wrinkle severity: before **(a)** and 2 weeks after **(b)**. Touch-up injection at the medial subcanthal wrinkle.

The needle is also oriented away from the orbit to prevent diffusion into the orbit and diplopia. Periorbital and sentinel veins are susceptible to rupture; thus, to prevent bruising, it is recommended that a superficial intradermal injection be administered in good lighting. The inferolateral perioral wrinkles are caused by contraction of not only the orbicularis oculi muscle but also the zygomaticus major muscle; therefore, vigorous treatment of this inferolateral wrinkle can result in the drop of a mouth corner, which leads to difficulty smiling or an asymmetric smile. In elderly people, malar edema can develop after crow's feet injection and this can persist for a few months. Xerophthalmia can develop or worsen either by reduced blinking or decreased lacrimal gland secretion. If only the lateral canthal lines are treated, medial subcanthal wrinkles can be exaggerated due to compensatory contraction; thus, 0.5- to 1-U injection is also necessary in the medial sides. Weakening of the orbicularis oculi muscle can occur if an excess amount is administered near the palpebral fissure resulting in the disappearance of eyelid roll or the appearance of scleral show and infraorbital fat bulging. These adverse events are more common when BoNT is injected into the lower eyelid to widen the eye aperture.[44]

15.3 Midface and Lower Face

Besides traditional upper face treatment, many new indications are being treated in the midface and lower face, either with BoNT alone or combined with fillers. In these areas, careful patient selection with full exploration of risks and benefits, a comprehensive aesthetic assessment, and an understanding of the functional anatomy of each patient are crucial. Owing to the risk of functional impairment and expression change, the principle is to start with a minimal dose, avoid overtreatment, and reevaluate at the 2-week follow-up. An exact placement with a higher concentration to minimize diffusion is important.

15.3.1 Bunny Lines

Bunny lines are nasal oblique lines on both sides of the nose dorsum that appear when smiling and when

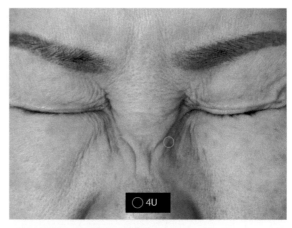

Fig. 15.5 Injection for bunny line.

frowning. They may occur following treatment of the glabellar or orbital regions due to compensatory activation. Bunny lines are caused by the transverse part of the nasalis and the levator labii superioris alaeque nasi (LLSAN). Intracutaneous injection of 4 U into the lines on each side can smooth wrinkles (▶ Fig. 15.5).

15.3.2 Nasal Flare

Some patients are bothered by flaring nostrils when talking. Usually, this habitual contraction of the dilator nasalis exacerbates with time. A 4- to 8-U injection into each dilator naris can prevent this occurrence. As nasal ala injection is quite painful, a small volume at a high concentration (8 U/0.1 mL) is recommended (▶ Fig. 15.6). Patients tend to also complain that the nostril widens when smiling, which is a result of the lateral and upward pulling of LLSAN. LLSAN originates from the frontal process of the maxilla and the maxillary process of the frontal bone. It inserts into the mid-central region of the orbicularis oris and nasal ala skin. A 0.5- to 1-U injection into LLSAN at the pyriform aperture or apical triangle of the upper lip can further reduce nostril widening.

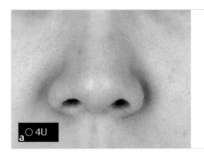
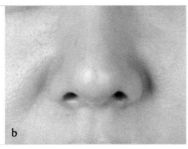

Fig. 15.6 Before **(a)** and 2 weeks after **(b)** nasal ala injection.

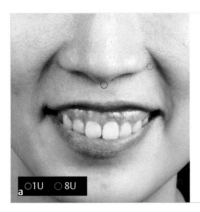
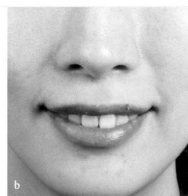

Fig. 15.7 **(a, b)** Injection into the depressor septi nasi and levator labii superioris alaeque nasi (LLSAN) treats gummy smile and plunging nose.

15.3.3 Nasal Tip Elevation of Plunging Nose Tip

In some patients, action of the depressor septi nasi (DSN) muscle leads to nasal tip drooping and shortened upper lip during smiling and talking. The depressor septi is a paired muscle in the columella, which originates from the incisive fossa of the maxilla and inserts into the nasal septum. Relaxing the DSN by a deep periosteal injection of 4 to 8 U at the subnasale allows the tip of the nose to be lifted and is often ancillary to filler rhinoplasty.[45] The DSN muscle usually works together with the LLSAN to widen the nostrils to make an arrow-shaped nose (▶ Fig. 15.7).

15.3.4 Gummy Smile

Excessive gingival display, known as gummy smile, occurs due to hyperactivity of the lip elevators while smiling. The DSN, LLSAN, levator labii superioris (LLS), zygomaticus minor (ZMi), and sometimes levator angularis oris (LAO) play a role in the creation of a gummy smile.[46] The three lip elevator muscles—LLS, LLSAN, and ZMi—converge on the area lateral to the ala and a single injection of 0.5 to 2 U at this converging point effectively reduces gingival display (▶ Fig. 15.7). In some patients with the ZMi fibers attached to the nasal alae, this injection can result in bulging in the paranasal area. Subcutaneous injection of 0.5 U into this bulging area can

smoothen this ala band. The medial part gingival display requires DSN injection of 2 to 4 U. Lateral gingival display by LAO or zygomaticus major contraction requires deep injection of approximately 1 U at the most contracting insertion site. Excessive paralysis of lip elevators can result in upper lip ptosis and the formation of a sad look; therefore, initial dose should be conservative.[47]

15.3.5 Asymmetric Lip and Asymmetric Smile

Asymmetric lip or nasolabial fold and asymmetric smile can be caused by muscle habit or a medical condition such as stroke, facial nerve palsy, or marginal mandibular nerve palsy. Asymmetry tends to worsen with time because muscles on the normal side tend to overcontract. Small doses of BoNT, usually 0.5 to 2 U, is subdermally injected into the hyperactive muscles on the normal side to restore symmetry[48,49] (▶ Fig. 15.8).

15.3.6 Nasolabial Fold and Marionette Fold

The nasolabial folds and Marionette folds are static wrinkles with soft-tissue volume depletion; some dynamic components also play a role here.[50] BoNT combination can be useful in patients with strong dynamic components, especially in the cases where fillers tend to migrate or easily disappear by strong muscle pulling. For

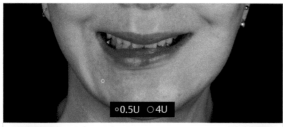

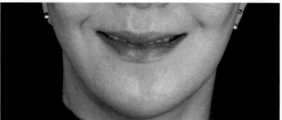

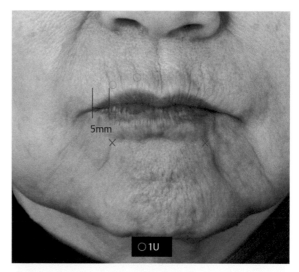

Fig. 15.8 Lip asymmetry by left marginal mandibular nerve palsy by laser liposuction (*upper*). Symmetry regained by botulinum neurotoxin (BoNT) injection into depressor angularis oris (DAO) and depressor labii inferioris (DLI) on the normal right side.

Fig. 15.9 Injection for perioral wrinkles.

a nasolabial fold, 1 to 2 U is deeply injected into the upper end of the nasolabial fold and 0.5 to 1 U is subdermally injected at a few points along the nasolabial fold. For each Marionette fold, 3 to 4 U is injected into the depressor angularis oris (DAO), usually 1 cm lateral and 1 cm inferior to the mouth corner.[51] For DAO, superficial injection, intradermal or subdermal, and symmetry in the dose, depth, and needle direction are important to prevent diffusion to the depressor labii inferioris (DLI), which can result in asymmetry or lower lip inversion. If asymmetry occurs, 0.25 to 0.5 U to the DLI on the unaffected site will help restore symmetry.

15.3.7 Perioral Wrinkle (Smoker's Line)

In select patients, perioral BoNT can ameliorate perioral rhytides (smoker's wrinkles). Vertical perioral rhytides appear with aging and are accentuated by repeated action of the orbicularis oris muscle. Patients with deep static wrinkles caused by photodamage and smoking require adjunctive treatments such as fillers, laser resurfacing, or chemical peeling. A 4- to 8-U injection into four points at the upper lip vermillion border, sparing 5 mm from the oral commissures, is performed (▶ Fig. 15.9). Injection at a proximity to the commissure may compromise functional patency and result in drooling, whereas injections medial to the philtral columns may cause flattening of Cupid's bow.[52] Superficial symmetrical injection is important to prevent asymmetrical lip movement. BoNT treatment of radial perioral wrinkles in the lower lip is not recommended because of the high risk of lip asymmetry or lip inversion (Fig. 15.9). Other complications include difficulty controlling the lip, especially

while drinking and pronouncing "*p*"s and "*b*"s. Patients who require tight control of the lips, such as public speakers, singers, and musicians, are not considered good candidates for BoNT therapy. In addition, perioral BoNT injection can induce some degree of lip eversion and is a good adjunct with lip filler treatment.

15.3.8 Cobblestone Chin

Cobblestone chin is caused by a hyperactive mentalis muscle. Hypertonic mentalis is common in patients with small chin, malocclusion, or habitual mouth frown. Hypertonic mentalis exacerbates recession of the chin with time, which together with volume loss in the lateral lip compartment, disturbs the smooth V line depicting youth and aggravates jowling. The mentalis muscle fibers originate from the alveolar bone of the mandible inferior to the lateral incisor. The fibers cross together, insert into the skin, and intertwine with DLI and the orbicularis oris. To relax the mentalis, 4 to 5 U is injected in each protuberance in a wide chin (▶ Fig. 15.10). For a small chin, a single-point deep periosteal injection of 8 to 10 U in the midline is safe to prevent diffusion into DLI and the resulting asymmetry.

15.3.9 Mouth Corner Elevation in Mouth Frown

Lip elevator and lip depressor muscles form an equilibrium of strength in the modiolus. Therefore, if lip depressors are relaxed with BoNT, mouth corner lifting can be achieved by a rebalance between lip elevators and depressors.[53] The target muscles are the DAO and mentalis, which work together to create a mouth frown. In patients with hypertonic mentalis, mouth corners are constantly pulled downward, aggravating Marionette folds and even nasolabial folds, giving the impression of a mouth frown. An 8- to 10-U deep injection into the mentalis and 3- to 4-U superficial injection into each DAO allow lifting of the mouth corners and smoothening of the folds (▶ Fig. 15.11). Sometimes, lip asymmetry can develop after treatment and this sudden asymmetry can be very distressing, lasting for a few months. Regain of symmetry should be achieved quickly by adding BoNT to the less relaxed side. In some patients, relaxation of the platysma muscles, another strong lip depressor, enables further lifting of the mouth corners.

15.3.10 The Nefertiti Lift, Platysmal Bands, Horizontal Neck Lines

The platysma acts as a major depressor in the lower face. It originates inferiorly from the pectoralis and deltoid

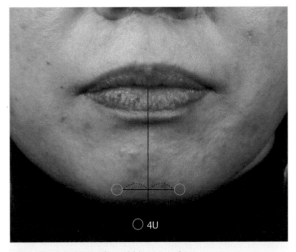

Fig. 15.10 Injection for cobble stone chin.

fascia and ascends upward, partially inserting directly under the mandible. The remaining fibers then move upward, blending into the modiolus, DLI, lower lip, DAO, and finally continuing upward to blend into the superficial musculoaponeurotic system (SMAS) and the skin of the cheeks. These insertions permit the platysma to pull the cheek skin and mouth corners downward. The Nefertiti lift technique is used to target the platysma muscle to redefine the jawline and raise the mouth corners. On average, 20 U per side is injected along the mandibular border and the upper half of the posterior platysma band.[54] Mandibular injection should be lateral to the medial margin of the DAO to prevent diffusion into the DLI (▶ Fig. 15.12a). The ideal candidate of Nefertiti lift is a patient whose jaw line is obscured by contracting platysma. Saying "eee" while clenching the teeth effectively contracts the platysma. Increased resting tone and hypertrophy with aging makes anterior and posterior platysmal bands visible even at rest, which leads to a senescent look. Lifting and grasping the bands, three to five intradermal injections of 2 to 4 U at each injection site are performed in each band. Horizontal neck lines can also be smoothened by BoNT injections along the neck lines by an intradermal injection of approximately 10 U into each line (▶ Fig. 15.12b). Although less effective than when used for bands, this injection serves as a good adjunct for fillers. To avoid dysphagia and dysphonia, a total dose of 50 U for the neck region should not be exceeded in one session.[52]

15.4 Facial Contouring and Body Contouring

15.4.1 Benign Masseteric Hypertrophy

Slimming of the square jaw using BoNT has gained great popularity in Asia where masseteric hypertrophy

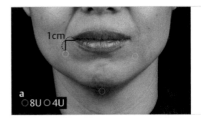
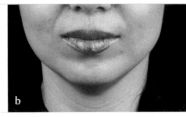

Fig. 15.11 Mouth corner lifting with botulinum neurotoxin (BoNT): before **(a)** and 2 weeks after **(b)**.

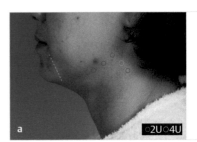
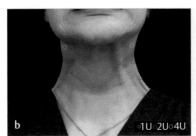

Fig. 15.12 **(a)** Nefertiti lift. **(b)** Injection for platysmal bands and horizontal neck lines.

is common due to racial characteristics and dietary habits. The masseter muscle originates from the zygomatic arch, runs downward, and inserts into the mandibular angle and the ramus. The masseter muscle consists of three heads: superficial, middle, and deep. The inferior half where all three heads merge is not only the thickest but also the ideal injection point. The line connecting the mouth angle and tragus roughly divides the masseter muscle into halves and is the upper border of the injection. Anterior and posterior borders of the masseter can be checked by clenching the teeth; the mandibular border defines the lower border. Injection should be confined to the lower and posterior three-quarters of this rectangle and delivered deep into each masseter at four to five points using a half-inch long needle (▶ Fig. 15.13). On average, 20 U per side is recommended for females with a muscle width of 3 to 5 cm and 28 to 40 U for males or patients with a muscle width greater than 5 cm. Evident reduction in the masseter volume starts 2 to 4 weeks after the injection and reaches maximal reduction at 3 months. This volume reduction progresses much faster in a previously treated patient. The duration of the effect is affected by few factors such as chewing habits, bruxism, and teeth clenching. Muscle volume may not fully recover 1 year after treatment, and repeated injection could result in long-term effects of muscle atrophy and fibrosis.[55] BoNT-induced muscle atrophy can also decrease the pulling on the underlying bone and prevent underlying bony flaring after anguloplasty.[56,57] If existent, pain and symptoms of grinding and clenching are improved. Paradoxical superficial masseter bulging on mastication can occur 1 to 2 days after injection when untreated superficial parts overly contract in cases of severe hypertrophy. This perplexing complication may disappear after a few weeks but can be resolved more quickly by injecting an additional 5 to 10 U in the bulging area. Other complications include sunken cheek in patients with insufficient cheek fat, jowling, and sagging by rapid volume reduction in the posterior cheek, loss of full smile, or an asymmetric smile due to diffusion into the risorius and zygomaticus major muscle by superficial and anterior injection.[58]

15.4.2 Salivary Gland Enlargement: Parotid Gland and Submandibular Gland

Salivary gland enlargement is common among Asians, affecting the contour of the lower face. Salivary gland enlargement can be observed in patients with various medical conditions such as eating disorders or alcoholism, and human immunodeficiency virus positive (HIV +) patients. Parotid gland enlargement creates a second facial contour in patients who have achieved masseteric atrophy after BoNT treatment. As BoNT blocks all cholinergic transmission, including that of the autonomous nervous system in neuroglandular junctions, it is increasingly used to treat sialorrhea. In addition, good clinical results of BoNT have been reported for the treatment of salivary gland enlargement.[59] Enlarged parotid glands can be identified by palpating diffuse round swelling that extends beyond the posterior border of the mandibular angle, giving patients a rounded toadlike face (▶ Fig. 15.14). Submandibular gland enlargement is often mistaken for submental fat accumulation and can be revealed due to increased laxity of the neck after facial bone surgery and liposuction. Before injection, imaging studies and workup should be performed to find any malignancy or underlying condition such as Sjögren's syndrome. The injection dose is 20 to 60 U per parotid gland and 20 to 40 U per submandibular gland. An intraglandular injection penetrating the gland fascia is important to prevent diffusion to surrounding neck muscles, which can cause difficulty when swallowing. Other possible complications include transient xerostomia, infection, and hematoma. An evident decrease in gland volume begins 1 to 2 weeks after injection and reaches the maximal reduction at 2 to 3 months. Treatment can be repeated until the desired volume is acquired, and the duration of effect is 6 months or more.

15.4.3 Botox Lifting or Mesobotox

Mesobotox has been widely performed in Asia, under various names such as skin botox, microbotox, botox lifting, or dermotoxin. Mesobotox is BoNT treatment of the whole face mostly using intradermal injections. The

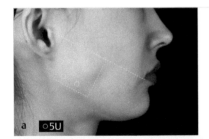 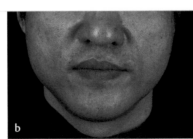 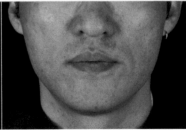

Fig. 15.13 (a) Injection for masseteric hypertrophy. (b) Before (*left*) and 3 months after injection of 30 U per masseter (*right*).

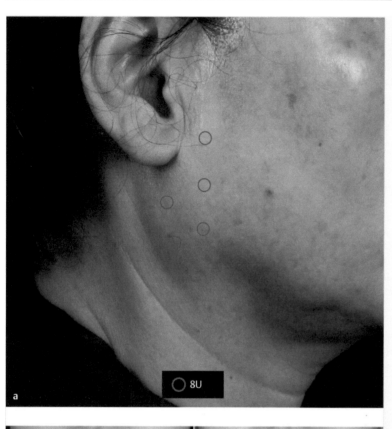

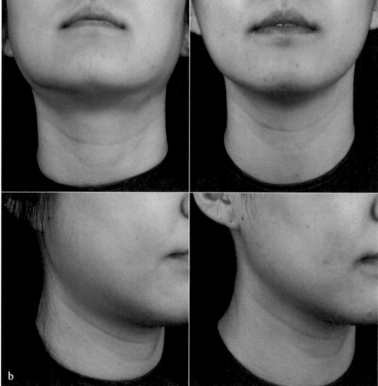

Fig. 15.14 **(a)** Injection for parotid gland enlargement. **(b)** Before (*left*) and 3 months after (*right*) botulinum neurotoxin (BoNT) injections into the enlarged parotid gland and submandibular gland.

purpose of this treatment is to reduce wrinkles and create a facial contour of a lifted look; overall improvement of skin quality is observed such as reduced fine wrinkles, pore tightening, and a shiny look to the skin. The mechanism under this improvement appears to result from lymphatic insufficiency, decreased seborrhea, and dermal remodeling.[60,61,62] BoNT may have a direct or indirect effect on fibroblast activity, stimulating collagen production and a reorganization of the collagen network within the extracellular matrix.[63] Injection dose is 40 to 80 U per session and the technique encompasses all previously mentioned areas. Conventional deep injections can be used for the corrugator, mentalis, and masseter or parotid gland. For other areas, a superficial intradermal injection of a higher dilution with 1 to 2 U/0.1 mL is used. The result is more natural and balanced without the effect of complete paralysis and lasts for approximately 3 months.

15.4.4 Body Contouring

Muscular atrophy induced by BoNT can be used to contour areas of the body such as the calves, thighs, shoulders, and upper arms. By controlling injection site and dose, it is possible to create the desired contours. When injecting big body muscles, the rule is to inject, intramuscularly, large volumes with lower concentrations (1–2 U/0.1 mL) for diffusion and smooth contouring. It is convenient to design muscle and injection points before injection. Based on muscle size, total dose is determined and divided by the number of points. Trigger points or most hypertrophied areas require more doses (▶ Table 15.4).

Trapezius hypertrophy is increasing due to prolonged crouching posture from excessive use of smartphones and computers, leading to shorter neck and even myofascial pain syndrome.[64,65] The recommended dose for trapezius hypertrophy is 20 to 40 U per side. BoNT injection at the most affected area of the upper trapezius creates a more beautiful shoulder line and reduces shoulder pain. Care should be exercised to avoid injecting medial to the neckline as this will prevent weakening of the neck muscles. For calf muscles, 50 to 100 U is injected into the gastrocnemius and soleus. Injection in the standing position can lead to vasovagal syncope; therefore, injection in the prone position is recommended. A boost injection at 3 months after the first injection, when atrophy is maximal and muscle regeneration occurs, can result in long-lasting results. At 1 to 2 weeks after injection, impaired foot rolling and falling may occur.[66] Hypertrophied quadriceps and deltoid muscle can also be treated in selected cases. It is noteworthy that the duration of muscle atrophy is increased with subsequent treatments, and muscle strength and volume may not fully recover.[67] Toxicity and distant paralysis from high-dose usage should be monitored.

15.5 Other Indications of Botulinum Toxin

The BoNT receptors and intracellular targets are not unique to neurotransmission as they have been found in both neuronal and non-neuronal cells. Non-neuronal cells that express BoNT-A binding proteins and/or cleavage target SNAP-25 include the following: epidermal keratinocytes; mesenchymal stem cells from subcutaneous adipose; nasal mucosal cells; neutrophils; macrophages, urothelial cells; intestinal, prostate, and alveolar epithelial cells; and breast cell lines. Serotype BoNT-A can elicit specific biological effects in dermal fibroblasts, sebocytes, and vascular endothelial cells. BoNTs have a much wider range of applications than what has been originally understood, and individual cellular responses to cholinergic impacts of BoNTs could provide fertile grounds for future studies.[68]

15.5.1 Hyperhidrosis

Primary focal hyperhidrosis is a common autonomic disorder that significantly impacts quality of life. This disorder is characterized by excessive sweating confined to circumscribed areas such as the axillae, palms, soles, and face. Less frequent types of focal hyperhidrosis that is secondary to underlying causes include gustatory sweating in Frey's syndrome, and after sympathectomy. Approval of BoNT for severe axillary hyperhidrosis in 2004 revolutionized the treatment of this indication.[69] To validate the injection area, the starch-iodine test can be used. The recommended doses for hyperhidrosis include 100 U per palm, 150 U per sole, 50 U per axilla, 20 U for the forehead, 16 U for the nose, and 200 U for the entire scalp. The injection is administered intradermally or subdermally and a BoNT-A dilution of 2 U/0.1 mL is commonly used. The duration of effect is usually 6 months and differs considerably at different sites. Treatment of palmar and plantar hyperhidrosis requires the mastering of nerve block. Complications include weakness of underlying muscles and impaired hand dexterity. Compensatory hyperhidrosis in other areas is possible but is much milder than in sympathectomy.

15.5.2 Pain and Pruritus

BoNT has recently been used to treat various types of neuropathic pain such as trigeminal neuralgia, postherpetic neuralgia, diabetic neuropathy, and intractable neuropathic pain such as poststroke pain and spinal cord injury.[70] BoNT acts on neuropathic pain by inhibiting the release of inflammatory mediators and peripheral neurotransmitters from sensory nerves such as substance P, calcitonin gene-related peptide (CGRP), and glutamate. Retrograde axonal transport and transcytosis of BoNT from the site of uptake at the sensory nerve ending into the dorsal root ganglion and the spinal cord is also

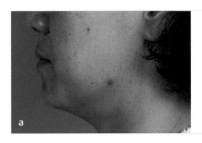
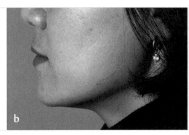

Fig. 15.15 Before **(a)** and 2 weeks after combination treatment of Nefertiti lift and IPL **(b)**.

believed to play a role in BoNT activity during pain. Indirectly, a change in the sensory cortex in the brain may occur following peripheral reduction of afferent input. The ability of BoNT to attenuate transmitter release from afferent sensory nerve terminals has made BoNT available for the treatment of localized recalcitrant pruritus. BoNT reduces mast cell degranulation and induces long-lasting antipruritic effects.[71]

15.5.3 Scar

BoNT treatments exert a positive effect on wound healing and scar appearance. This is accomplished by decreasing dynamic tension on the wound through the weakening of the underlying muscle. Time to immobilization of muscle is a key factor in the improvement of wound healing based on this technique.[72] BoNT injected before scar revision surgery resulted in the wound being stabilized, better wound healing, and the prevention of wound widening during healing.[73] BoNT may control hypertrophic scarring by inhibiting the proliferation of keloid fibroblasts and reducing transforming growth factor-$\beta 1$ (TGF-$\beta 1$) expression.[74]

15.5.4 Other Delivery Methods and Uses of Botulinum Toxin

Recently, there have been reports that BoNT can be safely delivered with minimal pain using various drug delivery devices such as jet nebulizer, microneedle, ablative fractional laser, nanoemulsion, and cell-penetrating peptide.[75,76] For example, BoNT delivered through nanomicroneedles not only reduced periorbital dynamic wrinkles but also treated static wrinkles by increasing skin elasticity, collagen content, and hydration.[77] The combination of various transdermal delivery tools and new BoNT drugs with low antigenicity can widen the scope of therapeutics for many indications. Delivery of BoNT has been shown to reduce signs and symptoms of acne, erythema/rosacea, psoriasis, localized cold intolerance or Raynaud's phenomenon from underlying vascular compromise, and to result in significant improvements in many rare diseases caused or exacerbated by hyperhidrosis.[78,79,80,81]

15.5.5 Botulinum Toxin Use as an Adjunct

BoNTs and fillers work together as a great duo to defeat aging by causing relaxation and reflation. This combination has shown superior efficacy and has improved patient satisfaction when used to treat deep static wrinkles and create facial contour. When given 2 weeks before filler treatment, BoNT decreases the dynamic component of targeted wrinkles, leading to increased efficacy and longevity of the filler. This BoNT combination is particularly valuable when used to treat glabellar frown lines, nasolabial folds, Marionette folds, and horizontal neck lines, and to contour the nose, chin, or forehead. BoNT combination before laser resurfacing contributes to improved aesthetic results and reduced wrinkle recurrence.[82] The effect of skin tightening by microfocused ultrasound or radiofrequency and treatment of pigmentation and texture with intense pulsed light (IPL) are enhanced by a combination with BoNT treatment (▶ Fig. 15.15).

References

[1] Brin MF. Development of future indications for BOTOX. Toxicon. 2009; 54(5):668–674

[2] Zhang S, Masuyer G, Zhang J, et al. Identification and characterization of a novel botulinum neurotoxin. Nat Commun. 2017; 8:14130

[3] Matarasso SL. Comparison of botulinum toxin types A and B: a bilateral and double-blind randomized evaluation in the treatment of canthal rhytides. Dermatol Surg. 2003; 29(1):7–13, discussion 13

[4] Flynn TC, Clark RE, II. Botulinum toxin type B (MYOBLOC) versus botulinum toxin type A (BOTOX) frontalis study: rate of onset and radius of diffusion. Dermatol Surg. 2003; 29(5):519–522, discussion 522

[5] Dressler D, Bigalke H, Benecke R. Botulinum toxin type B in antibody-induced botulinum toxin type A therapy failure. J Neurol. 2003; 250 (8):967–969

[6] Rasetti-Escargueil C, Lemichez E, Popoff MR. Variability of botulinum toxins: challenges and opportunities for the future. Toxins (Basel). 2018; 10(9):E374

[7] Davies JR, Liu SM, Acharya KR. Variations in the botulinum neurotoxin binding domain and the potential for novel therapeutics. Toxins (Basel). 2018; 10(10):E421

[8] Rogozhin AA, Pang KK, Bukharaeva E, Young C, Slater CR. Recovery of mouse neuromuscular junctions from single and repeated injections of botulinum neurotoxin A. J Physiol. 2008; 586(13):3163–3182

[9] Kutschenko A, Manig A, Reinert MC, Mönnich A, Liebetanz D. In-vivo comparison of the neurotoxic potencies of incobotulinumtoxinA, onabotulinumtoxinA, and abobotulinumtoxinA. Neurosci Lett. 2016; 627:216–221

[10] Frevert J. Content of botulinum neurotoxin in Botox®/Vistabel®, Dysport®/Azzalure®, and Xeomin®/Bocouture®. Drugs R D. 2010; 10 (2):67–73

[11] Frevert J. Pharmaceutical, biological, and clinical properties of botulinum neurotoxin type A products. Drugs R D. 2015; 15(1):1–9

[12] Kane MA, Gold MH, Coleman WP, III, et al. A randomized, double-blind trial to investigate the equivalence of incobotulinumtoxinA and onabotulinumtoxinA for glabellar frown lines. Dermatol Surg. 2015; 41(11):1310–1319

[13] Rappl T, Parvizi D, Friedl H, et al. Onset and duration of effect of incobotulinumtoxinA, onabotulinumtoxinA, and abobotulinumtoxinA in the treatment of glabellar frown lines: a randomized, double-blind study. Clin Cosmet Investig Dermatol. 2013; 6:211–219

[14] Kane MA, Monheit G. The practical use of AbobotulinumtoxinA in aesthetics. Aesthet Surg J. 2017; 37 suppl_1:S12–S19

[15] Kerscher M, Roll S, Becker A, Wigger-Alberti W. Comparison of the spread of three botulinum toxin type A preparations. Arch Dermatol Res. 2012; 304(2):155–161

[16] Seo K, Bae GY. Neuronox and Innotox. In: Carruthers A, Carruthers J, eds. Botulinum Toxin: Procedures in Cosmetic Dermatology. 4th ed. Toronto: Elsvier; 2018:57–63

[17] Carruthers JD, Fagien S, Joseph JH, Humphrey SD, et al. DaxibotulinumtoxinA for injection for the treatment of glabellar lines: results from each of two multicenter, randomized, double-blind, placebo-controlled, phase 3 studies (SAKURA 1 and SAKURA 2). Plast Reconstr Surg. 2020; 145(1): 45–58

[18] Hardas B, Brin MF. Topical botulinum toxin type A. In: Carruthers A, Carruthers J, eds. Botulinum Toxin: Procedures in Cosmetic Dermatology. 4th ed. Toronto: Elsvier; 2018:81–84

[19] Toth SI, Smith LA, Ahmed SA. Extreme sensitivity of botulinum neurotoxin domains towards mild agitation. J Pharm Sci. 2009; 98(9): 3302–3311

[20] Hsu TS, Dover JS, Arndt KA. Effect of volume and concentration on the diffusion of botulinum exotoxin A. Arch Dermatol. 2004; 140(11): 1351–1354

[21] Hexsel DM, De Almeida AT, Rutowitsch M, et al. Multicenter, double-blind study of the efficacy of injections with botulinum toxin type A reconstituted up to six consecutive weeks before application. Dermatol Surg. 2003; 29(5):523–529, discussion 529

[22] Parsa AA, Lye KD, Parsa FD. Reconstituted botulinum type A neurotoxin: clinical efficacy after long-term freezing before use. Aesthetic Plast Surg. 2007; 31(2):188–191, discussion 192–193

[23] Aranda MA, Herranz A, del Val J, Bellido S, García-Ruiz P. Botulinum toxin A during pregnancy, still a debate. Eur J Neurol. 2012; 19(8): e81–e82

[24] Tzou CH, Giovanoli P, Ploner M, Frey M. Are there ethnic differences of facial movements between Europeans and Asians? Br J Plast Surg. 2005; 58(2):183–195

[25] Carruthers A, Carruthers J. Prospective, double-blind, randomized, parallel-group, dose-ranging study of botulinum toxin type A in men with glabellar rhytids. Dermatol Surg. 2005; 31(10):1297–1303

[26] Dailey RA, Philip A, Tardie G. Long-term treatment of glabellar rhytides using onabotulinumtoxinA. Dermatol Surg. 2011; 37(7): 918–928

[27] Bai L, Peng X, Liu Y, et al. Clinical analysis of 86 botulism cases caused by cosmetic injection of botulinum toxin (BoNT). Medicine (Baltimore). 2018; 97(34):e10659

[28] Naumann M, Boo LM, Ackerman AH, Gallagher CJ. Immunogenicity of botulinum toxins. J Neural Transm (Vienna). 2013; 120(2):275–290

[29] Dressler D, Pan L, Adib Saberi F. Antibody-induced failure of botulinum toxin therapy: re-start with low-antigenicity drugs offers a new treatment opportunity. J Neural Transm (Vienna). 2018; 125 (10):1481–1486

[30] Moon IJ, Chang SE, Kim SD. First case of anaphylaxis after botulinum toxin type A injection. Clin Exp Dermatol. 2017; 42(7):760–762

[31] Rosenfield LK, Kardassakis DG, Tsia KA, Stayner G. The first case report of a systemic allergy to onabotulinumtoxinA (Botox) in a healthy patient. Aesthet Surg J. 2014; 34(5):766–768

[32] Yiannakopoulou E. Serious and long-term adverse events associated with the therapeutic and cosmetic use of botulinum toxin. Pharmacology. 2015; 95(1–2):65–69

[33] Shaari CM, Sanders I. Quantifying how location and dose of botulinum toxin injections affect muscle paralysis. Muscle Nerve. 1993; 16(9):964–969

[34] Shetty R. Dynamic relaxers of the face. J Cutan Aesthet Surg. 2018; 11 (2):47–50

[35] Kruger TH, Wollmer MA. Depression: an emerging indication for botulinum toxin treatment. Toxicon. 2015; 107 Pt A:154–157

[36] Finzi E. Update: botulinum toxin for depression: more than skin deep. Dermatol Surg. 2018; 44(10):1363–1365

[37] Isse NG, Elahi MM. The corrugator supercilii muscle revisited. Aesthet Surg J. 2001; 21(3):209–215

[38] Park JI, Hoagland TM, Park MS. Anatomy of the corrugator supercilii muscle. Arch Facial Plast Surg. 2003; 5(5):412–415

[39] Huilgol SC, Carruthers A, Carruthers JD. Raising eyebrows with botulinum toxin. Dermatol Surg. 1999; 25(5):373–375, discussion 376

[40] Ascher B, Talarico S, Cassuto D, et al. International consensus recommendations on the aesthetic usage of botulinum toxin type A (Speywood Unit): part I—upper facial wrinkles. J Eur Acad Dermatol Venereol. 2010; 24(11):1278–1284

[41] Keaney TC, Alster TS. Botulinum toxin in men: review of relevant anatomy and clinical trial data. Dermatol Surg. 2013; 39(10):1434–1443

[42] Anido J, Arenas D, Arruabarrena C, et al. Tailored botulinum toxin type A injections in aesthetic medicine: consensus panel recommendations for treating the forehead based on individual facial anatomy and muscle tone. Clin Cosmet Investig Dermatol. 2017; 10: 413–421

[43] Jun JY, Park JH, Youn CS, Lee JH. Intradermal injection of botulinum toxin: a safer treatment modality for forehead wrinkles. Ann Dermatol. 2018; 30(4):458–461

[44] Flynn TC, Carruthers JA, Carruthers JA. Botulinum-A toxin treatment of the lower eyelid improves infraorbital rhytides and widens the eye. Dermatol Surg. 2001; 27(8):703–708

[45] Redaelli A, Limardo P. Minimally invasive procedures for nasal aesthetics. J Cutan Aesthet Surg. 2012; 5(2):115–120

[46] Hwang WS, Hur MS, Hu KS, et al. Surface anatomy of the lip elevator muscles for the treatment of gummy smile using botulinum toxin. Angle Orthod. 2009; 79(1):70–77

[47] Polo M. Botulinum toxin type A (Botox) for the neuromuscular correction of excessive gingival display on smiling (gummy smile). Am J Orthod Dentofacial Orthop. 2008; 133(2):195–203

[48] Sadiq SA, Khwaja S, Saeed SR. Botulinum toxin to improve lower facial symmetry in facial nerve palsy. Eye (Lond). 2012; 26(11):1431–1436

[49] Haykal S, Arad E, Bagher S, et al. The role of botulinum toxin a in the establishment of symmetry in pediatric paralysis of the lower lip. JAMA Facial Plast Surg. 2015; 17(3):174–178

[50] Snider CC, Amalfi AN, Hutchinson LE, Sommer NZ. New insights into the anatomy of the midface musculature and its implications on the nasolabial fold. Aesthetic Plast Surg. 2017; 41(5):1083–1090

[51] Pessa JE, Garza PA, Love VM, Zadoo VP, Garza JR. The anatomy of the labiomandibular fold. Plast Reconstr Surg. 1998; 101(2):482–486

[52] Carruthers J, Carruthers A. Aesthetic botulinum A toxin in the mid and lower face and neck. Dermatol Surg. 2003; 29(5):468–476

[53] Goldman A, Wollina U. Elevation of the corner of the mouth using botulinum toxin type a. J Cutan Aesthet Surg. 2010; 3(3):145–150

[54] Levy PM. Neurotoxins: current concepts in cosmetic use on the face and neck—jawline contouring/platysma bands/necklace lines. Plast Reconstr Surg. 2015; 136(5) Suppl:80S–83S

[55] Kim NH, Chung JH, Park RH, Park JB. The use of botulinum toxin type A in aesthetic mandibular contouring. Plast Reconstr Surg. 2005; 115 (3):919–930

[56] Tsai CY, Shyr YM, Chiu WC, Lee CM. Bone changes in the mandible following botulinum neurotoxin injections. Eur J Orthod. 2011; 33 (2):132–138

[57] Libouban H, Guintard C, Minier N, Aguado E, Chappard D. Long-term quantitative evaluation of muscle and bone wasting induced by botulinum toxin in mice using microcomputed tomography. Calcif Tissue Int. 2018; 102(6):695–704

[58] Wu WT. Botox facial slimming/facial sculpting: the role of botulinum toxin-A in the treatment of hypertrophic masseteric muscle and parotid enlargement to narrow the lower facial width. Facial Plast Surg Clin North Am. 2010; 18(1):133–140

[59] Bae GY, Yune YM, Seo K, Hwang SI. Botulinum toxin injection for salivary gland enlargement evaluated using computed tomographic volumetry. Dermatol Surg. 2013; 39(9):1404–1407

[60] Dessy LA, Mazzocchi M, Rubino C, Mazzarello V, Spissu N, Scuderi N. An objective assessment of botulinum toxin A effect on superficial skin texture. Ann Plast Surg. 2007; 58(5):469–473

[61] Pessa JE, Nguyen H, John GB, Scherer PE. The anatomical basis for wrinkles. Aesthet Surg J. 2014; 34(2):227–234

[62] Shah AR. Use of intradermal botulinum toxin to reduce sebum production and facial pore size. J Drugs Dermatol. 2008; 7(9): 847–850

[63] Humphrey S, Jacky B, Gallagher CJ. Preventive, cumulative effects of botulinum toxin type A in facial aesthetics. Dermatol Surg. 2017; 43 Suppl 3:S244–S251

[64] Zhou RR, Wu HL, Zhang XD, et al. Efficacy and safety of botulinum toxin type A injection in patients with bilateral trapezius hypertrophy. Aesthetic Plast Surg. 2018; 42(6):1664–1671

[65] Kim DY, Kim JM. Safety and efficacy of prabotulinumtoxinA (Nabota®) injection for cervical and shoulder girdle myofascial pain syndrome: a pilot study. Toxins (Basel). 2018; 10(9):E355

[66] Wanitphakdeedecha R, Ungaksornpairote C, Kaewkes A, Sathaworawong A, Vanadurongwan B, Lektrakul N. A pilot study comparing the efficacy of two formulations of botulinum toxin type A for muscular calves contouring. J Cosmet Dermatol. 2018; 17(6):984–990

[67] Durand PD, Couto RA, Isakov R, et al. Botulinum toxin and muscle atrophy: a wanted or unwanted effect. Aesthet Surg J. 2016; 36(4): 482–487

[68] Grando SA, Zachary CB. The non-neuronal and nonmuscular effects of botulinum toxin: an opportunity for a deadly molecule to treat disease in the skin and beyond. Br J Dermatol. 2018; 178(5):1011–1019

[69] Weinberg T, Solish N, Murray C. Botulinum neurotoxin treatment of palmar and plantar hyperhidrosis. Dermatol Clin. 2014; 32(4): 505–515

[70] Park J, Park HJ. Botulinum toxin for the treatment of neuropathic pain. Toxins (Basel). 2017; 9(9):E260

[71] Boozalis E, Sheu M, Selph J, Kwatra SG. Botulinum toxin type A for the treatment of localized recalcitrant chronic pruritus. J Am Acad Dermatol. 2018; 78(1):192–194

[72] Dhawan A, Dhawan S, Vitarella D. The potential role of botulinum toxin in improving superficial cutaneous scarring: a review. J Drugs Dermatol. 2018; 17(9):956–958

[73] Shome D, Khare S, Kapoor R. An algorithm using botox injections for facial scar improvement in Fitzpatrick type IV-VI skin. Plast Reconstr Surg Glob Open. 2018; 6(8):e1888

[74] Hao R, Li Z, Chen X, Ye W. Efficacy and possible mechanisms of botulinum toxin type A on hypertrophic scarring. J Cosmet Dermatol. 2018; 17(3):340–346

[75] Iannitti T, Palmieri B, Aspiro A, Di Cerbo A. A preliminary study of painless and effective transdermal botulinum toxin A delivery by jet nebulization for treatment of primary hyperhidrosis. Drug Des Devel Ther. 2014; 8:931–935

[76] Kim WO. Treatment of focal hyperhidrosis with needleless injections of botulinum toxin into sites other than the axilla, palm, and sole. Dermatol Surg. 2017; 43 Suppl 3:S367–S369

[77] Cao Y, Yang JP, Zhu XG, et al. A comparative in vivo study on three treatment approaches to applying topical botulinum toxin A for crow's feet. BioMed Res Int. 2018; 2018:6235742

[78] Friedman O, Koren A, Niv R, Mehrabi JN, Artzi O. The toxic edge- a novel treatment for refractory erythema and flushing of rosacea. Lasers Surg Med. 2019; 51(4):325–331

[79] Schlessinger J, Gilbert E, Cohen JL, Kaufman J. New uses of abobotulinumtoxinA in aesthetics. Aesthet Surg J. 2017; 37 suppl_1: S45–S58

[80] Kim MJ, Kim JH, Cheon HI, et al. Assessment of skin physiology change and safety after intradermal injections with botulinum toxin: a randomized, double-blind, placebo-controlled, split-face pilot study in rosacea patients with facial erythema. Dermatol Surg. 2019; 45(9): 1155–1162

[81] Boukovalas S, Mays AC, Selber JC. Botulinum toxin injection for lower face and oral cavity Raynaud phenomenon after mandibulectomy, free fibula reconstruction, and radiation therapy. Ann Plast Surg. 2019; 82(1):53–54

[82] Zimbler MS, Holds JB, Kokoska MS, et al. Effect of botulinum toxin pretreatment on laser resurfacing results: a prospective, randomized, blinded trial. Arch Facial Plast Surg. 2001; 3(3):165–169

16 Soft-Tissue Augmentation with Dermal Fillers

Andreas Boker

Summary

Soft-tissue augmentation with injectable fillers is a procedure being performed with increasing popularity. Knowledge of the available materials and their properties, a solid understanding of relevant facial anatomy, and proper injection technique are all crucial to ensure safe treatments and optimize patient outcomes.

Keywords: soft tissue augmentation, facial contouring, dermal fillers, hyaluronic acids gels, calcium hydroxyapatite, poly-L-lactic acid

16.1 Introduction

The public awareness and demand for minimally invasive aesthetic procedures such as soft-tissue augmentation with dermal fillers has risen exponentially over the past 10 years. In 2017 alone, 2.6 million dermal filler treatments were performed in the United States, a 300% increase since 2000.[1,2] Since the introduction of bovine collagen-based dermal fillers during the 1980s, the quest for the ideal dermal filler, mainly, a safe, biocompatible, nonimmunogenic product that yields reproducible and appropriately long-lasting results has been ongoing.

Currently in the United States, the most commonly used fillers materials are nonpermanent hyaluronic acid (HA) gels, followed by "semi-permanent" calcium hydroxylapatite (CaHA) gel and poly-L-lactic acid (PLLA) suspension.

Over the past two decades, a greater understanding of the mechanisms responsible for the aging of the human face has led to a shift in the approach to facial rejuvenation. With the knowledge that age-related subcutaneous fat loss, gravitational fat compartment repositioning, and dermal collagen degradation are mainly responsible for facial senescence, the restitution of volume has become one of the principal goals of aesthetic facial rejuvenation and is now favored over sole resuspension of redundant skin via a rhytidectomy. In fact, over 80% of facelifting procedures currently being performed by plastic surgeons in the United States are executed in conjunction with volumizing procedures such as fat grafting and/or soft-tissue augmentation with filler gels.[3]

16.2 Commercially Available Devices

16.2.1 Hyaluronic Acid Gels

Background and Chemistry

Naturally occurring endogenous HA is a high-molecular-weight, polysaccharide that is an essential component of the extracellular matrix. It is found in abundance in all animal tissues including the skin, joints, vitreous humor, vascular tissue, and cartilage. In the skin, it is found predominantly in the papular and reticular dermis where it is organized in supermolecular networks capable of distending and maintaining the extracellular space as well as regulating tissue hydration.[4] As such, dermal HA plays a key role in cutaneous water balance, osmotic pressure, and ion flow regulation. It is also found in the basal layer of the epidermis where it facilitates critical epithelial repair functions. With age, the synthesis, quality, and performance of dermal HA declines, mostly as a result of fibroblast senescence, leading to an altered extracellular matrix.[5]

As a result, synthetic injectable HA gels have been bioengineered to emulate critical hydration and volumizing properties, with the aim of restoring age-related dermal and subcutaneous tissue atrophy. These products are glycosaminoglycan polymers composed of cross-linked glucuronic acid and N-acetyl glucosamine disaccharide units. The cross-linking of HA units yields a stable and biocompatible molecule with extended longevity in the human dermis. Individual manufacturers use proprietary cross-linking technology to yield gels with different physical properties used for a variety of indications.

There are multiple commercially available injectable HA gels currently approved for soft-tissue augmentation by the U.S. Food and Drug Administration (FDA; ▸ Table 16.1).[6] All available products in the U.S. market consist of the newer generation, nonanimal stabilized hyaluronic acids (NASHA), which are bioengineered via bacterial (mainly streptococcal) expression systems.

Table 16.1 FDA-approved implantable devices[a]

Name	Material	Manufacturer	FDA indication(s)
Restylane Restylane-L	Hyaluronic acid, lidocaine	Galderma	Correction of moderate-to-severe facial wrinkles/folds Lip augmentation
Restylane Silk	Hyaluronic acid, lidocaine	Galderma	Lip augmentation and dermal implantation for correction of perioral rhytids

(Continued)

Table 16.1 (*Continued*) FDA-approved implantable devices

Name	Material	Manufacturer	FDA indication(s)
Restylane Lyft	Hyaluronic acid, lidocaine	Galderma	Correction of moderate-to-severe facial folds and wrinkles, such as nasolabial folds. Subcutaneous to supraperiosteal implantation for cheek augmentation and correction of age-related midface contour deficiencies Dorsal hand to correct volume deficit
Restylane Refyne	Sodium hyaluronate	Galderma	Correction of mild-to-moderate to facial wrinkles and folds (such as nasolabial folds)
Restylane Defyne	Sodium hyaluronate	Galderma	Correction of moderate-to-severe deep facial wrinkles and folds (such as nasolabial folds)
Restylane Kysse	Hyaluronic acid, lidocaine	Galderma	Lip augmentation and correction of the upper perioral rhytids
Juvèderm Ultra XC, Juvèderm Ultra Plus XC	Hyaluronic acid, lidocaine	Allergan	Correction of moderate-to-severe facial wrinkles and folds (such as nasolabial folds)
Juvèderm Voluma XC	Hyaluronic acid, lidocaine	Allergan	Deep (subcutaneous and/or supraperiosteal) injection for cheek augmentation to correct age-related volume deficit in the midface
Juvèderm Volbella XC	Hyaluronic acid, lidocaine	Allergan	Injection into the lips for lip augmentation and for correction of perioral rhytids.
Juvèderm Vollure XC	Hyaluronic Acid	Allergan	Correction of moderate-to-severe facial wrinkles and folds (such as nasolabial folds)
Captique	Hyaluronic acid	Genzyme Biosurgery	Correction of moderate-to-severe facial wrinkles and folds (such as nasolabial folds)
Belotero Balance	Hyaluronic acid	Merz Pharmaceuticals	Injection into facial tissue to smooth wrinkles and folds, especially around the nose and mouth (nasolabial folds)
Prevelle Silk	Hyaluronic acid, lidocaine	Genzyme Biosurgery	Correction of moderate-to-severe facial wrinkles and folds (such as nasolabial folds)
Radiesse	Hydroxylapatite	Bioform Medical, Inc.	Correction of the signs of facial fat loss (lipoatrophy) in people with HIV Correction of moderate-to-severe facial wrinkles and folds (such as nasolabial folds) Subdermal implantation for hand augmentation to correct volume loss in the dorsum of the hands
Sculptra and Sculptra Aesthetic	Poly-L-lactic acid (PLLA)	Sanofi Aventis U.S.	Facial lipoatrophy in people with HIV Correction of shallow to deep nasolabial fold and other facial wrinkles or contour deficiencies
Elevess	Hyaluronic acid, lidocaine	Anika Therapeutics	Correction of moderate-to-severe facial wrinkles and folds (such as nasolabial folds)
Teosyal RHA 1, 2, 3, and 4	Hyaluronic acid, lidocaine	Teoxane	Correction of moderate-to-severe dynamic facial wrinkles and folds, such as nasolabial folds
Revanesse Versa	Hyaluronic acid, lidocaine	Prollenium Medical Technologies Inc.	Correction of moderate-to-severe facial wrinkles and folds, such as nasolabial folds
Bellafill (formerly Artefill)	Polymethylmethacrylate beads, collagen, and lidocaine	Suniva Medical	Correction of nasolabial folds and moderate-to-severe, atrophic, distensible facial acne scars on the cheeks

Abbreviation: FDA, Food and Drug Administration.
[a]Unless stated otherwise, all materials are approved for injection in patients over the age of 21 years.

Most products contain lidocaine to increase patient comfort during injection but all major manufacturers have lidocaine-free options for patients with a known hypersensitivity to lidocaine. Earlier products, which were manufactured from rooster combs, have been discontinued due to biosafety concerns.

Mechanical Properties/Rheology

Bioengineered HA gels possess different flow characteristics based on the concentration of HA they contain and the degree and type of cross-linking used during their manufacturing process.[7] When considering which filler to use to correct specific areas of the face, selecting the right gel with the ideal physical properties can lead to both superior results and fewer adverse outcomes. For example, when the treatment goal is volumization of the deep fat compartments of the midface, choosing a highly cross-linked, highly cohesive, more elastic (high G') "harder" material would be most appropriate, as this material would produce optimal vertical projection and offer higher resistance to shear deformity, maintaining its shape and size after injection. Conversely, when attempting to correct more superficial, fine dermal rhytids, a less elastic and low cohesive "softer" gel will allow for easier flow and molding within tissue. Facial animation, exterior mechanical stress (i.e., compression, stretching), and gravity are all forces that directly impact filler longevity and performance. Similarly, placement depth of the gel will also determine the degree of projection and contour achieved by individual injection boluses. The tighter dermal matrix will prevent the injected bolus from spreading laterally despite external vertical compression, whereas injection of the same material into the loser subcutaneous plane will allow the gel to spread more easily under similar mechanical stress. The concentration of HA also impacts the performance of individual products, with more concentrated gels (i.e., 20–24 mg/mL of HA) inducing significantly more rehydration and thus volumization after being implanted.

Safety and Contraindications

HA filler gels are almost universally well tolerated and due to absent species or tissue specificity are considered immunologically inert. True hypersensitivity reactions are rare but case reports have been published.[8,9,10]

Because exogenous HAs are mainly derived from *Streptococcus equi* bacteria, a known hypersensitivity to streptococcal or gram-positive bacteria should preclude the use of these gels in such patients. Similarly, a known hypersensitivity to lidocaine may be a contraindication for using lidocaine-containing gels. Most branded products like Restylane and are available without lidocaine. Furthermore, impurities in the manufacturing and/or handling process and improper or too frequent injections may potentially result in adverse inflammatory responses.

The safety of all injectable materials has not been studied during pregnancy or lactation and their use in both situations is therefore not recommended.

16.2.2 Calcium Hydroxyapatite

Radiesse is an injectable implant composed of smooth CaHA microspheres (diameter of 25–45 μm) suspended in a sodium carboxymethylcellulose gel carrier. After implantation, the carrier gel is resorbed over several months and is gradually replaced by an infiltrating fibrovascular stroma that gradually induces new type I collagen production around the microspheres.[11] It is thus considered a semi-permanent implant with an estimated longevity of 2 years or longer.[12]

It was first approved by the FDA for correction of HIV-related facial lipoatrophy but has since also received approval for correction of mild-to-moderate facial wrinkles and to correct volume loss in the dorsum of the hands. It is an opaque white gel that may become visible when placed too superficially in the dermis; so, it should be used as a deeper dermal filler. Due to its calcium content, it is radiopaque and may appear as high-attenuation linear streaks or clumps on computed tomography or hypermetabolic foci on fluorodeoxyglucose positron emission tomography (FDG-PET) scans.[13] This is an important consideration when placing the material around deep bony structures of the face and patients need to be informed of this pitfall so that future providers (i.e., dentists, radiologists) are aware of this potential artifact.

Inflammatory reactions and persistent nodularity have been reported as potential complications.[14]

16.2.3 Poly-L-Lactic Acid

Sculptra is an injectable implant that consists of microparticles of a biocompatible, biodegradable, synthetic polymer from the alpha hydroxy acid family. It is supplied as a sterile freeze-dried preparation containing PLLA, sodium carboxymethylcellulose (USP), nonpyrogenic mannitol (USP), which needs to be reconstituted prior to use by the addition of sterile water for injection (SWFI), USP to form a sterile, and nonpyrogenic suspension. Dilution standards vary, but most clinicians recommended adding 8 mL of sterile water and 1 mL of lidocaine to each vial at least 2 to 24 hours prior to injection to ensure complete hydration of the product. After injection, the PLLA microparticles induce an inflammatory reaction resulting in the formation of fibrous connective tissue and neocollagenesis.[15]

Injections are performed using larger bore (25- to 26-gauge) needles to prevent clogging and longer ones (1.25 inches) to facilitate reach within the deep subcutaneous plane. When treating the midfacial region, a common treatment method is to first place a set of intradermal 1% lidocaine local anesthetic blebs at the lateral malar cheeks and 1 cm lateral to each oral commissures as entry points. This is followed by insertion of the needle and retrograde injection of the suspension in a fanning pattern based at each of the injection points, with the aim of depositing a perpendicular cross-hatched uniform lattice across the entire treatment region. The decision of how many vials to inject depends on the degree of subcutaneous soft-tissue atrophy and should be made together with each patient. After injection, manual massage is performed against the bone to ensure even distribution of the product. As significant volumes of the suspension are injected, patients will notice an initial dramatic volumization or "overcorrection" of the treated areas. It is important to explain to patients that initial inflation is the result of the reconstitution fluid used for hydrating the product and that this will be resorbed within 1 to 3 days. Furthermore, patients need to be counseled of the delayed "filling effect" of the product and that series of monthly treatment sessions will be required to achieve the full result.[16]

16.2.4 Polymethylmethacrylate Beads, Collagen, and Lidocaine

Bellafill is an implant composed of nonresorbable polymethyl methacrylate (PMMA) microspheres, 30 to 50 µm in diameter, suspended in a water-based carrier gel composed of 3.5% bovine collagen, 92.6% buffered, isotonic water for injection, 0.3% lidocaine hydrochloride, 2.7% phosphate buffer, and 0.9% sodium chloride. Following implantation, immediate correction is achieved by the collagen in which the microspheres are suspended. As resorption of collagen begins, a foreign body inflammatory reaction composed of macrophages, fibroblasts, and capillaries is mounted against the microspheres, inducing neocollagenesis and filling the interstitial spaces between the microspheres. As the residual PMMA microspheres are nonbiodegradable, this device is considered permanent with longevity in human tissue demonstrated up to 20 years.[17]

PMMA is indicated for the correction of nasolabial folds and moderate-to-severe atrophic, distensible facial acne scars on the cheeks in patients older than 21 years.[18] It is contraindicated for patients with a history of allergies to any bovine collagen products, including but not limited to injectable collagen, collagen implants, hemostatic sponges, and collagen-based sutures. It is also contraindicated for lip augmentation.

Adverse reactions include injection site reactions, erythema, nodularity, hypersensitivity reactions, persistent edema, and granuloma formation.[19,20]

16.2.5 Liquid Injectable Silicone

The injection of highly purified medical-grade silicone (polydimethylsiloxane) has been performed for body contouring and soft-tissue augmentation for decades, but the practice remains controversial in the United States. Only two products (AdatoSil and Silikon1000) are FDA approved for the treatment of retinal detachment and any use for cosmetic intradermal injection is considered "off-label." The most acceptable injection method is a serial microdroplet puncture technique by which less than 0.01 mL of liquid silicone is placed into the subdermal plane at 2- to 4-mm intervals.[21] Despite its perceived inert character, impurities in various products used (some nonmedical grade) and improper injection techniques have been implicated in a variety of adverse inflammatory reactions including persistent erythema, edema, the formation of papules, nodules, abscesses, and granulomas.

16.3 Clinical Uses and Technique

16.3.1 Preoperative Care

Obtaining a thorough medical history, including comorbidities and current medications as well as a focused physical examination, should be part of every patient's preoperative evaluation. The patients are advised to avoid alcohol consumption for 24 hours prior to treatment. Patients with a history of herpes simplex labials seeking enhancement of their lips and/or perioral region should be given prophylactic antiviral treatment as per established protocols.

Written informed consent and high-quality, standardized preoperative photographs should be obtained prior to treatment. The informed consent should be tailored to each patient and specifically highlight the intended use of the filler and whether the area to be treated is considered to be an off-label indication. If the products to be used will be diluted with lidocaine to change their rheological properties, it should also be noted as this is also considered an "off-label" use.

Potential risks particular to the area to be injected should be discussed verbally with the patient.

The target area should be rinsed off with a gentle soap and water to remove any makeup or cosmeceutical product. The skin should be cleansed with an alcohol wipe and some injectors will additionally use an antiseptic agent such as chlorhexidine gluconate 4% or povidone iodine to further decrease the risk of bacterial inoculation during injection. Patients should be advised to avoid undergoing dental procedures or oral surgery for 2 weeks prior and after treatment with fillers given the risk of bacteremia and the resulting potential for infection and/or biofilm formation.

Patients should be injected in an upright sitting position with their head supported and under bright illumination.

16.3.2 Midfacial Rejuvenation

The pathophysiology of the aging face is a complex interplay of intrinsic/genetic and extrinsic/environmental factors. First, the facial skeleton undergoes chronological changes, mainly due to bone resorption and muscular stress on osteotendinous attachments with lead to a structural shift in the shape and angle of the facial bones. Second, weakening and thinning of facial muscles and supporting ligaments such as the SMAS or zygomatic ligament results in loss of support and downward displacement of subcutaneous fat compartments. Finally, loss of fat volume of important midfacial soft-tissue structures like the suborbicularis oculi fat (SOOF) pad ultimately leads to an overall haggard and atrophied appearance of the midface.[22]

Soft-tissue augmentation with filler gels and/or fat grafting has become the preferred method for addressing midfacial volume loss. The primary goal is restoration of the malar prominence and upper cheek with a natural convexity that then softly transitions down toward the mid-cheek hollow in the shape of an ogee curve. The projection achieved on the malar cheek will help reorient the inferior-pointing vectors of the sagging face, which in turn results in "lifting" and support of the inferior third of the face. As a result, this approach leads to softening of the appearance of the nasolabial folds, and prejowl sulci and an overall more youthful appearance[23] (▶ Fig. 16.1). This technique has been described as part of the popularized "Y-lift," aimed at accentuating the lateral malar prominences in concert with redefinition of the mandibular angle, jawline, and chin.

Rejuvenation of the midface should start by injecting fillers with increased stiffness (high elastic modulus, G′) into the deep midfacial fat compartments. Injection of these "harder" gels should be performed as single boluses

placed supraperiostially and should be done only after retraction of the plunger to ensure extravascular placement. Some injectors prefer to use blunt-tip cannulas to flow the gel into the deeper tissue planes and utilize a single injection point positioned lateral to the malar prominence or at the base of the lower cheeks to fan the gel in different directions radially.[24] Commonly used fillers for this purpose include Restylane Lyft, Restylane Defyne, Juvèderm Voluma, Juvèderm Ultra Plus, and Radiesse.

If necessary, following deeper volumization of the cheeks, a less viscous gel may then be injected more superficially directly underneath the nasolabial folds either via small-bolus serial puncture or linear threading techniques with a needle or cannula. Certain products like Restylane Defyne and Restylane Refyne have been specifically formulated for treating areas under constant motion from muscular stretch and compression and are thus ideally suited for correction of nasolabial folds and marionette lines. They have been shown to adapt to facial movement, resulting in a sustained natural correction during facial animation.[25] Restylane Defyne is typically indicated for deeper folds and Restylane Refyne for more superficial lines.

The amount of filler material needed to achieve the desired result depends on the degree of subcutaneous soft-tissue dystrophy and volume lost, the patient's age, and individual anatomical features. In patients with severe midfacial atrophy such as that seen in HIV-associated lipoatrophy, the use of semi-permanent implants such as calcium CaHA or repeat injections of PLLA every 4 to 6 months yields excellent and lasting aesthetic results[26,27] (▶ Fig. 16.2).

16.3.3 Periorbital Region

Loss of subcutaneous fat along the nasojugal groove leads to the emergence of formerly concealed infraorbital fat pads, which will also protrude as a result of gravity and lack of support from the orbital retaining and tear trough ligaments. Furthermore, the downward displacement of infraorbital fat compartments over a weakened orbital septum creates a deeper and wider orbit and a double convex deformity of the lower eyelid.[28] The result is a curvilinear trough starting at the medial canthus and extending laterally and parallel to the inferior orbital rim, imparting patients with a "tired" look and "hollowed out" appearance.

Correction of this deformity with injectable filler materials often requires concomitant augmentation of the malar cheek region to evenly blend both anatomical subunits in a seamless transition. Injections should be placed supraperiostially in small individual boluses and after retraction of the plunger to ensure extravascular placement. The use of a blunt-tip cannula inserted at the lateral malar or lower cheek affords easy access to the space beneath the orbicular oculi muscle and may thus result in less tissue trauma and ecchymosis. In patients with

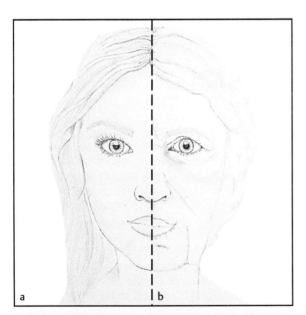

Fig. 16.1 Anatomy of facial aging. (Reproduced from Cotofana S, Fratila A A, Schenck T L et al. The Anatomy of the Aging Face: A Review. Facial Plastic Surgery 2016; 32(03): 253–260.)

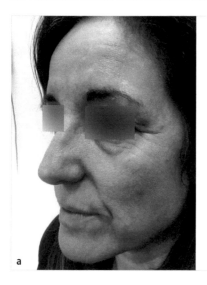
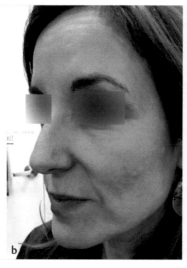

Fig. 16.2 Midfacial augmentation. (a) Before. (b) After.

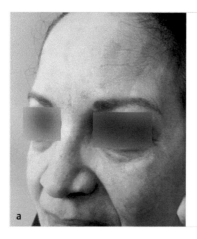
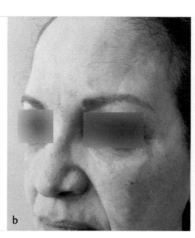

Fig. 16.3 Periorbital augmentation. (a) Before. (b) After.

severe volume loss and a prominent tear trough deformity, injection at multiple depth levels and a combination of "harder" and "softer" gels may be required to attain a full and even correction of all anatomical subunits.

The lateral tails of the eyebrows may be injected with small amounts of filler to enhance protrusion and "lifting" of the eyebrows. Injections are placed supraperiostially and very small volumes are required to achieve desired results (▶ Fig. 16.3).

16.3.4 Upper Face

Loss of subcutaneous fat of the mid to lower forehead in patients who have a flattened or slightly concave frontal bone may lead to accentuation of the supraorbital ridges, imparting patients with a "skeletonized" appearance. This region may be injected with filler gels to restore a more convex contour and soothe the transition onto the midface and ocular region. Injections are placed submuscularly as small, evenly spaced boluses using a serial puncture technique in a horizontal line along the depression or by using

a blunt-tip cannula inserted at the upper third of the forehead. This is then followed by firm digital massage to evenly distribute the implanted material.

The glabellar creases are sometimes injected to correct the vertical depression between the medial eyebrows caused by long-standing engagement of the procerus and corrugator muscles. This region is considered a "high-risk" area for filler injections given its high vascularity, specifically the positioning and trajectory of the supratrochlear artery and its anastomosis with the ophthalmic artery.[29] Thus, correction of volume deficits in this anatomic subunit should only be performed by experienced injectors.

The author recommends using a low-viscosity gel such as Belotero Balance or Restylane Silk injected very slowly and under extremely low pressure in very small aliquots into the deep dermal plane. Retraction of the plunger is always performed prior to advancement of the gel to ensure extravascular implantation. It is also recommended to first treat the dynamic rhytids with botulinum toxin injections into the corrugator and procerus muscle groups before considering correction of residual furrows with a filler material.

This approach serves two purposes: first, at a follow-up visit, the glabellar rhytids may appear shallower, requiring less volume of filler to attain full correction, and, second, decreased muscular action may prevent dynamic displacement of the injected gel, improving its longevity.

The temporal region is also subject to age-related subcutaneous volume loss including atrophy of the temporal fat pad and temporalis muscle, resulting in hollowing out of the temporal fossa. The surrounding zygomatic process and lateral orbital rim become more pronounced, imparting an "angular" or "sharp" look to the upper midface. Off-label injection of filler materials into this area restores the natural convexity of the region and imparts a more rounded contour to the lateral forehead as it transitions into the malar prominences. High G' HA gels and PLLA have shown good results when used in this region. Injections may be safely placed at three distinct levels: (1) the subcutaneous plane where often low G' gels are favored, (2) deep to the temporoparietal fascia, and (3) deep below the temporalis muscle on the periosteum. At the latter, slowly injecting a single depot of a higher G' gel leads to an even projection of the entire temporal fossa.[30]

The ear lobes are sometimes injected with dermal fillers in elderly women who have lost volume and desire rejuvenation for easier earring use. Gravity, especially with long-term use of heavy earrings, results in a stretch deformity and thinning of the ear lobe. Off-label injection of HA gels into the subcutaneous plane is an excellent method to restore lost volume and reshaping the earlobes.

16.3.5 Lower Face

With increasing age, progressive laxity and dehiscence of the mandibular septum, descent of the malar and perioral fat compartments, and resorption of the alveolar bone all lead to loss of definition of the jawline and accentuation of the prejowl sulci.[31]

Downward-pointing oral commissures often referred to as "marionette lines" are a common concern for patients as they impart a "sad face" appearance to the lips. Mild cases of jowling can be improved with soft-tissue augmentation alone, but more severe deformities with complete obliteration of the jawline are best addressed with a surgical rhytidectomy and fat repositioning with or without liposuction.[32] The use of soft-tissue fillers is an excellent noninvasive option but is considered an off-label indication for all commercially available products.

As mentioned earlier, restoring volume to the midface (i.e., malar cheeks) will "lift" the lower cheeks and should ideally be performed prior to addressing specific rhytids of the lower face. By doing so, less volume of filler will likely be needed to fully correct the prejowl sulci and result in a more natural appearance.

The chin is a common target for soft-tissue augmentation and/or mentoplasty in patients with varying degrees of chin retrusion. Although the ideal aesthetic chin proportions vary based on gender and ethnicity, a spherical, narrower, and slightly more projecting chin is generally considered a more aesthetically pleasing shape in women, whereas a more rectangular, broader, and flatter chin is considered more attractive in men. Filler gels can be employed using different injection techniques and depths to reshape the mental contour.[33]

In addition, redefining the jawline by injecting serial or linear depots along the mandibular angle will accentuate its length and sharpen the inferior edge of the face to a more youthful appearance.[34]

16.3.6 Lips

Volumization of the lips is a sought-after indication especially with advancing age as the mucosal lips deflate, the cutaneous portion of the upper lip lengthens, and the vermillion of the lip loses its shape.

In women in particular, restoring the forward and slightly upward projecting vermillion border or "ski slope" at the junction of the cutaneous and mucosal lip and replacing lost volume of both the upper and lower mucosal lips lead to a more youthful and attractive appearance.[35,36] The "ideal" ratio of upper to lower lip volume is subject to individual interpretation and personal or cultural preference. Some injectors advocate for slightly higher volumes of the lower lip compared to the upper lip and suggest aiming for a 1.6:1 volume ratio, respectively. Other injectors express preference for more equivalent lip ratios and patient themselves have shown in surveys that their volume preferences often vary depending on their age.[37] As with other cosmetic subunits of the face, rejuvenation of the lips and perioral region must often be accompanied by volumetric restoration of the lower third of the face to restore the structural support of the chin and jawline.

Medium G, small particle HA gels such as Restylane or Juvèderm Volbella can be safely used to restore volume to the mucosal lips, whereas thinner gels are often injected to redefine and sharpen the vermillion border and the philtrum columns.

The upper and lower cutaneous lips also suffer dermal and epidermal volume loss due to intrinsic and extrinsic aging and develop radially oriented rhytids. These may be corrected by injecting small boluses of less viscous, small particle HA gels. Some injectors recommend further dilution of commercially available HA products with varying amounts of lidocaine or bacteriostatic saline solution to decrease their viscosity and facilitate flow into smaller more superficial rhytids. There is conflicting evidence, however, on the benefit of diluting HA gels since the added hydration will invariably affect the materials' G' and its inherent ability to "lift"[38] (▶ Fig. 16.4).

16.3.7 Neck

With advancing age, accelerated collagen degradation and constant motion of the neck muscles will result in

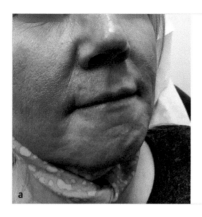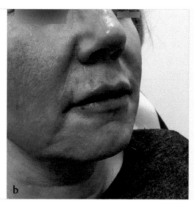

Fig. 16.4 (a, b) Before and after lip augmentation.

skin laxity and horizontal wrinkling of the skin. These superficial lines can be traced by injecting a lower G' "softer" gel in a serial puncture or linear treading fashion until full correction is attained.

16.3.8 Hands

Subcutaneous fat loss of the dorsal hands imparts a "skeletonized" appearance to aging hands with prominence of digital extensor tendons and superficial veins. There are two products approved by the FDA for injection into dorsal hands: Radiesse and Restylane Lyft. Both are injected in a retrograde linear threading fashion parallel to the digital extensor tendons in a subcutaneous plane. Injection may be performed with a needle or a cannula through a single or multiple injection points typically located over the base of the metacarpophalangeal joints and pointing the delivery device proximally.[39] After delivery of the material, firm manual massage is performed perpendicular to the extensor tendons to ensure an even spread. Given the thin subcutaneous and dermal plane, it is not uncommon for papules and nodules to become visible after treatment. As with other highly vascular anatomic regions, retraction of the syringe plunger prior to injection is recommended to ensure extravascular placement of the material. To prevent complications including nodularity, pain, excessive edema, and difficulty forming a fist, a maximum volume of 1.6 mL is recommended for injection into each hand.

16.3.9 Scars

Atrophic scars, especially those resulting from old acne lesions, are commonly corrected with injection of dermal fillers. Slightly depressed scars such as the "rolling" type respond very well to small boluses of thin HA gels injected directly underneath the depression.[40] Care should be exercised not to inject too superficially to avoid visible bluish papules due to the Tyndall effect. As mentioned previously, the PMMA collagen gel has gained FDA approval for semi-permanent correction of atrophic acne scars on the cheeks.[17]

16.3.10 Other Off-Label Uses

Due to their versatility and perceived safety and ease of use, fillers are being injected into an increasing number of areas where volume enhancement is desired. Nonsurgical augmentation of the nasal bridge and definition of the dorsal nose, especially in Asian patients seeking to sharpen their side profile, is a popular procedure. However, due to a wide anatomic variation of the dorsal nasal artery, injection into its vicinity is considered to be "high risk" for vascular complications and is therefore best avoided altogether.[41] Body contouring of the abdominal and gluteal region has also been attempted using soft-tissue augmentation with PLLA, HA gels, PMMA microspheres, and liquid silicone. These procedures are all off-label and are often performed by physicians as well as nonlicensed providers practicing outside the United States, mostly in South America. Due to the larger volumes of material needed to obtain visible enhancement of these areas, there is also a higher rate of complications associated with these injections including cellulitis, biofilm and abscess formation, myositis, subcutaneous nodules and/or granulomas, skin fibrosis necrosis, ulceration, fistula formation, embolization, and even death.

Enhancement of the male and female external genitalia with injectable fillers has also been reported.[42,43]

16.4 Pitfalls and Complications

16.4.1 Postoperative Care

Immediately following injection, the treatment area should be iced and pressure applied to minimize the risk of edema and ecchymosis. Patients should be instructed to avoid strenuous exercise and nonsteroidal anti-inflammatories for 2 to 3 days after undergoing filler injections to further minimize the risk of bruising. If possible, instruct patients to sleep in a face-up supine position with their head slightly elevated to minimize edema. It is also recommended to avoid facial massages or manipulating the treated area to prevent deformation or displacement of implanted gels. For postinjection pain control, the patients are recommended to take acetaminophen as needed and continue application of ice packs for 10 to 20 minutes four to five times daily for a few days. Use of sunblock, makeup, and other cosmetics is allowed the day after the procedure.

16.4.2 Edema

Injection of any foreign material into the human body will elicit a certain degree of inflammation resulting in swelling, but most currently used filler implants are designed to be fairly inert. HAs in particular are vastly hydrophilic and will naturally cause edema within the first 1 to 2 days after injection. It is helpful to reassure patients of this normal and transitory reaction and explain that it will resolve with elevation, application of cold packs, and avoidance of salty food consumption during the first few days after the injection. Severe edema is unusual and tends to occur more often in areas with thinner dermal planes such as the lips or the periorbital region or when more concentrated HA gels are used. For severe cases, a 1- to 3-day course of oral corticosteroids may be necessary to help the patient recover faster.

16.4.3 Ecchymosis

Mild and pinpoint ecchymoses at the site of needle insertion are normal and expected and will usually resolve within 5 to 7 days. Patients with an underlying bleeding diathesis or patients who routinely take anticoagulants including vitamins and herbal supplements (vitamin E, omega-3-fatty acids, *Ginkgo biloba*, ginseng, or garlic) or daily prophylactic low-dose aspirin or other nonsteroidal anti-inflammatory drugs may experience more pronounced ecchymosis following injection. The risk also correlates with the vascularity and anatomy of the treated sites, the number of needle sticks performed, and the injection technique. Whenever possible, it is recommended to stretch the skin and use proper illumination to help visualize vascular structures prior to needle insertion. Posttreatment digital compression and/or use of cold packs will also help induce hemostasis and prevent ecchymoses. The decision of whether to recommend discontinuation of anticoagulants prior to soft-tissue augmentation is based on physician experience and comfort level but may also be dictated by the targeted site. For example, the author recommends avoiding anticoagulants and oral supplements with known anticoagulant effects for a 7-day period before treating the periorbital area if feasible, given the highly vascular anatomy of the site, the thin dermal plane, and superficial location of the orbicularis oculi muscle.

Some physicians recommend the use of posttreatment topical or oral *arnica montana* to help minimize ecchymosis. In more severe cases, a pulsed dye laser or intense pulsed light may be used to accelerate resolution of ecchymoses.[44]

16.4.4 Vascular Occlusion

With the rapidly increasing number of filler procedures being performed each year, the number of vascular complications has also risen in parallel. Vascular compromise may result from direct intravascular injection of a gel or from external arterial compression by an adjacent bolus. Clinical manifestations of vascular occlusion depend on the injected site and compromised blood vessel. When a cutaneous arterial branch suffers embolization, patients may experience immediate onset of pain and blanching of the skin, which may then progress to erythematous or violaceous reticular patches. Skin necrosis with desquamation or ulceration may ensue and may result in permanent scarring.

The most feared vascular complication of filler injections, however, is ocular compromise resulting in blindness. This occurs from retrograde embolization of the ophthalmic artery due to injection of one of its branches or anastomoses. Arteries at highest risk of injection include the supratrochlear, dorsal nasal, supraorbital, and angular arteries. Patients may experience sudden ocular pain, headaches, nausea, and altered mental status. To date, 143 cases of ophthalmologic complications have been reported in the literature, with the majority of cases resulting from injection of autologous fat or HA into the glabellar, forehead, or nasal regions.[45,46]

It is crucial to recognize these potentially devastating complications early and initiate prompt management. General measures include stopping the injection immediately, massaging the area, applying warm compresses and nitroglycerin paste, injecting the area with hyaluronidase (if HA gel was used), and administering aspirin daily for 7 days. The two most widely used commercial formulations of hyaluronidase in dermatology include a human recombinant agent (Hylenex, concentration of 150 U/1 mL) and an ovine testicular hyaluronidase (Vitrase, concentration: 200 U/1 mL). Their use for dissolving injected HA gels is considered off-label and there are several proposed treatment protocols, including daily versus high-dose hourly injections depending on the surface area and/or vessel size suspected to be compromised. The goal is to flood the entire tissue block with enough enzyme to break down any intravascular HA particles and relieve the obstruction.[47] Given the potential for cross-sensitivity to hyaluronidase present in bee venom, a careful history should identify patients at risk of developing a hypersensitivity reaction to therapeutic hyaluronidase, and skin testing may be warranted in individuals with documented previous anaphylactic reactions to bee stings. In emergent situations and when faced with a potentially catastrophic vascular compromise from HA injection, the decision to use hyaluronidase in such a patient will depend on a careful risk–benefit assessment.[48]

If an ocular ischemic event is suspected, prompt transfer to an inpatient setting and/or emergent ophthalmology

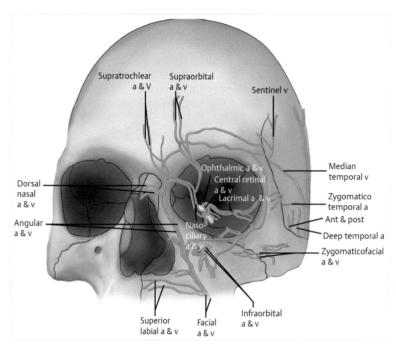

Fig. 16.5 High-risk area anatomy.

consultation is crucial. Some authors advocate immediate retrobulbar injection of hyaluronidase in an attempt to flood the optic nerve/vascular bundle and allow the hyaluronidase to diffuse into the occluded central retinal artery.[49] There is evidence, however, that hyaluronidase does not cross the dura of the optic nerve, resulting in a failure to reach the central retinal artery.[50]

As mentioned earlier, certain highly vascular areas of the face are at increased risk of intravascular injection and should be avoided if possible or approached with extreme care (▶ Fig. 16.5). It is paramount for injectors to have a thorough understanding of the vascular anatomy of the face and to practice conservative injection techniques to avoid complications. For example, it is recommended to avoid forceful or rapid injection of large boluses of material at a single static injection point as this may increase the risk of adjacent external blood vessel compression, especially in tight spaces framed by harder structures like cartilage or bone. It is also recommended that prior to each injection, a slight retraction ("pull test") of the syringe plunger be performed after needle insertion or needle-tip repositioning to assure the absence of blood in the anterior needle hub. This technique, however, is no guarantee of extravascular injection as re-aspiration of blood may be impeded by the viscous gel in the needle lumen.[51] Identifying and palpating known arteries at risk of injection is crucial before treatment. Some authors recommend digital external occlusion of such vessels as an additional safeguard to prevent retrograde flow of injected gels. An example is holding a finger on the supratrochlear artery before and during injection of the glabellar creases.[29] Another approach is keeping the needle or cannula tip in constant micromotion while slowly injecting the gel with low pressure to prevent intraluminal deposition.

16.4.5 Tyndall Effect

Translucent gels like HAs may cause a bluish discoloration of the overlying skin when injected too superficially in the dermal plane. This results from scattering of shorter (blue and violet) wavelengths when visible light passes through the pool of HA particles. It is a particular risk when more particulate dermal fillers are injected and it is often mistaken for a "bruise." Depending on the longevity of the HA gel used, the bluish discoloration may be long lasting and lead to significant patient anxiety and dissatisfaction with treatment.[52]

This complication can be avoided by injecting the gel into the deeper subcutaneous plane and injecting only small aliquots, especially in high-risk areas such as the periorbital or perioral regions. Treatment includes firm massage, a stab incision and drainage of the undesired gel, and, if necessary, dissolution of the gel with injection of hyaluronidase.

16.4.6 Nodularity

Injection of any material too superficially or in excessive quantities may result in visible contour irregularities. This is especially true when harder (higher G') gels are injected and these should therefore not be used to correct superficial rhytids. Gentle manual massage may help flatten and spread visible nodules, but for persistent lesions, a stab incision with extraction or injection of hyaluronidase, if applicable, may be necessary. The risk of persistent nodularity is greater with injection of semi-permanent gels like calcium CaHa or PMMA. A recent animal study showed promising results with dissolution of CaHa particles using intralesional injection of sodium thiosulfate or topical application of sodium metabisulfite.[53] Granulomatous reactions resulting in chronic recalcitrant nodules are rare and have been mostly reported after injection of silicone and PMMA.

16.4.7 Inflammatory Reactions and Biofilms

Inflammatory reactions to injected filler materials, especially HA-based gels, are uncommon. When they occur, they may represent sterile immune reactions to antigens inherent to the material or be the result of bacterial infections. Inoculation of skin flora during injection may account for most infectious granulomas; however, they may also develop from contiguous spread of a nearby infection or from systemic hematogenous spread. The presentation varies from asymptomatic, indolent, indurated papules, or nodules to warm, tender suppurating abscesses.[54] Reactions are more commonly reported after use of permanent fillers such as PMMA, polyacrylamide, or polymethylsiloxane,[55] and semi-permanent fillers like CaHa[56] and PLLA,[57] and have increasingly been reported after use of certain injectable HA gels.[58]

The formation of bacterial biofilms has been reported to occur in response to all injected filler materials. Their hallmark is resistance to antibiotics and chronic recurrences, making the management of such cases challenging. Treatment depends on the type of material injected, the severity of the reaction, and the results of laboratory analyses such as bacterial cultures and/or biopsies. For mild cases, intralesional injection of corticosteroids or a short course of prednisone 0.5 to 1 mg/kg/d × 7 to 14 days may resolve the inflammation. When HA gels are the culprit, injection of recombinant hyaluronidase may be effective and sufficient for reversing noninfectious granulomas. When infectious biofilms are suspected, prompt institution of a broadspectrum oral antibiotic combination such as a fluoroquinolone along with a tetracycline or macrolide for a period of 3 to 6 weeks is recommended[59] with or without incision and drainage or surgical debridement for more severe cases. More recently, the use of intralesional 5-fluorouracil has proved effective in chronic, persistent nodules.[60]

16.5 Pearls

To best manage patients' expectations and optimize outcomes, a preoperative conversation with the patient should emphasize a detailed treatment plan including the number of syringes the injector deems necessary to achieve the mutually agreed-upon goals. If a patient has a set budget, it is often most beneficial to aim for full correction of one particular area alone instead of attempting

rejuvenation of the entire face. Patients expect visible results and will be pleased if at least one of their concerns has been treated fully. These patients can then be provided with a detailed treatment schedule and budget outlining areas to be addressed at a later time. Patients should be allowed to express their areas of concern or desired correction, and physicians should point out to them and document any preexisting asymmetries in the target areas to optimize treatment outcome and patient satisfaction.

References

[1] Hojjat H, Raad R, Lucas J, et al. Public perception of facial fillers. Facial Plast Surg. 2019; 35(2):204–209

[2] American Society of Plastic Surgeons. Plastic Surgery Statistics Report. Arlinton Heights, IL: American Society of Plastic Surgeons National Clearinghouse; 2018

[3] Sinno S, Mehta K, Reavey PL, Simmons C, Stuzin JM. Current trends in facial rejuvenation: an assessment of ASPS members' use of fat grafting during face lifting. Plast Reconstr Surg. 2015; 136(1):20e–30e

[4] Kablik J, Monheit GD, Yu L, Chang G, Gershkovich J. Comparative physical properties of hyaluronic acid dermal fillers. Dermatol Surg. 2009; 35 Suppl 1:302–312

[5] Tzellos TG, Klagas I, Vahtsevanos K, et al. Extrinsic ageing in the human skin is associated with alterations in the expression of hyaluronic acid and its metabolizing enzymes. Exp Dermatol. 2009; 18(12):1028–1035

[6] U.S. Food and Drug Administration. Dermal Fillers Approved by the Center for Devices and Radiological Health. 2018. Available at: https://www.fda.gov/MedicalDevices/ ProductsandMedicalProcedures/CosmeticDevices/ ucm619846.htm#approved

[7] Santoro S, Russo L, Argenzio V, Borzacchiello A. Rheological properties of cross-linked hyaluronic acid dermal fillers. J Appl Biomater Biomech. 2011; 9(2):127–136

[8] Lupton JR, Alster TS. Cutaneous hypersensitivity reaction to injectable hyaluronic acid gel. Dermatol Surg. 2000; 26(2):135–137

[9] Artzi O, Loizides C, Verner I, Landau M. Resistant and recurrent late reaction to hyaluronic acid-based gel. Dermatol Surg. 2016; 42(1): 31–37

[10] Bhojani-Lynch T. Late-onset inflammatory response to hyaluronic acid dermal fillers. Plast Reconstr Surg Glob Open. 2017; 5(12):e1532

[11] Berlin AL, Hussain M, Goldberg DJ. Calcium hydroxylapatite filler for facial rejuvenation: a histologic and immunohistochemical analysis. Dermatol Surg. 2008; 34 Suppl 1:S64–S67

[12] Shumaker PR, Sakas EL, Swann MH, Greenway HT, Jr. Calcium hydroxylapatite tissue filler discovered 6 years after implantation into the nasolabial fold: case report and review. Dermatol Surg. 2009; 35 Suppl 1:375–379

[13] Feeney JN, Fox JJ, Akhurst T. Radiological impact of the use of calcium hydroxylapatite dermal fillers. Clin Radiol. 2009; 64(9):897–902

[14] Kadouch JA. Calcium hydroxylapatite: a review on safety and complications. J Cosmet Dermatol. 2017; 16(2):152–161

[15] Gogolewski S, Jovanovic M, Perren SM, Dillon JG, Hughes MK. Tissue response and in vivo degradation of selected polyhydroxyacids: polylactides (PLA), poly(3-hydroxybutyrate) (PHB), and poly(3-hydroxybutyrate-co-3-hydroxyvalerate) (PHB/VA). J Biomed Mater Res. 1993; 27(9):1135–1148

[16] Bartus C, William Hanke C, Daro-Kaftan E. A decade of experience with injectable poly-L-lactic acid: a focus on safety. Dermatol Surg. 2013; 39(5):698–705

[17] Lemperle G, Knapp TR, Sadick NS, Lemperle SM. ArteFill permanent injectable for soft tissue augmentation: I. Mechanism of action and injection techniques. Aesthetic Plast Surg. 2010; 34(3):264–272

[18] Joseph JH, Shamban A, Eaton L, et al. Polymethylmethacrylate collagen gel-injectable dermal filler for full face atrophic acne scar correction. Dermatol Surg. 2019; 45(12):1558–1566

[19] Medeiros CC, Cherubini K, Salum FG, de Figueiredo MA. Complications after polymethylmethacrylate (PMMA) injections in the face: a literature review. Gerodontology. 2014; 31(4):245–250

[20] Woodward J, Khan T, Martin J. Facial filler complications. Facial Plast Surg Clin North Am. 2015; 23(4):447–458

[21] Orentreich DS. Liquid injectable silicone: techniques for soft tissue augmentation. Clin Plast Surg. 2000; 27(4):595–612

[22] Cotofana S, Fratila AA, Schenck TL, Redka-Swoboda W, Zilinsky I, Pavicic T. The anatomy of the aging face: a review. Facial Plast Surg. 2016; 32(3):253–260

[23] Glaser DA, Lambros V, Kolodziejczyk J, Magyar A, Dorries K, Gallagher CJ. Relationship between midface volume deficits and the appearance of tear troughs and nasolabial folds. Dermatol Surg. 2018; 44(12): 1547–1554

[24] Hexsel D, Soirefmann M, Porto MD, Siega C, Schilling-Souza J, Brum C. Double-blind, randomized, controlled clinical trial to compare safety and efficacy of a metallic cannula with that of a standard needle for soft tissue augmentation of the nasolabial folds. Dermatol Surg. 2012; 38(2):207–214

[25] Percec I, Bertucci V, Solish N, Wagner T, Nogueira A, Mashburn J. An objective, quantitative, dynamic assessment of hyaluronic acid fillers that adapt to facial movement. Plast Reconstr Surg. 2020; 145(2):295e–305e

[26] Carruthers A, Carruthers J. Evaluation of injectable calcium hydroxylapatite for the treatment of facial lipoatrophy associated with human immunodeficiency virus. Dermatol Surg. 2008; 34(11):1486–1499

[27] Bassichis B, Blick G, Conant M, et al. Injectable poly-L-lactic acid for human immunodeficiency virus-associated facial lipoatrophy: cumulative year 2 interim analysis of an open-label study (FACES). Dermatol Surg. 2012; 38(7, Pt 2):1193–1205

[28] Wong CH, Hsieh MKH, Mendelson B. The tear trough ligament: anatomical basis for the tear trough deformity. Plast Reconstr Surg. 2012; 129(6):1392–1402

[29] Scheuer JF, III, Sieber DA, Pezeshk RA, Gassman AA, Campbell CF, Rohrich RJ. Facial danger zones: techniques to maximize safety during soft-tissue filler injections. Plast Reconstr Surg. 2017; 139(5): 1103–1108

[30] Breithaupt AD, Jones DH, Braz A, Narins R, Weinkle S. Anatomical basis for safe and effective volumization of the temple. Dermatol Surg. 2015; 41 Suppl 1:S278–S283

[31] Reece EM, Pessa JE, Rohrich RJ. The mandibular septum: anatomical observations of the jowls in aging-implications for facial rejuvenation. Plast Reconstr Surg. 2008; 121(4):1414–1420

[32] Rohrich RJ, Rios JL, Smith PD, Gutowski KA. Neck rejuvenation revisited. Plast Reconstr Surg. 2006; 118(5):1251–1263

[33] Vanaman Wilson MJ, Jones IT, Butterwick K, Fabi SG. Role of nonsurgical chin augmentation in full face rejuvenation: a review and our experience. Dermatol Surg. 2018; 44(7):985–993

[34] Juhász MLW, Marmur ES. Examining the efficacy of calcium hydroxylapatite filler with integral lidocaine in correcting volume loss of the jawline: a pilot study. Dermatol Surg. 2018; 44(8):1084–1093

[35] Beer K, Glogau RG, Dover JS, et al. A randomized, evaluator-blinded, controlled study of effectiveness and safety of small particle hyaluronic acid plus lidocaine for lip augmentation and perioral rhytides. Dermatol Surg. 2015; 41(Suppl 1):S127–S136

[36] Klein AW. In search of the perfect lip: 2005. Dermatol Surg. 2005; 31 (11, Pt 2):1599–1603

[37] Heidekrueger PI, Juran S, Szpalski C, Larcher L, Ng R, Broer PN. The current preferred female lip ratio. J Craniomaxillofac Surg. 2017; 45(5): 655–660

[38] Smith KJ. Should hyaluronic acid fillers be diluted? J Drugs Dermatol. 2014; 13(12):1437–1438

[39] Goldman MP, Moradi A, Gold MH, et al. Calcium hydroxylapatite dermal filler for treatment of dorsal hand volume loss: results from a 12-month, multicenter, blinded trial. Dermatol Surg. 2018; 44(1):75–83

[40] Dierickx C, Larsson MK, Blomster S. Effectiveness and safety of acne scar treatment with nonanimal stabilized hyaluronic acid gel. Dermatol Surg. 2018; 44 Suppl 1:S10–S18

[41] Sito G, Marlino S, Santorelli A. Use of Macrolane VRF 30 in emicircumferential penis enlargement. Aesthet Surg J. 2013; 33 (2):258–264

[42] Hexsel D, Dal'Forno T, Caspary P, Hexsel CL. Soft-tissue augmentation with hyaluronic acid filler for labia majora and mons pubis. Dermatol Surg. 2016; 42(7):911–914

[43] Tansatit T, Apinuntrum P, Phetudom T. Facing the worst risk: confronting the dorsal nasal artery, implication for non-surgical procedures of nasal augmentation. Aesthetic Plast Surg. 2017; 41(1): 191–198

[44] DeFatta RJ, Krishna S, Williams EF, III. Pulsed-dye laser for treating ecchymoses after facial cosmetic procedures. Arch Facial Plast Surg. 2009; 11(2):99–103

[45] Beleznay K, Carruthers JD, Humphrey S, Jones D. Avoiding and treating blindness from fillers: a review of the world literature. Dermatol Surg. 2015; 41(10):1097–1117

[46] Beleznay K, Carruthers JDA, Humphrey S, Carruthers A, Jones D. Update on avoiding and treating blindness from fillers: a recent review of the world literature. Aesthet Surg J. 2019; 39(6):662–674

[47] DeLorenzi C. New high dose pulsed hyaluronidase protocol for hyaluronic acid filler vascular adverse events. Aesthet Surg J. 2017; 37(7):814–825

[48] Keller EC, Kaminer MS, Dover JS. Use of hyaluronidase in patients with bee allergy. Dermatol Surg. 2014; 40(10):1145–1147

[49] Chesnut C. Restoration of visual loss with retrobulbar hyaluronidase injection after hyaluronic acid filler. Dermatol Surg. 2018; 44(3): 435–437

[50] Paap MK, Milman T, Ugradar S, Silkiss RZ. Assessing retrobulbar hyaluronidase as a treatment for filler-induced blindness in a cadaver model. Plast Reconstr Surg. 2019; 144(2):315–320

[51] Carey W, Weinkle S. Retraction of the plunger on a syringe of hyaluronic acid before injection: are we safe? Dermatol Surg. 2015; 41 Suppl 1:S340–S346

[52] Douse-Dean T, Jacob CI. Fast and easy treatment for reduction of the Tyndall effect secondary to cosmetic use of hyaluronic acid. J Drugs Dermatol. 2008; 7(3):281–283

[53] Robinson DM. In vitro analysis of the degradation of calcium hydroxylapatite dermal filler: a proof-of-concept study. Dermatol Surg. 2018; 44 Suppl 1:S5–S9

[54] Ibrahim O, Overman J, Arndt KA, Dover JS. Filler nodules: inflammatory or infectious? A review of biofilms and their implications on clinical practice. Dermatol Surg. 2018; 44(1):53–60

[55] Kadouch JA, Kadouch DJ, Fortuin S, van Rozelaar L, Karim RB, Hoekzema R. Delayed-onset complications of facial soft tissue augmentation with permanent fillers in 85 patients. Dermatol Surg. 2013; 39(10):1474–1485

[56] Goulart JM, High WA, Goldenberg G. Evidence of calcium hydroxylapatite migration: distant nodule formation in the setting of concurrent injection with nonanimal stabilized hyaluronic acid. J Am Acad Dermatol. 2011; 65(2):e65–e66

[57] Vleggaar D, Fitzgerald R, Lorenc ZP. Understanding, avoiding, and treating potential adverse events following the use of injectable poly-L-lactic acid for facial and nonfacial volumization. J Drugs Dermatol. 2014; 13(4) Suppl:s35–s39

[58] Sadeghpour M, Quatrano NA, Bonati LM, Arndt KA, Dover JS, Kaminer MS. Delayed-onset nodules to differentially crosslinked hyaluronic acids: comparative incidence and risk assessment. Dermatol Surg. 2019; 45(8):1085–1094

[59] Artzi O, Cohen JL, Dover JS, et al. Delayed inflammatory reactions to hyaluronic acid fillers: a literature review and proposed treatment algorithm. Clin Cosmet Investig Dermatol. 2020; 13:371–378

[60] Aguilera SB, Aristizabal M, Reed A. Successful treatment of calcium hydroxylapatite nodules with intralesional 5-fluorouracil, dexamethasone, and triamcinolone. J Drugs Dermatol. 2016; 15 (9):1142–1143

17 Procedural Hair Restoration: Platelet-Rich Plasma for Hair Loss and Hair Transplant

Benjamin Curman Paul

Summary

This chapter reviews the most common procedures performed by clinicians treating hair loss. Procedural hair restoration includes the injection of platelet-rich plasma (PRP) to improve the growth and health of the hair and hair transplantation. PRP is an autologous liquid derived from the patient's blood during an office visit. PRP is rich with growth factors that are used to stimulate the growth and health of the scalp. The major forms of hair transplantation described in this chapter are follicular unit transfer (FUT, strip method) and follicular unit extraction (FUE, dot excision) methods. In each method of hair transplant, the single unit of hair growth, the follicle, is isolated and implanted to create a result that is natural and lasting. Overall, technological advancements are now fully available to clinicians and have opened a new and exciting chapter in hair restoration.

Keywords: platelet-rich plasma, hair restoration techniques, hair transplant, follicular unit extraction, follicular unit transfer

17.1 Introduction to Modern Procedure of Hair Restoration

Hair loss is common, with up to 80% of men and 40% of women showing visible thinning throughout life. The loss of one's hair can have a damaging emotional impact.[1] Fortunately, hair restoration has come a long way in the past two decades. The major advances in hair restoration include improvements in technology as well as a dedicated focus on the restoration of hair in women.

In the recent past, the most common cause of hereditary hair loss was termed "androgenic alopecia" describing the impact of genetics and androgens on hair loss. No longer is the term "androgenic alopecia" universally described for male and female patients who display miniaturization and patterned loss. The terms "male pattern hair loss" (MPHL) and "female pattern hair loss" (FPHL) are now used to better appreciate that the underlying biology for patterned hair loss is different between the sexes and extends past simply genetics and androgens. Recent discoveries in the molecular pathways of the hair cycle have identified the importance of microcirculation, inflammation, and additional external factors in patterned hair loss in both men and women.[2] These additional targets have allowed exploration into harvest and application of growth factors to influence hair with a treatment known as platelet-rich plasma (PRP) therapy.

This chapter will focus on two procedural treatments, PRP therapy and hair transplant, both of which are used in the treatment of MPHL and FPHL.

17.2 Platelet-Rich Plasma

17.2.1 Introduction

Within our blood circulate platelets, cells that are rich with growth factors. Utilizing the patient's growth factors to reduce inflammation and stimulate healing and repair is now being performed in many areas of the body such as the skin, eyes, joints, heart, and hair.[3] Given the enormous amount of publicity and treatment potential, patients are now inquiring frequently about PRP for hair loss.

PRP is an autogenous platelet concentrate that is isolated after centrifugation from a patient's peripheral blood. Because the PRP is autologous, the risk of growth factor rejection, viral transmission, and hypersensitivity/allergy is virtually zero. From within the platelets, growth factors are isolated and concentrated to a level that the body has never seen. The platelet solution can be activated in vitro (turning into a gelatinous state) or injected as a liquid for in vivo activation.[3] Activation leads to the release of alpha granules containing many growth factors, and there has been much interest in the use of these growth factors to stimulate hair growth and repair.[4] Platelets contain several chemotactic and mitogenic proteins that influence the hair follicle as listed in ► Table 17.1.

Overall, these growth factors may influence the hair growth cycle by stimulating differentiation, proliferation, and hair follicle growth.

17.2.2 Indications

A comprehensive diagnostic approach and evaluation to hair loss must be completed prior to the selection of a treatment plan. The majority of research to date has evaluated the efficacy of PRP with the presumptive diagnosis of androgenic alopecia (MPHL and FPHL); however, additional studies are being performed in patients with alopecia areata and scarring alopecias such as frontal fibrosing alopecia. In patients with MPHL and FPHL, the most common complaints include shedding, miniaturization, and poor growth with a widened part. Although studies have shown positive trends, the use of PRP is often off-label, which has delayed robust standardized clinical trials.[3]

17.2.3 Patient Selection

The selection of a patient for PRP is based on the discretion of the physician as there are no accepted guidelines.

Table 17.1 Growth factors derived from PRP

Growth factors in PRP	Role of growth factors in the hair cycle
FGF	Induction and maintenance of anagen from telogen[5]
TGF-β	Helps develop follicular placode and architecture,[6] regulates chemotaxis and angiogenesis within endothelium[7]
VEGF	Secreted by dermal papilla cells and thought to promote angiogenesis,[7] essential for anagen phase for follicle
PDGF	Helps with development and proliferation of dermal papilla from the endothelium[6]
IGF-1	DHT has been shown to block IGF-1, so the addition of IGF-1 may signal downstream to the block from DHT[4]

Abbreviations: DHT, dihydrotestosterone; FGF, fibroblast growth factor; IGF-1, insulinlike growth factor 1; PRP, platelet-rich plasma; RDGF, platelet-derived growth factor; TGF-β, transforming growth factor-β; VEGF, vascular endothelial growth factor.

Table 17.2 Relative contraindications to PRP for hair loss

Concern	Notes
Hematologic concern	Coagulopathy, platelet disorder/dysfunction, thrombocytopenia, hemodynamic instability
Infectious	Scalp infection, folliculitis, local infection at site of harvest or graft injection site
Autoimmune disease	Avoid concentration of autoantibodies in plasma that would negatively impact hair
Pregnancy	
Active malignancy	
Alopecia universalis	There must be some hair to perform PRP. Unclear use on a bald scalp
Concern with healing	Prone to keloid formation

Abbreviation: PRP, platelet-rich plasma.

The physician should weigh the risks and benefits of treatment with each patient. The patient must have a reasonable underlying cause for hair loss that may respond to treatment. The most common patient to have PRP performed has either MPHL or FPHL. The most common goals of treatment are to reduce shedding, improve hair growth, and attempt to stimulate new growth from a dormant follicle. The patient must be able to tolerate phlebotomy. The patient should not have a contraindication to PRP as discussed in the following section.

17.2.4 Contraindications

▶ Table 17.2 describes relative contraindications to PRP.

17.2.5 Technique

PRP treatment for hair loss is performed during an office visit. Prior to arrival, patients are counseled to avoid any medicine that may influence the cyclooxygenase signaling pathway such as steroid, ibuprofen, or aspirin as this may influence the result. Patients should not put hair powder or hair product prior to the procedure. Patient is encouraged to eat prior to the visit.

After the patient is consented, phlebotomy is performed. Care is taken to use a large-bore needle (larger or equal to a 21-gauge butterfly) to prevent accidental hemolysis. Accidental platelet injury may unintentionally activate platelets prematurely.[8] The patient's blood is collected in vials, which vary greatly in volume depending on the system used to assist in the isolation of PRP.

The clinician must make a decision on the method of preparation of PRP. At this time, there is a lack of standardization in protocol in the medical literature. Between practices, there are variations in the kit or system used to aid in extraction and thus in the composition and volume of PRP produced. Options for PRP systems include manual systems with single spin and activation with 10% calcium chloride, manual two-step centrifugations to improve platelet yield, and automated kits, which have become increasingly popular since 2009.[9] There are numerous studies comparing the bioactive yields and composition of growth factors isolated with each kit, and the method of PRP production rests in the hands of the clinician.[10]

Often following phlebotomy, low-force centrifugation is performed. The duration of spin is at least 6 minutes, though it varies widely between systems. After centrifugation, the tube will have a supernatant of platelet-poor plasma, a buffy coat central layer that is rich in platelets and white blood cells, and a lowest red blood cell layer. There is then a second step in centrifugation in some protocols to further separate and eliminate the red blood cells and buffy coat layers. Under high centrifugal force, the platelet-rich layer and plasma supernatant may be further separated. A patient's PRP vial after centrifugation is displayed in ▶ Fig. 17.1. The final platelet suspension is four to six times more concentrated than blood, thus having roughly 1 to 1.5 million platelets per microliter to best induce mesenchymal stem cell proliferation.[11] There are concerns that concentrations above 1.5 million platelets per microliter may be deleterious to angiogenesis.[12]

Once separated, the concentrated PRP may then be activated, often with the addition of calcium chloride or calcium citrate to ensure degranulation of the growth factors prior to injection. An additional variable in technique is the addition of adjuvants and grafts to the PRP to improve platelet stability and prevent degranulation. Practices have attempted to add anticoagulants, scaffold extracellular matrix, and ultrafiltration techniques to improve outcome.[3] As of 2019, these adjuvants are of unclear value.

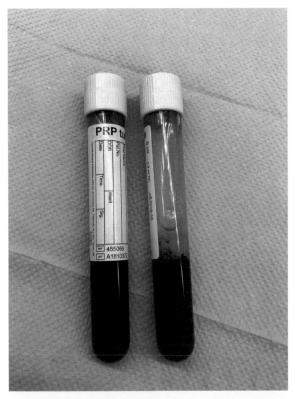

Fig. 17.1 Platelet-rich plasma (PRP) after centrifugation. Notice that the PRP is the *yellow liquid* at the top of the vial.

Once ready, the growth factor–rich PRP liquid is then injected into the areas of hair thinning. Prior to injection, the scalp should be cleansed with alcohol. Many practices perform a ring block with local anesthesia prior to injection to reduce discomfort. The goal of PRP injection is to bathe the hair follicle in the regions of hair loss with growth factors. A 30-gauge needle is used to inject PRP in a hypodermic plane at the level of the hair follicle. The endpoint to injection is determined by the clinician. The average amount of PRP injected ranges from 6 to 8 mL. The goal of treatment is to distribute the PRP across all areas of need.

17.2.6 Postoperative Care

At the conclusion of PRP, the scalp is rinsed with saline. Patients are cautioned that they will have small amounts of dried PRP and blood in the hair, which washes out easily with water. The patient should shower but not shampoo or condition at home following the procedure. The patient may exercise the next day and apply any hair product they wish. A minor headache is not uncommon, and patients should take Tylenol for pain.

In the long term, patients are counseled that 7 of 10 patients report improvement in hair quality, thickness, and appearance. Often, the first physical finding to confirm improvement is a reduction in shedding and consequent hair loss. There may be a delay of 2 to 4 months prior to the observation of improvement. On microscopic analysis, there is an improvement in hair shaft diameter, and on pull test, there is a reduction in hair loss 3 to 12 months following treatment with negative pull tests in roughly 70% of patients.[13]

The patient depicted in ▶ Fig. 17.2 had three PRP treatments with the Selphyl system every 2 months. The before photo on the right shows a widened part. The after photo on the left is taken after 6 months and shows a more narrow part.

Fig. 17.2 Before and 6 months after three sessions of platelet-rich plasma (PRP). Notice the part is no longer widened.

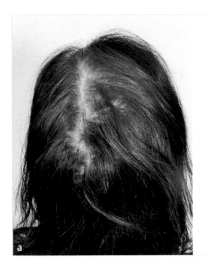
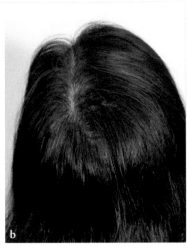

There has been significant debate about whether PRP should be repeated and if so at what time interval. Interestingly, all studies except for two have shown that PRP may be used to help with hair loss. The only two studies that failed to show that PRP works have a variable in common: they only performed the PRP once.[14,15] Both of these negative studies provide the suggestion that multiple injections are necessary to obtain a measurable improvement in hair restoration. The majority of the literature that has shown the strongest positive effects have used a series of at least three treatments. Treatments should be spaced anywhere from 4 to 12 weeks apart for the first three treatments, then the result is judged after 6 to 9 months. PRP responders should continue with maintenance of two to three times per year.[16,17,18]

Patients are counseled that PRP is one aspect of treatment for MPHL and FPHL. PRP is rarely used as monotherapy as the inflammatory pathways that PRP impacts most directly are just one component of the biologic pathways involved in hair loss. Results appear to be synergistically enhanced when PRP is combined with an antiandrogenic treatment such as minoxidil and finasteride.[18] There is also interest in the combination of PRP and hair transplant, and the early literature suggests a benefit in the combination of these procedures.[19]

17.2.7 Complications

In general, PRP is very well tolerated. Rare side effects include scalp erythema, headaches, mild pain, and scalp sensitivity. Temporary scalp and forehead swelling is uncommon. Even if it occurs, it often resolves within 24 hours. Rarely, visible swelling may descend following gravity and lymphatics from the forehead into the face. This swelling can take up to 1 week to resolve. There have been no reports of bacterial, viral, or mycobacterial infection or folliculitis. There are no reports of shock loss when PRP is injected without the addition of an adjuvant.[3]

17.2.8 Pearls/Pitfalls

- MPHL and FPHL may be safely improved with the injection of autologous growth factors derived from platelets within plasma.
- PRP for hair loss has many different kits available. More research is required to better elucidate an optimal treatment protocol. In general, the results appear better when the platelet is "activated" allowing for degranulation of growth factors.
- Patients with MPHL or FPHL should be counseled that multiple treatments will likely be required for improvement.
- PRP works best in concert with the other available treatment options for hair loss such as minoxidil, finasteride, and hair transplant.

17.3 Hair Transplant

17.3.1 Introduction

For decades, the gold standard of hair restoration has been hair transplantation. From relatively crude beginnings, advances in hair restoration now allow patients to receive lasting natural results with a much more comfortable recovery. Hair transplant is one of the most rapidly growing surgical procedures with over 600,000 transplants performed in 2016 alone.[20]

No longer are groups or plugs or flaps of hair moved en bloc; rather hair transplant is now performed by moving the fundamental unit of hair growth, known as the follicular unit. The follicular unit is an organelle and contains one, two, three, or four hairs as depicted in ▶ Fig. 17.3 as well as a sebaceous gland and arrector pili muscle. The shape of the follicular unit is cylindrical and each unit can be placed in such a way that the hair exits the scalp in a specified angulation. A single follicular unit is termed a micrograft when it has one to two hairs and a minigraft when it has three to eight hairs. Micrografts and small minigrafts with up to 4 hairs are the most commonly utilized follicular units. With follicular unit hair restoration, the surgeon has total control

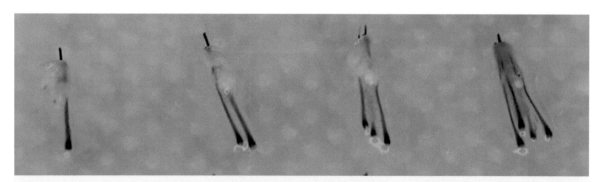

Fig. 17.3 Follicular units, hair follicle. Notice that some follicles have one hair and others have two, three, and four hairs.

of the density, direction, follicle property, and angulation when designing the result, all of which culminate in much more natural and beautiful results.[21]

A hair transplant is chosen when there are areas of hair loss that the patient wishes replenished with new hair follicles. The area of loss is termed the recipient zone. For

thinning to become cosmetically noticeable, at least 50% of the hairs must have fallen out in a particular area. In MPHL and FPHL, the common recipient regions have been "zoned" as pictured in ► Fig. 17.4.

The donor follicular units are most often harvested from the occipital hair, where the hair is biologically distinct. Occipital hair is often androgen insensitive and delayed in senescence. In most instances, donor hair grows for life. Upon transfer, the genetics of the transplanted follicle remain intact, and the hair will grow for life in the recipient zone.

In men, the Norwood classification scale is used to categorize the typical progression of hair loss as shown in ► Fig. 17.5. It is helpful to understand the small donor zone of a Norwood 7 as compared to a Norwood 5. In women, the Ludwig classification scale shows diffuse hair loss at the top of the scalp, while the hairline is maintained as pictured in ► Fig. 17.6.[22] Interestingly, regardless of Ludwig classification, the donor fringe on women is often similar in location to a Norwood 7 male patient, located in the low occiput, often below the nuchal ridge.[23]

The outcome is that hair transplant is a reliable, maintenance-free form of hair restoration for men and women. Hair transplants can be used to rebuild or reinforce the hairline and improve density in zones of hair loss that are not limited to just the scalp but may also include the eyebrows, sideburns, goatee, or body.

17.3.2 Indications

Patients interested in hair transplantation must have an adequate donor site from which to harvest, a recipient

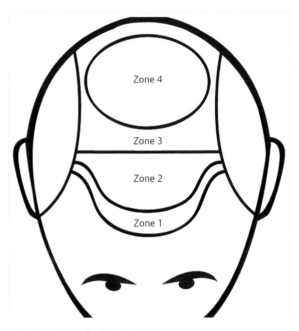

Fig. 17.4 Zones for hair transplant.

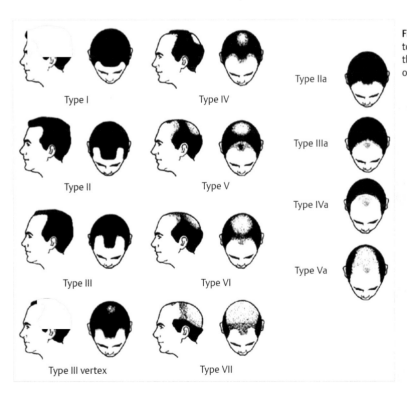

Fig. 17.5 Norwood scale. This scale is used to grade male hair loss. Note that even in the most advanced forms of hair loss, the occipital hair remains.

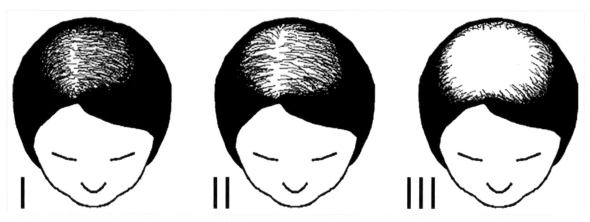

Fig. 17.6 Ludwig scale. This scale is used to grade female hair loss. Note the hairline is retained.

zone that can accept the transplant, and realistic expectations regarding outcome. Aesthetic indications for a hair transplant include lowering the hairline, reinforcing the hairline, and improving density on the scalp as well as the eyebrows, goatee, sideburns, or other areas of hair loss.[24]

The most common underlying diagnosis for which hair transplant is performed is MPHL or FPHL, both previously termed androgenic alopecia. There are other forms of alopecia that may benefit from transplant such as postsurgical or traumatic scarring, traction alopecia, and scarring after trichotillomania.

Results of hair transplantation are usually most dramatic when the procedure is performed on individuals with advanced degrees of hair loss. In general, the amount of hair transplanted is directly proportional to the degree of loss, with more grafts transplanted in patients with more loss and thus greater need.

17.3.3 Patient Selection

Hair transplantation is an elective and cosmetic procedure to restore hair to regions of loss. The procedure is rarely, if ever, covered by insurance. As with all aesthetic procedures, the patient's motivation and expectations must be understood and must be reasonable. A long-term plan must be outlined that includes hair transplant as a part of the greater treatment plan. Patients must understand that a rare minority of patients have enough donor hair to re-cover the entire scalp, and so there is often a role for concurrent medical therapy to help keep and support the original hair that remains. A patient must be informed that hair loss is progressive and multiple hair transplants may be required.[25] The patients must be able to understand the risks and participate in the recovery.

17.3.4 Procedure Selection

A major decision in the restoration is the method of harvest. Currently, the two most common methods are

known as follicular unit transfer (FUT) and follicular unit extraction (FUE). As of 2017, the term FUE may now be written as follicular unit excision, though it represents the same technique as FUE.

Both FUE and FUT result in the isolation of follicular units, the fundamental organelle from which hair grows. There are distinct advantages to both FUT and FUE, though at this time, FUT is considered the gold standard of harvest as the follicles are dissected by hand under direct visualization virtually eliminating the risk of accidental follicle transection.

▶ Table 17.3 helps explain the differences in harvest technique between FUT and FUE.

17.3.5 Contraindications

In order to perform a hair transplant, the patient must have an adequate donor site. An inadequate donor site may exist when there are insufficient follicles to harvest, possibly because of alopecia in the donor zone or because of prior harvest depleting the donor site. Similarly, if the recipient site is unable to accept donor hair, hair transplant should not be performed. Recipient site failure may exist if there is active psoriasis or infection. Relative contraindications include therapeutic anticoagulation, immunosuppression, scarring, patient unwilling or unable to remain still for the duration of the procedure, patient unwilling to cut hair to reveal the donor site for the procedure, and unrealistic expectations. The patient must be able to understand and accept the goals and risks of transplant as well as the progressive nature of hair loss. All patients are counseled that half of hair transplant patients seek a second transplant, and thus there is a possibility for additional transplant in the future.

17.3.6 Technique

Preoperative Planning

To optimize surgery, all patients are given directions in advance of their procedure that outlines the pre- and

Table 17.3 Comparing FUT and FUE as harvest techniques for hair transplant

	FUT	FUE
Technique	A strip of skin is removed from the donor site and the follicular units are dissected under magnification	A microdrill is used to extract single follicular units. The follicular units are then prepped under magnification
Healing	A running suture is used to close a linear incision line. The suture is removed after 1 wk	Sutureless; may heal with punctate, white dots from where follicles were extracted
Early evidence	The hair above the donor sites is kept long enough to hide the incision line. No early evidence of donor harvest	The hair in the donor site is cut short. After 1 wk, there is little evidence of surgery if neighboring hair is also short
FU limit	Limited by the laxity of the scalp	Limited by the area of the safe donor zone
Viability	Excellent	Excellent, though up to 10% of follicles may be transected
Time	Rapid extraction	Variable pending number of FU needed
Postoperative limits	No heavy exercise for 1 mo	Return to exercise sooner (no sutures)
Cost	Less expensive	More expensive; increased time and labor
Scalp laxity	Important: can only perform if laxity present	Unimportant: Can perform even after a prior FUT (strip)
Eyebrows, goatee, and beard	Acceptable	Excellent: Can hand select the most appropriate hairs for the recipient zone
If patient wears hair < 2 mm	Possible to see the linear incision line	Preferable
Curly hair	Gold standard	Concern of follicle transection
White hair	Gold standard	Concern of follicle transection

Abbreviations: FUE, follicular unit extraction; FUT, follicular unit transfer.
Source: Adapted from www.haircaremd.com.

postoperative plan. As with any procedure under local anesthesia, most healthy patients do not require a dedicated medical clearance. Medical clearance is reserved for those undergoing general anesthesia or those with a medical comorbidity that could require a change in medication management or might interfere with the procedure. Patients are asked to stop blood-thinning agents 2 weeks prior to surgery. Depending on the method of donor harvest, hair cutting may be indicated or restricted prior to the procedure. Patients are asked to avoid dyeing the hair and to stop the use of hair powder 4 days prior to the transplant.

Day of the Procedure

Prior to arrival, the patient is asked to eat breakfast if they are not receiving general anesthesia. The patient is asked to shower and rinse their hair prior to arrival.

Prior to the start of surgery, the aesthetic goals are reoutlined and the plan is confirmed. The hair is rinsed with alcohol prior to the application of markings in the recipient site. The patient is required to confirm the markings. It is valuable to have the patient's significant other or family member present to understand the plan.

Recipient Design

The recipient zone for hair transplant may start at the hairline, though it may be limited to patches of thinning on the scalp. At times, the recipient zone may involve the eyebrows or beard/goatee.

The design between male and female scalp hair loss varies greatly.[25] When creating the hairline, care is taken to ensure the hairline best frames the face with a recognition that further hair loss is likely and the hair transplant is likely to remain.[26] As such, care is taken to avoid overlowering the hairline and creating an unnatural line. The most aesthetically appealing results come when the patient's own hairline are used as a guide. The result is often a wavy hairline that is "irregularly irregular" with both macro- and micro-irregularities as shown in ▶ Fig. 17.7. The lowest point in the center of the hair is termed the trichion and can be identified using the horizontal rule of thirds.[25] Alternatively, the widow's peak can be placed 8 to 10 cm above the nasion (root of the nose). Another

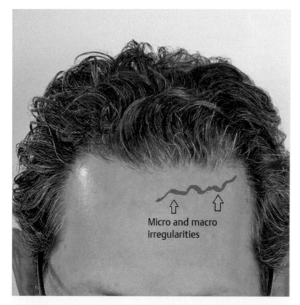

Fig. 17.7 This patient is 1 year post-hair transplant by the author (BP). Notice that the hairline has an irregularly irregular design. There are micro- and macro-irregularities to produce the most natural hairline possible.

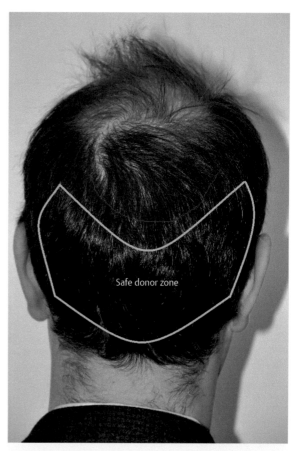

Fig. 17.8 The *area outlined in pink* is the safe donor zone. The *red line* represents the predicted transition zone of hair loss.

point of focus is known as the frontotemporal angle. The angle of the frontal and temporal hairline must be placed with caution and not over-lowered or fully erased. In summary, when designing the hairline, the most common errors that can lead to an unnatural result include (1) a line that is too straight, (2) perfect symmetry, (3) a hairline that is too low, and (4) blunting of the frontotemporal angles.

When transplanting the crown and vertex, a conservative approach is most valuable. The transplant hairs may remain centrally with a rim of thinning, then a rim of hair known as a bull's eye deformity. Patients must be counseled they may need further transplantation anytime the vertex is transplanted. In summary, the goal in the vertex is often to avoid a shiny scalp, rather than to provide dense coverage.

In women, the majority of transplants are focused on reinforcing the anterior one-third of the scalp in the region of the frontal core as well as the frontotemporal angle. As the surface area of the recipient site expands, the density of transplant is diminished. The goal is to provide the most aesthetic enhancement with each procedure.

Donor Preparation

The preparation of the donor site depends on whether FUT (strip) or FUE (dots) is chosen.

For FUT, the most important decision is the size of the strip to be harvested. The strip dimensions depend on the surface area of the recipient site one is trying to cover,

the density of the hair follicles, and, finally and most importantly, the laxity of the scalp, which is the limiting reagent in the harvest. The donor site is often near the nuchal ridge (not at the inferior aspect of the hairline). The goal is to ensure the harvest stays covered by hair. The harvest is thus performed from within the safe donor zone where the hair above the line will not senesce and therefore will provide adequate camouflage for life (▶ Fig. 17.8). In general, on a primary FUT, up to 2 cm of vertical height may be taken and closed safely. When less vertical height is taken, there is less tension and potential for widening of the scar. The ellipse of skin taken must allow for an adequate number of follicles to be harvested. A densiometer may be used to measure the amount of hairs available. As a rule of thumb, roughly 75 follicular units are present in a square centimeter. For example, a 15 cm × 1 cm strip will produce 15 × 1 × 75 = 1,125 grafts. The area of harvest will be clipped to 1 to 2 mm in length with an unguarded electric razor prior to incision. The area above and below the size of harvest is not clipped and will come together in closure to hide the donor site.

For FUE, the goal of donor evaluation is to identify the "safe zone" of harvest. The "safe zone" represents the hairs that will grow for life and are located in the low parietal and occipital scalp. In many cases, a 20 × 6 cm zone of occipital hair is shaved to allow for enough surface area to distribute harvest to avoid overthinning. In general, 1.2 mm of follicular length is ideal for harvest. If the hair is too long, the hair may twist or tangle in the microdrill. If the hair is too short, it can be difficult to judge the angulation of the exit and may increase the transection rate.

Oral Medications

For most patients, a cocktail of oral medications are required. The standard medications used include an anxiolytic such as diazepam, an anti-inflammatory such as methylprednisolone or prednisone 20 mg orally thrice a day × 3 days, gastrointestinal prophylaxis with a proton pump inhibitor, and an oral antibiotic (ether doxycycline or a first-generation cephalosporin). During the surgery, oral diazepam is re-dosed depending on need. Patients are often given 500 mg of Tylenol for pain control and are rarely given opioids. Advil and blood-thinning agents are avoided. For patients with significant anxiety, an anesthesiologist may accompany the procedure and dose medicines accordingly to sustain monitored anesthesia care. If a patient is already on propecia (finasteride), this is continued during the time of the transplant. For those using Rogaine (minoxidil), this topical is held on the day of the procedure and restarted 2 weeks later.

Local Anesthesia

Prior to the institution of local anesthesia, the skin is wiped with both alcohol and betadine (unless allergic). The local anesthesia used is 2% lidocaine with 1:100,000 epinephrine and is dosed based on weight and surface area. Care must be taken to avoid local anesthesia toxicity. The amount of lidocaine with epinephrine is limited to 7 mg/kg with a maximum dose of 500 mg. If epinephrine is not used, the amount of lidocaine is reduced to 4 mg/kg. After 90 to 120 minutes, there is value to reinforce the lidocaine with longer acting 0.5% bupivacaine with 1:100,000 epinephrine, limiting the dose to 3 mg/kg, with a maximum dose of 200 mg. There is often a benefit to performing an occipital block in the donor site as well as a V1 supraorbital and supratrochlear block as less local may be required. There is also benefit to infiltration with a ring block at the hairline.[27]

In addition, 0.9% saline with 1:100,000 epinephrine is kept separate to be used as tumescent during the procedure in areas that require either more skin turgor or additional hemostasis. These zones are already anesthetized and thus do not need more lidocaine.

Positioning

Patients are placed in the seated position for the initial haircut to expose the donor site. The hairs above and below the donor site are place in rubber bands. The boundaries of the donor harvest are marked with a surgical marking pen (ellipse for FUT, a rectangle for FUE) as shown in ▶ Fig. 17.9. The patient is then brought into a prone position. Care is taken to ensure the patient can breathe comfortably and is well padded. After the conclusion of the harvest, the patient is rotated to the supine or a semi-recumbent position for implantation.

Intraoperative Details: Donor Site

With the patient in the prone position, the skin is cleansed with alcohol and then betadine, and local anesthesia is injected slowly.

For FUT, approximately 10 mL of additional tumescent is added in the subcutaneous and supragaleal plane to lift the donor site off of the galea (and deep nerves), improve hemostasis, and improve skin turgor. A no. 10 blade is used to incise through the dermis in the subcutaneous fat. The incision is beveled to avoid transection to the hair. Next the strip is lifted in a subcutaneous plane. The

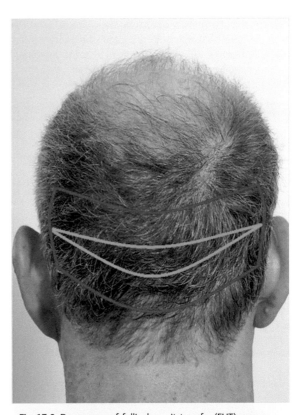

Fig. 17.9 Donor area of follicular unit transfer (FUT) versus follicular unit extraction (FUE). In FUT, an ellipse of hair is removed as shown in *red*. In FUE, the donor zone is shaved widely as shown in *blue*.

dissection must remain deep to the follicles and superficial to the galea. Hemostasis is performed with monopolar cautery with care to limit cautery to the skin edges and hair follicles. In the cases where the vertical height of the harvest is less than 1.1 cm, the donor site may be closed without deep sutures with 4-0 prolene or 4-0 plain gut. In larger harvests, deep 3-0 and 4-0 sutures may be placed to reduce tension and resultant widening of the scar during healing. ▶ Fig. 17.10 shows the progression of marking, to deep suturing, to closure.

In the case of secondary FUT with a prior scar, the surgeon must decide whether to include the prior scar when taking the next strip so as to leave the patient with a single incision line or create a second incision line. The major thought points include whether the location of the first strip was proper, what is the laxity above and below the prior scar, and how wide is the first scar, and whether a scar revision is necessary. In general, it is ideal to excise the old scar in the second strip to reduce the number of scars.

Once the strip is removed, it is "slivered" into rows of follicular units. This process is done delicately under magnification to avoid transection of the follicular units. The slivers are then hand dissected with a straight blade into follicular units. This is performed on a Teflon block that is placed over an LED light source. The 1-, 2-, 3-, and 4-haired follicular units are separated and stored in saline over ice. Care is taken when "prepping" the follicles to remove unnecessary skin and fat to reduce the metabolic demand and improve the survival of the graft.

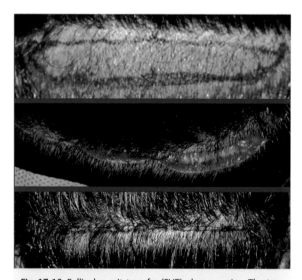

Fig. 17.10 Follicular unit transfer (FUT) closure series. The *top* photo shows the planned ellipse. The *middle* photo shows the value of deep sutures to remove tension off the closure. Note, because a trichophytic incision was performed, the hair follicles along the incision are intact. The *bottom* photo shows the 4-0 prolene running interrupted closure. Note, the hair above the incision is kept long to hide the donor site during healing.

In FUE, the patient is placed supine and the donor area is visualized using loupe magnification. Tumescence is used to provide skin turgor and the patient's head is placed in slight flexion to better place the occipital skin on stretch. A coring device that is either manual or powered is used to isolate and separate a cylindrical follicular unit from the surrounding skin. The surgeon must estimate the number of single-, double-, and triple-haired units needed for the recipient area and plan to harvest each accordingly. During extraction, a hair technician assists in separating and keeping count of the follicular units. The surgeon should NOT harvest adjacent grafts as this may lead to scarring as well as a spot of alopecia. Up to half the hairs in a given zone may be extracted before there is visual thinning. In most cases, 20 to 25% of the hairs in a zone are extracted during a session. This will allow for future harvest. ▶ Fig. 17.11 shows an immediate postoperative appearance of the patient after FUE as well as the appearance of the patient 1 year later with minimal evidence of FUE, if any.

There are many details and nuances regarding the FUE technique that may be optimized. The ideal punch is small enough in diameter to avoid unnecessarily large punctures and resultant large polka dot scars. The punch should not be so small that the rate of transection is high. The most common sizes for punches range from 0.8 to 1.0 mm in diameter. Larger punches are used when the follicular units are very large, have hairs that splay widely, are curved, or are very delicate. The speed and timing of rotation of the drill must be calibrated in each case, as some patients will have very thick skin requiring a faster spin. Often, the drill is rotated faster as time progresses as during the case it is expected that the drill will dull slightly. If the drill bit is deemed dull, it will be replaced. Care is taken not to spin too quickly as there is an increased potential to transect the follicle, twist the follicle, and create unnecessary thermal transfer that may increase scarring or reduce follicular viability. Once the follicular unit is separated from the surrounding skin, forceps are most often used to extract the follicle. Ultimately, there are many devices that aid in extraction, each with differing properties and some with advanced automation. Some of the variables include a contra-angle handpiece, the addition of suction to aid in extraction (Smartgraft, Neograft), fully robotic punch (Artas), modes that change from rotation of the drill to oscillation and vibration at programmed intervals to avoid twisting the graft (Mamba), and sensors to autorotate the microdrill without foot pedal or hand switch activation (Mamba).[28] The drill bits themselves come in many varieties with blunt, hexagonal, sharp, and trumpeted designs being the most common. With increased familiarity and technological advancement, each surgeon develops his or her own preferences for FUE.

In both FUT and FUE, the ultimate goal of the procedure is to harvest viable follicles. As such, a delicate touch is

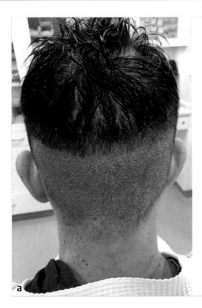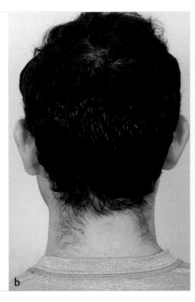

Fig. 17.11 Follicular unit extraction (FUE) after harvest **(a)** and 1 year later **(b)**. In most cases, 20 to 25% of the hairs in a zone are extracted during a session.

required when handling and prepping the follicles to avoid damage. In general, a viable follicle should have a small amount of skin, a cylindrical or tear-dropped dermal section that includes soft tissue, a bulb, continuity of the hair shaft, and may have a small amount of subcutaneous fat.[29]

Intraoperative Details: Recipient Site

The recipient zone surface area must be known prior to the start of the operation. The location of the recipient zone will determine if many single-hair units or no single-hair units are required. Both FUE and FUT create follicular units; however, in FUE, there is control on the number of single-hair units harvested. In FUT, the number of single-hair grafts depends on the number within the strip. Regardless of harvest technique, the recipient creation is the same.

The design of the recipient site is fully individualized. The patient's original hairline must be considered. The asymmetries and shape may be used to guide the design. The goal for many patients is to look natural, so macro- and micro-irregularities should be designed. In addition to the shape of the design, the density and angulation of graft exits are critical to consider. The single-haired grafts must be more densely packed (~30 grafts/cm^2), the multiunit grafts may be placed further apart. Overly dense packing risks a limitation to blood supply and failure.[30] There are written guides to help guide angulation throughout the scalp, but in almost all cases, the most natural results occur when the surgeon is able to follow the angulation of the patient's existing hair.[31] In the cases where there are few guide hairs, it is safe to angle the hair toward the widow's peak in the frontal zone, and the hair is more angled in the exit from the scalp near the hairline (moving anteriorly). The hair in the temporal zone tends

to point anteroinferiorly. The vertex tends to spin counterclockwise in a circular whorl.

There are many clinics around the world that require patients to shave their recipient zone prior to transplant. This aids in placement as long hair does not obstruct the recipient sites, though it is not essential. It is the author's preference and routine to never shave the recipient site. By keeping the recipient hair long, the patients can better camouflage the recipient site during healing, and the angulation of the original hairs are better visualized, allowing for the most natural result possible.

To prepare the recipient site, the skin is wiped with alcohol and injected with local anesthesia. Care is taken to avoid anesthetizing the donor and recipient zones at the same time at the start of the case to avoid local anesthesia toxicity. The recipient site must be fully anesthetized so the patient feels pressure but not pain.

Once the recipient site is ready, a series of slits are made that act as a pocket into which the cylindrical follicular unit is placed. Care is taken when making the slits not to damage exiting hair, as this may lead to telogen or loss of existing hair. Recipient sites can be made with small (< 2.0 mm) slits or as holes with an 18- or 19-gauge hypodermic needle. Using a needle driver, the hypodermic needle can be bent to set the depth of insertion as depicted in ▶ Fig. 17.12. In comparison between slits and holes, it appears the holes avoid overcompression of the multiunit grafts and lead to a more natural result. Additionally, there are some who argue more density can be created with holes. Some consider mixing slits and holes to be advantageous.[30]

When creating the recipient zone, there are two basic approaches to workflow. The first is known as stick and place, where a graft is placed as soon as the site is made. The other option is to make all the sites first, then place all the grafts. A jeweler's forceps is used to handle and

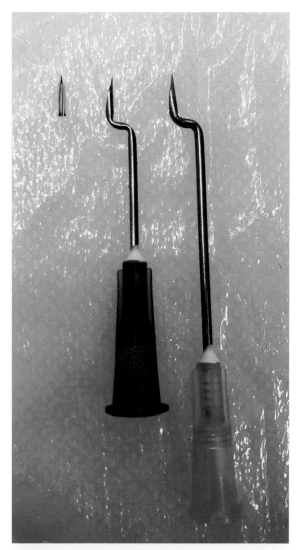

Fig. 17.12 This image shows that 18-gauge (*pink*) and 19-gauge (*tan*) needles may be bent to limit penetration when creating sites for transplant. The bend is customized to match the length of the patient's follicular unit, which is pictured alongside the needles.

place the grafts delicately. Care is taken to only grasp the subcutaneous tissue around the graft and not to disturb the hair shaft or bulb. Recently, more automated implantation devices have been developed to assist in placement, though they require significant handling and preparation of the grafts into loading canisters and are thus not necessarily faster or less traumatic at this time. In general, two hair technicians can place hair simultaneously and the amount of time required for placement depends on the number of hairs that need to be placed and the ease of placement.

Regardless of the technique, the grafts must be handled delicately and cared for cautiously. The less time the graft spends out of the body, the better the viability. While out of the body, the graft experiences a relative hypoxia and may suffer from depletion of adenosine triphosphate (ATP) and nutrients. There are nutrient-rich solutions that have ATP as well as antioxidants, and nutrients are being investigated as storage mediums for the grafts for the time between donation and placement.

The average hair transplant of 1,500 to 2,000 grafts takes a skilled team 6 to 8 hours. A smaller hair transplant with limited grafts may only take a few hours. In some clinics, recipient sites may be created a day prior to the procedure, allowing for just harvest and placement to occur on the second day.

At the end of the hair transplant surgery, the patient has bacitracin placed over the donor site. The patient may have bacitracin and telfa with a kerlix gauze wrap placed over the head or the recipient site may be left bare. The patient is brought home by an escort.

17.3.7 Posterative Instructions and Follow-Up

The patient is able to return home after hair transplant. The gauze wrap, when placed, is removed the following morning. The patient is asked to apply a thin coat of bacitracin to the donor site twice daily for 5 days after the wrap comes off. Patients routinely take Tylenol for pain as discomfort is mild for most, though some of them are given an opioid for breakthrough pain. Unless contraindicated, oral steroids may be given for 3 days to greatly reduce forehead swelling. Oral antibiotics are discontinued after postoperative day 1. Patients are asked to spray the recipient zone with normal saline with a spray bottle hourly while awake for 5 days. The saline helps reduce scabbing and itching.

The day following the transplant, the patient may shower and wash his or her body. The hair is washed the next day with great care to avoid direct spray of the shower over the grafts. A gentle shampoo is mixed in a cup with water and poured over the grafts. Additional water is then gently poured to avoid shampoo residue. Patients are encouraged to wash the hair daily for at least the first 2 weeks to reduce bacteria and loosen scabs.

The patients are routinely seen on day 10 when sutures are removed. At this visit, the transplanted hairs are slightly longer than when transplanted, indicating growth and health of the follicle. The majority of the scabs have dislodged. There is possibly slight erythema the recipient site. The patient is cautioned to avoid sunburns to the scalp in the first 6 weeks. Patients are asked to avoid sweating on the head for 3 weeks and to avoid the pool and ocean for 4 weeks, though some physicians allow for an earlier return to these activities.

The transplanted hairs are expected to experience telogen after the transplant and begin to shed on day 15 and onward. After shed, the hair follicle will rest for 3 to 4 months. The result begins to appear 4 to 5 months after transplant and continues to improve over the following 1 to 2 years. There are suggestions that the addition of minoxidil as well as finasteride helps the hair return faster.[32] For most, once 9 to 12 months have passed, the results become significant as many of the hairs are growing. ▶ Fig. 17.13, ▶ Fig. 17.14, and ▶ Fig. 17.15 show a male and two female patients who each underwent hair transplant. There is significant improvement in thinning at 1 year posttransplant.

The overall survival of a hair transplant depends on the type of surgery (FUT vs. FUE) and certain patient variables. Overall, FUT is considered the gold standard for survival with rates exceeding 95% in most cases. FUE may have a survival ranging from 80 to 90% on average, although it may be higher in skilled hands and favorable circumstances. The patient variables that most directly impact survival include the inherent nature of the hair (white hair, fine hair, and curly hair have lower survival rates) and recipient site variables (scar tissue, poor blood supply, smoking all reduce survival).

In the long term, roughly 50% of patients undergo a second hair transplant at some point in the future. The reasons for a second transplant vary from wishing for improved density to wishing for more coverage. As hair loss progresses, additional transplants may be indicated to fill in new regions of thinning. The delay between procedures may be years or even decades.

17.3.8 Complications

A properly performed hair transplant results in an incredible aesthetic improvement that is both natural and lasting. Complications may result from errors in planning, errors in execution, and errors in healing.[33]

Poor aesthetic result can occur from a number of factors. Most commonly, errors occur when the design of the transplant is too straight, overly lowered, or if large grafts are placed at the hairline. If the angle of the grafts is incorrect, the result can be unnatural with improperly angled or crisscrossing hairs. If all the angles of hair exit are the same, the result may be unnatural, with a picket fence appearance.

The perioperative risks of hair transplant include and are not limited to bleeding, reaction to anesthesia, infection, ingrown hair, cyst, suture granuloma, scar, keloid, alopecia, telogen, persistent pain, scarring in the recipient site (much reduced with micrograft technique), hyperpigmentation, hypopigmentation, or rippling/ridging/cobblestoning/pitting of the skin.[34]

Poor hair growth may be due to poor technique in handling and preparing the grafts. Lack of growth is very uncommon as the donor hairs have "donor dominance" and tend to survive transplant. Sometimes there is delayed growth, and the final result may take up to 18 months to mature.

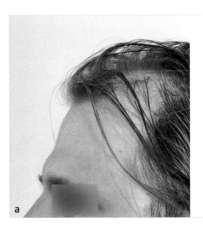
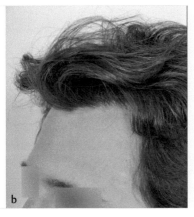

Fig. 17.13 (a, b) A male patient before and 1 year after hair transplant. This transplant was performed to reinforce the hairline.

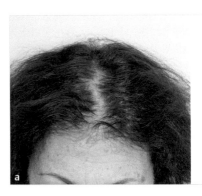
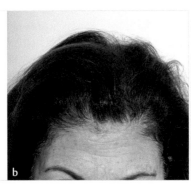

Fig. 17.14 (a, b) A female patient before and 1 year after hair transplant. This transplant was performed to replenish a depleted frontal core and to narrow a widened part.

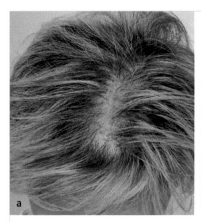
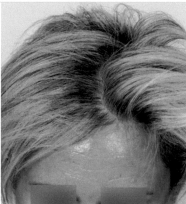
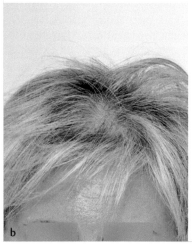
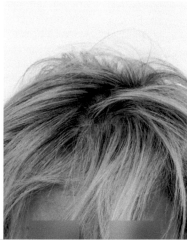

Fig. 17.15 (a, b) This female patient with androgenic alopecia (female pattern hair loss) underwent hair transplant and began minoxidil. The after photo is 1 year later and the patient is thrilled that her part is narrower, her hair is thicker, and her result is completely natural appearing.

Delayed aesthetic errors may occur when planning for the future is overlooked. Over time, most patients with MPHL or FPHL will have progressive loss or recession. In these cases, there is ideally a reserve of hair from the donor site to harvest to fill in new regions of loss. Over time, the most common delayed aesthetic concerns are a lack of continuity from the temporal peaks to the frontal hair as well as a transplant to the crown followed by circumferential balding, leading to a bullseye appearance with central hair, then a bald zone, and then more hair.

Fortunately, many undesirable results in hair transplant can be remedied through reparative techniques. Examples of repair include the following: Hair plugs from yesteryears can be redistributed via modern FUE techniques; anterior hairline scars from hairline lowering surgery can be shadowed by placing single hairs into and in front of the scar; and discontinuities between the frontal hair and temporal hair can be filled in.

17.3.9 Pearls/Pitfalls

- To date, hair transplant is the only permanent, maintenance-free form of hair restoration.

- When planning a hair transplant, an understanding of not only current loss but also future loss is essential to craft a long-term, natural result.
- The major forms of hair transplant are FUT and FUE. Both techniques result in the isolation of the follicular unit, which is the fundamental growth unit of hair.
- The major advantage to FUT is that the scar allows for the harvest of delicate hair that may be transected with FUE such as gray or curly hair. The process of FUT does not require any shaving of the head and so the donor site is well hidden immediately.
- The major advantage of FUE is the lack of scalpels, sutures, and linear scars. The surgeon can choose exactly the number of single-, double-, and triple-hair follicles to harvest. Healing is quick with little pain. FUE generally requires a large zone of the donor site to be shaved, which may be a problem for some patients.
- A natural design is as much an art as a science. The patient's hair is the best guide to create a natural result in both distribution and angulation.
- Patients should be counseled about the timeframe of healing prior to the operation and should expect a period of postoperative telogen with no result at 3 to 4 months after the hair transplant.

References

[1] Davis DS, Callender VD. Review of quality of life studies in women with alopecia. Int J Womens Dermatol. 2018; 4(1):18–22

[2] Ioannides D, Lazaridou E. Female pattern hair loss. Curr Probl Dermatol. 2015; 47:45–54

[3] Badran KW, Sand JP. Platelet-rich plasma for hair loss: review of methods and results. Facial Plast Surg Clin North Am. 2018; 26(4):469–485

[4] Gentile P, Garcovich S, Bielli A, Scioli MG, Orlandi A, Cervelli V. The effect of platelet-rich plasma in hair regrowth: a randomized placebo-controlled trial. Stem Cells Transl Med. 2015; 4(11):1317–1323

[5] Lin WH, Xiang LJ, Shi HX, et al. Fibroblast growth factors stimulate hair growth through β-catenin and Shh expression in C57BL/6 mice. BioMed Res Int. 2015; 2015:730139

[6] McElwee K, Hoffmann R. Growth factors in early hair follicle morphogenesis. Eur J Dermatol. 2000; 10(5):341–350

[7] Dhurat R, Sukesh M. Principles and methods of preparation of platelet-rich plasma: a review and author's perspective. J Cutan Aesthet Surg. 2014; 7(4):189–197

[8] Dohan Ehrenfest DM, Pinto NR, Pereda A, et al. The impact of the centrifuge characteristics and centrifugation protocols on the cells, growth factors, and fibrin architecture of a leukocyte- and platelet-rich fibrin (L-PRF) clot and membrane. Platelets. 2018; 29(2):171–184

[9] Leitner GC, Gruber R, Neumüller J, et al. Platelet content and growth factor release in platelet-rich plasma: a comparison of four different systems. Vox Sang. 2006; 91(2):135–139

[10] Dhillon RS, Schwarz EM, Maloney MD. Platelet-rich plasma therapy: future or trend? Arthritis Res Ther. 2012; 14(4):219

[11] Marx RE. Platelet-rich plasma (PRP): what is PRP and what is not PRP? Implant Dent. 2001; 10(4):225–228

[12] Giusti I, Rughetti A, D'Ascenzo S, et al. Identification of an optimal concentration of platelet gel for promoting angiogenesis in human endothelial cells. Transfusion. 2009; 49(4):771–778

[13] Bayat M, Yazdanpanah MJ, Hamidi Alamdari D, Banihashemi M, Salehi M. The effect of platelet-rich plasma injection in the treatment of androgenetic alopecia. J Cosmet Dermatol. 2019; 18(6):1624–1628

[14] Puig CJ, Reese R, Peters M. Double-blind, placebo-controlled pilot study on the use of platelet-rich plasma in women with female androgenetic alopecia. Dermatol Surg. 2016; 42(11):1243–1247

[15] Mapar MA, Shahriari S, Haghighizadeh MH. Efficacy of platelet-rich plasma in the treatment of androgenetic (male-patterned) alopecia: a pilot randomized controlled trial. J Cosmet Laser Ther. 2016; 18(8):452–455

[16] Gupta AK, Versteeg SG, Rapaport J, Hausauer AK, Shear NH, Piguet V. The efficacy of platelet-rich plasma in the field of hair restoration and facial aesthetics: a systematic review and meta-analysis. J Cutan Med Surg. 2019; 23(2):185–203

[17] Stevens J, Khetarpal S. Platelet-rich plasma for androgenetic alopecia: a review of the literature and proposed treatment protocol. Int J Womens Dermatol. 2018; 5(1):46–51

[18] Gupta AK, Cole J, Deutsch DP, et al. Platelet-rich plasma as a treatment for androgenetic alopecia. Dermatol Surg. 2019; 45(10):1262–1273

[19] Rose PT. Advances in hair restoration. Dermatol Clin. 2018; 36(1):57–62

[20] Avram MR, Finney R, Rogers N. Hair transplantation controversies. Dermatol Surg. 2017; 43 Suppl 2:S158–S162

[21] Joshi R, Shokri T, Baker A, et al. Alopecia and techniques in hair restoration: an overview for the cosmetic surgeon. Oral Maxillofac Surg. 2019; 23(2):123–131

[22] Piraccini BM, Alessandrini A. Androgenetic alopecia. G Ital Dermatol Venereol. 2014; 149(1):15–24

[23] Unger RH. Female hair restoration. Facial Plast Surg Clin North Am. 2013; 21(3):407–417

[24] Umar S. Body hair transplant by follicular unit extraction: my experience with 122 patients. Aesthet Surg J. 2016; 36(10):1101–1110

[25] Rodman R, Sturm AK. hairline restoration: difference in men and woman-length and shape. Facial Plast Surg. 2018; 34(2):155–158

[26] Sirinturk S, Bagheri H, Govsa F, Pinar Y, Ozer MA. Study of frontal hairline patterns for natural design and restoration. Surg Radiol Anat. 2017; 39(6):679–684

[27] Lam SM. Hair transplant and local anesthetics. Clin Plast Surg. 2013; 40(4):615–625

[28] Rose PT, Nusbaum B. Robotic hair restoration. Dermatol Clin. 2014; 32(1):97–107

[29] Buchwach KA. Graft harvesting and management of the donor site. Facial Plast Surg Clin North Am. 2013; 21(3):363–374

[30] Farjo B, Farjo N. Dense packing: surgical indications and technical considerations. Facial Plast Surg Clin North Am. 2013; 21(3):431–436

[31] Rose PT. The latest innovations in hair transplantation. Facial Plast Surg. 2011; 27(4):366–377

[32] Adil A, Godwin M. The effectiveness of treatments for androgenetic alopecia: a systematic review and meta-analysis. J Am Acad Dermatol. 2017; 77(1):136–141.e5

[33] Lam SM. Complications in hair restoration. Facial Plast Surg Clin North Am. 2013; 21(4):675–680

[34] Konior RJ. Complications in hair-restoration surgery. Facial Plast Surg Clin North Am. 2013; 21(3):505–520

18 Blepharoplasty, Lower Facelift, and Brow Lift

Robert Blake Steele, Rawn Bosley, and Cameron Chesnut

Summary

Facelift, blepharoplasty, and browlift are minimally invasive surgical approaches to facial rejuvenation. This chapter provides the background, anatomy, and detailed surgical methods to familiarize readers with cutting-edge facial cosmetics.

Keywords: facelift, blepharoplasty, browpexy, facial rejuvenation

18.1 Facelift: Introduction and Modalities

As the popularity of rejuvenating the aging face increases, the evolution of one of our most classic tools, rhytidectomy, accelerates. Today, novel techniques benefit from over 100 years of past experience. Publications describing the facelift can be found as early as the beginning of the 20th century.[1] In its earliest stages, the procedure consisted primarily of interrupted skin excisions and sutures along the hairline. Without discounting minor improvements such as the addition of continuous skin incisions and skin undermining, the skin-focused procedure remained relatively unchanged until the 1970s when the "Skoog-type" rhytidectomies emerged. This new generation of facelift procedures was spurred by a better understanding of facial anatomy, particularly the superficial musculoaponeurotic system (SMAS), the fascia separating the superficial and deep adipose layers.

Drs. Vladimir Mitz and Martine Peyronie coined the term SMAS in 1976, shortly after its original description and dissection by Swedish physician Dr. Torg Skoog. The SMAS is an inelastic, unified fascial layer that enables the muscles of facial expression to function together as a cohesive unit. Whereas previous skin-only rhytidectomies could not withstand tension or time, dissection of the deeper SMAS allowed for increased durability and a more natural look.

"Skoog-type" or low-SMAS rhytidectomies address the lower face and neck. These techniques include SMAS plication, SMAS imbrication, and lateral SMASectomy. The SMAS plication involves folding the SMAS on itself and suturing it in place without any additional cutting or undermining of the SMAS itself. It is useful in mini-lifts as it can be done through small incisions and can strategically preserve and stack volume. A similar but more durable method, the SMAS imbrication involves undermining of the SMAS, followed by elevating and overlapping the SMAS in a diagonal direction, which can also strategically stack volume. Finally, the lateral SMASectomy involves excising a small amount of SMAS and suturing it back

together, helping in this case to limit the amount of volume suspended. Although significantly better than skin-only facelifts, low-SMAS rhytidectomies do not address the nasolabial folds and midface. The inability to address the midface can result in a "lateral sweep," where an unsuspended, aged cheek sits on top of, and starkly contrasts with a SMAS-corrected, tight lower face.

In the 1980s, a new form of rhytidectomy known as extended SMAS rhytidectomies was developed to address the midface. Popularized by Dr. Sam Hamra and Dr. Fritz Barton, the deep plane rhytidectomy and high SMAS rhytidectomy involve release of the zygomatic and masseteric retaining ligaments, allowing for vertical suspension of the midface and correction of the nasolabial folds. Modifications of techniques to address the SMAS are constantly evolving, striving for less invasive approaches with durable and natural results.

In contrast to extended SMAS techniques, another subset of rhytidectomy modifications has focused on minimally invasive approaches through limited incisions and limited dissection. The short scar and mini-lifts, as the names suggest, employ smaller incision points and typically utilize some combined form of minimal skin and SMAS manipulation. Minimal access cranial suspension (MACS) lifts are characterized by small incisions, a vertical vector of tension that attempts to minimize lateral tension. Sutures are placed into the SMAS resulting in more longevity than skin-only procedures, but the SMAS is not undermined. The finger-assisted malar elevation (FAME) lift is a procedural technique that involves SMAS elevation utilizing digital dissection and manipulation of the lateral orbicularis oculi muscle and malar fat pad, attempting to address the midface.

The procedures noted above do not comprise a comprehensive list; moreover, most procedures can be performed in a myriad of ways with many modifications. Ultimately, the procedure of choice will depend on patient needs. As a best practice, the method chosen should be catered and modified according to each individual patient's anatomy, needs, and desires.

18.1.1 Anatomy and Indications: Facelift

"Rhytidectomy" etymologically breaks down to the removal of rhytids and dates back to the procedure's skin-focused roots, but the facelift's current applications and benefits extend well beyond wrinkle removal. In fact, patients who are only concerned with wrinkles may actually benefit more from nonsurgical cutaneous resurfacing techniques. Selecting the correct modality depends on the patient's goals and expectations, anatomic needs, and budget. Almost universally, patients present with some combination of skin change, volume loss, and soft-tissue redistribution presenting as pendulous gravitational descent from soft-tissue laxity and bony remodeling. Rhytidectomy can offer limited improvements to focal aspects of cutaneous change and volume loss, but its benefits are much more robust in the correction of facial laxity and pendulous tissue descent. Mixing modalities to address the gravitational, volumetric, and cutaneous aspects of facial aging is common and yields the most natural and durable results.

Understanding facial anatomy and how facial structure changes with time allows surgeons to appropriately address aging changes and correctly identify facelift candidates. Facial anatomy is intricate due to its complex functionality. The soft tissue of the face is dynamic; it must accommodate movement to cover orifices and create facial expressions while also maintaining firmness in the resting state. Surgical rejuvenation of the face requires intimate knowledge of anatomy, which can best be understood in terms of interconnected layers. Each area of the face serves a unique purpose and the facial layers reflect these differences. Similarly, functional anatomical variation of these layers can offer insight into what causes aging changes.

From superficial to deep, the first layer is the skin, which covers the entire face but is thinner, and thus more susceptible to aging in the more mobile areas of the face such as the eyelids.[2] The next layer is the subcutaneous layer, which is comprised of subcutaneous fat and retinaculum cutis in varying proportions depending on the area of the face. In the eyelids and lips, there is no fat present, whereas the nasolabial region has an accumulation of subcutaneous fat large enough to garner its own name, the malar fat pad. The retinaculum cutis is actually the subcutaneous portion of ligaments that traverse all layers of the face, including connection of the periosteum to the dermis. The positioning of the retinaculum cutis in the subcutaneous tissue depends on the layers below. If there is a space in a layer below, then the fibers will be horizontally oriented as the fibers will not be able to extend vertically from the periosteum to the dermis.[2]

The third layer is the musculoaponeurotic layer. As the name suggests, this layer is composed of fascia and muscle. Most facial muscles are contained in this layer. Depending on location, the name of this third layer is also known as the galea, temporoparietal fascia, orbicularis muscle/fascia, and the SMAS. In the scalp, the top three layers are easily recognizable as they dissect from the periosteum as a composite unit to easily form scalp flaps.[2] Utilizing these three layers on the scalp to manipulate tissue is analogous to and the basis for SMAS procedures in the lower face.[2]

The fourth layer of the face is predominantly composed of ligaments and spaces. Dissection of this layer must be done cautiously as important structures such as the temporal and mandibular branches of the facial nerve and the sentinel vein are housed in the ligamentous portion of this layer, outside of the spaces. Ligaments form the boundaries of the adjacent spaces, and these spaces do not contain important structures, and thus can easily be dissected with a blunt instrument.

Because the spaces contain soft tissue, they are more susceptible to the gravitational effects of aging. As the ligaments forming the boundaries of the face become lax, particularly the zygomatic and masseteric ligaments, distention of facial spaces becomes apparent. Fullness in the superolateral face near the lateral canthus slowly moves inferomedially in a pendulous motion revealing stigmata of aging including the following: lower lid bags from the preseptal space, malar mounds from the prezygomatic space, nasolabial folds from the vestibule of the oral cavity, jowls from the premasseter space, and labiomandibular folds from the masticator space.[2] The perioral and periocular areas are notable as they experience significant movement with repetitive opening and closing of the mouth and eyes. The additive effects of time, gravity, and movement cause the soft tissue of the midcheek and lower face to congregate in bony cavities and around ligaments that are not apparent in younger individuals. As the midface continues to sag, previously concealed ligaments and bony tissue become more visible. In the midface, the palpebromalar, nasojugal, and midcheek grooves become more prominent.

18.1.2 Layers of Traction and Dissection

Aging occurs at a variable rate and distribution in each layer. Understanding these layers allows surgeons to address the manifestations of aging more directly, specific to the patient's needs. In order to correct the pendulous movement of tissues in an inferomedial direction, traction must be applied to the tissue in a primarily vertical vector. Traction can be applied to skin, SMAS, or periosteum. The layer immediately inferior to the layer of traction is the layer of dissection, which provides a plane whereby the layer of traction can glide. Ideally, the layer of traction should be applied immediately beneath the layer of laxity. Applying traction to the skin in individuals with significant subcutaneous tissue laity, the layer *below* the skin, does not address the problem directly and can impose excessive tension on the skin resulting in suboptimal and unnatural long-term results. Skin-only lifts are rarely appropriate. Traction on the periosteum can be used to move all the layers; however, because a large portion of facial laxity occurs above the SMAS, several layers above the periosteum, periosteal lifts require overcorrection to have any appreciable effects as a result of "lift lag."

Using the SMAS for traction allows surgeons to most directly correct subcutaneous laxity in a durable fashion because the SMAS lies directly below the lax tissue. The layer beneath the SMAS must be dissected to create a plane of movement for the SMAS layer during the facelift. As mentioned earlier, the layer below the SMAS is composed of spaces with boundaries of ligaments that contain important structures such as the facial nerve. Although the boundaries of these spaces must be dissected carefully, the spaces themselves provide "predissected" areas that allow for quick and easy blunt dissection as no important structures lie within these spaces.[2] A posterior, subcutaneous approach until reaching the border of the chosen space allows for a convenient entry point into the space, where blunt dissection of the underlying deeper space can continue. These spaces can be used to navigate the deeper planes of the face in a safe manner without disrupting important structures.

18.1.3 Preoperative/Patient Selection

No two patients will present identically. It is important to evaluate each patient on a case-by-case basis. A thorough examination of each patient's anatomy, skin, bony structural changes, soft-tissue volume, and distribution is necessary to determine which combination of primary and adjuvant interventions is most appropriate. The ideal rhytidectomy depends on the nature and extent of a patient's aging. A young patient with minimal deep tissue migration may benefit from a minimally invasive approach, whereas an older patient with significant tissue change will require more aggressive intervention. Tissue movement naturally creates distortion and redundancy, and these changes need to be planned and accounted for. Thus, when large amounts of tissue are mobilized, more access and areas for distributing and discarding this distortion and redundancy are necessary.

Addressing the SMAS and its variations serve as the foundation for modern rhytidectomy and the senior author's practice. The senior author's primarily vertical vector deep plane SMAS technique aims to restore youthful contour without any pulling or stretching, create a crisp jawline including resolution of jowls, reduce heaviness in the perioral region, elevate the cheeks, efface the nasolabial folds, produce natural transitions around the eyes, and volumize the gonial angle and cheeks. SMAS repositioning restores contour to the midface by raising the cheek into a more youthful position and the lower face by restoring jowl descent and jawline definition. Selecting the proper SMAS technique is key to maximizing results and procedural satisfaction. For instance, if a patient requires specific midface improvement, principles from an extended procedure, such as the high SMAS, could be utilized to address the midface and avoid additional or revision procedures. The decision to pursue a plication or imbrication should be made preoperatively with points and anchors marked accordingly. Before the first incision, be familiar with key anatomic danger zones such as the frontal branch of the facial nerve and great auricular

nerve. Proper SMAS techniques will avoid these structures as the plane of manipulation is superficial to SMAS where no named vessels or nerves will be encountered. Deep plane maneuvering exposes more facial nerve branches but is still safe when performed properly. Neck dissection can be superficial to the SMAS or include platysma as a deep plane, which can also allow submandibular gland ptosis to be addressed. Midline platysmaplasty, subplatysmal fat resection, and direct or suction-assisted lipectomy can be performed as ancillary procedures if needed for redundant platysmal bands or excess adiposity. If fat grafting is to be done simultaneously, it should be done before the lift; otherwise, fat tends to gravitate into planes postsurgically.

Additionally, it is important to obtain a thorough history as prior lifting procedures, as other nonsurgical treatments such as poly-L-lactic acid, fat transfer, and deoxycholic acid injections may alter preoperative planning and surgical approach. As with all procedures, cardiopulmonary, bleeding, and medication history need to be obtained. Any medications that interfere with hemostasis will need to be discontinued early enough to allow normal clotting function during surgery.

18.1.4 Incision Considerations

Prior to cutting the skin, thorough evaluation and planning are necessary. Proper marking must be done before local anesthesia, as injection volumetrically distorts anatomy. We advise against intraoperative revision of skin markings for this reason.

Several calculated incisions will need to be made in order to both gain access to deeper tissues and provide an anchoring point to suture the eventual repositioned skin or SMAS flap. The goal of the incisions is to provide adequate access to deep tissue with minimal scarring. When incisions are made at the hairline, care must be taken to minimize scarring and alopecia. Avoiding cautery as it may destroy hair follicles and using crenated or beveled incisions to conceal the scar and give more incision length to distribute distortion may improve long-term incision outcomes.

The incision in front of the ear can be done as a retrotragal or pretragal incision. Retrotragal incisions are advantageous and most commonly used because the subsequent scar is concealed, but it should only be used in the appropriate patients. With retrotragal incisions, cheek skin will eventually replace the skin on the tragus. If cheek skin is bearded or otherwise appreciably different from the native tragal skin, the outcome may not be ideal. In general, pretragal incisions are better suited for men with thick facial hair, but laser can be used to remove tragal hair if a retrotragal approach is used. Great care must be taken with a retrotragal incision to maintain the definition of the tragus by maintaining the thin cartilage and potentially thinning a thick flap placed over this cartilage.

The pretragal or retrotragal incision is hidden in pre-auricular folds and grooves wherever possible before extending to the inferior portion of the lobule. Care must be taken to maintain an identical look of preoperative lobule adhesion, avoiding the telltale "pixie ear" deformity. The anterior access is continuous with the incision posterior to the ear in the retroauricular groove that travels superiorly to at least the level of the external auditory canal. From here, the ensuing incisions will depend on each patient's presentation. If the patient has excess neck skin, this incision may subsequently travel to hair-bearing scalp in the occipital region to accommodate excess soft tissue and avoid bunching while taking care to keep the posterior hairline smooth. The exact location of this extension can vary from the inferior hairline to a number of other more vertical incisions. Notably, on secondary or revision facelifts, the posterior hairline is more easily distorted and extra care needs to be afforded (▶ Fig. 18.1).

The temporal incision can be placed at the inferior portion of the temporal tuft, in the hairline, or as a combination of the two. Placement will depend on the amount of anticipated tissue removal and the patient's baseline temporal tuft position. Incisions within the hair create less visible scars; however, excessive skin laxity can result in a superiorly shifted temporal tuft. Altering the hairless strip of skin between the tragus and sideburn may create an unnatural look and is a telltale sign of a facelift. Incisions below the temporal hair tuft will not result in sideburn shifts; however, this may cause the scarring to be more visible as compared to the other positioning options.

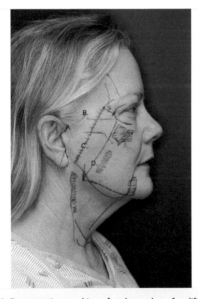

Fig. 18.1 Preoperative markings for deep plane facelift. A, retrotragal incision marking; B, Temporal tuft incision marking; C, Pitanguy's line; D, deep plane entry point.

18.1.5 Senior Author's Surgical Technique in a Female Patient

The senior author prefers using a primarily vertical vector deep plane SMAS technique as follows. Prior to surgery, an outline over the cheek and neck of the area to be undermined should be clearly demarcated. This area is based on individual needs, and these preplanned areas of dissection are not changed once anesthesia has tumesced. Pitanguy's line is marked from the infralobular region to the midpoint of the zygomatic arch extending to a point 1.5 cm lateral to the brow region to delineate the path of the temporal branch of the facial nerve. The deep plane entry point is marked by drawing a line from the lateral canthus to the angle of the mandible, roughly the demarcation of where the concavity of the face turns into a convexity. Next, we mark the temporal incision. Mirroring the temporal hair tuft, the incision line should be abutted against the area of thickest, most dense hair, not where small wispy hairs are, as the incision will be more visible there. The extent of the incision will depend on the amount of redundancy we have when we redrape the skin vertically. This incision continues to the anterior ear at the junction of helical root and facial skin, where there is most often a fold and concavity. The incision is taken retrotragal with great care to the contour of the tragus at the time of skin redraping. At the inferior portion of the lobule, 1 mm of skin can be maintained outside of the natural crease to avoid blunting the ear lobe during redraping. The incision continues behind the ear to hide at the junction of the concha and the neck, but the incision should not extend on to the concha to avoid an unnatural skin position after redraping the skin. The incision line then curves posterior, most often along the hairline as opposed to curving it back into the hair, to maintain hairline contour perfectly. The apex of postauricular incision should be at the level of the triangular fossa so that it is high enough to be hidden if the female patient wears her hair up (▶ Fig. 18.2).

Once incision planning is done, injection of local anesthesia can be started. The senior author prefers using local anesthesia along with sedation, whether oral or intravenous (IV), depending on patient needs and preference. One percent lidocaine with 1:100,000 epinephrine and bicarbonate 1:10 buffer is used for incision lines, whereas 0.2% lidocaine with 1:500,000 epinephrine is used in planned areas of dissection as tumescent anesthesia. Postoperatively, liposomal bupivacaine is utilized along suture lines, in the sternocleidomastoid (SCM) muscle, under the flap, at drain sites, and as regional nerve blocks in the infraorbital nerve totaling no more than 20 mL on both sides. This postoperative regimen has shown a strong reduction to elimination of narcotic use in the senior author's practice.[3]

After adequate anesthesia, a 2- to 3-cm incision is made at the posterior portion of the submental crease

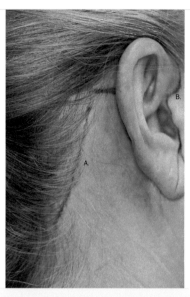

Fig. 18.2 Preoperative markings for deep plane facelift. A, postauricular incision marking; B, retrotragal incision marking.

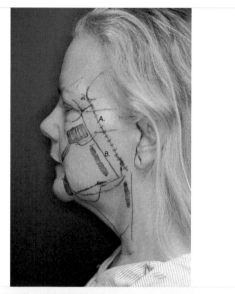

Fig. 18.3 Deep plane entry marking. A, Pitanguy's line approximates the course of the frontal branch of facial nerve; B, deep plane entry point drawn from the lateral canthal skin to the angle of the mandible.

with a no. 15 blade. A submental flap is raised with facelift scissors using blunt, spreading dissection. Care is taken to leave approximately 5 mm of fat on the deep undersurface of the skin. Dissection is usually carried to the level of the thyroid cartilage. If lipectomy is needed, it should be taken from the deeper surface of the platysma as opposed to the deep surface of the skin, where fat is purposefully left to hide deep contour changes. The subplatysmal plane can be entered by elevating the medial edges of the platysma with scissors spreading dissection to the level of the thyroid cartilage. Laterally, the dissection should expose subplatysmal fat and the anterior bellies of the digastric muscles. Subplatysmal fat can be excised at this point very conservatively and should be removed to the caudal surface of the digastric muscle to prevent a submental depression, or "cobra neck" deformity from forming. Various types of a corset platysmaplasty can be performed to tighten the midline platysmal decussation and eliminate platysmal banding. The author prefers using 3–0 PDS in a running fashion from the thyroid cartilage to submental crease, which can be a difficult task with a small access point, requiring precise headlamp usage or a fiberoptic retractor. It is tempting to overtighten the midline platysmal flaps, but the surgeon must be aware of submental skin redundancy that can form, with a full release of mandibulocutaneous ligaments necessary to mobilize and eliminate this redundancy. Before closing the submental region, the lateral portions of the facelift are performed to allow small midline adjustments before closure.

Next, a no. 10 or 15 blade is used to make incisions along all premarked areas. Incisions are made parallel to the direction of the hair follicles, as opposed to against

them, to maximize postoperative hair growth and incision camouflage. A wide, thick subcutaneous flap is raised deep to the subdermal plexus, extending to the level of the deep plane entry point, previously marked from the lateral canthus to the angle on mandible. Dissection is performed with spatulated-tipped facelift scissors and with a no. 10 blade, belly facing up to the underside of the flap to maintain flap thickness and plane of dissection. The postauricular dissection elevates the flap off of the SCM muscle and extends anteriorly to the area where a previous submental flap was created. The mandibulocutaneous ligaments are released along the inferior border of the mandible if not already performed via a midline incision (▶ Fig. 18.3).

Once dissection of the flap to the deep plane entry point is complete, the deep plane is entered sharply with the facelift scissors. After incision into the platysma muscle, the glistening tissue of the parotideomasseteric fascia is encountered immediately beneath the muscle. Vertical spreading is utilized to open up this fascial plane, staying deep to the platysma and protecting the marginal mandibular branch of the facial nerve. As long as dissection occurs atop the parotideomasseteric fascia, the nerve branches will be safe deep to the dissection plane. The dissection is continued superiorly near the lateral canthal region. Visualization of the orbicularis muscle will signal the beginning of the deep plane entry point superiorly.

Next, dissection continues inferiorly to the SMAS and platysma from the angle of mandible to the chin. Once this dissection is complete, an index finger is used to perform a finger-assisted malar elevation (FAME). To do this, the finger is inserted into the superiorly dissected area.

The finger will slide anteriorly and inferiorly toward the nasolabial fold into the prezygomatic space. When downward pressure is applied with the finger, the zygomaticocutaneous ligaments will restrict the finger from moving downward any further. At this point, two pockets separated by the zygomaticocutaneous ligaments are formed: the prezygomatic space superiorly and the sub-SMAS pocket inferiorly.

Next, the zygomaticocutaneous ligaments need to be dissected. Dissection of the zygomaticocutaneous ligaments extends from superior to inferior using blunt dissection, making sure to stay on top of the zygomaticus musculature. At this point, there is a complete release of the midface. The deep plane has been dissected extending to the nasolabial fold under the malar fat pad. thus, when this flap is repositioned, the whole cheek mass is free and can be repositioned superiorly. Of note, high SMAS procedures sometimes only release a focal area of the SMAS, but the descended midcheek remains fixated. The zygomaticocutaneous ligaments need to be released to appropriately address the midface. Also, of note, the deep plane entry point along the jaw is where most SMAS procedures end; however, the senior authors extend to the deep plane in order to directly address the more anterior areas of midface descent (▶ Fig. 18.4).

In the neck and postauricular areas, a platysma flap is created to add contour to the neck. Blunt dissection is carried deep to the platysma at the beginning of the edge of the sternocleidomastoid muscle to form a pocket extending near the jaw. The marginal mandibular branch of the facial nerve is located in the superficial cervical fascia, so the nerve will remain intact by staying superficial to this and directly under the platysma muscle.

With the dissection completed, it is now time to suspend the flap. The flap is a composite with the skin and subcutaneous tissue. The SMAS is not repositioned as a separate tissue. The overall vector of lift for the face parallels the zygomaticus muscles obliquely and more vertically; too much

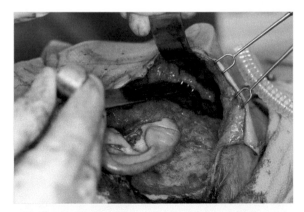

Fig. 18.4 Deep plane dissection and development of deep plane flap.

posterior vector puts tension on the skin and does not volumize the cheek. Lifting more vertically will bring volume up over the cheek area. Although the zygomaticus muscle can be used as a guideline, one must understand that the tissues will settle naturally into place. Next, suspension of the flap occurs at the deep plane entry point, which extends from the lateral canthus to the angle of the mandible. This is in contrast to suspending the SMAS from a more lateral position such as in a traditional high SMAS procedure. Care is taken to take full advantage of the release of the midface, with the ability to suspend the midface over deeper tissue.

To suspend the SMAS, a suture is placed at the inferior aspect of the jaw, through the composite flap at the deep plane entry point in a horizontal mattress fashion. Multiple suspension sutures are placed along the deep plane entry line through the deep fibrous fascia in the preauricular region usually with a 3–0 PDS or polyglactin 910. Fortunately, with the superior extent of the deep tissue area adjacent to the lateral canthus, the procedure also provides vertical support for the inferior lid margin. The most superior suture is placed into the deep temporal fascia, yet it is unnecessary to expose the fascia before suturing. Suspension for the most superior flap suture is high and lateral and should be about 1.5 cm above the zygomatic arch. While the entry to the deep plane is medial, the suspension of the deep plane flap is high and lateral to dramatically rejuvenate the midface. A common misconception is that the lateral SMAS must be entered to have a lateral effect, but this is unnecessary with release of the midface. Interestingly, this suspension is actually higher and more lateral than many high or lateral SMAS facelifts because release of the midface allows for more mobility. Approximately six sutures are placed in total in the midface. Because the midface is released, the sutures simply need to hold the flap in place and thus do not need to be high-tension.

Next, the platysma flap is grasped with forceps and extended toward the angle of the jaw allowing it to transpose under the jawline. Using a 3–0 suture, the flap is directed towards the mastoid fascia and sutured in place. The platysma flap effectively turns into a hammock that muscularly supports the submandibular gland and keeps it in place. The authors generally prefer not to remove the submandibular gland or attempt to put a suture directly in the gland's capsule. However, at times, sculpting of the submandibular gland is necessary to have optimal outcomes. Repositioning of the deep plane flap over the gonial angle gives the jaw contour and creates a submandibular concavity (▶ Fig. 18.5).

Next, the excess skin from the flap needs to be addressed. The apex of the turn from where the helix meets the temporal incision is marked. If there is continued laxity extending superiorly, the temporal incision may need to be extended slightly, which adds no burden as the tension is on the deep plane of the flap and not on the skin. A small amount of skin is removed posteriorly to inset the earlobe, taking care to not pull the earlobe forward. The

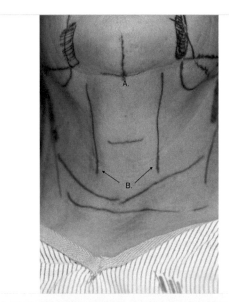

Fig. 18.5 Preoperative markings for deep plane necklift. A, Submental incision marking; B, platysmal band dehiscence marking.

neck skin flap is tacked back into the fascia area to prevent any tethering or pulling of the earlobe. This will alleviate any tension on the tragus and minimize bunching in the temporal area while keeping the incisions hidden along the hairline. Wider undermining superior to the incision point in the temple region will allow the skin to redrape without bunching when using a more vertical vector. It is helpful to utilize cardinal sutures at the helical root, inferior lobule, and postauricular sulcus. As a note of fine detail, one should take care to appropriately thin the new tragal portion of the flap and ensure proper concavity is created anterior to the tragus. Postauricular closure should be anchored to the mastoid fascia in order to prevent flap descent and migration. Suture or staples can be used in the hair-bearing areas of skin. All suture lines in glabrous skin, including the small submental incision, are closed with 5–0 polyglactin 910 and 5–0 polypropylene.

18.1.6 Postoperatively

Liposomal bupivacaine is performed at the conclusion of the procedure as described earlier. If desired during closure, drains may be inserted. The senior author prefers passive window drains with 14-gauge IV catheters. Other drains that can be used are fenestrated JP or Blake drains placed under bulb negative pressure suction. A light compressive wrap is placed to provide both compression and support, as well as immobilize the freshly raised flap. Great care should be taken to ensure the compression is not tight enough to limit vascular flow to the distal portions of the flap.

Patients should use ophthalmic ointment and artificial tears as needed. Sutures should be removed 5 to 7 days after surgery. Light exercise can begin 2 to 3 weeks after surgery, but strenuous activities including heavy lifting and intense aerobic exercise should be avoided for at least 1 month.

18.1.7 Adjuvant Modalities

Sagging tissues often require surgical intervention for repositioning and excision. Surgical lifts boast the ability to restore facial contour, but patients who require rhytidectomy almost universally need resurfacing and volume restoration as well. The use of resurfacing techniques and volume in conjunction with rhytidectomy provides a multifaceted approach that can more comprehensively address the aging face. It is important to note that mid and lower face changes are most often accompanied by concurrent periorbital and brow aging. It is possible to disrupt facial balance with overcorrection of one area. Thus, it may be in the patient's best interest to consider multiple surgical modalities, such as blepharoplasty and brow lift, for optimum balance in facial rejuvenation.

Fat grafting can be done to help move volume superiorly, creating a heart-shaped face without overvolumizing the cheeks. The facelift itself can eliminate the need for fat grafting in the midface if the facelift corrects the descent of a volumized malar fat pad. Fat can be grafted into the upper eyelid, tear trough, temples, forehead, earlobes, cupid's bow, lips, mental region, and philtral columns. Fat grafting can also address the orbital rim, nasojugal groove, and the lid cheek area where the orbitomalar retaining ligaments cause depression. Temporal fat grafting is an option to soften the transition from the forehead to the zygoma where a concavity is formed as a natural part of aging. Temporal fat grafting is placed with a cannula beneath the deep temporal fascia and the area is massaged after fat placement to avoid contour irregularity. Place the fat over the periosteum perpendicular to the area requiring volumization in order to prevent worming or blebs of fat from superficial placement. It is important not to excessively graft fat and overcorrect, as it is harder to remove fat than to add it. Fat grafting should occur before the facelift to avoid fat migration.

A lip lift can be done at the same time as the facelift. A long upper lip can make a patient look continually aged, despite the facelift; thus, lip lifting can be an excellent concurrent procedure.

18.1.8 Complications

Hematomas can occur during surgery and are best avoided by discontinuation of anticoagulation and careful dissection and hemostasis. Infections are a risk with any surgery, but quite low with the excellent facial tissue vascularization. Flap necrosis is a feared complication that can result from a variety of causes including improper flap dissection, excessive tension during wound closure, or inappropriate ligation and cauterization of blood vessels; excessive and expanding bleeding leading to a malignant hematoma can also compromise vascularity and is a true surgical emergency. Other complications are those inherent to the surgery but can be exacerbated by inadequate technique, including exposed scars and shifted hairlines. A windswept appearance or lateral sweep can form with lower face correction when the midface is not addressed. This can be corrected by concomitant midface procedures or extended SMAS approaches. The most feared complication of any rhytidectomy is motor nerve damage, which most commonly affects the frontal or marginal mandibular branches of the facial nerve. Involvement of these nerves most commonly results in temporary neuropraxia and long-term deficits are rare. The great auricular is the most commonly injured nerve in rhytidectomy, and this injury is exclusively sensory in nature.

18.1.9 Pearls and Pitfalls

The face ages in multiple ways, as a single unit. Rejuvenation of the aging face must account for this harmony to maintain facial balance. Multiple modalities are often necessary to achieve the best results.

Pearls: Facial aging occurs differently for each individual, yet it consistently affects all areas of the face in some capacity. Patients undergoing rhytidectomy will likely need intervention with other aspects of facial aging that rhytidectomy does not address, such as eyes, brows, neck, and cutaneous aging. These deficiencies should be addressed in conjunction with rhytidectomy using surgical adjuncts, skin resurfacing, and/or volume replacement. It is up to the surgeon to determine the most appropriate interventions.

Pitfall: Failing to address the many factors that contribute to aging may leave patients with less than desirable results. Focusing on individual areas rather than paired cosmetic units may reveal that a cosmetic surgery was performed. For example, failing to address ptotic brows while undergoing a facelift may result in an obvious demarcation of the treated areas juxtaposed to laxity at the temple-cheek junction.

18.2 Blepharoplasty and Brow Lift Introduction

The perception of facial beauty plays a vital role in social interactions. Investigation into the attributes that comprise facial beauty, and the social impact these factors have on our species' evolution, has historically focused on holistic traits such as facial symmetry.[4] More recently, however, research has indicated that certain isolated facial features may also play more significant roles in the perception of facial beauty.[5] Although men and women process facial features differently to determine beauty, there is a commonality: both men and women view the eyes as one of the most attractive facial features.[5] It is quite well described that the eyes are a key to facial and emotional recognition and the perception of beauty. Thus, recognition of changes in the periorbita is hardwired into humans. Perhaps this innate hyperawareness of the eyes' appearance can partially explain the increasing desire to maintain a youthful periorbital region. The eyebrows and eyelids are one intimately related unit, and they both contribute to periorbital appearance.

Over time, the cumulative effects of sun exposure, gravity, facial muscle use, inherent skin thickness, and periorbital tissue quality contribute to accelerated aging in the periorbital tissues characterized by vertical elongation of a youthful orbit.[6,7] Soft tissues deteriorate, lose elasticity, and become lax. This leads to downward movement of several structures including the eyebrow, especially laterally where there are fewer fibrous adhesions and limited temporalis muscle attachment; the lid–cheek junction, which leads to more prominent bony tissue and both the upper and lower eyelid.[8,9,10] Fat on the face is held in place by ligamentous boundaries, but over time these boundaries become lax and allow fat migration. The orbicularis retaining ligament and orbital septum weaken resulting in herniation or pseudoherniation of periorbital fat causing the infamous "bags" beneath the eyes.[11,12] The malar fat pad descends and the nasolabial fold deepens, forming a tear trough or nasojugal groove and orbitomalar groove.[10] Brow lift and blepharoplasty aim to restore a youthful appearance in the periorbital region by improving upper eyelid aesthetics and creating a seamless transition from the eyelid to the cheek, respectively. These procedures are often performed simultaneously and thus will be discussed together. In addition to brow lift and blepharoplasty, which will be discussed at length, ancillary procedures that are beneficial include upper lid medial fat pad transposition and repositioning for hollow A-frame deformities, brassiere suture lateral brow fat pad suspension, ptotic lacrimal gland repositioning, lower fat pad repositioning, lower lid skin removal, and lateral canthal tightening procedures including canthopexy and canthoplasty.

18.2.1 Brow Lift Modalities

Many approaches to the brow lift procedure have been described and the appropriate method ultimately comes down to individual patient needs and goals. Surgical intervention of the periorbital region must be done on an individualized basis; this point cannot be overemphasized. Proper brow position varies according to gender, ethnicity, anatomy, and patient preference. thus, a cookie-cutter approach to the brow lift is inappropriate. Incision access to the brow can be achieved from multiple locations, each offering distinct advantages and disadvantages. Brow lifting methods include direct, midforehead, temporal, pretrichial, coronal, endoscopic, and transblepharoplasty browpexy. Brow lift innovation seeks to provide long-lasting results in the least invasive manner possible. In general, incision sites farther away from the brow cannot lift as durably, especially in the most lateral area of the eyebrow, but offer less visible scars. Conversely, the direct method provides the most durable lift but is accompanied by the most visible scar. The focus of this section will be on the temporal approach and transblepharoplasty browpexy approach—two methods that are proven to offer both lasting results and minimal invasiveness.

18.2.2 Indications/Patient Selection

The ideal eyebrow position is dependent on several factors including preference, gender, ethnicity, and facial proportions. Additionally, the perceived ideal positioning of the eyebrow has evolved with time. For example, synophrys, or connection of the eyebrows at the midline, was once considered attractive. The ideal position today is inseparably dependent on a multitude of interrelated factors that depend on the uniqueness of each individual. Advanced metrics have been used to determine ideal brow positioning. In general, both men and women prefer the highest point of the brow just medial to the lateral canthus, but a flatter overall arc to the brow is a more masculine shape.[13] It is the senior author's strategy to pay careful attention to a patient's individual, ideal shape, which takes precedent in surgical planning over pure brow height (▶ Fig. 18.6).

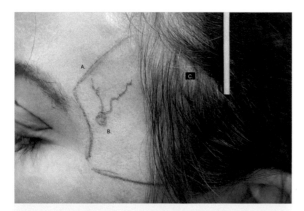

Fig. 18.6 Preoperative markings of deep plane temporal brow lift. A, boundaries of the superior temporal fossa (superior temporal lines and upper border border of zygomatic arch); B, zygomaticotemporal (sentinel) vein; C, marking for incision posterior to the temporal hair line.

18.2.3 Technique for Deep Plane Temporal Brow Lift

Marking key surface anatomy should occur prior to lidocaine infiltration, in the upright position. Important structures to mark include the temporal line of fusion or conjoint tendon, zygomaticotemporal (sentinel) vein, and the desired vectors of lift. The zygomaticotemporal vein is an excellent marker for the overlying branches of the superficial temporal branch of the facial nerve, which remain untouched from the deep plane. The deep branch of the supraorbital nerve runs between 0.5 and 1.5 cm medial to the temporal line of fusion. The planned point of incision and access occurs at least 1 cm behind the hairline and is up to 6 cm in length. After completion of marking, tumescent lidocaine with epinephrine solution is used to infiltrate the planned area of dissection and allow at least 10 minutes for vasoconstriction to take effect. Intraoperative marking changes should not be made at this time as local anesthesia infiltration will distort the patient's anatomy. The incision is made in a premarked area posterior to the hairline after forethought in managing untrimmed hairs with tape or other retraction. The incision is carried through the subcutaneous fat to the level of the superficial temporal fascia. After hemostasis is achieved, the superficial temporal fascia is removed as an ellipse with a Colorado microdissection needle. A plane is identified and developed between the superficial temporal fascia and the superficial leaflet of the deep temporal fascia. With facelift scissors, down to the glistening white deep temporal fascia, blunt dissection is carried inferiorly in a plane between the superficial and deep temporal fascia in the temple down beyond the zygomatic arch releasing the inferior temporal septum; carried medially releasing the superior temporal septum in a plane above the periosteum. One should take care to avoid the marked out supraorbital nerve and its deep neurovascular branch along with the temporal branch of facial nerve near the sentinel vein. The conjoint tendon is fully released as well as the arcus marginalis at the lateral orbital rim. The periosteum overlying the frontal bone is then scraped using a periosteal elevator. After a full release, within the temporal incision points, the superficial temporal fascia is then anchored to the deep temporal fascia in the direction of the desired vector of lift with 3-0 absorbable suture in a mattress fashion. In the author's experience, a 3-0 PDS is preferred. The remainder of the incision is closed with 4-0 vicryl or other absorbable suture via buried vertical mattress sutures followed by running 5-0 prolene or nylon suture, under minimal tension.

Supraorbital notch regional nerve blockade is performed using liposomal bupivacaine for the supraorbital nerve. This step can be done preoperatively as well, depending on surgeon preference, to limit operative pain.

Apply light dressing after the procedure. Postoperative narcotics are generally avoided to manage postoperative pain.

18.3 Blepharoplasty

Eyelid rejuvenation can be achieved via nonsurgical or surgical means. For those who are not surgical candidates or who do not desire surgery, hyaluronic acid filler can be injected into the lower lid depressions to smooth the lid–cheek junction. In the hands of an expert, it can also be used to fill the hollows above the eyes. This can be done with a needle or a microcannula. The latter tends to reduce bruising and swelling as compared to a needle. Fillers do not correct fat pad malpositioning, the actual underlying anatomic issue with most eye bags, and thus can be suboptimal even in skilled hands and require repeat treatment for sustained results. Laser resurfacing can also be utilized to address aging skin in the upper and lower lids, with variably appreciable tightening and skin change. However, deeper, more causative tissue changes are not as well addressed with a superficial modality.

18.3.1 Technique: Upper Blepharoplasty

Today, the most commonly used modality to address the upper lid is upper lid surgery with fat pad transfer and repositioning. First, the upper lid blepharoplasty incisions are carefully marked. The initial markings are made with the patient in an upright position. The upper eyelid crease is marked on the preexisting tarsal crease, with a series of dots. In women, this crease is approximately 8 to 10 mm above the lash line and in men 6 to 8 mm above the lash line. Once the patient is in a supine position, the superior aspect of the incision is drawn approximately 10 to 15 mm below the glabrous skin in women and in men, 10 mm below the glabrous skin.

Pinch testing the planned resection with nontoothed forceps helps ensure an appropriate surgical plan, leaving enough skin to allow complete eyelid closure. The amount of skin removed must be customized for each patient and should be conservatively done to avoid lagophthalmos. At least 20 mm of skin should be left behind to avoid lagophthalmos (▶ Fig. 18.7).

Upper eyelid crease is approximately 8 to 10 mm above the lash line in women and in men 6 to 8 mm above the lash line. Forceps are used to pinch excess skin along the surgical markings to evaluate for potential lagophthalmos.

18.3.2 Medial Fat Pad Repositioning

Incision along the premarked lines using a no. 15 blade or a Colorado microdissection needle is performed and skin is removed with curved blepharoplasty scissors and fine

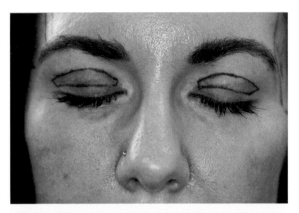

Fig. 18.7 Preoperative markings for upper blepharoplasty.

forceps. One should take care to leave the orbicularis oculi muscle intact during skin excision. Next, dissection down through the orbicularis to access the medial and central fat pads is performed. To augment upper lid hollowing, the medial fat pad as a vascular pedicle is isolated and transposed over the central, preaponeurotic fat pad. The repositioned medial fat pad is fixed to the orbital rim with a 6-0 polyglactin 910 suture or similar, often at multiple points.

18.3.3 Internal Browpexy

The lateral aspect of the orbicularis oculi is incised just inferior to the lateral orbital rim. The dissection is carried superiorly under the orbicularis oculi to access the retro orbicularis oculi fat or ROOF. Subsequently, the arcus marginalis is released at the orbital rim to continue the dissection in the subgaleal plane lateral to the supraorbital neurovascular bundle. The desired area of fixation is marked percutaneously at the level of the brow with a 32G needle. The underside of the orbicularis oculi muscle and the retro orbicularis oculi fad pad are grasped with a 5-0 prolene suture and tacked to the periosteum of the frontal bone.

Next, the lateral brow fat pad and orbicularis muscle are re-approximated with a 6-0 polyglactin 910 using a buried vertical mattress tacking technique or "brassiere" suture passed through the periosteum of the orbital rim. Finally, the skin incision is closed with 6-0 Prolene in a running fashion. It is always a good idea to ensure proper upper and lower lid position at the end of the case as adjustments become more difficult with time.

18.3.4 Modalities: Lower Blepharoplasty

Although a common procedure, a standard approach to the lower lid blepharoplasty remains debatable; indeed, the evolution of the procedure continues today. The effective transcutaneous skin–muscle flap was commonly employed from the 1970s through the 1990s. During the 1990s, the transconjunctival approach with fat resection and postoperative CO_2 laser gained popularity for its ability to avoid certain deficiencies of the skin–muscle flap such as denervation atrophy and lid malposition.[14] However, as with the skin–muscle flap, early transconjunctival approaches with excessive fat removal often resulted in a hollow appearance postoperatively.[15] Current blepharoplasty innovation is driven by a better long-term understanding of facial aging and aims to rejuvenate the face via fat preservation and soft-tissue repositioning instead of simple skin and fat removal. The transcutaneous and transconjunctival approaches are the two commonly utilized approaches, yet they are quite different.

The transcutaneous approach requires cutting into the skin, muscle, and orbital septum, which can lead to lower lid malposition, orbicularis denervation atrophy, and frank ectropion.[16,17,18] In patients with markedly excessive skin, or individuals with lower lid laxity, the transcutaneous approach is still desirable. Over the past couple of decades, the transconjunctival approach has gained favor over the transcutaneous method, in part, for its less invasive nature. The transcutaneous method was previously desirable for the surgical access it offered for simultaneous midface lift procedures; however, many of these can now be achieved via the transconjunctival approach. The transconjunctival approach was initially utilized for patients with fat pseudoherniation and without excess skin. Its favorability in a variety of circumstances is growing among surgeons, especially with increased use of adjuvant modalities, such as concurrent laser resurfacing. The author prefers the transconjunctival approach with liberal use of adjuvant procedures whenever possible.

18.3.5 Transconjunctival Blepharoplasty with Fat Repositioning and Directed Fat Transfer

Improved methods for the transconjunctival lower lid blepharoplasty are continually being developed. Although there are many methods in use, certain dynamic approaches yield superior outcomes. The senior author prefers the retroseptal approach over the preseptal approach because it avoids disruption of the septum near the tarsal plate. The inlet to the premaxillary space through the orbicularis muscle is avoided with the retroseptal approach, which is one of the at-risk areas for motor nerve damage. Thus, the risk of bleeding and nerve damage is mitigated. A submuscular plane is the safest and is more easily afforded by the retroseptal approach.[19] The senior author prefers the preperiosteal approach over the subperiosteal approach due to decreased downtime, edema, and risk of ptosis.[20]

This technique aims to create a safer procedure for patients and improve surgical recovery and outcomes. This can be performed utilizing exclusively local anesthesia, avoiding the complications associated with general anesthesia. Local infiltration into each fat pad helps improve patient comfort as manipulation of fat pad pedicles may cause some discomfort. The senior author favors fat pad transposition alone or in combination with fat grafting over fat pad resection and pure fat grafting alone, when possible, as blood supply is not disrupted to the fat pedicle as compared to free fat grafts. This increases fat pad survival, is more predictable, and may avoid lipogranuloma formation.[21]

Standard technique involves transposition of the medial and middle fat pads. The lateral fat pad is typically trimmed or not addressed.[22] Although technically difficult due to location and increased septa within the fat pad itself, lateral fat pad redistribution or transposition is superior to debulking lipectomy in the senior author's hands. Volume loss inferior to herniation of orbital fat almost universally contributes to the aesthetic of lower lid aging. The senior author uses the analogy of a mountain next to a valley, making each look more prominent. With this technique, we metaphorically use the mountaintop to fill the valley. Many surgeons shy away from lateral fat pad repositioning because of potential surgical pitfalls including significant bleeding from disruption of the zygomaticofacial neurovascular bundle and permanent facial drooping secondary to facial nerve damage and disruption of the zygomatic retaining ligament, all of which can be avoided with meticulous release of the inferior orbital rim structures.

18.3.6 Preoperatively

The initial evaluation of surgical candidates includes a thorough examination. Patients should be informed of the potential complications. The eyes should be examined for baseline visual acuity, including visual fields, as any change postoperatively will need to be addressed early. Evaluate the patient for eye dryness, which will transiently worsen after surgery, Bell's phenomenon, lid laxity, preexisting ptosis or lagophthalmos, and use of contact lenses. Medications that interfere with blood clotting should be discontinued as appropriate. Similarly, blood pressure should be appropriately managed before surgery. It is important to examine the periorbital tissues and be intimately familiar with the surrounding anatomy. Pay attention to upper lid hollowness preoperatively; it can be masked by excess skin, the correction of which can reveal the concealed hollowness, automatically resulting in a poor outcome.

Transconjunctival lower eyelid blepharoplasty is indicated to address herniated orbital fat, which manifests as lower lid fullness. Aging follows the general trend of vertical lengthening; however, specific age-related changes vary from person to person and an individual approach is again necessary. Often, even a single patient will present with variation in their two eyes.

18.3.7 Surgical Technique Exposing the Fat Pads

With a Jaeger lid plate protecting the globe and providing inferior traction in the conjunctival fornix, the transconjunctival incision is made with a needle tip on cutting cautery, starting inferior to the tarsal plate and vascular arcade, around 7 mm inferior to the lid margin, extending from the punctum medially to the canthus laterally. One to three traction sutures are then placed through the inferior free edge of the conjunctiva and lower lid retractors secured superiorly with a hemostat to a surgical towel. This conjunctiva acts as an eye shield, effectively utilizing the conjunctiva to cover the entire exposed globe while simultaneously providing traction to increase functional workspace for dissection and fat pad manipulation.

Once through the conjunctiva and underlying, adherent capsulopalpebral fascia, a combination of cautery and blunt dissection with cotton tips is utilized to dissect inferiorly and anteriorly toward the orbital rim, exposing the medial, middle, and lateral fat pads. To increase fat pad exposure, an assistant applies traction inferiorly on the lid with fingers, a double skin hook, or insulated retractor. With all three lower fat pads visible and separated, they are carefully dissected from the lower lid retractors and inferior oblique muscle, which separates the medial and middle fat pads. The more septate lateral fat pad is specifically addressed to a level determined preoperatively to avoid the common issue of a noticeable postoperative bulge at the lateral aspect of the lower lid (▶ Fig. 18.8).

Creating the Premaxillary Pocket for Pedicles

With the fat pads exposed and separated, a Freer periosteal elevator or spatulated tip curved blepharoplasty scissor is used to dissect and gain access to the preperiosteal space of the mid-cheek. Next, extending from the medial lacrimal crest to the lateral orbital rim, the tear trough ligament, also known as the orbital retaining ligament, is released from its preperiosteal connection, which lies 3 to 4 mm directly inferior to the arcus marginalis. Complete release of these structures allows for full transposition of the fat pad pedicles and releases the binding and groove-forming periosteal connections of the tear trough and malar skin. Bleeding can occasionally occur at this stage due to the proximity of the orbicularis to the arcus marginalis and insertion of the levator labii superioris at the medial infraorbital margin. Great care is taken to avoid the infraorbital neurovascular bundle medially, the zygomaticofacial neurovascular bundle laterally, and the

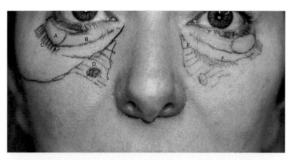

Fig. 18.8 Preoperative marking for lower blepharoplasty. A, lateral orbital fat pad; B, central and medial orbital fat pads; C, palpebromalar groove; D, deep medial cheek volume deficit; E, tear trough ligament; F, orbital retaining ligament.

origins of the lip elevators inferiorly and posteriorly. After this key releasing step, one continuous pocket exists in the premaxillary space that is available for fat repositioning and repurposing.

Pedicle Preparation

Preoperative planning includes assessment of the amounts of excess fat in the lid and the amount needed to drape over the orbital rim. Prior to any pad manipulation, the fat pads are directly re-anesthetized with lidocaine and epinephrine to increase hemostasis and comfort. The fat pads are thoroughly released from surrounding fascia to ensure easy and tensionless transposition. Rarely, fat pad sculpting is employed, with care to leave enough length and bulk in the pedicle to achieve these predetermined needs while not leaving any excess bulk or bag in the lid. All excised, sculpted fat is placed in cooled normal saline for potential use as free grafts.

Pedicle Transposition and Fixation

After the three fat pads are fully dissected and shaped, they are turned into transposable fat pedicles that will be used as "aprons" to be draped over the orbital rim into the premaxillary space hollowing. The most distal end of that first apron is secured with a figure-eight suture bites using a 4–0 polyglactin 910 on a PS-2 needle or 2-0 PDO Quill suture on a SKI 23 needle. The freer periosteal elevator is then placed from the conjunctival incision into the most inferior point of the pocket created in the premaxillary space, with its distal tip marking the desired inferior point of fat transposition. This is aimed into the specific part of the pocket desired, depending on which fat pad is being transposed. Notably, at this point, if the pedicle does not have adequate length to reach the distal or desired region of the pocket, the portions of sculpted fat that were saved in saline can be shaped into 2- to 3-mm free fat grafts that can be strung along the suture to reach those distal regions, which we have termed a "shish-ka-bleph."

Fat grafts can also be placed freely under direct visualization into the pocket, but the authors note more fat movement and extrusion at later stages of the procedure than with the shish-ka-bleph stringing of the grafts.

With the elevator tip in the distal pocket retracting the lower lid and mid-cheek anteriorly, the PS-2 SKI 23 needle tip can slide down the posterior part of the retractor's flat spatula and precisely penetrate from the premaxillary space anteriorly to the skin surface. Once the needle is grasped at the skin surface, the suture can be fixed with steri-strips, or if a concurrent laser procedure is to be performed, knots can be tied over small squares of nonadherent pad about 1 cm from the skin surface to allow any postoperative swelling to expand while placing light traction on the sutures. If a quill suture is used, there is no need for use of a nonadherent pad or knot tying, as the quill can simply be clipped at the skin surface allowing for no visible suture to be present. The process is repeated five more times to ensure placement of all three pads on each side. Importantly, it is visually verified that the inferior oblique is not incarcerated between the medial and middle pads, which can lead to postoperative diplopia. Care is taken with placement of these sutures to ensure that the six are symmetrically spaced on the face around the premarked landmarks such as the infraorbital nerve. A portion of this symmetric spacing is simply for patient perception during the recovery period. This method allows exact placement of the inferior extent of the pedicle in the dissected space.

The free edges of the conjunctiva are released from suture traction, and they are approximated with forceps; no sutures are necessary to close the conjunctiva, but they can be used as interrupted, buried fast gut sutures if the conjunctiva is not aligning as desired.[23]

The presence of aprons transposed after fat transposition prevents tissue re-adherence along the orbital rim.[24] Although uncontrolled damage to the orbicularis retaining ligament may result in ectropion or prolonged swelling and chemosis,[25] controlled release of the tear trough ligament, which runs in continuity with the orbicularis retaining ligament,[26] may be one of the most important aspects of the procedure to improve the tear trough deformity and palpebromalar groove.

Adjuvant Procedures

Blepharoplasty alone may insufficiently address certain deficiencies, including but not limited to excess, lax, and poor-quality lower eyelid skin and a negative maxillary vector. In these circumstances, additional interventions may be necessary to achieve aesthetically pleasing outcomes.

If there is excess lower eyelid skin, it needs to be planned for preoperatively, usually with either a skin pinch or laser. A subciliary skin pinch can take 2 to 3 mm of excess skin while leaving the orbicularis oculi fully intact. Fractional ablative laser resurfacing can be used to tighten lower lid skin and simultaneously improve skin quality and is thus the preferred adjuvant modality. The laser can also be employed simultaneously with the blepharoplasty procedure for treatment of full-face photodamage to multipurpose the patient's downtime.

Lower lid laxity, predetermined by symptoms or objective snap and distraction tests, can be managed simultaneously with canthoplasty or canthopexy. Canthopexy is more commonly used in cosmetic cases due to patient selection bias and utilization of the transconjunctival approach, which puts significantly less force on the lower lid compared to transcutaneous approaches.[27]

For patients with a negative or neutral maxillary vector who require maxillary support, structural fat grafting or filler support of the midface bony structure may be necessary to ensure proper lower lid function and aesthetic.[27] In severe or revision cases of prior lower lid surgery, transconjunctival midface lifting or posterior lamellar mucosal grafts may be required for support.[27] If portions of the mid-cheek or tear trough need additional volume augmentation not addressed by a pedicle, further filler or free fat grafts can be placed at the time of surgery in those specific locations.[22,27]

Finally, in step with the evolution of the senior author's practice, the utilization of platelet-rich plasma intradermally has expanded to include nearly every patient, especially when laser or fat grafting is utilized adjuvantly with lower lid blepharoplasty.

18.3.8 Postoperatively

Ideally, this procedure is done primarily under local anesthesia with addition of a mild oral or IV sedative if needed. It is important to test ocular movements to ensure there is no nerve entrapment and to verify normal visual function. It is imperative to inform the patient to expect swelling and bruising in the postoperative period. Cold compresses and head elevation can be used to minimize swelling. If the patient is experiencing discomfort, the pain can be managed with mild analgesics. The patient should contact the physician in the presence of significant pain as this is abnormal. Eye drops or ophthalmic ointment can be used if the patient reports dry eyes. Proper sun protection is always important, and if laser resurfacing was performed, the necessity of sun avoidance is magnified. Vigorous activity is avoided for several weeks and sutures are removed at day 5 to 7.

18.3.9 Complications

Brow lift complications are uncommon with appropriate preoperative evaluation but can occur. Damage to the frontal branch of the facial nerve is a common, but avoidable complication with proper understanding of anatomy. Hematoma can also occur. Hollowing out of the upper eyelid, as mentioned previously, is also common and problematic.

When done correctly, the transconjunctival blepharoplasty is a safe procedure; however, there are pitfalls to avoid. Retrobulbar hematoma is the most feared complication, believed to be caused by traction and rupture of vessels within posterior orbital fat during sculpting and removal of the anterior orbital fat.[28] This complication can be prevented by avoiding excessive traction or aggressive manipulation of the anterior orbital fat. In the event of a retrobulbar hematoma, lateral canthotomy and cantholysis are necessary.

Chemosis, or transudative edema of the bulbar and fornical conjunctiva, is a common complication of blepharoplasty procedures and has several causes, which include irritation and decreased fluid drainage.[29] These can be avoided, in part, by minimizing total dissection and keeping the patient's head elevated during and after the procedure.[29]

Lower lid malposition is a problem that can be avoided by a proper understanding of each patient's anatomy and a systematic preoperative evaluation. Tepper et al's recommendation of a preoperative evaluation includes a checklist of seven important anatomical findings: vector analysis, tarsoligamentous integrity, scleral show, canthal tilt, lateral canthus-to-orbital rim soft-tissue distance, midface position, and vertical restriction.[30] Lower lid malposition can be fixed with canthopexy. Residual bags occur in lower lid blepharoplasty procedures when there is a failure to adequately address the fat pads, most often the lateral pad, skin laxity, or orbicularis hypertrophy and laxity.[31]

Diplopia during the initial postoperative period can be caused by the local anesthetic, but persistent diplopia may indicate inferior oblique entrapment. This is avoided following fat pad transposition and fixation with confirmation that the inferior oblique is free from entrapment.[32]

Damage to the inferior rectus can occur with an excessively posterior dissection vector.[33] Damage to lip elevators and neurovascular bundles during the creation of premaxillary pockets for pedicle placement can be avoided by meticulous yet delicate dissection.[34] The lateral fat pad is near the zygomaticofacial neurovascular bundle, disruption of which can lead to significant bleeding. Direct visualization of the zygomaticofacial neurovascular bundle and lateral fat pad helps mitigate bleeding risk. Fat pad infiltration with local anesthetic helps differentiate the lateral fat pad from the surrounding connective tissue.

Damage to the midface retaining ligaments, for example, the zygomatic retaining ligament, should be avoided. The zygomatic retaining ligament, commonly referred to as McGregor's patch, is centered on the zygomaticotemporal suture at the anterior end of the zygomatic arch where it supports the tissues of the of the upper lateral cheek.[35,36] Disruption of this tissue can lead to permanent facial drooping from direct ligament damage or through disruption of the facial nerve, which is particularly vulnerable due its proximity to McGregor's patch. A thorough understanding of facial anatomy with careful dissection can avoid these complications.

18.3.10 Pearls and Pitfalls

The early methods of blepharoplasty often involved transection of fat from fat pads, but we now know it is better to transpose fat whenever possible. In most cases, facial rejuvenation involves restoration of volume. In fact, hollowing of the face, which can inadvertently be caused by fat transection, is an indication for facial rejuvenation. Oftentimes, adequate revolumization can be achieved by transposing all three orbital fat pads. When correctly repositioned, the often ignored lateral fat pad can provide a subtle yet important enhancement to the lateral canthal region including volumization of the palpebromalar groove. Concomitant laser resurfacing with blepharoplasty can enhance overall aesthetic outcomes by tightening the lower eyelid skin as well as improving the skin's tone and quality.

Excess fat removal will have a counterproductive outcome with regard to facial rejuvenation as, over time, this may result in periorbital hollowing. Although advancements in cosmetic surgery have been remarkable in recent years, it is still imperative for surgeons to instill realistic expectations in their patients prior to surgery. All patients have anatomical and age-related limitations that must be discussed prior to surgery. Overly aggressive surgical interventions often result in inferior outcomes that can be discernible even to the inexperienced eye.

References

[1] Rousso DE, Brys AK. Minimal incision face-lifting. Facial Plast Surg. 2012; 28(1):76–88

[2] Mendelson BC. Facelift anatomy, SMAS, retaining ligaments and facial spaces. In: Aston SJ, Steinbrech DS, Walden JL, eds. Aesthetic Plastic Surgery. Philadelphia, PA: Saunders Elsevier: 2009:53–72

[3] Chen P, Smith H, Vinciullo C. Bupivacaine as an adjunct to lidocaine in mohs micrographic surgery: a prospective randomized controlled trial. Dermatol Surg. 2018; 44(5):607–610

[4] Gangestad SW, Thornhill R, Yeo RA. Facial attractiveness, developmental stability, and fluctuating asymmetry. Ethol Sociobiol. 1994; 15:73–85

[5] Gill D. Women and men integrate facial information differently in appraising the beauty of a face. Evol Hum Behav. 2017; 38(6):756–760

[6] Rohrich RJ, Coberly DM, Fagien S, Stuzin JM. Current concepts in aesthetic upper blepharoplasty. Plast Reconstr Surg. 2004; 113(3): 32e–42e

[7] Hester TR, Jr, Codner MA, McCord CD, Nahai F, Giannopoulos A. Evolution of technique of the direct transblepharoplasty approach for the correction of lower lid and midfacial aging: maximizing results and minimizing complications in a 5-year experience. Plast Reconstr Surg. 2000; 105(1):393–406, discussion 407–408

[8] Hamra ST. Arcus marginalis release and orbital fat preservation in midface rejuvenation. Plast Reconstr Surg. 1995; 96(2):354–362

[9] Baker SR. Orbital fat preservation in lower-lid blepharoplasty. Arch Facial Plast Surg. 1999; 1(1):33–37

[10] Hester TR, Jr, McCord CD, Nahai F, Sassoon EM, Codner MA. Expanded applications for transconjunctival lower lid blepharoplasty. Plast Reconstr Surg. 2001; 108(1):271–272

[11] Rohrich RJ, Arbique GM, Wong C, Brown S, Pessa JE. The anatomy of suborbicularis fat: implications for periorbital rejuvenation. Plast Reconstr Surg. 2009; 124(3):946–951

[12] Rohrich RJ, Pessa JE. The fat compartments of the face: anatomy and clinical implications for cosmetic surgery. Plast Reconstr Surg. 2007; 119(7):2219–2227, discussion 2228–2231

[13] Sclafani AP, Jung M. Desired position, shape, and dynamic range of the normal adult eyebrow. Arch Facial Plast Surg. 2010; 12(2):123–127

[14] Roberts TL, III. Laser blepharoplasty and laser resurfacing of the periorbital area. Clin Plast Surg. 1998; 25(1):95–108

[15] Hidalgo DA. An integrated approach to lower blepharoplasty. Plast Reconstr Surg. 2011; 127(1):386–395

[16] Baylis HI, Long JA, Groth MJ. Transconjunctival lower eyelid blepharoplasty. Technique and complications. Ophthalmology. 1989; 96(7):1027–1032

[17] McGraw BL, Adamson PA. Postblepharoplasty ectropion. Prevention and management. Arch Otolaryngol Head Neck Surg. 1991; 117(8):852–856

[18] McCord CD, Jr, Ellis DS. The correction of lower lid malposition following lower lid blepharoplasty. Plast Reconstr Surg. 1993; 92(6):1068–1072

[19] Korchia D, Braccini F, Paris J, Thomassin J. Transconjunctival approach in lower eyelid blepharoplasty. Can J Plast Surg. 2003; 11(3):166–170

[20] Marshak H, Morrow DM, Dresner SC. Small incision preperiosteal midface lift for correction of lower eyelid retraction. Ophthal Plast Reconstr Surg. 2010; 26(3):176–181

[21] Goldberg RA. Transconjunctival orbital fat repositioning: transposition of orbital fat pedicles into a subperiosteal pocket. Plast Reconstr Surg. 2000; 105(2):743–748, discussion 749–751

[22] Miranda SG, Codner MA. Micro free orbital fat grafts to the tear trough deformity during lower blepharoplasty. Plast Reconstr Surg. 2017; 139(6):1335–1343

[23] Goldberg RA, Lessner AM, Shorr N, Baylis HI. The transconjunctival approach to the orbital floor and orbital fat. A prospective study. Ophthal Plast Reconstr Surg. 1990; 6(4):241–246

[24] Marten TJ. Closed, nonendoscopic, small-incision forehead lift. Clin Plast Surg. 2008; 35(3):363–378, discussion 361

[25] Chan NJ, et al. Orbicularis retaining ligament release in lower blepharoplasty: assessing efficacy and complications. Ophthal Plast Reconstr Surg. 2018; 34(2):155–161

[26] Wong C-H, Hsieh MKH, Mendelson B. The tear trough ligament: anatomical basis for the tear trough deformity. Plast Reconstr Surg. 2012; 129(6):1392–1402

[27] Wong C-H, Mendelson B. Extended transconjunctival lower eyelid blepharoplasty with release of the tear trough ligament and fat redistribution. Plast Reconstr Surg. 2017; 140(2):273–282

[28] Wolfort FG, Vaughan TE, Wolfort SF, Nevarre DR. Retrobulbar hematoma and blepharoplasty. Plast Reconstr Surg. 1999; 104(7):2154–2162

[29] Weinfeld AB, Burke R, Codner MA. The comprehensive management of chemosis following cosmetic lower blepharoplasty. Plast Reconstr Surg. 2008; 122(2):579–586

[30] Tepper OM, Steinbrech D, Howell MH, Jelks EB, Jelks GW. A retrospective review of patients undergoing lateral canthoplasty techniques to manage existing or potential lower eyelid malposition: identification of seven key preoperative findings. Plast Reconstr Surg. 2015; 136(1):40–49

[31] Warren RJ. International Textbook of Aesthetic Surgery. 2017:NP129–NP130

[32] Ghabrial R, Lisman RD, Kane MA, Milite J, Richards R. Diplopia following transconjunctival blepharoplasty. Plast Reconstr Surg. 1998; 102(4):1219–1225

[33] Sniegowski M, Davies B, Hink E, Durairaj VD. Complications following blepharoplasty. Expert Rev Ophthalmol. 2014; 9(4):341–349

[34] Yoo DB, Peng GL, Massry GG. Transconjunctival lower blepharoplasty with fat repositioning: a retrospective comparison of transposing fat to the subperiosteal vs supraperiosteal planes. JAMA Facial Plast Surg. 2013; 15(3):176–181

[35] Tyers AG, John ROC. Colour atlas of Ophthalmic Plastic Surgery. Philadelphia, PA: Elsevier Health Sciences; 2008

[36] Furnas DW. The retaining ligaments of the cheek. Plast Reconstr Surg. 1989; 83(1):11–16

19 Devices and Treatment Options for Axillary Hyperhidrosis

Cameron Rokhsar and Austin Lee

Summary

Primary hyperhidrosis, or uncontrollable sweating, is a condition that affects the social and psychological well-being of millions of people worldwide. It can present in several focal, eccrine-dense areas, with the axillae being one of the most common. Following diagnosis and an assessment of severity, patients can choose from several treatment options for axillary hyperhidrosis. These include topical, injectable, and systemic pharmacological treatments, and devices such as lasers and microwave energy delivery systems. We explain here the effectiveness and techniques involved in these treatment options, postoperative care, and management of potential complications.

Keywords: primary hyperhidrosis, axillae, pharmacological treatment, topical, injectable, systemic, devices, lasers, microwaves

19.1 Introduction

Sweating is an important mechanism for regulating body temperature. However, a condition called *hyperhidrosis* is characterized by excessive, uncontrollable sweating, and is classified as either primary or secondary. Primary hyperhidrosis is most common, and usually presents in a focal, eccrine-dense area such as the axillae, palms, soles, and/or the craniofacial region.

Secondary hyperhidrosis is usually caused by an underlying condition or medication, and more often has a unilateral, asymmetrical, and generalized distribution. This chapter will focus on primary focal hyperhidrosis; however, the importance of differentiating and identifying the condition warrants a discussion of the secondary hyperhidrosis first.[1]

There are several causes of secondary hyperhidrosis. Hyperhidrosis is associated with several metabolic and endocrine disorders, such as diabetes mellitus, hyperthyroidism, hyperpituitarism, and pheochromocytoma. It can also be caused by stimulation of the hypothalamus in response to temperature elevations, which are common in febrile illnesses (i.e., infections and lymphoma). Drugs can also cause hyperhidrosis, such as cholinomimetic agents, cholinesterase inhibitors, adrenomimetic agents, hypoglycemic agents, central nervous system (CNS) stimulants, antidepressants, opioids, and others. Gustatory hyperhidrosis can occur normally while eating or drinking, typically affecting the cheeks or the upper lip. It can also occur in response to nerve injury, such as in Frey's syndrome, which often develops after undergoing surgery in patients who have lesions on the parotid gland with facial nerve damage. Gustatory sweating can also be hereditary, or compensatory in diabetic patients. Genodermatoses, or genetic skin disorders, can cause hyperhidrosis in the palmoplantar regions as well as autonomic neuropathies, damage to the nerves that control everyday functions such as sweating. Hyperhidrosis in one region can result from diminished sweating, or hypohidrosis, in another. Secondary hyperhidrosis can also result from non-neural conditions, such as menopause, or through direct, localized stimulation of eccrine glands.[1,2,3,4]

It is important to distinguish primary and secondary hyperhidrosis because treatment of secondary hyperhidrosis is possible through suppression of the cause. Additionally, identification of associated causes in patients with secondary hyperhidrosis can point to an underlying condition, such as systemic disease.

The remainder of this chapter will concentrate on primary focal hyperhidrosis.

19.2 Prevalence

Current prevalence measurements of this disease vary widely. In one survey of American households, an estimate of 2.8% was found.[5] A second, estimated U.S. prevalence at 1.0 and 1.6% in the United Kingdom, with a consistent range from 0.1 to 0.3% during the study.[6] Hyperhidrosis has also been approximated at 4.6% in Germany,[7] 5.5% in Sweden, 12.3% in Vancouver,[8] 12.8% in Japan,[9] and 14.5% in Shanghai.[8] Despite the variation in prevalence estimates, which can be attributed to different criteria and subjective assessment, it is clear that primary hyperhidrosis is a significant clinical issue.

19.3 Assessment and Diagnosis

19.3.1 Diagnostic Criteria

Correct diagnosis is required before considering treatment. Primary hyperhidrosis can be diagnosed in patients with a duration of excessive sweating of ≥ 6 months, and four or more of the following[1]:

- Bilateral and symmetric area affected.
- Nocturnal absence.
- Episodes at least weekly.
- Onset at or before the age of 25 years.
- Positive family history.
- Impairment of daily activities.

19.3.2 Assessment of Severity and Response to Treatment

Several criteria can be used to measure the extent of the disorder and treatment response. One, the hyperhidrosis

Table 19.1 Hyperhidrosis disease severity scale

Score	Patient response
1	My axillary sweating is never noticeable and never interfered with my daily activities
2	My axillary sweating is tolerable but sometimes interferes with my daily activities
3	My axillary sweating is barely tolerable and frequently interferes with my daily activities
4	My axillary sweating is intolerable and always interferes with my daily activities

Table 19.2 Axillary Sweating Daily Diary (ASDD)

ASDD	
Item 1 (gatekeeper)	During the past 24 h, did you have any underarm sweating? *Yes/No* (When item 1 is answered "no," item 2 is skipped and scored as zero)
Item 2	During the past 24 h, how would you rate your underarm sweating at its worst? *0 (no sweating at all) to 10 (worst possible sweating)*
Item 3	During the past 24 h, to what extent did your underarm sweating impact your activities? *0 (not at all), 1 (a little bit), 2 (a moderate amount), 3 (a great deal), 4 (an extreme amount)*
Item 4	During the past 24 h, how bothered were you by your underarm sweating? *0 (not at all bothered), 1 (a little bothered), 2 (moderately bothered), 3 (very bothered), 4 (extremely bothered)*
Axillary Sweating Daily Diary-Children (ASDD-C)	
Item 1 (gatekeeper)	Thinking about **last night and today**, did you have any underarm sweating? *Yes/No* (When item 1 is answered "no," item 2 is skipped and scored as zero)
Item 2	Thinking about last night and today, how bad was your underarm sweating? *0 (no sweating at all) to 10 (worst possible sweating)*

disease severity scale (HDSS), is a four-question scale in which patients rate tolerability and degree to which hyperhidrosis hinders their daily activities[10] (see ▶ Table 19.1). In the starch–iodine or minor test, iodine is applied to the surface of the affected area and allowed to dry. Cornstarch is then applied, and when sweat is detected, a dark blue color appears. Although the test is qualitative, semi-quantitative scales can be used to measure the total area affected. Gravimetry is the most quantitative assessment, in which preweighed pads or pieces of filter paper are placed in the affected areas, then weighed again after a length of time.[11] Other subjective numerical scales are used as well, such as the Dermatology Life Quality Index (DLQI).

19.4 Treatment of Hyperhidrosis

19.4.1 Drugs

Topical, injectable, and systemic agents are pharmacologic treatment options.

Aluminum Chloride

Aluminum salts are considered a first-line treatment for hyperhidrosis due to their low cost and quick effectiveness. Aluminum chloride is used in cosmetic antiperspirants, and is the partially neutralized form, whereas aluminum chloride hexahydrate is used in prescription treatments, often used as a 20% solution in more severe cases. Over-the-counter aluminum chloride antiperspirants may be effective in less severe hyperhidrosis.[12] The salts are believed to function by forming a plug in the distal sweat duct through interaction between the metal ions and mucopolysaccharides. Hölzle and Braun-Falco also found necrosis of epidermal cells lining the ducts within the acrosyringium of eccrine glands. Other changes reported after treatment with aqueous aluminum chloride included intra- and intercellular vacuolization of secretory cells, conspicuous dilation of the secretory portion, irregular appearance of acini accompanied by loss of structural integrity, and widening of the lumina of eccrine acini and dermal ducts. Some of the widened acini were filled with periodic acid–Schiff

(PAS) positive, diastase-resistant, amorphous material. Long-term treatment led to atrophy of secretory cells as well. Loss of sweat correlated with these changes in most patients. The study concluded that treatment could lead to degeneration of the eccrine acini by forming blockages in the distal acrosyringium.[13] Other metal salts such as zirconium, vanadium, and indium are believed to work using a similar mechanism, although aluminum chloride remains more common due to its availability, low cost, and nontoxicity.

Skin irritation is a possible adverse effect when using aluminum chloride treatments. To avoid this effect and for better efficacy, antiperspirants should be applied on dry skin at night, right before bed, and should remain on the skin for 6 to 8 hours. Overnight application is recommended due to lack of active sweating during sleep, which can prevent diffusion of the ions into the sweat gland.[12,14]

Glycopyrronium Tosylate

Recently, a topical anticholinergic agent called glycopyrronium tosylate (GT) was approved by the U.S. Food and

Drug Administration (FDA) for treatment of axillary hyperhidrosis in patients aged ≥ 9 years. GT is applied to the axillae once a day using a premoistened towelette. Glycopyrronium cloth, 2.4% was tested in in two replicate, phase 3, randomized, double-blind, vehicle-controlled, parallel-group, 4-week trials by Glaser et al.[15] Three hundred and thirty patients with primary axillary hyperhidrosis as measured by at least a 3 or 4 on the HDSS and 50 mg of sweat in 5 minutes were randomized in a 2:1 ratio to treatment or vehicle groups. Patients applied the product once daily to clean, dry skin of both axillae for 4 weeks and were not allowed to wash the area for 4 hours after application. Response was measured by the Axillary Sweating Daily Diary (ASDD), a four-item patient-reported outcome (PRO) measure to be completed daily by patients age ≥ 16 years (▶ Table 19.2), the ASDD-C item 2, the first two items from an 11-point numeric rating scale of severity of sweating for subjects older than 9 years but younger than 16 years (▶ Table 19.2), and by mean absolute change from baseline (CfB) in sweat production in both axillae. A positive response was defined as at least a ≥ 4 average in weekly average responses from baseline. In each trial, the ASDD/ASDD-C item 2 responder rates were significantly higher for GT versus vehicle at week 4, with 52.8 versus 28.3% in trial 1 and 66.1 versus 26.9% in trial 2 ($p < 0.001$ for both). Statistically significant differences favoring GT for CfB at week 4 were also seen in both trials, after the exclusion of an extreme outlier in trial 1. Differences favoring the GT group were observed in both ASDD/ASDD-C item 2 and CfB as early as week 1. Secondary efficacy responses, an HDSS score improvement of ≥ 2 and sweat production rate reduction of ≥ 50% from baseline, were also significantly higher in the GT group than in the vehicle group in week 4 ($p < 0.001$ in both trials).

Topical application of GT can minimize but not completely eliminate its anticholinergic side effects, such as blurry vision, trouble urinating, and dry mouth. Most treatment emergent adverse effects cited in the trials were transient and reversible, and manageable by modifying frequency of the agent. The study noted that subjects who did not carefully wash their hands following application could have transferred it to other areas of the body, such as the eye, leading to blurry vision and mydriasis. Other adverse effects, such as trouble urinating and dry mouth, were likely due to systemic exposure due to prolonged absorption of the drug.

Botulinum Toxin Type A

Botulinum toxin type A (onabotulinumtoxin A) is a safe, effective neurotoxin produced by the anaerobic bacterium *Clostridium botulinum* for treatment of primary axillary hyperhidrosis. It works by temporarily inhibiting acetylcholine release in neurons, preventing stimulation of the eccrine gland. The treatments must be provided by a physician. Small injections are made into the subcutis

of the axilla. Experiments have shown an average efficacy of 6 to 9 months, depending on the condition's severity and location. The treatment is FDA approved for axillary hyperhidrosis in patients age ≥ 18 years, but is considered off-label for treating craniofacial and palmoplantar hyperhidrosis. Treatment of palmoplantar hyperhidrosis may require local anesthesia due to the high density of nerve endings. A regional block (e.g., Bier's block) can minimize pain effectively, but nerve damage is possible, and not all physicians can reliably perform this procedure. Placement of ice packs on the treated area for 15 minutes prior is a sufficient method in many patients. Vibration using a handheld massager or other device as well as lidocaine cream can be applied if needed.[16] Botulinum toxin weakens muscles, and weakened grip is a possible side effect of palmar treatment that patients should be cautioned about. Weakness is temporary and typically lasts a few weeks after treatment. Typically, 50 U of botulinum toxin are injected per axilla, 150 U/sole, and 50 to 100 U into each palm typically at a density of 1 injection/m².

Two randomized, multicenter, double-blind, placebo-controlled studies are cited on the product packaging to describe safety and efficacy. In one study, 50 U, 75 U, or placebo were administered in a 1:1:1 ratio in the axilla of 322 subjects with axillary hyperhidrosis. Fifty-five percent of those receiving 50 U and 49% of those receiving 75 u experienced an improvement of at least 2 HDSS scores. Only 6% of the placebo group responded by this criterion. Eighty-one percent of the 50-u group, 86% of the 75-u group, and 41% of the placebo group experienced at least 50% in gravimetric reduction in sweating 4 weeks after treatment. Median duration of response (the number of days between injection and first visit at which patients return to 3 or 4 on the HDSS scale) was 197, 205, and 96 days in the 75-U group, 50-U group, and placebo group, respectively.[17]

In the second study,[18] 320 adults were randomized to receive 50 u of botulinum toxin or placebo. Ninety-one percent of the treatment group and 36% of the placebo group experienced a reduction of at least 50% in axillary sweating 4 weeks after injection as measured by gravimetry ($p < 0.001$).

Multiple studies have demonstrated the efficacy of all commercially available botulinum toxin type A products in treatment of hyperhidrosis, such as abobotulinumtoxin, onabotulinumtoxin, and incobotulinumtoxin.

Systemic Treatments

Oral medications can be beneficial when first-line, focally targeted therapies are ineffective or unavailable, or if multiple areas of the body are affected. The most common category of systemic agents used for hyperhidrosis is anticholinergics. Anticholinergic agents work by competitive inhibition of acetylcholine, the primary neurotransmitter of nerves in the sweat glands, at the muscarinic receptor. Side effects can be compounded when patients use other anticholinergic medications at the same time. Anticholinergic therapy may be contraindicated in patients with glaucoma, obstructive uropathy, obstructive disease of the gastrointestinal (GI) tract, paralytic ileus, severe ulcerative colitis, and myasthenia gravis. Glycopyrrolate, which comes in oral and topical form, is favored over other anticholinergics because it does not cross into the CNS through the blood–brain barrier, which causes fewer systemic side effects. Glycopyrrolate is usually taken in 1- to 2-mg doses once or twice daily, and patients are asked to increase the dosage by 1 mg/d at 2-week intervals depending on response and side effects.

In a study by Walling,[19] a total of 71 patients (59 of which completed the study with at least 2 months of follow-up data) were prescribed systemic agents. Before starting the medications prescribed in the study, most patients had previously failed other treatments, including topical aluminum chloride, iontophoresis, and other oral medications. Palmoplantar and/or axillary hyperhidrosis was most common (71%), followed by generalized (15%) and craniofacial (14%) hyperhidrosis. Of these, 45 patients were glycopyrrolate, with a response rate of 67% (30/45). About one quarter of the patients prescribed glycopyrrolate used it as their only treatment, whereas three-quarters took glycopyrrolate in combination with another form of therapy, including topical aluminum chloride, botulinum toxin, and iontophoresis. Fourteen of the 30 indicated a degree of improvement: 6 of 14 (42%) stated improvement was "great," "excellent," or "> 75%"; 8 of 14 (59%) noted "some," "moderate," or "> 50%" improvement. Oxybutynin, another anticholinergic drug, is a tertiary amine that is used to treat hyperhidrosis. Due to its structure, it can penetrate the blood–brain barrier more than glycopyrrolate, but has still been used successfully. For oral administration, a typical dose is 5 to 10 mg daily, but doses up to 15 to 20 mg may be required.

Other drugs include beta blockers and alpha-adrenergic agonists. Beta blockers have traditionally been used to suppress symptoms related to social phobias and performance anxiety, which sometimes produce sweating. The use of beta blockers such as propranolol can treat hyperhidrosis in low, infrequent doses. A typical propranolol dose would be 10 to 20 mg/h before an anxiety-inducing "performance" such as a meeting or speech. Smaller doses such as 5 mg can be used initially in patients with low blood pressure, slower baseline heart rate, or a smaller body index. Due to the numerous contraindications, a thorough patient history is required prior to prescription, including the patient's resting blood pressure and heart rate.[20] Clonidine is an alpha-adrenergic agonist traditionally used to treat hypertension and some anxiety disorders that has also been used as a treatment for hyperhidrosis. The study by Walling[19] prescribed 0.1 mg of clonidine twice daily to 13 patients, with a response rate

of 46%. There have been case reports for other systemic treatments, but these are beyond the scope of this chapter.[20]

19.4.2 Devices

Microwave Destruction of Sweat Glands

Microwave-based treatment of axillary hyperhidrosis was approved by the FDA in 2011. After application of local anesthetic, energy at 5.8 GHz is delivered to the skin. The differences in the properties between dermal and underlying adipose tissue lead to a large reflection of the energy at the dermal–hypodermal interface, close to where the eccrine and apocrine glands are located. The antenna in the device takes the reflected energy to create an optimal interference pattern, leading to constructive interference near the dermal–hypodermal interface and destructive interference at the epidermis. The larger microwave conductivity in dermal tissue makes it more absorptive than the adipose layer. This absorption causes dielectric heating and destruction of the dermal tissue. The epidermis is protected due to the destructive interference and due to application of a contact cooling system consisting of a circulating layer of water and a ceramic cooling plate.[21]

Glaser et al[22] conducted a multicenter, randomized, sham-controlled study with 120 adults affected by primary axillary hyperhidrosis. Subjects were required to have an HDSS score of 3 or 4 and baseline sweat production greater than 50 mg/5 min as measured by gravimetry. The protocol planned two treatment sessions spaced 2 weeks apart, but subjects could opt out if only one session was effective or if further treatment was declined. Subjects were randomized in a 2 to 1 ratio for the first session to a treatment group ($n = 81$) and sham group ($n = 39$). At 30 days, 89% of the active group and 54% of the sham group recorded an HDSS score of 1 or 2 ($p < 0.001$). At 6 months, these scores were achieved by 69% of the active group and 44% of the sham group ($p = 0.02$). Efficacy was statistically significantly greater for the treatment group than for the sham group, in all time points with data from both groups as measured by the HDSS. Gravimetry revealed a reduction of ≥ 50% in sweat at the 30-day follow-up visit in 80% of the treatment group and 67% of the sham group ($p = 0.07$). No other difference in later time points was close to statistical significance, although there was a greater reduction in the treatment group. Side effects in the treatment group included persistent pain and swelling, pustules, and/or blisters, resulting in seven subjects receiving only one treatment. The frequency of these complications has decreased as a result of protocol improvements, most notably the use of tumescent anesthesia prior to treatment. The anesthesia is particularly useful because the fluid protects underlying nerves that lie beneath the subcutaneous space from the heat of the microwaves. As a result, the incidence of sensory and motor nerve complications has decreased substantially.

In the author's experience, whereas some patients receive satisfactory results after one treatment session, a majority require two sessions spaced 3 months apart for long-term reduction. Five percent require three sessions, and are typically patients whose condition is most severe and unresponsive to other treatment options. Fifty percent to 60% improvement is typically reported after one treatment session, and 70 to 90% after two sessions. The nonresponder rate is very low, estimated to be less than 1%. Tumescent anesthesia allows application of microwave treatment at the highest energy settings, improving efficacy while minimizing discomfort and previously documented side effects. Patients may experience temporary side effects, including edema that typically resolves within a week, and hard nodules that disappear after a few weeks up to 3 months. Numbness in the axillae as well as inner arms is an alarming side effect for patients, which should be discussed prior to procedure. This usually resolves within months. In the authors' opinion,

microwave technology has revolutionized treatment of axillary hyperhidrosis and should be considered the gold standard.

Patients are told to shave their axillae 2 to 3 days before treatment, as shaving too soon prior to treatment could increase the incidence of infection. The area is marked with a grid, then numbed with 120 to 240 mL of tumescent fluid containing saline, epinephrine, sodium bicarbonate, and lidocaine. The applicator is used to treat the underlying armpit, and treatment typically takes 30 to 45 minutes. Although the machine usually starts at the lowest energy setting and gradually increases in energy throughout treatment, the authors recommend starting at the highest energy, level 5, for stronger results. However, it is recommended that patients with less subcutaneous fat start at lower energy settings to avoid complications. Following treatment, patients are advised to apply ice to the axillae for the remainder of the day, but not longer due to the possibility of reduced healing. Patients are also instructed to take nonsteroidal anti-inflammatory drugs (NSAIDs) with food (▸ Fig. 19.1, ▸ Fig. 19.2, ▸ Fig. 19.3).

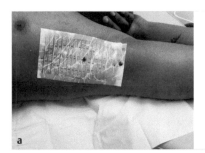
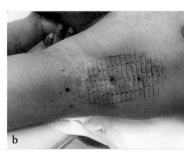

Fig. 19.1 (a, b) The axillae are first marked with a grid to provide an outline of the treatment zones.

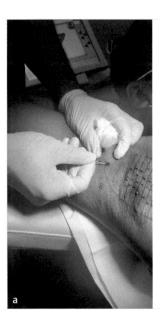
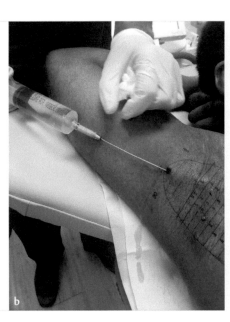

Fig. 19.2 (a, b) A Nokor needle is used to provide an entry point for the cannula through which tumescent fluid is injected in the treatment area.

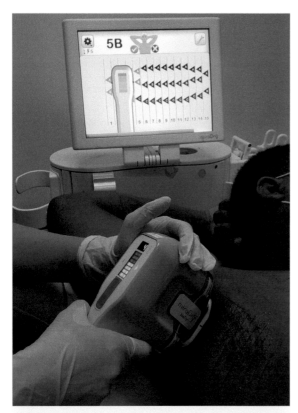

Fig. 19.3 The operator applies microwave energy, positioning the applicator of the device onto the treatment zones indicated by the grid. The whole process takes from 30 to 45 minutes per axilla.

Microfocused Ultrasound

A high-intensity microfocused ultrasound device with visualization (MFU-V) commonly used for skin tightening of the face and neck was tested in two randomized, double-blind, sham-controlled pilot studies conducted by Nestor and Park.[23] The device produces small thermal lesions (~1 mm³) or coagulation points within the dermis at depths of the sweat glands, up to 4.5 mm, effectively destroying them. The ultrasound focuses the energy delivery to specific soft tissue within subcutaneous layers behind the superficial dermis, whereas the visualization component ensures consistent energy delivery as well as avoidance of other anatomical structures, such as bone. In the first study, each subject received two MFU-V treatments in one axilla 30 days apart, and two sham treatments in the other axilla 30 days apart. Each treatment consisted of two passes set at the maximum allowable energy for the given transducer, one using 4 MHz at a focal depth of 4.5 mm, followed by the other pass of 7 MHz with a depth of 3 mm. Energy was set to 0 J on the sham side. Positive response was defined as a spontaneous axillary sweat reduction greater than 50% on the treated axilla 90 days after the second treatment (day

120 of the study overall) as measured by gravimetry. Fourteen patients completed this study, with more than 50% reporting a positive response.

The second study randomized 20 subjects to 2 bilateral MFU ultrasound treatments ($n = 12$) or 2 bilateral sham treatments ($n = 8$), 30 days apart. Positive treatment response was defined as a reduction in the HDSS score from 3 or 4 to 1 or 2 30 days following the second treatment (day 60 of the study). Secondary positive responses included changes in HDSS scores and gravimetric reduction of at least 50% at each follow-up visit, and changes in the starch–iodine test and patient satisfaction questionnaire (PSG) scores. On days 7, 14, and 30 after the first treatment, efficacy was assessed through the HDSS, gravimetry, and starch–iodine tests. Efficacy assessments were made on days 37, 44, 60, 90, 120, and 365 after the second treatment. Patients also completed a PSQ on days 60, 90, 120, and 365 after the second treatment. At 30 days after the second treatment (day 60), a positive HDSS response rate of 67% was achieved by the MFU-V group ($p = 0.005$), with positive response rates above 50% for all time points. Zero percent was reported in the sham group at 30 days ($p = 0.005$), and for all of the other time points. Gravimetry revealed reduction in baseline sweat production by ≥ 50% at all time points in the MFU-V group, but not the sham group. All percent reductions from baseline were significantly greater in the MFU-V group than in the sham group, regardless of study visit ($p > 0.0001$). Ten of 12 (83%) patients in the MFU-V group (none in the sham group) experienced a median ≥ 50% sweat reduction from baseline over all time points after the second treatment. According to the PSQ responses at all time points, most patients in the MFU-V group reported satisfaction or high satisfaction, whereas all patients in the sham group reported dissatisfaction or high dissatisfaction with their treatment results ($p = 0.0001$ for the day 60 comparison). A 12-month follow-up was provided for some of the subjects. Five of six in the MFU-V group continued to report noticeable clinical improvement and remained satisfied with the treatment, whereas five maintained a positive response based on gravimetric measurement.

Laser Treatment

Minimally Invasive Laser

Leclère et al[24] conducted a randomized prospective controlled trial with an experimental laser on 100 axillary hyperhidrosis patients divided into four groups with different conditions applied for about 40 minutes including anesthetization: laser alone at 975 nm (group 1), laser alone at 924/975 nm simultaneously (group 2), curettage alone (group 3), and laser at 924/975 nm followed by curettage (group 4). Curettage was applied to the level of the subcutaneous fat and deep dermis, where sweat glands are found. The diode laser system tested consisted of two lasers, one emitting at 924 nm

Table 19.3 Results from minimally invasive surgery study

Group	HDSS mean (standard deviation) at: Baseline 1 mo 12 mo	Starch–iodine mean (standard deviation) at: Baseline 1 mo 12 mo	GAIS mean (standard deviation) at: 1 mo 12 mo
975 nm	3.88 (±0.33) 3.40 (±0.50) 3.44 (±0.51)	2.60 (±0.48) 2.48 (±0.51) 2.76 (±0.44)	1.04 (±0.35) 0.92 (±0.28)
975 and 924 nm	3.84 (±0.37) 1.96 (±0.68) 1.96 (±0.61)	2.60 (±0.60) 1.36 (±0.49) 1.48 (±0.51)	2.36 (±0.49) 2.72 (±0.46)
Curettage	3.85 (±0.37) 2.20 (±0.41) 2.32 (±0.48)	2.58 (±0.48) 1.56 (±0.51) 1.76 (±0.60)	2.28 (±0.46) 2.64 (±0.49)
975 and 924 nm, curettage	3.88 (±0.33) 1.24 (±0.44) 0.48 (±0.51)	2.64 (±0.49) 0.40 (±0.50) 0.44 (±0.51)	3.72 (±0.54) 3.76 (±0.44)

Abbreviations: GAIS, Global Aesthetic Improvement Scale; HDSS, hyperhidrosis disease severity scale.

and the other one at 975 nm, built into the same device. Laser parameters used were a 1.5-mm diameter/27-cm cannula and emission power of 20 W, and treatment was applied in a back and forth motion in the subdermal space. Assessments were performed 1 month and 1 year following treatment using the HDSS, starch–iodine test, and the Global Aesthetic Improvement Scale (GAIS), and a semi-quantitative 4-point scale was used to measure improvement on the starch–iodine test. Minimal improvement was reported in group 1 (975-nm laser alone), but improvement was notable in groups 2 and 3. The 924-/975-nm laser followed by curettage was found to be the optimal treatment, with the greatest improvement reported in group 4. Quantitative scores were reported, but did not include significance values (see ▶ Table 19.3).

Goldman and Wollina[25] studied treatment using a subdermal 1,064-nm Nd:YAG (neodymium:yttrium aluminum garnet) laser in 17 patients with axillary hyperhidrosis. Laser energy was directed to the subcutaneous tissue through a 300-mm fiberoptic delivered by an 18-gauge Tuohy disposable epidural needle.

A 100-ms pulsed laser at 40 Hz of frequency and 15 mJ of energy (working at 6 W) was used for all patients after tumescent anesthesia. The needle and fiber were moved back and forth around the level of the dermal/subdermal junction. Twelve of 17 patients reported "excellent results," 3 reported "good," and 2 reported "fair" using patient global assessment. Physician global assessment in pre- and postsurgery photographs based on estimated

percentage reduction in hyperhidrosis area was excellent in 10, good in 4, and fair in 3 patients.

Noninvasive Laser

In a 21-subject study (19 of whom completed) by Bechara et al,[26] a long-pulsed 800-nm diode laser at 50 J/cm^2 was used for a total of five treatments on one axilla for 30 ms, whereas the other served as a control. Sweat rates were measured and compared before therapy and 4 weeks after the last treatment using gravimetry. Subjects used visual analog scales (VAS) at 4 weeks and 12 months after the last laser treatment to estimate their decrease in sweating and rate their satisfaction. Sweat rate measured on the treated side was significantly reduced after treatment, with a decrease from a median of 89 mg/min (range: 42–208) to a median of 48 mg/min (range: 17–119; $p < 0.001$). However, a decrease was also observed in the control side, from a median of 78 mg/min (25–220) to a median of 65 mg/min (range: 24–399 mg/min; $p = 0.04$). The difference in sweat rate reduction between the treatment and control axilla was not statistically significant ($p = 0.10$). Patient satisfaction was rated 5.9 at 4 weeks and 4.1 at 12 months after the last treatment. However, the appearance of apocrine and eccrine glands did not significantly change, as shown by skin biopsies before and after treatment. The authors concluded that the reduction in hyperhidrosis could not be attributed to the treatment, possibly resulting from inadequate statistical power.

Aydin et al[27] researched axillary hair removal using a 1064 nm Nd:YAG laser in a 38-patient study. Patients received a total of 6- to 10-monthly treatments in both axillae until desirable hair removal results were achieved, at fluences and pulse durations suitable for skin type. Room temperature and time of day were controlled for in the study. Results were measured using the iodine–starch test before treatment as well as 1 month and 1 year after the final treatment. Total area with active sweating was recorded as number of active pixels in photos analyzed by computer. Additionally, a 10-point VAS was used to assess intensity of patient sweat production. Compared to the pretreatment values, a significant increase in sweat area was found 1 and 12 months after final treatment in both axillae. In the right axilla, involved area *increased* from 579.5 ± 1,582.5 before treatment to 8,822.5 ± 1,6761.8 at 1 month and 7,001.961 ± 12,688.3 at 12 months after final treatment. Left axilla values were 593.5 ± 1,140.4, 7,748.5 ± 1,4051.8, and 6,864.7 ± 11,056.9, respectively. VAS scores also increased from 4.55 ± 1.05 to 6.15 ± 1.66 at 1 month and 5.81 ± 1.37 at 12 months.

Hair reduction using a 1,064-nm Nd:YAG laser was also investigated by Letada et al[28] in six adults with severe hyperhidrosis unmanageable with standard treatments. One axilla was treated, whereas the other served as a control. The laser was prepared with a spot size of 12 mm and pulse duration of 20 ms, and fluences ranged from 24 to 56 J/cm², dependent on Fitzpatrick skin type. Five or six treatments were performed for each subject. The Global Assessment Questionnaire (GAQ) was used to assess efficacy on a scale of 0 to 3 based on level of improvement, as well as the starch–iodine test. Subjective improvement following each treatment and good to excellent subjective improvement 1 month after final treatment were reported. Significant changes in sweat gland density or morphology were not revealed by pre- and posttreatment histologic analysis.

Fractionated Microneedle Radiofrequency

Fractional microneedle radiofrequency (FMR) devices, traditionally used to reduce wrinkles, acne scars, and pores, utilize insulated microneedles to deliver energy to the deep dermis, where sweat glands are located, without destroying the epidermis. In a study by Kim et al,[29] 20 subjects with primary axillary hyperhidrosis were treated with two sessions of FMR treatment at 4-week intervals. The areas were treated with six passes each session, with the needles placed 0.5 to 3.5 mm below the skin surface. The HDSS and starch–iodine test were used to qualitatively measure severity, whereas transepidermal water loss (TEWL) was used to measure amount of sweat. Mean HDSS scores were 3.5, 1.5, 1.8, and 2.3 at baseline, 4 weeks after the first treatment, 4 weeks after the second treatment, and 8 weeks after the second treatment, respectively ($p < 0.05$ after repeated measures analysis of variance [ANOVA]). A decrease in TEWL was also observed after the first session, but an increase after the second and in the 2-month follow-up visit. The authors attributed this to environmental variations and damage to the epidermal barrier as a result of the device. Histological analysis of samples after the first treatment session demonstrated atrophy and necrosis of glands at high magnification. One month after the first session, a decrease in density and size of apocrine and eccrine glands compared to baseline was observed as well. The authors concluded that FMR causes direct heat damage to destroy sweat glands, effectively reducing hyperhidrosis.

Fatemi Naeini et al[30] tested FMR in 25 patients with severe primary axillary hyperhidrosis in a single-blind, sham-controlled comparative study. The patients went through three sessions of FMR at 3-week intervals at a depth of 2 to 3 mm below the skin with one axilla serving as the treatment side and the other serving as a sham control. The patients were evaluated at baseline and posttreatment at 3, 6, and 9 weeks and 3 months using the HDSS, a 10-point sweating intensity VAS (0 being no sweating to 10 being the worst), and a 6-point patient satisfaction measure. The follow-up evaluation revealed that 79% of the patients showed a decrease of 1 or 2 scores in HDSS. In total, 80% of patients reported more than 50% satisfaction at the end of the study. VAS sweating intensity score also decreased for the treatment side

at 21 weeks relative to that of control, with a mean score of 3.92 ± 1.31 vs. 8.44 ± 1.55 ($p < 0.001$). Histopathologic analyses 30 days after the last treatment corroborated those of Kim et al's, demonstrating atrophy and decrease in number of sweat glands, but the study did not provide quantitative information. A longer-term follow-up study at 1 year posttreatment[31] demonstrated significant difference in HDSS score in the treatment versus control side (mean score of 2.50 vs. 3.38; $p < 0.001$). Ten patients had no relapse after 1 year (41.6%), whereas 11 patients relapsed and 3 patients did not respond. One patient did not complete the long-term follow-up.

Schick et al[32] treated 30 adult patients with pronounced axillary hyperhidrosis using a microneedle fractional RF system for three treatments, spaced 6 weeks apart. After subcutaneous local anesthesia, the axillae were treated at a depth of 3 mm for two consecutive passes, followed by a single pass at 2-mm depth using a 5 × 5 array of noninsulated microneedles. Response was measured using the HDSS, DLQI, and gravimetry. Average HDSS score declined from 3.5 pretreatment to 2.1 at 6 months after the third session ($p < 0.05$). DLQI score improved from an average baseline level of 16 to a final level of 7 ($p < 0.05$). Gravimetry showed a reduction from 221 mg/min at baseline to a final level of 33 mg/min ($p < 0.05$).

19.5 Conclusion

Primary focal hyperhidrosis affects the quality of life for millions of people. However, a variety of pharmacological and device-based treatments exist to respond to this difficult condition. Although axillary hyperhidrosis is the most frequently studied, many options (which may be off-label) show promise to treat palmoplantar hyperhidrosis. Patient compliance, cost of materials and devices, and insurance coverage can be significant though not insurmountable problems. Patients should be made aware that treatment options include topical and oral medications, treatment with devices and injections. No cases of compensatory sweating have been reported in the studies of treatments mentioned (▶ Table 19.4). Microwave energy–based treatment remains the only FDA-cleared device-based treatment for axillary hyperhidrosis with the most experience among clinicians and should be considered the gold standard among the device-based treatments.

19.6 Pearls and Pitfalls

- Proper treatment modality as well as expectations should be discussed to ensure more successful and satisfactory results.
- Due to its efficacy in reducing axillary hyperhidrosis, use of microwave thermolysis of sweat glands in other

Table 19.4 Summary of studies

Study	Device tested	Study design	No. of subjects	Primary outcome measure(s)	Outcome
Nestor and Park[23]	Microfocused ultrasound w/ visualization	Two treatments in one axilla vs. sham treatments in other axilla	14	≥ 50% reduction in baseline spontaneous axillary sweat production measured gravimetrically on day 120	> 50% of subjects achieved the primary outcome measure
Nestor and Park[23]	Microfocused ultrasound w/ visualization	Two treatments in both axillae vs. two sham treatments in both axillae	20 (12 received treatment and 8 received sham)	Reduction in HDSS score by 2 points on day 60	67% response in the treatment group and 0% in the sham group
Leclère et al[24]	Minimally invasive laser (cannula introduced into subdermal space)	*Single treatment* Four groups: 975 nm alone 975/924 nm curettage alone 975/924 nm + curettage	102 25 in group 1, 26 in group 2, 26 in group 3, and 25 in group 4	HDSS, starch–iodine test (semi-quantitative 4 point scale), GAIS (Global Aesthetic Improvement Scale)	Summarized in ▶ Table 19.3
Goldman and Wollina[25]	Minimally invasive laser (300-µm optic fiber inserted into subdermal space)	Single treatment in bilateral axillae	17	Patient global assessment and physician global assessment	*Patient global assessment:* 12 subjects: "excellent" 3 subjects: "good" 2 subjects: "fair" *Physician global assessment:* 10 subjects: "excellent" 4 subjects: "good" 3 subjects: "fair"
Bechara et al[26]	800-nm diode laser	5 treatments in one axilla vs. untreated contralateral control	19	Gravimetry at 4 wk, patient evaluation of sweat reduction at 4 wk and 12 mo (VAS), and patient satisfaction at 4 wk and 12 mo (VAS)	**Gravimetry:** *Treated side:* 89 mg/min (range: 42–208) > 48 mg/min (17–119) at 4 wk *Untreated side:* 78 mg/min (range: 25–220) > 65 mg/min (rang: 24–399) at 4 wk *Subjective perception of reduction in hyperhidrosis:* 32.4% at 4 wk, 25% at 12 mo *Patient satisfaction:* 5.9 at 4 wk, 4.1 at 12 mo
Letada et al[28]	1,064-nm laser	5–6 treatment in one axilla vs. untreated contralateral control	6	Global assessment questionnaire (efficacy rated 0–3 for "poor," "fair," "good," and "excellent")	All patients reported some improvement after each treatment, and all reported good to excellent improvement at 1 mo after final treatment
Aydin et al[27]	1,064-nm laser	6–10 treatments in both axillae	38	Starch–iodine test and patient scoring using VAS. Measured at baseline and at 1 and 12 mo following treatment	Significant increase in sweating at 1 and 12 mo for both starch–iodine test and patient scoring

(Continued)

Table 19.4 (*Continued*) Summary of studies

Study	Device tested	Study design	No. of subjects	Primary outcome measure(s)	Outcome
Kim et al[29]	Fractionated microneedle radiofrequency	Two treatments separated by 4 wk	20	HDSS and TEWL (transepidermal water loss) at baseline, 4 wk after first treatment, 4 wk after second treatment, and 8 wk after second treatment	*HDSS* 3.5 (baseline) > 1.5 (4 wk after first treatment) > 1.8 (4 wk after second treatment) > 2.3 (8 wk after second treatment) *TEWL* Significant decrease at 4 wk, but steady rise thereafter
Fatemi Naeini et al[30]	Fractionated microneedle radiofrequency	Three treatments at 3-wk intervals in one axilla vs. sham treatment in contralateral control	25	HDSS at baseline, 3 wk, 6 wk, 9 wk, and 3 mo. Response defined as 2-point reduction in HDSS	*HDSS* Significant decrease in treatment vs. control starting after second treatment
Schick et al[32]	Fractionated microneedle radiofrequency	Three treatment sessions at 6-wk intervals	30	HDSS, DLQI, gravimetry at baseline and at 6 mo following third treatment	HDSS: 3.5 > 2.1 DLQI: 16 > 7 Gravimetry: 221 mg/min > 33 mg/min All $p < 0.05$

Abbreviations: DLQI, Dermatology Life Quality Index; HDSS, hyperhidrosis disease severity scale; VAS, visual analog scale.

areas has been investigated. Treatment of the groin area can be successful as an off-label use of this procedure.

- Treatment of hands and feet with microwave thermolysis should be avoided. Botulinum injections remain the treatment of choice for this area.
- Proper tumescent anesthesia of the treatment area renders the microwave thermolysis procedure virtually painless while protecting the underlying axillary plexus, increasing the margin of safety.
- A thorough patient history, as well as a clear understanding of medication instructions, is essential to avoid any adverse effects of pharmacologic treatments.
- Surgery may be considered as a final resort if other treatment options have been unsuccessful. These include surgical removal of sweat glands, and sympathectomy, which is the interruption of signals transmitted to the sweat glands through the cutting or destruction of certain nerves. However, all surgeries involve some risk, and can lead to permanent side effects.

References

[1] Walling HW. Clinical differentiation of primary from secondary hyperhidrosis. J Am Acad Dermatol. 2011; 64(4):690–695

[2] Schlereth T, Dieterich M, Birklein F. Hyperhidrosis: causes and treatment of enhanced sweating. Dtsch Arztebl Int. 2009; 106(3):32–37

[3] Miller JL. Diseases of the eccrine and apocrine sweat glands. In: Bolognia JL, Jorizzo JL, Schaffer JV, eds. Dermatology. 3rd ed. Philadelphia, PA: Elsevier; 2012

[4] Hornberger J, Grimes K, Naumann M, et al. Multi-Specialty Working Group on the Recognition, Diagnosis, and Treatment of Primary Focal Hyperhidrosis. Recognition, diagnosis, and treatment of primary focal hyperhidrosis. J Am Acad Dermatol. 2004; 51(2): 274–286

[5] Strutton DR, Kowalski JW, Glaser DA, Stang PE. US prevalence of hyperhidrosis and impact on individuals with axillary hyperhidrosis: results from a national survey. J Am Acad Dermatol. 2004; 51(2): 241–248

[6] Ricchetti-Masterson K, Symons JM, Aldridge M, et al. Epidemiology of hyperhidrosis in 2 population-based health care databases. J Am Acad Dermatol. 2018; 78(2):358–362

[7] Augustin M, Radtke MA, Herberger K, Kornek T, Heigel H, Schaefer I. Prevalence and disease burden of hyperhidrosis in the adult population. Dermatology. 2013; 227(1):10–13

[8] Liu Y, Bahar R, Kalia S, et al. Hyperhidrosis prevalence and demographic characteristics in dermatology outpatients in Shanghai and Vancouver. PLoS One. 2016; 11(4):e0153719

[9] Fujimoto T, Kawahara K, Yokozeki H. Epidemiological study and considerations of primary focal hyperhidrosis in Japan: from questionnaire analysis. J Dermatol. 2013; 40(11):886–890

[10] Kowalski JW, Eadie N, Dagget S, Lai P. Validity and reliability of the Hyperhidrosis Disease Severity Scale (HDSS). J Am Acad Dermatol. 2004; 50(3):51

[11] Stefaniak TJ, Proczko M. Gravimetry in sweating assessment in primary hyperhidrosis and healthy individuals. Clin Auton Res. 2013; 23(4):197–200

[12] Pariser DM, Ballard A. Topical therapies in hyperhidrosis care. Dermatol Clin. 2014; 32(4):485–490

[13] Hölzle E, Braun-Falco O. Structural changes in axillary eccrine glands following long-term treatment with aluminium chloride hexahydrate solution. Br J Dermatol. 1984; 110(4):399–403

[14] Hölzle E. Topical pharmacological treatment. Curr Probl Dermatol. 2002; 30:30–43

[15] Glaser DA, Hebert AA, Nast A, et al. Topical glycopyrronium tosylate for the treatment of primary axillary hyperhidrosis: results from the ATMOS-1 and ATMOS-2 phase 3 randomized controlled trials. J Am Acad Dermatol. 2019; 80(1):128–138.e2

[16] Doft MA, Hardy KL, Ascherman JA. Treatment of hyperhidrosis with botulinum toxin. Aesthet Surg J. 2012; 32(2):238–244

[17] Lowe NJ, Glaser DA, Eadie N, Daggett S, Kowalski JW, Lai PY, North American Botox in Primary Axillary Hyperhidrosis Clinical Study Group. Botulinum toxin type A in the treatment of primary axillary hyperhidrosis: a 52-week multicenter double-blind, randomized, placebo-controlled study of efficacy and safety. J Am Acad Dermatol. 2007; 56(4):604–611

[18] Naumann M, Lowe NJ. Botulinum toxin type A in treatment of bilateral primary axillary hyperhidrosis: randomised, parallel group, double blind, placebo controlled trial. BMJ. 2001; 323 (7313):596–599

[19] Walling HW. Systemic therapy for primary hyperhidrosis: a retrospective study of 59 patients treated with glycopyrrolate or clonidine. J Am Acad Dermatol. 2012; 66(3):387–392

[20] Glaser DA. Oral medications. Dermatol Clin. 2014; 32(4):527–532

[21] Johnson JE, O'Shaughnessy KF, Kim S. Microwave thermolysis of sweat glands. Lasers Surg Med. 2012; 44(1):20–25

[22] Glaser DA, Coleman WP, III, Fan LK, et al. A randomized, blinded clinical evaluation of a novel microwave device for treating axillary hyperhidrosis: the dermatologic reduction in underarm perspiration study. Dermatol Surg. 2012; 38(2):185–191

[23] Nestor MS, Park H. Safety and efficacy of micro-focused ultrasound plus visualization for the treatment of axillary hyperhidrosis. J Clin Aesthet Dermatol. 2014; 7(4):14–21

[24] Leclère FM, Moreno-Moraga J, Alcolea JM, et al. Efficacy and safety of laser therapy on axillary hyperhidrosis after one year follow-up: a randomized blinded controlled trial. Lasers Surg Med. 2015; 47(2):173–179

[25] Goldman A, Wollina U. Subdermal Nd:YAG laser for axillary hyperhidrosis. Dermatol Surg. 2008; 34(6):756–762

[26] Bechara FG, Georgas D, Sand M, et al. Effects of a long-pulsed 800-nm diode laser on axillary hyperhidrosis: a randomized controlled half-side comparison study. Dermatol Surg. 2012; 38(5):736–740

[27] Aydin F, Pancar GS, Senturk N, et al. Axillary hair removal with 1064-nm Nd:YAG laser increases sweat production. Clin Exp Dermatol. 2010; 35(6):588–592

[28] Letada PR, Landers JT, Uebelhoer NS, Shumaker PR. Treatment of focal axillary hyperhidrosis using a long-pulsed Nd:YAG 1064 nm laser at hair reduction settings. J Drugs Dermatol. 2012; 11(1):59–63

[29] Kim M, Shin JY, Lee J, Kim JY, Oh SH. Efficacy of fractional microneedle radiofrequency device in the treatment of primary axillary hyperhidrosis: a pilot study. Dermatology. 2013; 227(3):243–249

[30] Fatemi Naeini F, Abtahi-Naeini B, Pourazizi M, Nilforoushzadeh MA, Mirmohammadkhani M. Fractionated microneedle radiofrequency for treatment of primary axillary hyperhidrosis: a sham control study. Australas J Dermatol. 2015; 56(4):279–284

[31] Abtahi-Naeini B, Naeini FF, Saffaei A, et al. Treatment of primary axillary hyperhidrosis by fractional microneedle radiofrequency: is it still effective after long-term follow-up? Indian J Dermatol. 2016; 61(2):234

[32] Schick CH, Grallath T, Schick KS, Hashmonai M. Radiofrequency thermotherapy for treating axillary hyperhidrosis. Dermatol Surg. 2016; 42(5):624–630

20 Thread Lifts

David J. Goldberg and Lindsey Yeh

Summary

Thread lifts have been used to provide a minimally invasive facelift for many years. The effectiveness, patient satisfaction, and side effect profile improved with the introduction of absorbable sutures. We review the long-term outcomes, effectiveness, and benefits of thread lifts and discuss identifying the best candidates and surgical techniques for thread lifts.

Keywords: barbed sutures, facelift, thread lift, antiaging, wrinkles/rhytides, rhytidectomy, jowls, marionette lines, absorbable suture lift, noninvasive lift

20.1 Introduction

Signs of aging are the result of several natural changes and environmental exposures that occur over time. Early signs of aging are due to loss of elasticity and collagen, although exposure to ultraviolet (UV) light leads to discoloration and decreased quality of skin over time. Thinning of subcutaneous fat, shifting fat pads, bone loss that manifests as skin laxity all lead to the appearance of skin laxity resulting in brow ptosis, deepening nasolabial folds, and jowl formation. The gold standard for treating skin laxity today is still rhytidectomies; however, the number of facelifts performed each year has been steadily decreasing. Between 2016 and 2017, the number of facelifts decreased by 4 and 6% since 2000, whereas the number of noninvasive procedures has increased dramatically.[1] This reflects increasing demand for and availability of minimally invasive cosmetic procedures such as filler, thread lifts, and energy-based devices. Patients prefer procedures that are more affordable with minimal pain, risks, recovery, and downtime. For comprehensive facial rejuvenation, a multifaceted approach is usually necessary. Thread lifts have become a viable option to safely improve the appearance of ptotic skin with minimal recovery time and are safe to use in conjunction with other cosmetic treatments.

Dr. Gregory Ruff and Dr. Marlen Sulamanidze first introduced the use of thread lifting for suspension separately in the late 1990s.[2] The concept of barbed sutures was first pioneered by Alcamo in 1964 to close wounds without the need to tie knots. In 1997, Sulamanidze created a barbed polypropylene thread designed to keep the tissue from sagging and aptly named the thread APTOS for antiptosis threads.[2] In 1999, Ruff cut barbs into polydioxanone (PDO) sutures (Ethicon Inc., Somerville, New Jersey, United States) and used it to lift brows, faces, and necks for cosmetic purposes.[2] He patented a cannulated device for single direction and later bidirectional insertion in 1994 and 2001, respectively.[3,4] Subsequently, Wu and Isse made alterations and new designs of threads by increasing the number of barbs and the direction the barbs pointed.[2] In 2004, the U.S. Food and Drug Administration (FDA) approved barbed sutures for aesthetic purposes.[2] FDA approval was quickly retracted in 2007 due to complications and patient dissatisfaction. Despite the loss of FDA clearance, thread lifts continued to grow in popularity among patients and practitioners. The use of thread lifts shifted with the introduction of resorbable sutures and more specifically the Silhouette Soft. This was introduced in Europe in 2013, which has guided the design for the now popular Silhouette Instalift (London, United Kingdom), which was approved for midface suspension in 2015.[5]

20.2 Modalities/Treatment Options Available

A variety of absorbable and nonabsorbable materials have been employed when designing thread lifts. Materials that are commonly used for threads include gold, poly-l-lactic acid, caprolactone, polypropylene, and PDO. Barbs are cut into the sutures in both unidirectional and bidirectional patterns. Some are designed with absorbable cones, which provide the ability to grip the tissue in all directions. The barbs are characterized by the depth and angle of the barbs. Decreasing the degree of the angle increases the tensile and holding strength. Bidirectional sutures have barbs in both directions and are self-anchoring. This eliminates the need to secure a knot, whereas unidirectional sutures need to be looped and secured. The Silhouette InstaLift uses a unique suture with cones oriented in a bidirectional pattern (▶ Fig. 20.1a, b). For the past three decades, thread lifts have undergone multiple evolutions and a number of techniques have been described. However, there is no clear consensus regarding the type of suture that provides the best traction and long-term outcomes.[6] Currently available thread lifts are listed in ▶ Table 20.1. The table is not comprehensive and is changing as new developments occur.

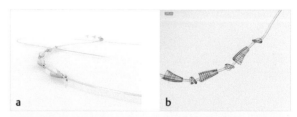

Fig. 20.1 (a) The Silhouette InstaLift absorbable suture and cones composed of 18% poly lactic-co-glycolic acid (PLGA) and 82% poly-L-lactic acid (PLLA). **(b)** Close-up view of the silhouette InstaLift absorbable suture and cones.

Table 20.1 Types of thread lifts

Thread	Suture type	Absorbable or nonabsorbable	Suture design
Aptos Thread	Polypropylene Polylactic acid Caprolactone	Nonabsorbable Absorbable Absorbable	Variable depending on area of treatment
Contour Thread Lift System	2–0 polypropylene	Nonabsorbable	25-cm length, central 10-cm segment of 50 unidirectional helicoidally configured barbs
Promo Italia Happy Lift	Polylactic caprolactone	Absorbable	Bidirectional barbs
Isse Endo Progressive Face Lift	2–0 polypropylene	Nonabsorbable	25-cm length, distal 10 cm containing 50 unidirectional barbs
NovaThreads	Polydioxanone	Absorbable	Smooth, twist, and barb threads
Silhouette InstaLift	82% poly-L lactic acid (PLLA), 18% poly lactic-co-glycolic acid (PLGA)	Absorbable	26.8- to 30-cm long with 12-cm 34-gauge needle on each end, bidirectionally oriented cones with a 2-cm space in the middle, 8- and 12-cone sutures available

Thread lifts offer a safe, minimally invasive tissue lifting, for repositioning and contouring the face and neck. It effectively improves uneven skin texture, slack midface, and minimal-to-moderate jowls. It can safely be used in combination with other cosmetic treatment modalities such as neuromodulators, fillers, microneedling, and energy-based devices. Off-label uses include use off the face and neck such as the abdomen, knees, and buttocks. It serves as a treatment option for those who do not wish to undergo a surgical facelift or neck lift. However, it does not replace a rhytidectomy. Expectations of the patient must be tempered and made clear that lifting benefits of this procedure are temporary and additional procedures will be needed in the future whether it is touch-ups or another surgical procedure. Patients will be disappointed if they expect the outcome of a thread lift to be comparable to a traditional surgical facelift.

20.3 Clinical Outcomes

The number of studies describing the benefits and outcome of thread lifts is somewhat limited; however, the studies that are available do support the effectiveness and benefits of thread lifts, while demonstrating a good safety profile. Lycka et al followed 350 female patients treated with barbed monofilament polypropylene produced by Aptos in both 3–0 and 2–0 suture sizes of various lengths. Of the 350 participants, 198 (57%) reported 80 to 100% reduction of ptosis, whereas 97 patients (28%) had a 60 to 80% reduction in ptosis and 47 patients had a 40 to 60% correction. One hundred and seventeen of the patients were followed for 12 to 24 months.[7] Seventy percent maintained their initial correction as determined by blinded photographic assessment.[7]

Ninety-six participants were followed for 3 years and maintained 60% of their initial correction.[7]

An early review of barbed sutures in 2008 primarily reviewed Aptos threads, Isse Endo Progressive Face Lift Sutures, and contour threads. The review found barbed sutures to be a promising, minimally invasive technique, but further research was still needed to clarify the long-term benefits and outcomes.[8] Gülbitti et al felt that not much had changed 11 years later, still citing that there was little to no substantial evidence supporting the effectiveness of thread lift sutures over the years.[9] The interest in thread lifts still remains high particularly due to the shift in focus from using nonabsorbable threads to designing thread lifts with absorbable sutures. This change has come largely due to the number of adverse events and because people were uncomfortable with the idea of having a permanent foreign body in their face. Recent studies on absorbable threads has been promising demonstrating effectiveness in improving laxity, high patient satisfaction, and good safety profile.

A study using two different types of absorbable threads (polylactic caprolactone and polylactic acid) were used to treat the jawline, midface, brows, and neck.[10] Two surgeons assessed the results and the patients based on the global aesthetic improvement scale (GAIS) score at 1 week, 1 month, 3 months, and 6 months.[10] Patient satisfaction level was highest at 6 months after the surgery with 99% of the patients reporting high or good satisfaction.[10] The surgeons rating GAIS scores also reported steadily increasing improvement from week 1 to month 6.[10] There was no follow-up beyond the 6-month period for this particular study. A separate study evaluating outcomes of Silhouette Instalift reported reduced lift at 12 months.[11] However,

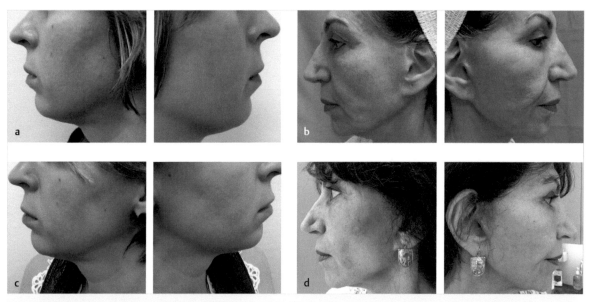

Fig. 20.2 (a–d) Pre- and posttreatment with Silhouette InstaLift. (These images are provided courtesy of Dr. Ron Shelton.)

patients continued to report a benefit distinct from lifting. The poly-L lactic acid (PLLA) induces a foreign body response and promotes collagen synthesis. As the physical lifting capacity of the suture itself diminishes, the new collagen provides re-volumization. Subjects described ongoing changes as "recontouring" and also noted remarkable changes in skin quality for 18 to 24 months after placement of the sutures[11] (▶ Fig. 20.2a, b). The improvement was reflected by both the investigator and subject in their GAIS and FACE-Q scores. At 12 months, there was ongoing improvement in patient satisfaction and patients generally did not require retreatment for 12 to 18 months.[11]

In a prospective study of 100 patients who underwent treatment of laxity in the face and neck with absorbable sutures only, 62% of the patients had 8 cone threads placed in the midface, 54% of the patients had 8 cone threads placed along the jawline, and 33% of patients had 12 cone threads placed in the neck.[12] Patient completed surveys regarding their general experience with the procedure, and photographs were evaluated both pre- and postprocedure both at 2 weeks and at 3- and 6-month follow-ups.[12] The Allergan Photometric Midface Volume Deficit Scale was used to assess pre- and postprocedure improvement. On average, facial volume deficits improved by 1 degree on the scale. Sixty-four patients (70.3%) experienced 1 degree of improvement, 12 patients (13.2%) experienced 2 degrees of improvement, and no patients experienced more than 2 degrees of improvement. Patients reported an overall satisfaction rate with absorbable suture suspension of 79%, with 83% reporting improvements in age-related changes and 82% being willing to recommend the procedure.[12]

Thread lifts are effective as a primary treatment for skin laxity, but superior results in lifting and patient satisfaction were found when thread lifts were used in combination with filler and neurotoxin. Abraham et al performed a retrospective review of patients who underwent a thread lift procedure with the Contour Thread lift system alone or in combination with procedures including lipotransfer, chemical peels, and/or rhytidectomies.[13] Aesthetic improvement scores were determined by four independent, blinded, board-certified facial plastic surgeons. Aesthetic improvement was deemed to be significantly better when thread lifts were combined with other procedures than when used alone.[13]

Combination treatments (filler/platelet-rich plasma [PRP]/onabotulinumtoxin A) with absorbable PDO sutures were also rated most highly in outcomes and patient satisfaction when compared to thread lift alone or filler/PRP/onabotulinumtoxin A only.[14] The combination group had the highest degree of lifting immediately and up to 24 months after treatment.[14] Immediately after the full treatment, all 100% of the patients reported a 6- to 10-mm lift.[14] By 24 months, the majority of the patients' lift had decreased to 3- to 6-mm lifts, but still saw changes.[14] The lifting score in this group peaked at 3 months when 76% of the patients had greater than 6- to 10-mm lifts.[14] Thread lifts alone were still superior to the filler/PRP/neurotoxin-only group.[14] The group that was not treated with any thread lifts showed no measurable skin lifting after just 6 months.[14] Even immediately after the procedures, patients only reported a 1- to 2-mm lift.[14] Immediately after the thread lifts, only 81% had a greater than 6- to 10-mm lift. This score improved to 100% at 3- and 6-month follow-ups.[14] After 2 years, 33.3% of the patients had a 3- to 6-mm lift, but the majority (57%) showed only a 1- to 2-mm lift.[14] Thread lifts used simultaneously with other treatments had the best short- and long-term outcomes when compared to thread lifts alone, with no increased adverse events.[14]

20.4 Histopathologic Findings

As demonstrated by the studies, absorbable thread lifts show long-term improvement in skin laxity, but it wanes with time. The procedure itself results in a high patient satisfaction rate.[15] Patient assessment of improvement was found to be greater than those of physicians. Even after the lifting benefits of thread lifts have waned, there is continued improvement of the texture and quality of the overlying skin.[15,16] This is supported by histopathological evidence suggesting the threads stimulate collagen and fibrosis formation.[17] A thick fibrous shell was seen around the permanent threads when Sulamanidze treated his patients with rhytidoplasty 1 to 1.5 years after initial placement of Aptos threads.[18] The threads remained situated in the areas they were initially placed without any changes to the structure of the thread itself suggesting that PLLA induces a foreign body response that promotes collagen synthesis.[18]

Animal models treated with synthetic absorbable threads had fibrous sheaths at 1 and 3 months after implantation.[19] The capsule consists of fibroblasts, extracellular collagen, inflammatory cells, and neovascularization.[20,21] After 7 months, the fibrous sheath was replaced by connective tissue and the tissue continued to produce collagen even after absorption.[19,21] Dermal layers directly above the threads had components of dense collagen and increase in collagen type I and transforming growth factor-β1 (TGF-β1).[19] PDO and PLA threads produced collagen (Col1α1, Col1α3) at 2 weeks after insertion. PDO threads produced more Col1α3 at 2 weeks than PLA threads. Multiple PDO filaments produced more collagen than spring type PDO.[19] In a recent study, biopsies of patients treated with PLLA/PGLA absorbable suspension sutures were taken at 1, 90, and 180 days. The biopsies showed progressive increase of collagen type I and III expression[16] (▶ Fig. 20.3a, b).

20.5 Adverse Events

Swelling and erythema are the common side effects of thread lift procedures. Lycka et al's study demonstrated effective lifting with polypropylene Aptos sutures and found that 42.9 and 13.7% of the patients reported edema and erythema, respectively.[7] All cases resolved without additional intervention. Fifty patients reported mild discomfort that resolved with nonsteroidal anti-inflammatory drugs (NSAIDs). Fifty-two procedures (15%) required touch-ups with additional threads or removal, but the authors found that the need for correction sharply declined with experience.[7] Two of the 350 patients did request

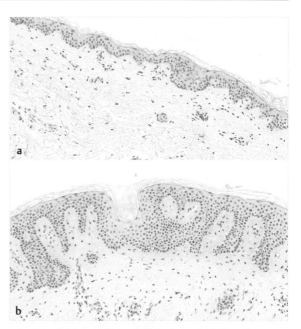

Fig. 20.3 (a) Human dermis before placement of the Silhouette InstaLift. **(b)** Increase of collagen in the dermis can be seen 6 months after placement of Silhouette Instalift.

removal because they did not like the outcome.[7] More troublesome complications such as visible threads, dimpling, and asymmetry were also reported.[7] Approximately 3% of the patients required the insertion of additional threads to treat asymmetry.[7] The frequency of dimpling ranged from 3.5 to 27.5%,[7,22,23] and 5 to 34% reported palpable threads.[22,23] Rachel et al reported three cases of paresthesias, whereas other studies did not report any cases.[22]

Although both absorbable and nonabsorbable threads have been demonstrated to be safe, the number of minor adverse events was off-putting to practitioners and consumers, which is what partially prompted the loss of FDA clearance in 2007 and the shift to the use of absorbable threads. Bruising and tumefaction are still the primary adverse outcomes with absorbable threads. The frequency of periprocedural edema ranged from 43.3 to 100%.[12,15,19] After 100 patients were treated with the Silhouette Instalift, there were no signs of dimpling, excessive skin bunching, or any complaints of palpability of cones at 1 week postprocedure.[12] Twenty of these patients were not satisfied with the improvement they saw after the procedure.[12] All of the inadequate responders were for neck concerns, and 16 underwent two additional suture placements.[12] The neck seems to be a difficult area to treat with thread lifts and multiple studies have found that the neck requires the most touch-up procedures.[10,12] Rezaee Khiabanloo et al found that pain was reported by 5.9% of patients and most commonly in the neck when compared to the jawline, midface, and eyebrow.[10] Dimpling was reported in 32.4% of patients, but least frequently reported in the neck. The frequency of asymmetry ranged from 0.6 to 6.5%.[10,24] Overall, patient survey results indicate that absorbable suture suspension was reported as tolerable in 96% of patients and manageable in 89% with mild pain that was manageable with acetaminophen.[12] The issues of paresthesias and thread extrusion seen with nonabsorbable sutures are not common with absorbable sutures. Although there is the theoretical risk of more severe adverse outcomes with thread lifts, these are not commonly reported in the literature.

20.6 Patient Selection

20.6.1 Good Candidates

As with any procedure, selecting the appropriate patient and setting patient expectations are crucial to achieving the best outcome and highest degree of patient satisfaction. The ideal candidate for thread lifts is a patient who does not have significant wrinkles or much redundant skin, but does have skin laxity such as visible marionette lines, nasolabial folds, jowls, and/or loss of definition along the mandibular border. The laxity requires tissue repositioning beyond what can be achieved by revolumization alone. Patients with excessive laxity or redundant skin would be better served with a rhytidectomy, but patients often wish to delay or are unwilling to undergo invasive procedures. Patients who previously underwent rhytidectomies are good candidates and thread lifts can serve as an easy touch-up or maintenance treatment. Strong underlying bone projects are needed to support the elevated tissue. The quality of the overlying skin is also crucial for good outcomes. Good skin quality and adequate thickness are necessary to prevent palpability of the sutures and visible implants.

20.6.2 Poor Candidates

Patients who are too thin and have no underlying fat or have excessive laxity and/or subcutaneous tissue would make poor candidates for thread lifts. Skin that is too thin, very thick, or immobile would not benefit from thread lifts. These qualities limit the ability of the sutures to lift the skin adequately. Thread lifts are not indicated for treatment of significant photoaging or very prominent wrinkles. For patients who may have excessive laxity that requires a facelift, if the patient prefers not to undergo invasive procedures, thread lifts can still be performed, but setting realistic expectations of the improvement that can be achieved.

20.6.3 Setting Expectations

Different manufacturers of threads claim different durations of results. Silhouette Instalift claims long-term results lasting up to 2 years. Novathreads state that the simulation of collagen synthesis and the skin structures created will hold for 12 to 15 months. Some manufacturers have claimed the duration of results for up to 5 years. In clinical practice, an estimation of continued lift of about 1 to 2 years, with further improvement of skin quality, is a realistic expectation to give to the patient. Duration and results of the treatment will vary depending on the degree of laxity of the patient prior to treatment, the number and type of threads used, as well as the location the threads are placed in. Patients should also be advised that the improvement is a natural and sometimes subtle lift and is not meant to replace the results that could be achieved with a surgical procedure.

20.7 Contraindications

There are relatively few contraindications for thread lifts. The procedure should not be performed when there is an active infection or in patients who are pregnant or nursing. It is contraindicated in those with a known allergy to the suture material, hemophilia, autoimmune diseases, and oncological diseases. Caution should be exercised in those at high risk of developing keloids.

20.7.1 Preoperative Instructions

Once a patient has been deemed a good candidate for thread lifts, patients should be advised to schedule the procedure at least 2 weeks before any important events. The procedure itself is an in-office procedure that takes less than an hour. Patients can resume normal daily activities, but will have swelling and bruising that can take up to 1 week to resolve. To minimize the risk of bruising, any unnecessary medications or supplements that increase the risk of bruising and bleeding (i.e., ibuprofen, aspirin, vitamin E, fish oil, ginkgo, St. Johns wort, etc.) should be stopped at least 1 week prior. It is not necessary to stop any medications that are medically needed.

If a patient has a history of cold sores, prophylactic valacyclovir should be started the day before the procedure and continued for 5 to 10 days. Dental procedures should be avoided 2 weeks before and after the thread lift. To ease any anxiety the day of the procedure, anxiolytics can be prescribed and taken 30 to 60 minutes before the procedure, but is typically not necessary. If anxiolytics are prescribed and taken, transportation after the procedure needs to be arranged beforehand.

20.8 Technique

Marking and measurement of the desired treatment area should be completed while the patient is in a fully upright position. The procedure itself is most easily performed while the patient is seated at a 45-degree angle. After the mobility of the skin is assessed, the insertion and exit points of the thread should be marked in a straight-line vector and placed perpendicular to the plane it is intended to elevate. The track the suture will take does not need to be marked. Typically, the exit point should be placed 1.5 cm past the point that one is attempting to lift. Each suture has one entry site in the middle of the vector and two exit sites at each distal end.

Multiple techniques for anchoring the threads have been described depending on the type of thread and location being treated. Use of linear, horizontal, and even U- and V-shaped vectors have been described, but straight-line vector planning (SLVP) has been found to provide maximal lifting capacity and longevity compared to the other methods. The placement of curved sutures undermines the design of the device and limits the lifting capacity of the sutures, leading to poor results. Placement of the suture should be perpendicular to the plane that is being elevated.

Although the treatment should be individualized for each patient, a minimum of three to four sutures per side of the midface is recommended for moderate-to-severe laxity and two to three sutures are recommended for mild-to-moderate laxity. Additional sutures can be placed along the jawline to address jowls. An adequate number of sutures are critical to providing good outcomes and enough support to advance the tissue and to stimulate collagen synthesis.

The skin should be thoroughly cleansed by removing all makeup, followed by hibiclens and alcohol or hypochlorous acid. Local anesthesia (lidocaine 1–2% with epinephrine) is administered intradermally to the entry and exit points. No anesthesia is needed in any other areas. The needles and thread come with two guiding needles attached at the center by the suture. An 18-gauge needle is inserted into an entry point to provide an opening for the insertion of the needle attached to the sutures. The needle is inserted perpendicularly at the entry point at a 5-mm depth. There is a marking at the tip of the needle to indicate the correct depth at which the needle should enter the skin to reach the ideal plane. Once the desired depth is reached, the needle is turned at a 90-degree angle and advanced in the subcutaneous plane above the superficial musculoaponeurotic system (SMAS) followed by the thread. There should be no significant resistance and patients should not experience any pain. Any pain or discomfort during the procedure is a sign that the needle is in the wrong plane and can be adjusted by slowly backing the needle until it is in the proper plane. Continue to advance the needle until the exit point is reached. A needle cap can be held above the marked exit point to catch the needle and minimize the risk of needle sticks. The thread is pulled through the exit point and countertraction is provided from the entry point. The same steps are repeated in the opposite direction through the same entry point. There should be no dimpling if the sutures are in the correct plane. After the suture is in place, apply tension to the inferior portion of the suture and advance the tissue over the cones in the desired direction. Massage the tissue over the superior cones to fully elevate the tissue.

Slowly adjust the tissue over the sutures as needed. Any puckering or gathering of tissue should resolve within 2 to 3 days. The protruding suture should be cut with suture scissors flush with the skin.

20.9 Postoperative Instructions

Apply ice to the treated areas for 30 minutes after the procedure and for 15 minutes three to four times a day for 48 hours after the treatment to minimize edema and pain. Caution should be advised to apply the ice gently. Patients often apply excessive pressure when icing and disrupt the suture. Petroleum-based ointments or silicone gels can be applied to the puncture sites. Patients may gently wash their face or apply makeup 24 hours after treatment. When leaving the office, the patients will have mild swelling and erythema.

20.10 Potential Complications and How to Manage

Patients may experience some degree of pain, swelling, temporary asymmetry, transient dimpling, ripples, bruising/hematoma, and inflammation. All these symptoms will resolve with time. Although the overall procedure is less invasive than a facelift, the downtime can potentially be longer than anticipated because it can take up to 2 weeks for the dimpling to resolve.

Swelling, erythema, and bruising are experienced by the majority of patients. Bruising and swelling can be easily managed with icing and is self-limiting. Less than half of the patients have erythema and this typically resolves in a week.[7,15] Other side effects include mild pain or soreness and skin dimpling. Studies have shown up to one-third of the patients experience dimpling and pain. Any discomfort is usually relieved with oral NSAIDs or acetaminophen. Narcotics are typically not needed. Skin dimpling resolves within 1 to 2 weeks if it does not, this may require soft-tissue massage, subcision, calcium hydroxylapatite injection lipoaugmentation or removal of the suture. Mild asymmetry has been reported in 6% of cases that were self-limited or were easily corrected.[15,25] The rate of complications was similar with the use of absorbable and nonabsorbable sutures.[10] Interestingly, females were significantly more likely to develop ecchymosis and dimples than men, but were not correlated with the site of lifting.[10]

Suture breakage is uncommon, but if this occurs, the suture can be left in place and replaced. Although allergic reactions, sensory/nerve injury, chronic pain, and infections are all potential complications, there are not many reports of these adverse events. There have been reports of partial extrusion of a polypropylene thread after facial rejuvenation with barbed suture lifting by Rachel at al.[22] Threads can be gently pulled out if one end of the thread is visible. If the thread is not visible, use of ultrasonography or a bright overhead light can help locate the thread and a small punch excision or blade overlying the tissue uncovers the thread allowing for easier removal.

The likelihood of side effects increased with the number of sutures that were placed. Experts also found that the number of adverse events declined with experience. Icing the treated areas and sleeping with two pillows at night for 1 week can help minimize swelling. Taking oral analgesics and prednisone can help with minor pain and swelling but are not needed regularly. There have been reported incidences of threads breaking from pressure and impact to the face. Patients should be advised to avoid rigorous application of makeup, cleansing, chewing, and distorting facial expressions such as grimacing or yawning for 1 week postprocedure. Patients should sleep on their back for a week and avoid face-down massages, dental procedures, and high -impact exercises for 2 weeks.

20.11 Combination Therapy

Treatment with a multifaceted approach will best address laxity that most patients who seek out or who are candidates for thread lifts have. This will result in the most dramatic and natural-appearing results. Laxity of skin is due to a combination of loss of collagen and elasticity in the skin as well as loss of volume. To address the issue of volume, treatments with dermal fillers or fat transfers will also provide additional subtle lift to the tissue in addition to thread lifts as well as restoring more youthful contours. Fillers can be placed the same day as thread lifts. It is suggested the filler be placed first as potential swelling from the thread lift may distort assessment of the face prior to treatment with fillers.

Neurotoxins can be injected in areas that are not being treated with threads on the same day. The concern is for diffusion of the neurotoxin to undesired areas leading to unwanted effects. To further address laxity, there are other noninvasive treatments that deliver radiofrequency or ultrasound energy into the skin to stimulate collagen production and contraction. These should not be performed immediately after a thread lift due to local anesthesia potentially interfering with the treatment.

20.12 Pearls and Pitfalls

Selecting a good candidate and setting patient expectations are crucial for a positive outcome for both the provider and the patient. Assessing the treatment area and placing the adequate number of sutures on each side of the area to fully lift and support the lax skin are crucial. Finding the proper depth to place the suture will allow

for seamless placement of the threads. As the studies have supported, using thread lifts in conjunction with other rejuvenation treatments significantly improves patient satisfaction. Touch-up treatments may be needed shortly after the procedure or years after the initial procedure.

20.13 Conclusion

The technology and design of thread lifts have been evolving and improving since its introduction 30 years ago. Thread lifts were previously criticized for the paucity of veracious studies evaluating the effectiveness and long-term outcomes of thread lifts. This has changed more recently with the more controlled and measured evaluations of absorbable threads. The adverse events are minor, primarily swelling and erythema with some asymmetry that is either self-limiting or can be easily corrected with the placement of additional threads. Otherwise, the risks are low and have demonstrated high patient satisfaction and long-term improvement of the quality of skin.

References

[1] American Society of Plastic Surgeons. 2017 Plastic Surgery Statistics Report. 2017. Available at: https://www.plasticsurgery.org/documents/News/Statistics/2017/plastic-surgery-statistics-report-2017.pdf. Accessed November 5, 2018

[2] Ruff GL. Inserting device for a barbed tissue connector. US patent 5,342,376. August 30, 1994

[3] Ruff GL. Barbed bodily tissue connector. US patent 6,241,747 B1. June 5, 2001

[4] Ruff GL. The history of barbed sutures. Aesthet Surg J. 2013; 33(3) Suppl:12S–16S

[5] Food and Drug Administration. FORM FDA 3881. Available at: https://www.accessdata.fda.gov/cdrh_docs/pdf14/K142061.pdf. Accessed November 15, 2018

[6] Park TH, Seo SW, Whang KW. Facial rejuvenation with fine-barbed threads: the simple Miz lift. Aesthetic Plast Surg. 2014; 38(1):69–74

[7] Lycka B, Bazan C, Poletti E, Treen B. The emerging technique of the antiptosis subdermal suspension thread. Dermatol Surg. 2004; 30(1):41–44, discussion 44

[8] Villa MT, White LE, Alam M, Yoo SS, Walton RL. Barbed sutures: a review of the literature. Plast Reconstr Surg. 2008; 121(3):102e–108e

[9] Gülbitti HA, Colebunders B, Pirayesh A, Bertossi D, van der Lei B. Thread-lift sutures: still in the lift? A systematic review of the literature. Plast Reconstr Surg. 2018; 141(3):341e–347e

[10] Rezaee Khiabanloo S, Jebreili R, Aalipour E, et al. Outcomes in thread lift for face and neck: a study performed with Silhouette Soft and Promo Happy Lift double needle, innovative and classic techniques. J Cosmet Dermatol. 2019; 18(1):84–93

[11] Mark Nestor MD. PhD; Personal Communication

[12] Ogilvie MP, Few JW, Jr, Tomur SS, et al. Rejuvenating the face: an analysis of 100 absorbable suture suspension patients. Aesthet Surg J. 2018; 38(6):654–663

[13] Abraham RF, DeFatta RJ, Williams EF, III. Thread-lift for facial rejuvenation: assessment of long-term results. Arch Facial Plast Surg. 2009; 11(3):178–183

[14] Ali YH. Two years' outcome of thread lifting with absorbable barbed PDO threads: Innovative score for objective and subjective assessment. J Cosmet Laser Ther. 2018; 20(1):41–49

[15] Suh DH, Jang HW, Lee SJ, Lee WS, Ryu HJ. Outcomes of polydioxanone knotless thread lifting for facial rejuvenation. Dermatol Surg. 2015; 41(6):720–725

[16] David J. Goldberg, MD, JD; Personal communication

[17] Shimizu Y, Terase K. Thread lift with absorbable monofilament threads. J Japan Soc Aesthetic Plast Surg. 2013; 35(2):1–12

[18] Sulamanidze MA, Fournier PF, Paikidze TG, Sulamanidze GM. Removal of facial soft tissue ptosis with special threads. Dermatol Surg. 2002; 28(5):367–371

[19] Kim J, Zheng Z, Kim H, Nam KA, Chung KY. Investigation on the cutaneous change induced by face-lifting monodirectional barbed polydioxanone thread. Dermatol Surg. 2017; 43(1):74–80

[20] Kurita M, Matsumoto D, Kato H, et al. Tissue reactions to cog structure and pure gold in lifting threads: a histological study in rats. Aesthet Surg J. 2011; 31(3):347–351

[21] Jang HJ, Lee WS, Hwang K, Park JH, Kim DJ. Effect of cog threads under rat skin. Dermatol Surg. 2005; 31(12):1639–1643, discussion 1644

[22] Rachel JD, Lack EB, Larson B. Incidence of complications and early recurrence in 29 patients after facial rejuvenation with barbed suture lifting. Dermatol Surg. 2010; 36(3):348–354

[23] Wu WT. Barbed sutures in facial rejuvenation. Aesthet Surg J. 2004; 24(6):582–587

[24] de Benito J, Pizzamiglio R, Theodorou D, Arvas L. Facial rejuvenation and improvement of malar projection using sutures with absorbable cones: surgical technique and case series. Aesthetic Plast Surg. 2011; 35(2):248–253

[25] Savoia A, Accardo C, Vannini F, Di Pasquale B, Baldi A. Outcomes in thread lift for facial rejuvenation: a study performed with happy lift™ revitalizing. Dermatol Ther (Heidelb). 2014; 4(1):103–114

21 Cosmeceuticals

Emily C. Murphy and Adam Friedman

Summary

This chapter discusses the mechanism, stability, topical penetration, and supporting clinical evidence of common cosmeceutical ingredients. The stability and penetration data for these ingredients were gathered under controlled laboratory conditions. Given these products will be exposed to oxygen during application and may be stored in nonideal conditions, the shelf lives are likely lower than advertised. Use of niacin, the peptide palmitoyl-lysine-threonine-threonine-lysine-serine (Pal-KTTKS), and some growth factors in clinical trials produced only small improvements in wrinkles, so their costs may outweigh the benefits. Oral collagen may improve wrinkles based on preliminary evidence, but over-the-counter products are diverse and may not have adequate quantity of active collagen peptides. Two retinoid derivatives, retinaldehyde and retinol, demonstrated more substantial antiwrinkle effects, but their efficacy may still be lower than prescription retinoids. On the contrary, retinoid esters were not effective in reducing wrinkles but can concentrate in the epidermis, offering protection from ultraviolet (UV) induced deoxyribonucleic acid (DNA) damage. Other agents that were efficacious in reducing photodamage include DNA repair enzymes and the antioxidants, vitamin C, vitamin E, and ferulic acid, in combination. These agents that protect the skin from DNA damage may be useful additions to moisturizers and sunscreens to reduce the risk of photoaging. Azelaic acid and hydroquinone both reduce hyperpigmentation in randomized, controlled trials and are recommended as first-line therapies. However, hydroquinone may be more beneficial in prescription formulations than over-the-counter products. Overall, some cosmeceuticals have evidence substantiating their claims, but many other product claims are unfounded. Patients may benefit from consulting their dermatologists for guidance on how to best treat their cosmetic needs rather than spending time and money determining which cosmeceuticals are effective.

Keywords: cosmeceutical, topical penetration, retinoids, hydroquinone, kojic acid, tranexamic acid, DNA repair enzymes, oral collagen, azelaic acid, curcumin

21.1 Introduction

Cosmeceuticals are nonprescription products with active ingredients that benefit the skin's appearance or function.[1,2] Many patients have turned to cosmeceuticals to avoid invasive procedures or prescriptions that require doctor appointments and insurance coverage hurdles, and in turn companies responded to this interest, offering a range of products. However, despite the claims made by these products, many provide little to no benefit. For a product to be effective, the active ingredient must remain stable in storage, penetrate the stratum corneum (SC), and reach adequate concentrations in the skin to produce its intended effect. In this chapter, we will discuss the stability and topical penetration of common cosmeceutical ingredients, and we will highlight clinical trials and animal studies examining the efficacy of these ingredients. All results reported as statistically significant have a *p* value of ≤ 0.05 compared to control. Many commonly used ingredients such as resveratrol, phloretin, and honey were excluded given the lack of published, peer-reviewed articles on these ingredients. Instead, this chapter will focus only on ingredients with published evidence-based information. Further, peeling agents, like glycolic acid, and filling agents, such as hyaluronic acid, are beyond the scope of this review.

21.2 Retinoids

Vitamin A and its synthetic and natural derivatives are known as retinoids. Over-the-counter (OTC) natural derivatives include retinol (ROL), retinaldehyde (RAL), and retinyl esters (REs, including retinyl palmitate [RPa], retinyl acetate [RAc], and retinyl propionate [RPr]).[3] All retinoids are converted to biologically active retinoic acid (RA) in the skin (▶ Fig. 21.1), but the efficacy of each derivative varies, with OTC retinoids having lower efficacy than prescription forms.[2,4,5] Lipophilic retinoids diffuse through cell membranes and into the nucleus, where they bind RA receptors and alter gene expression, leading to changes in epithelial cell proliferation, differentiation, and turnover.[2,3,6] Retinoids may also increase collagen synthesis, possibly leading to decreased wrinkles.[2] Finally, retinoids can decrease hyperpigmentation by stimulating keratinocyte turnover and inhibiting melanosome transfer.[7,8] Limiting their clinical utility are established adverse effects of topical retinoid use, including photosensitivity[9] and local reactions with burning, erythema, and scaling.[9] Irritation can be minimized by reducing application frequency or trying a different retinoid, especially OTC derivatives that may be less irritating.[10,11,12] Although systemic effects such as teratogenicity are possible, minimal systemic absorption makes these unlikely.[13] Despite case reports of suspected embryotoxicity from topical retinoids, three prospective trials failed to demonstrate this risk.[13,14,15,16]

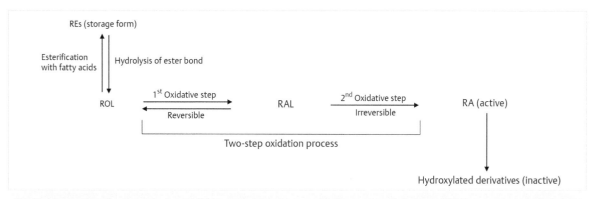

Fig. 21.1 Formation of active retinoic acid (RA) occurs via a two-step oxidation process. Retinyl esters (REs) can undergo hydrolysis to form retinol (ROL), which then undergoes oxidation to RA; this reaction can be reversed to store vitamin A. RA can be inactivated via conversion to hydroxylated derivatives. RAL, retinaldehyde.

21.2.1 Stability and Topical Penetration

Retinoids are difficult to formulate given their instability when exposed to light and oxygen.[1,17] This sensitivity will also reduce the amount of active agent present in OTC products, especially for ROL, the least stable of the OTC retinoids.[17,18] Retinoids are able to penetrate the epidermis, but after penetration, their activity depends on their efficiency of conversion to active RA.[2] The amount of RA in the skin is controlled by RA 4-hydroxylase (RA 4-OHase); so, retinoid activity can be assessed by measuring this enzyme.[19] Using this principle, Duell et al applied retinoid solutions to patients for 4 days and then biopsied the skin to measure the amount of RA 4-OHase using high-performance liquid chromatography (HPLC).[19] Compared to RA, higher concentrations of ROL (25-fold), RAL (10-fold), and RPa (600-fold) were needed to significantly induce RA 4-OHase.[19] So while RPa penetrates the skin, only a small amount is converted to RA, limiting its clinical value.

21.2.2 Evidence for Retinaldehyde

RAL is an intermediate metabolite formed during the conversion of ROL to RA.[7,20] To evaluate antiwrinkle efficacy in a randomized, double-blind trial, 125 patients applied 0.05% RAL cream, 0.05% RA cream, or vehicle nightly for 44 weeks.[10] Silicone replicas of patients' lateral canthi were taken and analyzed with optical profilometry. At weeks 18 and 44, RAL and RA significantly reduced wrinkling compared to baseline, but the vehicle did not produce significant changes. However, there were no significant differences in wrinkling between RAL and vehicle nor between RAL and RA. RAL was better tolerated than RA, possibly because RA "overloads" its biological pathway. As a precursor, RAL may prevent this overload by allowing a slower, more controlled conversion to RA.[10,20]

21.2.3 Evidence for Retinyl Esters

REs contain fatty acyl groups esterified to the hydroxyl terminus of ROL and exist as the body's retinoid storage form.[21] Although REs are stable[22] and have low irritancy potential,[11] they are considered the least effective retinoid.[22] Their ester bonds must be cleaved to obtain ROL, which then must be converted to RA via a two-step oxidative process (▸ Fig. 21.1).[22] These processes are limited in the skin, decreasing the efficacy of REs.[22] Yet, the desire to find less irritating, effective retinoids motivated the study of REs. One double-blind, randomized trial explored the photoaging effects of RPr.[11] Patients applied 0.15% RPr or placebo creams to their faces, forearms, and hands daily for up to 48 weeks ($n=75$ for 24 weeks; $n=59$ for 48 weeks). Assessments of overall skin aging, wrinkling, and other symptoms such as roughness and mottled pigmentation were done by two clinicians. Patient self-assessment of overall skin aging was also done. Clinician-rated overall aging and symptom scores as well as self-assessment scores did not differ between the RPr and control groups.[11]

RPa has also been explored for its antiaging properties. Aging is associated with dermal changes including reduced collagen, elastin, and microfibrils (including fibrillin-1), as well as increased matrix metalloproteinases (MMPs).[23] A study used these as markers of dermal repair to compare three moisturizers, basic, 2% total active complex (TAC; lipopentapeptide, white lupin peptides, antioxidants), and 6% TAC (same ingredients as 2% TAC with < 0.02% RPa; Boots, Nottingham, United Kingdom), to RA (0.025% Retin-A).[23] Patients ($n=9$) applied the moisturizers to their forearms under patch occlusion for 12 days, reapplying on days 4 and 8. RA was only applied on day 8 given its irritancy potential. Biopsies were done and immunohistochemistry (IHC) was used to assess levels of fibrillin-1, procollagen I, and MMP-1. Although the 2% TAC moisturizer did not change these levels compared to the basic moisturizer, the 6% TAC moisturizer increased dermal deposition of fibrillin-1 and procollagen I. RA only increased fibrillin-1 compared to the basic moisturizer, possibly because it was applied for a shorter duration than the 6% TAC (12 vs. 4 days). This combination of peptides and RPa induced dermal changes indicative of skin repair, but it is unknown whether it altered the skin's appearance.[23]

Given REs can concentrate in the epidermis and absorb ultraviolet (UV) radiation, RPa has additionally been used as a UV filter to protect against photodamage.[24] Two percent RPa, sun protection factor-20 (SPF20) sunscreen, and vehicle were applied to separate areas on six male participants under occlusion for 3 to 4 hours and for 30 minutes 24 hours later.[24] Patients were then exposed to 2 to 4 minimal erythema doses (MEDs) of UVB radiation and punch biopsies were taken 30 minutes later. DNA was extracted and the level of thymine dimers (these form when UVB radiation is absorbed by DNA) was quantified with immune dot blots. Erythema was also quantified 24 hours after irradiation using a chromameter. RPa and sunscreen similarly reduced thymine dimers and erythema compared to vehicle. Therefore, although REs may not have the same antiaging efficacy as other retinoids, their ability to concentrate in the epidermis may allow REs to protect the skin from UV damage and possibly the resulting photodamage.[24]

21.2.4 Evidence for Retinol

To examine the antiaging efficacy of 0.4% ROL compared to vehicle, Kafi et al performed a randomized, double-blind trial with 36 elderly patients.[25] ROL or vehicle was applied to one arm up to three times per week for 24 weeks (average 1.6 times/wk). Treatment was discontinued for one or more sessions if patients experienced irritation. Two blinded dermatologists assessed skin roughness, wrinkling, and overall aging, and biopsies were done at baseline and 24 weeks to perform IHC. Only 23 patients completed the study; these patients had statistically significantly reduced wrinkling with ROL compared to vehicle. Last observation carried forward analysis showed statistically significant reductions in wrinkling, roughness, and overall aging for ROL compared to vehicle. Further, ROL increased the levels of glycosaminoglycan and procollagen compared to vehicle. Most patients experienced only mild irritation from ROL, but three patients had severe reactions, necessitating withdrawal from the study. Although a large dropout rate may have introduced bias, this study shows that ROL may reduce skin atrophy and fragility, and offer antiwrinkle benefits in elderly populations.[25]

21.2.5 Evidence for Combination Products

A randomized, double-blind trial including 38 female patients with photodamage compared 1.1% tri-retinol cream (ROL, RAc, and RPa) to 0.025% tretinoin cream.[26] The products were applied for 3 months (2 times/wk for the first week, 3 times/wk for the second week, and then daily). Clinical evaluations showed that both tri-retinol and tretinoin significantly improved photodamage signs (wrinkles, firmness, tone, pigmentation, roughness) compared to baseline. Only mild adverse reactions were seen, but there was a small, significant increase in erythema and burning for tri-retinol compared to tretinoin.[26] Therefore, whereas OTC retinoids may offer reduced side effects compared to tretinoin when used alone, the combination of retinoids may actually increase irritation compared to tretinoin. Combination products have also been used to reduce hyperpigmentation. Tretinoin is more frequently used to treat hyperpigmentation, most effectively in combination with hydroquinone (HQ) and a topical steroid (triple combination).[8] As reviewed by Sheth and Pandya, a combination of HQ and ROL showed moderate efficacy, but the authors still recommend triple combination therapy as first line.[8]

Overall, the efficacy of OTC retinoids is variable. Although there is some evidence for RAL's and ROL's antiaging efficacy, RPr did not reduce wrinkles and RPa induced dermal changes indicative of skin repair, but its effect on the skin's appearance is unknown. Thus, REs may be better utilized to prevent photodamage given their ability to concentrate in the epidermis. Prescription retinoids offer an alternative to those unsatisfied with OTC formulations.

21.3 Tyrosinase Inhibitors: Hydroquinone and Kojic Acid

HQ is a phenolic compound that is considered the standard hyperpigmentation treatment.[27] By binding to and inhibiting tyrosinase, HQ prevents melanin production.[28] OTC formulations have 1.5 to 2% HQ, whereas prescriptions contain 3 to 4% HQ.[28] Twice daily application is recommended and improvement can take up to 6 months.[29] HQ causes mild skin irritation[29,30] and is associated with ochronosis, but this is rare in the United States with only 22 reported cases over 23 years of use.[31,32] Concerns have also been raised about the malignancy potential of HQ based on the risk of renal or hepatocellular adenomas and leukemia in murine models.[33] However, because of physiologic differences between humans and rodents, this risk does not apply to humans and consequently, there have been no reported cases of malignancy in over 50 years of HQ use.[31,33] Another tyrosinase inhibitor that is used less commonly than HQ as a skin-lightening agent is kojic acid; it is made by *aspergillus oryzae* fungus and used in concentrations of 1 to 4%.[34,35] Kojic acid is reported to be more stable than HQ but is also more expensive, has less evidence, and is more irritating compared to HQ.[34]

21.3.1 Stability and Topical Penetration

Patients applied 2% HQ to their foreheads ($n = 6$) or forearms ($n = 4$) for 24 hours. Their urine was collected for 96 hours to assess the penetration of HQ: 45.3% of the forehead dose and 24% of the forearm dose were detected.[36] Diffusion through human skin samples was also assessed using glass penetration slides. Two percent HQ was applied for 24 hours and the amount of HQ was quantified using thin-layer chromatography. Thirty-four percent of the sample penetrated through the skin into the receiver compartment and 9.3% remained in the skin.[36] Overall, HQ can effectively penetrate the skin; however, its stability is problematic as HQ is rapidly oxidized leading to yellow/brown discoloration and decreased biological activity.[27] Therefore, HQ must be packaged in opaque, airtight containers.[27,30] On the contrary, kojic acid is reported to be more stable and less likely to oxidize while in storage than HQ; however, limited data exist to substantiate this claim.[34] As a hydrophilic molecule that has low permeability and a short half-life in the circulatory system, kojic acid may have inadequate tyrosinase inhibitor activity. Kim et al showed that a kojic acid-tripeptide prepared from kojic acid was 15 times more stable and exhibited 100-fold greater tyrosinase inhibitory active compared to kojic acid,[37] so there are likely issues with kojic acid's stability and efficacy in OTC products. The absorption of this hydrophilic molecule could be improved with various carriers, for instance, the cutaneous absorption of kojic acid was improved by creating kojic acid solid lipid nanoparticles.[35]

21.3.2 Evidence for Hydroquinone

According to a comprehensive update by Sheth and Pandya, extensive research shows that HQ is effective in treating hyperpigmentation disorders.[8] One such study used results from multiple trials including 300 Hispanic patients with melasma where 2 to 5% HQ with or without 0.05 to 0.1% RA was applied twice daily for 3 months.[38] Formulations with 2% HQ and 0.05 to 0.1% RA were the most efficacious. Two percent HQ alone was nonirritating, but produced good results in only 18% of participants.[38] There are numerous products containing HQ, both OTC and by prescription, as summarized in a table by Gupta et al.[29] Although there is evidence for prescription formulations, many OTC products have not been tested; therefore, although patients can safely try these products, prescription HQ may be needed to reduce their symptoms.[8,27]

21.3.3 Evidence for Kojic Acid

Two studies compared the skin-lightening ability of kojic acid to HQ. Garcia and Fulton compared 2% kojic acid and 2% HQ in a split-face study of 39 participants with facial hyperpigmentation; 5% glycolic acid was also added to each formulation to decrease the SC barrier function and augment the penetration of the active ingredients.[34] The formulations were applied twice daily for 3 months.

Based on the evaluation by an investigator, there was no significant difference between kojic acid and HQ: 51% of participants responded equally, 28% had a more dramatic response to kojic acid, and 21% had a more dramatic response to HQ. Although kojic acid was shown to have similar efficacy to HQ for the treatment of hyperpigmentation, kojic acid was more irritating according to participants.[34] On the contrary, a study by Monteiro et al compared daily application of 0.75% kojic acid/2.5% vitamin C cream and 4% HQ cream in 60 patients with facial melasma for 12 weeks and found conflicting results.[39] Efficacy was assessed using the Melasma Area and Severity Index (MASI). Both kojic acid/vitamin C and HQ creams resulted in significant reductions in MASI scores from baseline, but HQ performed significantly better compared to kojic acid/vitamin C (change in MASI score 11.4 HQ vs. 2.4 kojic acid/vitamin C). Side effects were similar in both study groups and included only erythema and a mild burning sensation.[39] These studies are difficult to compare given different additives and concentrations of kojic acid used. Based on the results, kojic acid may perform similarly to OTC HQ (1.5–2%) but inferiorly to prescription HQ (3–4%), and glycolic acid may be a superior additive compared to vitamin C. Further studies are needed to evaluate the use of kojic acid compared to the standard tyrosinase inhibitor, HQ.

21.4 Azelaic Acid

Azelaic acid (Az) is a nine-carbon dicarboxylic acid obtained from *Pityrosporum ovale*. By inhibiting tyrosinase, Az is used twice daily for 2 to 3 months to treat hyperpigmentation.[8,40] Az may also be cytotoxic to melanocytes[41] and may decrease reactive oxygen species (ROS) generated by neutrophils.[42] Az is safe overall but can cause pruritus, burning, and tingling in 1 to 5% of patients; less common reactions include erythema, scaling, dryness, and contact dermatitis.[8,40]

21.4.1 Stability and Topical Penetration

Az has low stability and water solubility, making it difficult to incorporate into cosmetic products.[43] In one study, only 23% of Az remained in suspension after 8 weeks of storage.[43] Even within ethosomes (phospholipid vesicles with ethanol), only 62 to 69% of Az remained after 8 weeks.[43] Topical absorption of Az is also limited. Penetration of 20% Az was assessed in six male volunteers by collecting their urine for 4 days after application to measure the amount of Az using HPLC—only 2.2% of the dose was extracted.[44] Incorporation of Az into various carriers, including liposomes and microemulsions, has enhanced this limited penetration.[45,46]

21.4.2 Evidence

A review by Gupta et al summarized four 24-week randomized, double-blind, controlled (compared to vehicle or 2–4% HQ) trials of 20% Az for melasma or other facial hyperpigmentation.[40] Overall, Az improved melasma with 20% Az being more effective than 2% HQ and having similar efficacy to 4% HQ.[40] Therefore, a comprehensive update by Sheth and Pandya recommended Az as a first-line alternative agent for melasma, with a level A U.S. Preventive Services Task Force strength, indicating good evidence supports its use.[8]

21.5 Tranexamic Acid

Tranexamic acid (TA) inhibits plasminogen-binding sites, preventing the conversion of plasminogen to plasmin; oral TA is available as a prescription to prevent fibrinolysis and thus reduce bleeding risk. Oral (250 mg twice daily) and topical (2–5%) formulations of TA are also used in cosmetics as a treatment for melasma.[47,48] The mechanism of TA for treating hyperpigmentation is thought to be related to its plasmin inhibition.[47] UV radiation induces plasmin activity in keratinocytes, which increases levels of arachidonic acid and alpha-melanocyte-stimulating hormone. These two substances can in turn activate melanin synthesis.[47] Further, TA has a similar structure to tyrosine and can therefore inhibit tyrosinase activity.[47] As TA reduces bleeding risk, thromboembolic events are a potential side effect. However, thromboembolic events have not been reported at the doses used for melasma.[48,49] Regardless, patients should be screened for risk factors that further increase thromboembolism risk. As oral TA is available by prescription only, this chapter will focus on topical TA.

21.5.1 Stability and Topical Penetration

Limited studies exist on the stability and skin penetration of topical TA. In one study, Donnelly examined the stability of TA in mouth rinse.[50] After storage at room temperature (23 °C) for 31 days, 97.2% of the initial concentration of TA remained (measured using HPLC).[50] As for penetration through the skin, Vijayakumar et al observed that as a hydrophilic molecule, permeation of TA is limited.[51] To remedy this, the authors created a bead formulation of TA. Permeation through murine skin was 1.92 times higher for the TA beads compared to a commercial TA cream.[51]

21.5.2 Evidence

Taraz et al reviewed clinical studies using topical TA to treat melasma.[47] Three small, controlled, split-face studies were done where participants applied topical TA twice daily for 12 weeks and efficacy was assessed using MASI scores.[52,53,54] In one study comparing 5% TA and vehicle, 18 of 23 participants had reductions in MASI scores, but there were no significant differences between the two groups.[52] The other studies found similar reductions in MASI scores compared to HQ.[53,54] Ebrahimi and Naeini compared 3% TA and 3% HQ/0.01% dexamethasone

solutions ($n = 39$); MASI scores decreased significantly from baseline in both groups, but the scores did not vary between the TA (21 point difference) and HQ/dexamethasone (18 point difference) groups.[53] There were significant differences in side effects though, with HQ/dexamethasone resulting in significantly more side effects than TA, including erythema, irritation, xerosis, and hypertrichosis.[53] Similarly, in the third study, 5% liposomal TA was compared to 4% HQ cream; MASI scores were significantly reduced in both groups, but the differences between the two groups were not significantly different (8-point difference for TA and 7-point difference for HQ).[54] Overall, there is some evidence that TA may treat melasma to a similar degree as HQ; however, this was shown in only small studies[53,54] and one study failed to show a response with topical TA.[52]

Although oral TA is only available by prescription, one recent study should be briefly discussed. Del Rosario et al compared the efficacy of oral TA (250 mg twice daily) and placebo capsules for melasma using modified MASI scores ($n = 39$).[48] After 3 months, treatment with TA led to a 49% reduction in modified MASI score versus an 18% reduction in scores for the placebo. Three months after treatment ended, the difference between the two groups narrowed (26% reduction in TA group compared to 19% in the placebo group).[48] Although oral TA led to a large improvement in melasma, the results did not persist after treatment was stopped; topical TA could be a long-term treatment option to maintain treatment responses.

21.6 Vitamin B3 (Niacin)

Two forms of niacin are used in cosmeceuticals, niacinamide/nicotinamide (NIC) and nicotinic acid. Given nicotinic acid causes facial flushing, this review will focus on the more commonly used NIC.[2] NIC is a precursor to the cofactor niacinamide adenosine dinucleotide phosphate (NADPH), which functions in reduction–oxidation reactions. Thus, NIC may increase the skin's antioxidant capacity by increasing production of NADPH. NIC may also increase ceramide and collagen synthesis, improving the skin's barrier and reducing wrinkles.[2,55] The mechanisms of these effects are not fully elucidated but likely involve NADPH.[2] Finally, an in vitro study using a coculture of keratinocytes and melanocytes showed that NIC reduced melanosome transfer, indicating that it may be able to reduce hyperpigmentation.[56] Topical NIC can cause burning or stinging but is well tolerated otherwise.[57,58]

21.6.1 Stability and Topical Penetration

NIC is easy to formulate given its stability with light and oxygen exposure. However, an NIC microemulsion changes color at 45 °C, so storage at refrigerator or ambient temperatures is recommended.[59] Penetration was evaluated by applying carbon tracer–labelled NIC to the forearms of seven patients for 24 hours and their urine was collected for 5 days. NIC likely adequately penetrates the skin to exert its biological effects because 11.08% of the applied NIC dose was detected compared to only 0.34% for nicotinic acid.[60]

21.6.2 Evidence

Bissett et al performed a double-blind, randomized trial with 49 patients where 5% NIC moisturizer was applied to half of the face and placebo moisturizer to the other half twice daily for 12 weeks.[57] Based on computer analyses, blotchiness, yellowness, and hyperpigmentation increased with both products (expected based on the season change), but NIC statistically significantly prevented these increases compared to placebo moisturizer. Further, NIC moisturizer significantly decreased wrinkles compared to the placebo, but the overall reduction was small (5.5% reduction).[57] To examine NIC's effect on the epidermal barrier, Tanno et al performed a trial with 12 men who applied 2% NIC solution twice daily to one shin and vehicle solution to the other shin for 4 weeks.[55] NIC decreased transepidermal water loss by 27% compared to vehicle and increased ceramide (quantified after extraction from skin samples) by 34% compared to vehicle.[55] Therefore, NIC may increase ceramide synthesis, enhancing the epidermal barrier. NIC was also evaluated to treat melasma compared to placebo and HQ. Navarrete-Solís et al performed a split-face study of 27 patients with melasma, comparing daily use of 4% NIC cream to 4% HQ cream for 8 weeks along with sunscreen.[61] Using the MASI, NIC resulted in a 62% decrease in melasma severity compared to a 70% decrease for HQ (▶ Fig. 21.2). Colorimetry was also used to assess the lightening efficacy of these products; after 8 weeks, the results did not significantly differ between the two therapies.[61] A second study by Hakozaki et al compared 5% NIC moisturizer to vehicle in patients with facial hyperpigmentation (lentigines, melasma, or freckles).[56] After applying the moisturizers twice daily for 8 weeks, using both computer analysis and visual assessment of images, NIC resulted in statistically significant reduction in hyperpigmentation compared to vehicle ($n = 18$). Based on these two studies, NIC may reduce melasma and other forms of hyperpigmentation, but larger studies should be done to further explore the impact of NIC.

21.7 Vitamin C (Ascorbic Acid) and Vitamin E (Alpha-Tocopherol)

The active form of vitamin C, LAA, and vitamin E or alpha-TOC are two antioxidants that are commonly used in cosmetic products. These vitamins can prevent free radical generation that induces photodamage and photoaging.[62] Whereas sunscreens block UV radiation on top of the skin, antioxidants only work when inside the skin but can offer protection for days.[63,64] AA also increases the expression of type I and III collagen in cultured human fibroblasts meaning it may have antiwrinkle effects.[65,66] These vitamins work together to protect the skin: TOC is hydrophobic, protecting lipid structures including cell membranes, and AA is hydrophilic, protecting the aqueous environment.[62] Further, AA reduces the amount of TOC that is oxidized by free radicals,[67] so these vitamins are often used together. AA and TOC are safe overall, although low pH preparations of AA can be irritating[68] and TOC can cause contact dermatitis and pruritus.[69]

AA and TOC are also often combined with ferulic acid (FA), a phenolic phytochemical found in plants.[70] As an antioxidant, FA scavenges free radicals and inhibits ROS formation.[70] With these properties, FA stabilizes AA and TOC by limiting their oxidation while also acting as an active ingredient, offering further photoprotection.[70]

21.7.1 Stability and Topical Penetration

The stability of AA is affected by exposure to oxygen, high pH, and temperature changes.[71,72] Degradation can start within days to weeks, leading to brown discoloration. Various techniques have been employed to increase AA's stability such as exclusion of oxygen during formulation and encapsulation.[72,73] One study created an oil/water emulsion with 3% AA in the oil phase; 85 to 95% of AA remained in an airtight container for 6 months, although during real-life use, commercial products will be opened daily and exposed to oxygen during application.[71] More stable ester derivatives of AA, such as magnesium ascorbyl phosphate, have been created, but these are expensive, have lower efficacy given they must be converted to AA inside the skin, and may not penetrate the epidermis.[63,71,74] Overall, AA's stability varies depending on the formulation, packaging, and storage conditions. Similarly, TOC can be oxidized when exposed to air.[75] More stable esterified forms of TOC have also been developed, but these may not be metabolized to TOC when applied topically.[76] The stabilities of AA and TOC are enhanced when these vitamins are used together[62] and by the addition of FA.[77]

As for penetration, despite being hydrophilic, human ex vivo data have shown that AA can penetrate the skin, with optimal penetration occurring when the vehicle's pH is below AA's pKa (4.2), reducing its charge density.[63,72] In one study, the authors applied topical AA solutions at various pHs to pigs for 24 hours. Biopsies were then taken and the amount of AA was quantified using HPLC.[63] They found that the formulation must have a pH less than 3.5 to enter the pig's skin and that tissue levels increased with increasing AA concentrations up to 20%.[63] Overall, to exert biological effects, AA must be used at a concentration of at least 10% in acidic vehicles.[78] On the contrary, based on a murine model, TOC's lipophilic nature allows for absorption within minutes of application. Therefore, TOC is used at low concentrations of 1 to 5%.[78,79]

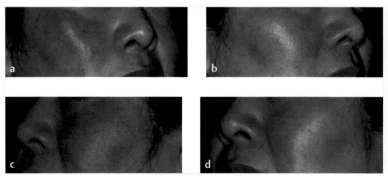

Fig. 21.2 *Top row*: Treatment of right side with nicotinamide (NIC). **(a)** Onset. **(b)** Eight weeks later. *Bottom row*: Treatment of left side with hydroquinone (HQ). **(c)** Onset. **(d)** Eight weeks later. (Copyright © 2011 Josefina Navarrete-Solís et al.)

21.7.2 Evidence

Lin et al applied a 15% AA/1% TOC solution to pig skin daily for 4 days and compared the photoprotection offered by this combination to AA or TOC alone.[62] On day 4, the pigs were irradiated with 1 to 5 MEDs. The combination solution offered fourfold protection against erythema measured with a chromameter compared to twofold protection with AA or TOC alone. Compared to controls, hematoxylin and eosin staining of biopsies showed decreased sunburn cells (keratinocytes with pyknotic nuclei and eosinophilic cytoplasm) for all treatments at 1 to 2 MEDs and only for the combination treatment at 3 to 4 MEDs. Using IHC, the combination solution was also protective against thymine dimer formation.[62] In the same model, adding 0.5% FA doubled the photoprotection offered by the combination solution.[77] Based on these results, Murray et al examined the ability of a 15% AA/1% TOC/0.05% FA solution (SkinCeuticals) to protect against UV radiation in a clinical trial.[64] Near identical methods as Lin et al[62] were used, except nine patients were treated, radiation doses ranged from 2 to 10 MEDs, and p53 activation, which is induced in response to DNA damage, was also measured with IHC. Compared to vehicle, the active formulation statistically significantly protected against erythema, p53 activation, and sunburn cell and thymine dimer formation.[64] Hence, inclusion of all three antioxidants, AA, TOC, and FA, is likely useful to maximize protection from UV-induced damage compared to products with only one or two of these antioxidants.

To explore the ability of these vitamins to reduce existing photodamage, a double-blind trial compared 10% AA/7% tetrahexyldecyl ascorbate (a lipid analog of AA) gel to vehicle gel.[68] Patients ($n = 12$) applied the active product to one half of their faces and the vehicle to the other half daily for 12 weeks. Based on clinical evaluations compared to baseline, the active agent significantly decreased cheek and perioral wrinkles, but the vehicle did not (13 vs. 4% reduction for cheeks and 15 vs. 2.5% for perioral skin). Both formulations significantly improved periorbital wrinkles (18.6% reduction for active and 14.5% for vehicle), whereas neither improved forehead wrinkles. Biopsies of four patients were taken at the end of the study (baseline staining not assessed) for in situ hybridization; probing for type I collagen mRNA showed higher staining for the active agent than the vehicle (+4 vs. +3 in 3/4 patients). Although AA reduced wrinkles compared to baseline in skin areas other than the forehead, the results were not compared to the control group, so it is unclear whether these results were statistically significant compared to vehicle.[68] Another study used AA alone to treat photodamage in a double-blind, randomized trial.[80] Five percent AA cream (Active C, La Roche-Posay) or a vehicle cream was applied to the upper chest and forearms by 19 female patients daily for 6 months. Clinical assessment demonstrated statistically significant improvement in global scores (including hydration, roughness, laxity, wrinkles, and suppleness) for the AA cream compared to the vehicle (6.7 to 4.4 for AA vs. 6.7 to 5.3 for vehicle). Silicone rubber replicas of treated skin were also taken at baseline and 6 months; a statistically significant increase in skin microrelief (wrinkle depth 0–10 µm) density and decrease in deep furrow (wrinkle depth >20 µm) density were seen for the AA cream compared to vehicle.[80] Although AA performed superiorly to the control, the global photoaging scores between these two groups were not vastly different, so the results may not be clinically significant.[68,80] Thus, AA/TOC/FA products may be better able to protect against photodamage rather than reduce existing photodamage.

21.8 Curcumin

Curcumin, the active agent of the spice turmeric, has anti-inflammatory, antioxidant, wound-healing, and antimicrobial activities through its direct and indirect modulation of numerous signaling molecules.[81] Within the skin, curcumin inhibits phosphorylase kinase, resulting in the downregulation of two pathways involved in photodamage (▶ Fig. 21.3).[81,82] Curcumin may also regulate hair growth and loss (▶ Fig. 21.4). A phase 1 trial showed oral curcumin to be nontoxic up to 8,000 mg per day ($n = 25$).[83] Topical curcumin was also well tolerated in clinical trials, although it can cause contact dermatitis and its yellow color can stain the skin.[84,85,86]

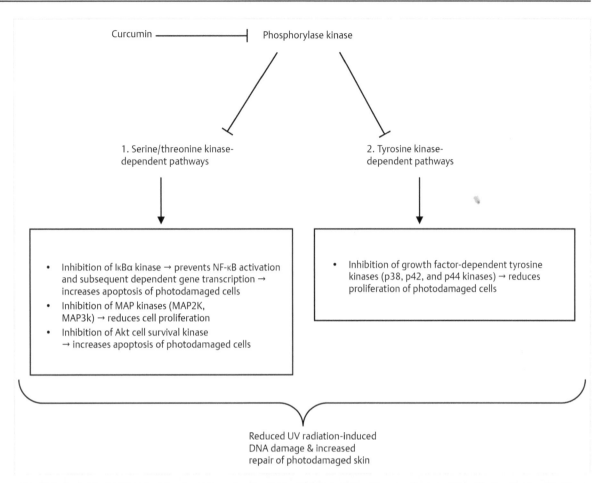

Fig. 21.3 Curcumin inhibits phosphorylase kinase, leading to the inhibition of two kinase pathways, which affect numerous signaling molecules involved in photoaging (summarized by Heng[82] and Gupta et al[81]).

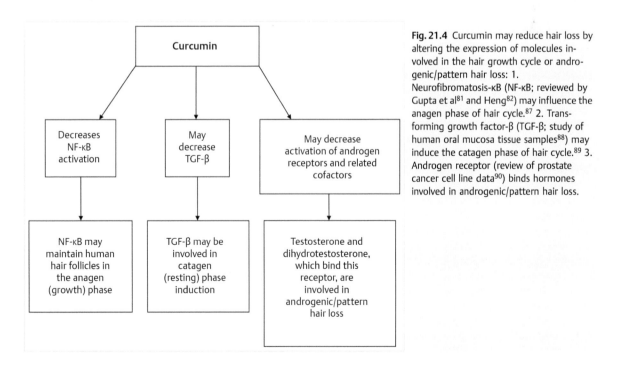

Fig. 21.4 Curcumin may reduce hair loss by altering the expression of molecules involved in the hair growth cycle or androgenic/pattern hair loss: 1. Neurofibromatosis-κB (NF-κB; reviewed by Gupta et al[81] and Heng[82]) may influence the anagen phase of hair cycle.[87] 2. Transforming growth factor-β (TGF-β; study of human oral mucosa tissue samples[88]) may induce the catagen phase of hair cycle.[89] 3. Androgen receptor (review of prostate cancer cell line data[90]) binds hormones involved in androgenic/pattern hair loss.

21.8.1 Stability and Topical Penetration

Curcumin's stability is reduced by high temperature and alkaline pH. It also has limited aqueous solubility, especially at acidic and neutral pHs.[91] Vehicle choice further affects curcumin's stability as demonstrated by Wang et al who incubated curcumin with various vehicles for 8 hours and then measured its concentration with HPLC. In phosphate buffer and serum-free medium, 90% of curcumin decomposed within 30 minutes. Curcumin was more stable in medium with serum and human blood, with 50% remaining after 8 hours.[92] Given its low absorption through the gut as well as rapid metabolism and elimination, curcumin also has poor oral bioavailability.[86] The average peak serum concentration after consuming 8,000 mg of oral curcumin was 1.8 mM (measured via HPLC) and urinary excretion was undetectable.[83] A number of delivery strategies including using liposomes, microemulsions, nanoparticles, and polymer micelles show promise for increasing curcumin's bioavailability.[93] Combination of curcumin with an intestinal/hepatic glucuronidase inhibitor, piperine (black pepper extract), also increased its bioavailability by 2,000% in a murine model.[94] Despite its low bioavailability, curcumin exerts numerous effects beyond the gut.[95] This paradox cannot be explained yet, but one theory is that curcumin's degradation products, vanillin, FA, and feruloylmethane, may contribute to its activity.[91] To explore curcumin's topical penetration, 1% curcumin gel was applied to 10 patients with psoriasis. Curcumin significantly decreased phosphorylase kinase activity compared to the control gel, indicating that curcumin sufficiently penetrated the skin to inhibit this enzyme.[96]

21.8.2 Evidence

In a randomized, double-blind study, Tricutan gel (Dermyn: 0.1% curcumin, 0.3% rosemary, 1% gotu kola) was applied to one side of the face and placebo gel to the other by 28 women (including 3 dropouts for contact dermatitis) twice daily for 4 weeks.[84] Tricutan gel significantly reduced ultrasound wave propagation speed through the skin, indicating increased firmness, compared to the placebo gel (184–164 for Tricutan vs. 183–210 for placebo). Additionally, compared to placebo gel, Tricutan gel–treated skin had significantly higher scores for overall skin appearance based on self-evaluations (4 vs. 2.7) and clinical evaluations by a dermatologist (3.2 vs. 2).[84] Further studies are warranted given these positive results; however, the high rate of contact dermatitis (3/28 patients) is problematic.

Another combination product with curcumin was studied for its ability to reduce hair loss. Nutrafol is an oral supplement with curcumin, ashwagandha, saw palmetto, tocotrienol, piperine, and capsaicin among other ingredients that claims to have anti-inflammatory, antioxidant, and DHT-inhibiting properties.[85] A randomized, double-blind study was done with women who took four

Nutrafol ($n = 26$) or placebo capsules ($n = 14$) daily for 6 months. Using phototrichograms, terminal and vellus hairs were counted in a 1 cm² area on the anterolateral triangle of the scalp. Nutrafol use significantly increased the number of terminal (142–156 Nutrafol vs. 137–141 placebo) and vellus (13–15 Nutrafol vs. 13–13 placebo) hairs compared to the control group. Investigators also completed Blinded Investigators Global Hair Assessments, which showed significant improvements in hair growth and quality for Nutrafol compared to the control group.[85] Although it shows promising results, the high cost of this product may be a concern for some patients. Further, the effects of curcumin alone cannot be deduced, but the results motivate the additional study of curcumin for hair loss.

21.9 DNA Repair Enzymes

UV radiation exposure produces DNA lesions such as cyclobutane pyrimidine dimers (CPDs)[97] that can induce photoaging and mutagenesis.[98] The skin has intrinsic DNA repair mechanisms, but these are incompletely efficient so topically applied DNA repair enzymes can serve as a supplement.[98] One enzyme, T4 endonuclease V (T4N5), was originally isolated from T4 bacteriophage-infected *Escherichia coli*[99] and another, photolyase, is derived from the cyanobacterium *Anacystis nidulans*.[100] No significant adverse effects have been reported with T4N5[99,101] or photolyase[100]; however, a thorough review of possible reactions has not been done.

21.9.1 Stability and Topical Penetration

DNA repair enzymes are included in liposomes to increase their percutaneous absorption; however, only T4N5 has been studied. The penetration of T4N5 liposomal lotion with fluorescently marked liposome membranes and enzymes was explored in a murine model.[102] After exposure to UVB radiation, the lotion was applied for 1 hour. Fluorescent microcopy showed that the liposomes penetrated the SC and localized in the epidermis and around hair follicles. Liposomes remained there for up to 18 hours with little dermal penetration. Using transmission electron microscopy, liposomes and T4N5 were also seen within the cytoplasm and nuclei of keratinocytes.[102]

21.9.2 Evidence

To examine the ability of T4N5 to repair DNA damage, Yarosh et al applied T4N5 liposome lotion or placebo liposome lotion to postmastectomy breast tissue.[97] Increased CPD loss, measured with an alkaline agarose gel assay, was observed with increasing doses up to 60% of control.[97] Given these results, 30 patients with xeroderma pigmentosum (XP) applied T4N5 liposome lotion or a placebo liposome lotion daily for 1 year in a double-blind, randomized study.[101] The rates of new actinic keratoses (AKs) and basal cell carcinomas (BCCs) were statistically significantly decreased with the T4N5 liposome lotion compared to placebo (68% reduction for AKs and 30% for BCCs). A review of additional in vitro and clinical studies concluded that T4N5 liposome lotion can repair DNA damage as well as reduce AKs and BCCs.[99]

Berardesca et al added photolyase liposomes to SPF50 sunscreen and examined CPD formation and apoptosis using enzyme-linked immunosorbent assay (ELISA) after three times MEDs of UV radiation for 4 days ($n = 10$ patients).[100] Test formulations (vehicle, sunscreen, photolyase liposomes/sunscreen) were applied to three sites 30 minutes before UV exposure and a fourth site was untreated. Based on biopsies 3 days after irradiation, photolyase liposomes/sunscreen prevented 93% of CPD formation, which was significantly more than sunscreen alone (62% prevention). Photolyase liposomes/sunscreen also reduced apoptosis significantly more than sunscreen alone (82 vs. 40% prevention).[100] Although the antiphotoaging efficacies of T4N5 and photolyase have not been examined, DNA damage contributes to photoaging, so these enzymes may also prevent photodamage signs.[98] Additional studies are needed to compare the effectiveness of photolyase and T4N5 and to examine the stability of these enzymes in commercial formulations.

21.10 Peptides and Proteins

Peptides are chains of amino acids added to cosmetic products for various indications, although their high costs necessitate the use of low levels.[1] Three types exist: carrier peptides, which facilitate transport of another agent (glycyl-L-histidyl-L-lysine-Cu^{2+} [GHK-Cu]); signal peptides, which are designed to increase collagen (palmitoyl-lysine-threonine-threonine-lysine-serine [pal-KTTKS]); and neurotransmitter (NT) peptides, which are theorized to inhibit acetylcholine release at the neuromuscular junction (NMJ), decreasing muscle movement that increases wrinkles. However, it is unknown whether NT peptides reach the NMJ in vivo.[1,73] This section will focus on the most well-characterized carrier and signaling peptides. Pal-KTTKS is a procollagen-I fragment that has been shown to stimulate the production of type I and III collagens in cultured fibroblasts and is thus used as an anti-wrinkle therapy.[73,103,104] Pal-KTTS was well tolerated by trial participants, producing no skin irritation.[73,103] GHK-Cu is a copper tripeptide complex that includes GHK to facilitate copper transport; this complex has not caused adverse effects in clinical trials.[105,106] In vitro studies and animal models summarized by Miller et al have shown that GHK-Cu stimulates collagen synthesis and angiogenesis.[107] GHK-Cu gel also increased plantar ulcer closure compared to the control group in a randomized trial.[105]

Consequently, GHK-Cu is used to reduce wrinkles and enhance healing after cosmetic procedures.

Large proteins are also used in cosmeceuticals, including growth hormones and cytokines. Products are often marketed for "skin rejuvenation" and include a single growth factor or a combination of numerous growth factors and cytokines.[108] These proteins were first studied in wound healing; their role in dermal repair and remodeling led to their use in cosmetics. Growth factors and cytokines are proposed to penetrate the skin and interact with cells in the epidermis, such as keratinocytes, causing these cells to produce cytokines that affect deeper cells in the dermis, like fibroblasts, ultimately increasing the growth of these cell types or leading to the production of proteins like collagen, which are decreased in aging skin.[108,109] Clinical trials using a variety of growth factors have shown these products to be well tolerated other than minor eye irritation, seborrheic dermatitis, or a possible study-related cutaneous viral infection.[109,110,111]

21.10.1 Stability and Topical Penetration

Choi et al assessed the stability and penetration of pal-KTTKS using a murine model.[112] Palmitate is a fatty acid included to increase KTTKS's lipophilicity and penetration. Skin extracts were incubated with the peptides for up to 120 minutes and the amount of protein remaining was quantified using liquid chromatography with tandem mass spectrometry (LC-MS/MS). Both KTTKS and pal-KTTKS were rapidly degraded, but pal-KTTKS was more stable with 11.2% remaining after 120 minutes compared to only 1.5% of KTTKS after 60 minutes. The stability of both peptides improved with protease inhibitor inclusion. To evaluate penetration, mouse skin samples were mounted on Franz diffusion cells. After 24 hours of application, the peptides were not found in the receptor compartment, meaning they did not permeate through the entire skin sample. KTTKS was not detected in the skin, but pal-KTTKS was detected in all skin layers (8.3% in SC, 5.6% in the epidermis, and 0.6% in the dermis).[112] Similar to pal-KTTKS, there is evidence that GHK-CU penetrates the skin. Using HPLC and mass spectrometry to identify degradation products, GHK-Cu was stable in water for at least 2 weeks, but was susceptible to hydrolytic cleavage at high and low pHs.[106] GHK-Cu's penetration was also studied using flow-through diffusion cells. GHK-Cu solution was applied to human cadaveric skin (SC, epidermis, or split-thickness: epidermis with dermis) for 48 hours.[113] Using mass spectrometry, copper was detected in the receptor fluid and in the skin samples (438x baseline for SC, 165x baseline for epidermis, and 31x baseline for split thickness).[113]

In nonphysiologic environments, growth factors and cytokines may not remain stable. Mehta et al examined the stability of a product with over 110 growth factors, cytokines, and soluble matrix proteins (TNS Recovery Complex, SkinMedica, Irvine, California, United States).[110] The authors extracted three proteins from the product, measured their concentrations after storage at room temperature with cytokine antibody array analysis, and found that the proteins remained at high levels.[110] However, the proteins in commercial products vary tremendously and real-world use would include opening the product and fluctuating temperatures. Unlike smaller peptides, the ability of larger proteins to penetrate the SC is questionable. Growth factors and cytokines can be more than 15,000 Da in molecular weight and molecules larger than 500 Da have limited penetration.[108] Although evidence is not yet available to substantiate this assertion, it is proposed that growth factors and cytokines penetrate the skin through hair follicles, sweat glands, or microtears.[108] Even if only a small amount of cytokine is able to infiltrate into the skin, it may be able to interact with other cells leading to a cascade effect, where these cells then produce other cytokines that can travel deeper into the dermis and interact with other dermal cells.[108]

21.10.2 Evidence for GHK-Cu

In a randomized, investigator-blinded trial after circumoral carbon dioxide laser resurfacing ($n = 13$), one group used a petroleum-based product with GHK-Cu until re-epithelialization, followed by moisturizers with GHK-Cu daily for 12 weeks (from ProCyte Corp).[107] Another group followed a similar regimen but used nonpeptide products (from La Roche-Posay). Erythema was evaluated by software and by clinical evaluators. The evaluators also assessed wrinkles and overall skin improvement. There were no significant differences in these factors between the groups. Patient satisfaction was significantly higher for the GHK-Cu products, although the participants were not blinded to treatment group.[107]

21.10.3 Evidence for Pal-KTTKS

Robinson et al performed a randomized, double-blind trial examining the antiwrinkle efficacy of pal-KTTKS.[103] Control moisturizer was applied to one side of the face and moisturizer with 3 ppm pal-KTTKS to the other side twice daily for 12 weeks by 93 women. Wrinkles were assessed by computer analysis and expert grading, which showed a small but significant decrease in wrinkles with pal-KTTKS compared to control (although $p < 0.10$ was used). Based on self-assessments, there was no difference in wrinkles between groups. The authors theorized that using more pal-KTTKS would increase the benefits, but this is not possible given its cost.[103] Similarly, Fu et al compared the antiwrinkle efficacy of a moisturizer regimen with NIC, Pal-KT, Pal-KTTKS, and 0.3% RPr (NPP) to a prescription regimen with 0.02% tretinoin (Rx) in an 8-week randomized, investigator-blinded study ($n = 196$).[114] In addition to daily moisturizers, the NPP formulation was applied twice daily to areas of concern and for the Rx regimen, tretinoin was applied to the entire face every other day for 2 weeks and then daily. Based on expert grader analysis, both regimens reduced wrinkles, but the NPP regimen significantly more. Similar results were obtained by computer analysis; however, the difference between the regimens was slightly above significance (17% NPP vs. 11% Rx improvement; $p = 0.06$). Based on self-assessments, the NPP regimen increased overall skin appearance more than the Rx regimen. Compared to baseline, erythema was significantly increased for both regimens at 2 weeks; this side effect disappeared for the NPP regimen after 2 weeks but continued for the Rx regimen. Thus, combination products may be useful to reduce costs compared to peptide-only products.[114]

21.10.4 Evidence for Growth Factors and Cytokines

The antiaging properties and melasma treatment efficacy of growth factor–based products will be reviewed. Mehta et al examined the ability of a product with over 110 growth factors, cytokines, and soluble matrix proteins secreted by cultured neonatal human dermal fibroblasts (TNS Recovery Complex, SkinMedica) to treat facial photodamage.[110] Participants ($n = 60$) applied the active gel or vehicle gel to their faces twice daily for 6 months. Based on optical profilometry using silicone impressions of subjects' lateral canthi, the active gel led to significant improvement in fine lines and texture shadows compared to vehicle at 3 months but not at 6 months; major fine lines did not significantly vary between groups at either time point. Further, review of photographs by three blinded dermatologists did not show any significant difference in photodamage scores between the active and vehicle gels.[110] In a second antiaging study, Gold et al studied a cream including a mixture of growth factors and cytokines cultured from fetal skin cells (PSP, Neocutis, Inc, San Francisco, California, United States).[109] Twenty volunteers with lateral canthi wrinkling applied the growth factor cream or placebo cream for 2 months. Clinical assessment of wrinkles by two independent investigators showed no significant difference between the groups at the end of the study. Skin topography was also assessed via three-dimensional optical imaging (Phase-shift Rapid in-vivo Measurement of Skin device). Several roughness parameters, including maximum roughness depth, were significantly improved for the active cream compared to placebo; however, there were no significant differences between the groups for average roughness and mean roughness depth. While Gold et al found some improvements in wrinkles using optical imaging, these differences were not appreciated by the investigators and thus may not be clinically significant.[109]

In contrast to the previous products that included numerous proteins, Lyons et al performed a split-face study to examine the efficacy of a serum with epidermal growth factor (EGF) for the treatment of melasma.[111] EGF promotes growth and has been used in cosmetics as a whitening agent, moisturizer, and to aid wound healing. Women ($n = 15$) applied either EGF serum or placebo serum to the designated side of their faces twice daily for 8 weeks. Improvement in melasma was assessed by two dermatologists using the Physician Global Aesthetic Improvement Scale. Scoring showed that melasma improved in 73% of subjects using the EGF serum compared to only 13% of those using the placebo serum (p-values not reported). This small pilot study showed promising results for the ability of EGF to treat melasma, and further testing should be done. Although there is some evidence that cosmeceuticals with growth factors may be able to minimally decrease skin wrinkling and treat melasma, OTC growth products vary tremendously in their ingredients and thus likely their efficacy. Given the high price of these cosmeceuticals, consumers may be more satisfied with more affordable, better-studied products.

21.11 Oral Collagen

As the most abundant component of the extracellular matrix, oral collagen supplements are marketed as having antiaging properties. Collagen is extracted from various sources, including porcine, bovine, or marine collagen.[115] Gelatin is formed when collagen is denatured; enzymatic hydrolysis of gelatin then forms collagen hydrolysates (CH).[115] These CH can be further degraded into collagen bioactive peptides, including collagen dipeptides (CDP), like proline–hydroxyproline and hydroxyproline–glycine, as well as collagen tripeptides (CTP), like proline–hydroxyproline–glycine.[115] Given how collagen is processed to various hydrolysates and peptides, OTC collagen products are very diverse; many products also include other ingredients such as vitamins and minerals.[115] Patients need to examine the concentration and composition of active collagen peptides within an OTC product and be advised that the purity of the active ingredients is unknown given the lack of cosmeceutical regulation.[115] Despite the diversity of active and inactive ingredients, a systematic review including over 805 patients observed no adverse effects from the consumption of collagen over 69.2 days on average.[115]

21.11.1 Stability and Systemic Absorption

Choi et al reviewed research on the human bioavailability of CDP and CTP; three studies showed that collagen peptides can be detected in the bloodstream after the oral consumption of CH.[115] After entering the bloodstream, collagen peptides then need to travel to the skin. Using a mouse model, Kawaguchi et al showed that radioactively labelled CH appeared in the skin 30 minutes after oral consumption.[116] Collagen was also detected in dermal fibroblasts using thin-layer chromatography.[116]

21.11.2 Evidence

Choi et al performed a systematic review of 11 randomized controlled trials ($n = 805$ in total) that evaluated dermatologic benefits of oral collagen.[115] Eight studies used an average of 10 g of CH, one study used 5 g of CDP, and two studies used 3 g of CTP on average. However, only three of these studies examined the antiaging effects of oral collagen. The other studies evaluated collagen's effects of various skin parameters including skin hydration, skin elasticity, and collagen density. Proksch et al completed an 8-week study where 114 women consumed 2.5 g of CH daily (bioactive collagen peptide, VERISOL, Gelita AG, Eberbach, Germany).[117] Wrinkle volume at the lateral canthus was measured using a three-dimensional optical instrument. Collagen consumption led to a 20.1% reduction in eye wrinkle volume compared to the placebo group ($p < 0.01$).[117] In a second study, Schunck et al used the same collagen product (VERISOL) to examine collagen's effect on thigh cellulite morphology in 105 female subjects over 6 months.[118] Cellulite morphology was assessed using the pinch test, where the skin of the subject's outer thigh is pinched and skin dimpling is graded from 0 (no cellulite) to 4 (severe dimpled surface while lying down and standing). After 6 months, daily collagen consumption led to a 9% reduction in mean cellulite scores compared to the placebo group.[118] The third antiaging study used CDP; Inoue et al performed an 8-week study that included 85 female participants who consumed a 5-g fish CH product with either a high ratio of CDP (proline–hydroxyproline, hydroxyproline–glycine; 2 g/kg) or low ratio of CDP (0.1 g/kg).[119] Wrinkles were assessed from the cheek to lateral canthus using a visual analysis device. After 8 weeks, the high CDP product led a statistically significant reduction in the number of wrinkles, wrinkle depth, and roughness compared to placebo; there was no difference between groups for wrinkle area. The low CDP product only significantly improved skin roughness.[119] Overall, preliminary results show that oral collagen consumption may have beneficial effects on skin wrinkles and cellulite. But the studies only examined short-term results and included only a small number of healthy women; so, larger studies with more diverse participants are needed.

21.12 Conclusion

This chapter discussed the stability, topical penetration, and supporting evidence of common cosmeceutical ingredients. Regardless of the results, the stability and penetration data are based on controlled conditions in a lab. Thus, the shelf lives of cosmeceutical products are likely lower than indicated given they will be exposed to oxygen with application and may be stored at nonrecommended, fluctuating temperatures. Although safe, many of these ingredients can cause skin irritation, especially topical curcumin, which caused contact dermatitis in 10% of patients.[84] The efficacy of these ingredients is variable. Niacin, pal-KTTKS, and growth hormone/cytokine products reduced wrinkles, but only marginally, so these ingredients may not be worth the high price. Oral collagen may improve wrinkles and reduce skin cellulite based on preliminary evidence, but OTC products are diverse and may not have sufficient active collagen hydrolysates or peptides to produce the desired effects. OTC retinoids, excluding REs, have a larger impact on wrinkles, but patients may experience more success with prescription retinoids. REs do not reduce wrinkling but can concentrate in the epidermis, offering photoprotection. DNA repair enzymes and AA/TOC/FA products also prevented photodamage; therefore, these ingredients may be useful additions to sunscreens and moisturizers to prevent photoaging. To reduce hyperpigmentation, Az, HQ, kojic acid, NIC, and TA all showed efficacy in clinical trials. However, similar to retinoids, prescriptions including higher concentrations of HQ are more effective. Use of EGF showed improvement in melasma in a small pilot trial, but given its high cost, this protein needs further study before it is added to our armamentarium of hyperpigmentation treatments. Overall, although some ingredients are efficacious, patients should be aware that many product claims are not substantiated. Given the crowded cosmeceutical market and the high number of non-evidence-based products, patients may be better served by asking their dermatologists for guidance rather than spending time and money determining which cosmeceuticals provide benefits.

References

[1] Draelos ZD. Cosmeceuticals: what's real, what's not. Dermatol Clin. 2019; 37(1):107–115

[2] Levin J, Momin SB. How much do we really know about our favorite cosmeceutical ingredients? J Clin Aesthet Dermatol. 2010; 3(2):22–41

[3] Babamiri K, Nassab R. Cosmeceuticals: the evidence behind the retinoids. Aesthet Surg J. 2010; 30(1):74–77

[4] Kedishvili NY. Retinoic acid synthesis and degradation. Subcell Biochem. 2016; 81:127–161

[5] Sorg O, Antille C, Kaya G, Saurat J-H. Retinoids in cosmeceuticals. Dermatol Ther. 2006; 19(5):289–296

[6] Lee C-M. Fifty years of research and development of cosmeceuticals: a contemporary review. J Cosmet Dermatol. 2016; 15(4):527–539

[7] Ortonne J-P. Retinoid therapy of pigmentary disorders. Dermatol Ther. 2006; 19(5):280–288

[8] Sheth VM, Pandya AG. Melasma: a comprehensive update: part II. J Am Acad Dermatol. 2011; 65(4):699–714

[9] Stratigos AJ, Katsambas AD. The role of topical retinoids in the treatment of photoaging. Drugs. 2005; 65(8):1061–1072

[10] Creidi P, Vienne MP, Ochonisky S, et al. Profilometric evaluation of photodamage after topical retinaldehyde and retinoic acid treatment. J Am Acad Dermatol. 1998; 39(6):960–965

[11] Green C, Orchard G, Cerio R, Hawk JL. A clinicopathological study of the effects of topical retinyl propionate cream in skin photoageing. Clin Exp Dermatol. 1998; 23(4):162–167

[12] Kang S, Duell EA, Fisher GJ, et al. Application of retinol to human skin in vivo induces epidermal hyperplasia and cellular retinoid binding proteins characteristic of retinoic acid but without measurable retinoic acid levels or irritation. J Invest Dermatol. 1995; 105(4):549–556

[13] Veraldi S, Rossi LC, Barbareschi M. Are topical retinoids teratogenic? G Ital Dermatol Venereol. 2016; 151(6):700–705

[14] Shapiro L, Pastuszak A, Curto G, Koren G. Safety of first-trimester exposure to topical tretinoin: prospective cohort study. Lancet. 1997; 350(9085):1143–1144

[15] Loureiro KD, Kao KK, Jones KL, et al. Minor malformations characteristic of the retinoic acid embryopathy and other birth outcomes in children of women exposed to topical tretinoin during early pregnancy. Am J Med Genet A. 2005; 136(2):117–121

[16] Jick SS, Terris BZ, Jick H. First trimester topical tretinoin and congenital disorders. Lancet. 1993; 341(8854):1181–1182

[17] Fu PP, Cheng S-H, Coop L, et al. Photoreaction, phototoxicity, and photocarcinogenicity of retinoids. J Environ Sci Health Part C Environ Carcinog Ecotoxicol Rev. 2003; 21(2):165–197

[18] Higgins S, Wesley NO. Topical retinoids and cosmeceuticals: where is the scientific evidence to recommend products to patients? Curr Dermatol Rep. 2015; 4(2):56–62

[19] Duell EA, Kang S, Voorhees JJ. Unoccluded retinol penetrates human skin in vivo more effectively than unoccluded retinyl palmitate or retinoic acid. J Invest Dermatol. 1997; 109(3):301–305

[20] Saurat JH, Didierjean L, Masgrau E, et al. Topical retinaldehyde on human skin: biologic effects and tolerance. J Invest Dermatol. 1994; 103(6):770–774

[21] O'Byrne SM, Blaner WS. Retinol and retinyl esters: biochemistry and physiology. J Lipid Res. 2013; 54(7):1731–1743

[22] Lupo MP. Antioxidants and vitamins in cosmetics. Clin Dermatol. 2001; 19(4):467–473

[23] Watson REB, Long SP, Bowden JJ, Bastrilles JY, Barton SP, Griffiths CEM. Repair of photoaged dermal matrix by topical application of a cosmetic "antiageing" product. Br J Dermatol. 2008; 158(3):472–477

[24] Antille C, Tran C, Sorg O, Carraux P, Didierjean L, Saurat J-H. Vitamin A exerts a photoprotective action in skin by absorbing ultraviolet B radiation. J Invest Dermatol. 2003; 121(5):1163–1167

[25] Kafi R, Kwak HS, Schumacher WE, et al. Improvement of naturally aged skin with vitamin A (retinol). Arch Dermatol. 2007; 143(5):606–612

[26] Ho ET, Trookman NS, Sperber BR, et al. A randomized, double-blind, controlled comparative trial of the anti-aging properties of nonprescription tri-retinol 1.1% vs. prescription tretinoin 0.025%. J Drugs Dermatol. 2012; 11(1):64–69

[27] Draelos ZD. Skin lightening preparations and the hydroquinone controversy. Dermatol Ther. 2007; 20(5):308–313

[28] Halder RM, Richards GM. Management of dyschromias in ethnic skin. Dermatol Ther. 2004; 17(2):151–157

[29] Gupta AK, Gover MD, Nouri K, Taylor S. The treatment of melasma: a review of clinical trials. J Am Acad Dermatol. 2006; 55(6):1048–1065

[30] Gao X-H, Zhang L, Wei H, Chen H-D. Efficacy and safety of innovative cosmeceuticals. Clin Dermatol. 2008; 26(4):367–374

[31] Levitt J. The safety of hydroquinone: a dermatologist's response to the 2006 Federal Register. J Am Acad Dermatol. 2007; 57(5):854–872

[32] Levin CY, Maibach H. Exogenous ochronosis. An update on clinical features, causative agents and treatment options. Am J Clin Dermatol. 2001; 2(4):213–217

[33] DeCaprio AP. The toxicology of hydroquinone–relevance to occupational and environmental exposure. Crit Rev Toxicol. 1999; 29(3):283–330

[34] Garcia A, Fulton JE, Jr. The combination of glycolic acid and hydroquinone or kojic acid for the treatment of melasma and related conditions. Dermatol Surg. 1996; 22(5):443–447

[35] Khezri K, Saeedi M, Morteza-Semnani K, Akbari J, Rostamkalaei SS. An emerging technology in lipid research for targeting hydrophilic

drugs to the skin in the treatment of hyperpigmentation disorders: kojic acid-solid lipid nanoparticles. Artif Cells Nanomed Biotechnol. 2020; 48(1):841–853

[36] Wester RC, Melendres J, Hui X, et al. Human in vivo and in vitro hydroquinone topical bioavailability, metabolism, and disposition. J Toxicol Environ Health A. 1998; 54(4):301–317

[37] Kim H, Choi J, Cho JK, Kim SY, Lee YS. Solid-phase synthesis of kojic acid-tripeptides and their tyrosinase inhibitory activity, storage stability, and toxicity. Bioorg Med Chem Lett. 2004; 14(11):2843–2846

[38] Yoshimura K, Sato K, Aiba-Kojima E, et al. Repeated treatment protocols for melasma and acquired dermal melanocytosis. Dermatol Surg. 2006; 32(3):365–371

[39] Monteiro RC, Kishore BN, Bhat RM, Sukumar D, Martis J, Ganesh HK. A comparative study of the efficacy of 4% hydroquinone vs 0.75% kojic acid cream in the treatment of facial melasma. Indian J Dermatol. 2013; 58(2):157

[40] Gupta AK, Gover MD, Nouri K, Taylor S. The treatment of melasma: a review of clinical trials. J Am Acad Dermatol. 2006; 55(6):1048–1065

[41] Fitton A, Goa KL. Azelaic acid. A review of its pharmacological properties and therapeutic efficacy in acne and hyperpigmentary skin disorders. Drugs. 1991; 41(5):780–798

[42] Akamatsu H, Komura J, Asada Y, Miyachi Y, Niwa Y. Inhibitory effect of azelaic acid on neutrophil functions: a possible cause for its efficacy in treating pathogenetically unrelated diseases. Arch Dermatol Res. 1991; 283(3):162–166

[43] Nugrahani HN, Iskandarsyah, Harmita. Stability study of azelaic acid proethosomes with lyoprotectant as stabilizer. J Adv Pharm Technol Res. 2018; 9(2):61–64

[44] Täuber U, Weiss C, Matthes H. Percutaneous absorption of azelaic acid in humans. Exp Dermatol. 1992; 1(4):176–179

[45] Gasco MR, Gallarate M, Pattarino F. In vitro permeation of azelaic acid from viscosized microemulsions. Int J Pharm. 1991; 69(3):193–196

[46] Burchacka E, Potaczek P, Paduszyński P, Karłowicz-Bodalska K, Han T, Han S. New effective azelaic acid liposomal gel formulation of enhanced pharmaceutical bioavailability. Biomed Pharmacother. 2016; 83:771–775

[47] Taraz M, Niknam S, Ehsani AH. Tranexamic acid in treatment of melasma: a comprehensive review of clinical studies. Dermatol Ther (Heidelb). 2017; 30(3):e12465

[48] Del Rosario E, Florez-Pollack S, Zapata L, Jr, et al. Randomized, placebo-controlled, double-blind study of oral tranexamic acid in the treatment of moderate-to-severe melasma. J Am Acad Dermatol. 2018; 78(2):363–369

[49] Bala HR, Lee S, Wong C, Pandya AG, Rodrigues M. Oral tranexamic acid for the treatment of melasma: a review. Dermatol Surg. 2018; 44 (6):814–825

[50] Donnelly RF. Stability of tranexamic acid mouth rinse. Int J Pharm Compd. 2018; 22(5):412–416

[51] Vijayakumar A, Baskaran R, Yoo BK. Skin permeation and retention of topical bead formulation containing tranexamic acid. J Cosmet Laser Ther. 2017; 19(1):68–74

[52] Kanechorn Na Ayuthaya P, Niumphradit N, Manosroi A, Nakakes A. Topical 5% tranexamic acid for the treatment of melasma in Asians: a double-blind randomized controlled clinical trial. J Cosmet Laser Ther. 2012; 14(3):150–154

[53] Ebrahimi B, Naeini FF. Topical tranexamic acid as a promising treatment for melasma. J Res Med Sci. 2014; 19(8):753–757

[54] Banihashemi M, Zabolinejad N, Jaafari MR, Salehi M, Jabari A. Comparison of therapeutic effects of liposomal tranexamic acid and conventional hydroquinone on melasma. J Cosmet Dermatol. 2015; 14(3):174–177

[55] Tanno O, Ota Y, Kitamura N, Katsube T, Inoue S. Nicotinamide increases biosynthesis of ceramides as well as other stratum corneum lipids to improve the epidermal permeability barrier. Br J Dermatol. 2000; 143(3):524–531

[56] Hakozaki T, Minwalla L, Zhuang J, et al. The effect of niacinamide on reducing cutaneous pigmentation and suppression of melanosome transfer. Br J Dermatol. 2002; 147(1):20–31

[57] Bissett DL, Miyamoto K, Sun P, Li J, Berge CA. Topical niacinamide reduces yellowing, wrinkling, red blotchiness, and hyperpigmented spots in aging facial skin. Int J Cosmet Sci. 2004; 26(5):231–238

[58] Otte N, Borelli C, Korting HC. Nicotinamide: biologic actions of an emerging cosmetic ingredient. Int J Cosmet Sci. 2005; 27(5):255–261

[59] Boonme P, Boonthongchuay C, Wongpoowarak W, Amnuaikit T. Evaluation of nicotinamide microemulsion on the skin penetration enhancement. Pharm Dev Technol. 2016; 21(1):116–120

[60] Feldmann RJ, Maibach HI. Absorption of some organic compounds through the skin in man. J Invest Dermatol. 1970; 54(5):399–404

[61] Navarrete-Solís J, Castanedo-Cázares JP, Torres-Álvarez B, et al. A double-blind, randomized clinical trial of niacinamide 4% versus hydroquinone 4% in the treatment of melasma. Dermatol Res Pract. 2011; 2011:379173

[62] Lin JY, Selim MA, Shea CR, et al. UV photoprotection by combination topical antioxidants vitamin C and vitamin E. J Am Acad Dermatol. 2003; 48(6):866–874

[63] Pinnell SR, Yang H, Omar M, et al. Topical L-ascorbic acid: percutaneous absorption studies. Dermatol Surg. 2001; 27(2):137–142

[64] Murray JC, Burch JA, Streilein RD, Iannacchione MA, Hall RP, Pinnell SR. A topical antioxidant solution containing vitamins C and E stabilized by ferulic acid provides protection for human skin against damage caused by ultraviolet irradiation. J Am Acad Dermatol. 2008; 59(3):418–425

[65] Geesin JC, Darr D, Kaufman R, Murad S, Pinnell SR. Ascorbic acid specifically increases type I and type III procollagen messenger RNA levels in human skin fibroblast. J Invest Dermatol. 1988; 90(4):420–424

[66] Tajima S, Pinnell SR. Ascorbic acid preferentially enhances type I and III collagen gene transcription in human skin fibroblasts. J Dermatol Sci. 1996; 11(3):250–253

[67] Chan AC. Partners in defense, vitamin E and vitamin C. Can J Physiol Pharmacol. 1993; 71(9):725–731

[68] Fitzpatrick RE, Rostan EF. Double-blind, half-face study comparing topical vitamin C and vehicle for rejuvenation of photodamage. Dermatol Surg. 2002; 28(3):231–236

[69] Tanaydin V, Conings J, Malyar M, van der Hulst R, van der Lei B. The role of topical vitamin E in scar management: a systematic review. Aesthet Surg J. 2016; 36(8):959–965

[70] Zduńska K, Dana A, Kolodziejczak A, Rotsztejn H. Antioxidant properties of ferulic acid and its possible application. Skin Pharmacol Physiol. 2018; 31(6):332–336

[71] Raschke T, Koop U, Düsing H-J, et al. Topical activity of ascorbic acid: from in vitro optimization to in vivo efficacy. Skin Pharmacol Physiol. 2004; 17(4):200–206

[72] Stamford NPJ. Stability, transdermal penetration, and cutaneous effects of ascorbic acid and its derivatives. J Cosmet Dermatol. 2012; 11(4):310–317

[73] Bissett DL. Common cosmeceuticals. Clin Dermatol. 2009; 27(5):435–445

[74] Austria R, Semenzato A, Bettero A. Stability of vitamin C derivatives in solution and topical formulations. J Pharm Biomed Anal. 1997; 15 (6):795–801

[75] Keen MA, Hassan I. Vitamin E in dermatology. Indian Dermatol Online J. 2016; 7(4):311–315

[76] Alberts DS, Goldman R, Xu MJ, et al. Disposition and metabolism of topically administered alpha-tocopherol acetate: a common ingredient of commercially available sunscreens and cosmetics. Nutr Cancer. 1996; 26(2):193–201

[77] Lin FH, Lin JY, Gupta RD, et al. Ferulic acid stabilizes a solution of vitamins C and E and doubles its photoprotection of skin. J Invest Dermatol. 2005; 125(4):826–832

[78] Burke KE. Interaction of vitamins C and E as better cosmeceuticals. Dermatol Ther. 2007; 20(5):314–321

[79] Steenvoorden DPT, Beijersbergen van Henegouwen G. Protection against UV-induced systemic immunosuppression in mice by a single topical application of the antioxidant vitamins C and E. Int J Radiat Biol. 1999; 75(6):747–755

[80] Humbert PG, Haftek M, Creidi P, et al. Topical ascorbic acid on photoaged skin. Clinical, topographical and ultrastructural evaluation: double-blind study vs. placebo. Exp Dermatol. 2003; 12 (3):237–244

[81] Gupta SC, Prasad S, Kim JH, et al. Multitargeting by curcumin as revealed by molecular interaction studies. Nat Prod Rep. 2011; 28 (12):1937–1955

[82] Heng MCY. Curcumin targeted signaling pathways: basis for anti-photoaging and anti-carcinogenic therapy. Int J Dermatol. 2010; 49 (6):608–622

[83] Cheng AL, Hsu CH, Lin JK, et al. Phase I clinical trial of curcumin, a chemopreventive agent, in patients with high-risk or pre-malignant lesions. Anticancer Res. 2001; 21 4B:2895–2900

[84] Sommerfeld B. Randomised, placebo-controlled, double-blind, split-face study on the clinical efficacy of Tricutan on skin firmness. Phytomedicine. 2007; 14(11):711–715

[85] Ablon G, Kogan S. A six-month, randomized, double-blind, placebo-controlled study evaluating the safety and efficacy of a nutraceutical supplement for promoting hair growth in women with self-perceived thinning hair. J Drugs Dermatol. 2018; 17(5):558–565

[86] Vaughn AR, Branum A, Sivamani RK. Effects of turmeric (Curcuma longa) on skin health: a systematic review of the clinical evidence. Phytother Res. 2016; 30(8):1243–1264

[87] Kloepper JE, Ernst N, Krieger K, et al. NF-κB activity is required for anagen maintenance in human hair follicles in vitro. J Invest Dermatol. 2014; 134(7):2036–2038

[88] Gupta S, Ghosh S, Gupta S, Sakhuja P. Effect of curcumin on the expression of p53, transforming growth factor-β, and inducible nitric oxide synthase in oral submucous fibrosis: a pilot study. J Investig Clin Dent. 2017; 8(4)

[89] Seiberg M, Marthinuss J, Stenn KS. Changes in expression of apoptosis-associated genes in skin mark early catagen. J Invest Dermatol. 1995; 104(1):78–82

[90] Shishodia S. Molecular mechanisms of curcumin action: gene expression. Biofactors. 2013; 39(1):37–55

[91] Salem M, Rohani S, Gillies ER. Curcumin, a promising anti-cancer therapeutic: a review of its chemical properties, bioactivity and approaches to cancer cell delivery. RSC Advances. 2014; 4(21): 10815–10829

[92] Wang Y-J, Pan M-H, Cheng A-L, et al. Stability of curcumin in buffer solutions and characterization of its degradation products. J Pharm Biomed Anal. 1997; 15(12):1867–1876

[93] Liu W, Zhai Y, Heng X, et al. Oral bioavailability of curcumin: problems and advancements. J Drug Target. 2016; 24(8):694–702

[94] Shoba G, Joy D, Joseph T, Majeed M, Rajendran R, Srinivas PS. Influence of piperine on the pharmacokinetics of curcumin in animals and human volunteers. Planta Med. 1998; 64(4):353–356

[95] Hatcher H, Planalp R, Cho J, Torti FM, Torti SV. Curcumin: from ancient medicine to current clinical trials. Cell Mol Life Sci. 2008; 65 (11):1631–1652

[96] Heng MC, Song MK, Harker J, Heng MK. Drug-induced suppression of phosphorylase kinase activity correlates with resolution of psoriasis as assessed by clinical, histological and immunohistochemical parameters. Br J Dermatol. 2000; 143(5):937–949

[97] Yarosh D, Alas LG, Yee V, et al. Pyrimidine dimer removal enhanced by DNA repair liposomes reduces the incidence of UV skin cancer in mice. Cancer Res. 1992; 52(15):4227–4231

[98] Kabir Y, Seidel R, Mcknight B, Moy R. DNA repair enzymes: an important role in skin cancer prevention and reversal of photodamage–a review of the literature. J Drugs Dermatol. 2015; 14 (3):297–303

[99] Cafardi JA, Elmets CA. T4 endonuclease V: review and application to dermatology. Expert Opin Biol Ther. 2008; 8(6):829–838

[100] Berardesca E, Bertona M, Altabas K, Altabas V, Emanuele E. Reduced ultraviolet-induced DNA damage and apoptosis in human skin with topical application of a photolyase-containing DNA repair enzyme

cream: clues to skin cancer prevention. Mol Med Rep. 2012; 5(2): 570–574

[101] Yarosh D, Klein J, O'Connor A, Hawk J, Rafal E, Wolf P, Xeroderma Pigmentosum Study Group. Effect of topically applied T4 endonuclease V in liposomes on skin cancer in xeroderma pigmentosum: a randomised study. Lancet. 2001; 357(9260):926–929

[102] Yarosh D, Bucana C, Cox P, Alas L, Kibitel J, Kripke M. Localization of liposomes containing a DNA repair enzyme in murine skin. J Invest Dermatol. 1994; 103(4):461–468

[103] Robinson LR, Fitzgerald NC, Doughty DG, Dawes NC, Berge CA, Bissett DL. Topical palmitoyl pentapeptide provides improvement in photoaged human facial skin. Int J Cosmet Sci. 2005; 27(3):155–160

[104] Katayama K, Armendariz-Borunda J, Raghow R, Kang AH, Seyer JM. A pentapeptide from type I procollagen promotes extracellular matrix production. J Biol Chem. 1993; 268(14):9941–9944

[105] Mulder GD, Patt LM, Sanders L, et al. Enhanced healing of ulcers in patients with diabetes by topical treatment with glycyl-l-histidyl-l-lysine copper. Wound Repair Regen. 1994; 2(4):259–269

[106] Badenhorst T, Svirskis D, Wu Z. Physicochemical characterization of native glycyl-l-histidyl-l-lysine tripeptide for wound healing and anti-aging: a preformulation study for dermal delivery. Pharm Dev Technol. 2016; 21(2):152–160

[107] Miller TR, Wagner JD, Baack BR, Eisbach KJ. Effects of topical copper tripeptide complex on CO_2 laser-resurfaced skin. Arch Facial Plast Surg. 2006; 8(4):252–259

[108] Mehta RC, Fitzpatrick RE. Endogenous growth factors as cosmeceuticals. Dermatol Ther. 2007; 20(5):350–359

[109] Gold MH, Goldman MP, Biron J. Human growth factor and cytokine skin cream for facial skin rejuvenation as assessed by 3D in vivo optical skin imaging. J Drugs Dermatol. 2007; 6(10):1018–1023

[110] Mehta RC, Smith SR, Grove GL, et al. Reduction in facial photodamage by a topical growth factor product. J Drugs Dermatol. 2008; 7(9):864–871

[111] Lyons A, Stoll J, Moy R. A randomized, double-blind, placebo-controlled, split-face study of the efficacy of topical epidermal growth factor for the treatment of melasma. J Drugs Dermatol. 2018; 17(9):970–973

[112] Choi YL, Park EJ, Kim E, Na DH, Shin Y-H. Dermal stability and in vitro skin permeation of collagen pentapeptides (KTTKS and palmitoyl-KTTKS). Biomol Ther (Seoul). 2014; 22(4):321–327

[113] Hostynek JJ, Dreher F, Maibach HI. Human skin retention and penetration of a copper tripeptide in vitro as function of skin layer towards anti-inflammatory therapy. Inflamm Res. 2010; 59(11): 983–988

[114] Fu JJJ, Hillebrand GG, Raleigh P, et al. A randomized, controlled comparative study of the wrinkle reduction benefits of a cosmetic niacinamide/peptide/retinyl propionate product regimen vs. a prescription 0.02% tretinoin product regimen. Br J Dermatol. 2010; 162(3):647–654

[115] Choi FD, Sung CT, Juhasz MLW, Mesinkovsk NA. Oral collagen supplementation: a systematic review of dermatological applications. J Drugs Dermatol. 2019; 18(1):9–16

[116] Kawaguchi T, Nanbu PN, Kurokawa M. Distribution of prolylhydroxyproline and its metabolites after oral administration in rats. Biol Pharm Bull. 2012; 35(3):422–427

[117] Proksch E, Schunck M, Zague V, Segger D, Degwert J, Oesser S. Oral intake of specific bioactive collagen peptides reduces skin wrinkles and increases dermal matrix synthesis. Skin Pharmacol Physiol. 2014; 27(3):113–119

[118] Schunck M, Zague V, Oesser S, Proksch E. Dietary supplementation with specific collagen peptides has a body mass index-dependent beneficial effect on cellulite morphology. J Med Food. 2015; 18(12): 1340–1348

[119] Inoue N, Sugihara F, Wang X. Ingestion of bioactive collagen hydrolysates enhance facial skin moisture and elasticity and reduce facial ageing signs in a randomised double-blind placebo-controlled clinical study. J Sci Food Agric. 2016; 96(12):4077–4081

22 Kybella/Deoxycholic Acid/Off-Label Uses

Sachin M. Shridharani, Teri N. Moak, Trina G. Ebersole, and Grace M. Tisch

Summary

Fat reduction for facial and body contouring continues to be one of the most sought-after aesthetic procedures. There continues to be a keen interest in permanent reduction of adipocyte deposition by less invasive methods. The introduction of injectable deoxycholic acid has had a profound impact on aesthetic facial and body contouring by offering both clinicians and patients an FDA-approved option to reduce the appearance of unwanted fat. This chapter serves as an overview to assist the clinician interested in incorporating this treatment into their practice and a top line summary of alternatives.

Keywords: Kybella, deoxycholic acid, DCA, kythera, fat-reduction, aesthetic facial contouring, liposuction

22.1 Introduction

The practice of aesthetic surgery seeks to provide patients with a youthful, healthy appearance via contouring of diverse areas in the face and body alike. Although bony structures may be targets for aesthetic improvement, this subspecialty of plastic surgery largely focuses on manipulation of soft tissues to achieve youthful beauty. Adipose tissue, in particular, has long been a target *and* vehicle for attaining an aesthetically improved appearance in multiple areas of the body. Specifically, removal of unwanted fat has historically been a means of creating a sleek, healthy contour in areas such as the thighs, abdomen, and arms. In more recent years, injection of fat has been recognized as an equally viable means of rejuvenation in areas such as the face and breast. As such, the evolution of adiposity tailoring plays a key role in modern-day aesthetics.

Removal of unwanted fat in multiple areas of the body was one of the first targets of aesthetic interventions. This technique is known today as liposuction, and it has become the gold standard for fat removal and the most popular procedure worldwide since its introduction in the latter half of the 20th century.[1] The first known attempt at removal of unwanted fat for cosmetic purposes was performed by the French surgeon Dr. Charles Dujarier in 1921. His technique involved excision of excess skin and subcutaneous tissue, unfortunately resulting in tissue necrosis and amputation secondary to overly aggressive tissue removal and compromised blood supply.[2,3] Multiple nuances in technique were developed and modified, though significant complications plagued direct adipose tissue excision.[3] In the 1970s, the German physician Dr. Josef Schrudde introduced the first semblance of liposuction as we know it today, employing a sharp uterine curette to excise subcutaneous adipose tissue. He later began using a "windshield wiper motion" with this sharp curette in the subcutaneous layers of fat to improve upon evenness of fat resection.[3] Dr Bahman Teimourian, a U.S. surgeon, implemented a tunneling technique around the same time as Schrudde with similar goals.[2] Unfortunately, these techniques were still complicated by excess bleeding and ecchymoses, contour irregularities, seroma, postprocedure loose and sagging skin, and even skin necrosis from overly aggressive fat resection, which compromised blood supply to superficial tissue layers.[2,3] In 1977, Drs Arpad and George Fisher described the use of suction to assist the removal of fat, though this was still performed with a sharp curette, and high complication rates persisted.[2] It was not until the introduction of technological advances by the French surgeon Dr Yves-Gerard Illouz that modern liposuction began to take shape. Illouz was the first to perform liposuction with a blunt-tip cannula and suction assistance via small access incisions with use of clear tubing to visualize fat removal for assessment of quantity and presence of blood in the aspirate.[2,3]

The evolution of liposuction has continued, resulting in multiple methodologies in use today, each with their distinct advantages and disadvantages. Although an exhaustive comparison is beyond the scope of this text, a brief synopsis is provided on the most commonly used mainstream liposuction techniques.

22.1.1 Ultrasound-Assisted Liposuction

Ultrasound-assisted liposuction (UAL), initially described by Zocchi, employs ultrasonic energy to allow for more selective lipolysis. Ultrasound energy is used to create large-scale cellular disruption of adipocytes and is removed in a second stage with the use of suction-assisted lipectomy (SAL). This method results in decreased blood loss and improved contour, particularly in areas with abundant fibrous tissue such as the back and chest. Disadvantages of this technique involve increased cost, larger access incisions, and increased thermal injury risk.[2,4,5]

22.1.2 Power-Assisted Liposuction

Power-assisted liposuction (PAL) utilizes a rapidly vibrating cannula to break up fibrous fat in a less labor-intensive procedure with decreased operative time. Disadvantages of this technique involve increased cost compared with SAL and a steep operator learning curve.[2]

22.1.3 Laser-Assisted Liposuction

Laser-assisted liposuction (LAL) was first described by Apfelberg in 1994 and exploits the principles of selective photothermolysis to preferentially lyse adipocytes without affecting surrounding tissues. Multiple lasers have been studied for laser lipolysis with each laser having its own unique advantages. However, as a whole, LAL boasts superior treatment of areas with large fat deposits with less bleeding and improved postprocedure skin elasticity. The potential for thermal injury, prolonged procedure time, and high equipment cost are the most significant disadvantages of this technique.[2,3,5]

22.1.4 Radiofrequency-Assisted Liposuction

Radiofrequency-assisted liposuction (RFAL) was developed to target the complication of loose and sagging skin following various fat reduction techniques. Radiofrequency not only dissolves adipocytes but also contracts the fibroseptal network, resulting in skin tightening via dermal collagen contraction, subdermal remodeling, and neocollagen formation. Theoretically with RFAL, there is a risk of thermal injury, though few instances have been reported. However, this remains a relatively new technology with longer-term data collection needed to assess the true incidence of this complication.[2]

22.1.5 Helium Plasma

Helium plasma, developed by Apyx Medical as Renuvion/ J-plasma, emerged from hepatobiliary surgery during its use for coagulation when it was noted that alteration in settings of this technology resulted in shortening of fibroseptal networks from dermis to muscle fascia, thus tightening skin. Unlike prior technologies on the market, helium plasma does not pose a risk of thermal injury to surrounding tissues.

Unfortunately, all of the above-listed methods of managing excess body fat involve an invasive, surgical procedure. Furthermore, the majority of these techniques aim to address unwanted fat in larger quantities over larger body surface areas. As such, these techniques have limitations in their ability to treat unwanted fat in small or finite areas such as the face and neck. Until recently, no effective, nonsurgical interventions were available to patients who did not want to incur the risk or downtime of surgery or who were not good surgical candidates for various reasons.

In the late 1990s and early 2000s, mesotherapy, developed by the Frenchman Dr Michel Pistor, emerged as one of the first nonsurgical means of addressing unwanted fat.[6] Mesotherapy is a technique that involves microinjections of pharmaceutical and homeopathic combinations of chemical compounds, plant extracts, vitamins, and other ingredients into areas of unwanted fat to induce lipolysis and cell death.[6] Unfortunately, mesotherapy was never approved by the Food and Drug Administration (FDA) secondary a lack of peer reviewed

data to support reproducible, reliable, and safe results. Although mesotherapy is not used in the United States, it is still widely available in Europe and South Africa.[6]

Further advances in nonsurgical fat reduction have built on the principles of surgical liposuction. For example, although LAL utilizes heat thermolysis to address adipose tissue, cryolipolysis or CoolSculpting involves the use of cooling tissue to a temperature that induces breakdown of adipose tissue without affecting surrounding tissue. Body FX has built on RFAL technology, delivering RF energy in a noninvasive manner to target subdermal fat and tighten overlying skin. Liposonix employs US technology similar to UAL to noninvasively reduce fat in unwanted areas. Whereas these methodologies have alleviated the surgical versus nonsurgical component of choosing an appropriate treatment, they remain limited in their ability to treat fat in small, targeted areas.

Continued interest in fat reduction in small areas not amenable to surgical intervention has resulted in the interest of creating an injectable molecule to address these problem areas. This interest has led to the recognition of deoxycholic acid (DCA). That DCA could safely stimulate adipocytolysis has resulted in this treatment being the current gold standard for nonsurgical fat reduction in small pockets.

22.2 Modalities/Treatment Options Available

Multiple modalities exist for targeting unwanted fat across multiple areas of the body. In general, the decision-making process should include the following considerations: surgical versus nonsurgical approach, large-volume versus small-volume fat reduction, and large versus small body surface area involved. A summary of many current technologies is discussed in the prior section. However, the focus of this chapter is tailored fat reduction in small-volume, small body surface areas. Specifically, this chapter aims to provide a thorough understanding of DCA, its uses, techniques for injection, and patient care including preprocedure patient selection and postprocedure care.

DCA is a secondary bile acid produced endogenously in the human gastrointestinal (GI) tract. This bile acid functions to emulsify and solubilize dietary fats as they undergo digestion and conversion to utilizable sources of energy.[7,8,9] Knowledge of DCA and its chemical properties has led to the adaptation of this molecule for aesthetic use in the form of ATX-101 (Kybella, United States; Belkyra, Canada; Kythera Biopharmaceuticals Inc., subsidiary of Allergan Inc., Westlake Village, California, United States).[7,8,9] ATX-101 is synthetic, sterile DCA with its chemical structure identical to human GI tract endogenous bile acid.

Prior to its use in aesthetics, ATX-101 has previously been used in the treatment of lipomas and in association with other substances such as influenza vaccines.[10,11,12,13,14] When injected into subcutaneous tissues, ATX-101 causes lysis of adipocytes via membrane destabilization with a subsequent reduction in fat volume. The injectable nature of this chemical compound makes it an ideal treatment for fat reduction in very small areas not amenable to treatment with large cannulas or applicators. Further, its predictability in dispersion, half-life, and results render it the treatment of choice for sensitive areas that require tailored treatment. In 2015, ATX-101 was approved by the FDA as the first injectable drug indicated for submental fat (SMF) reduction in the United States and Canada and has since become the gold standard for nonsurgical, small-volume fat reduction.[8,9]

22.3 Indications

Over $1.6 billion was spent on injectables according to the most recent American Society for Aesthetic Plastic Surgery (ASAPS) data from 2019.[15] Nonsurgical fat reduction, in particular, was among the top four most common nonsurgical procedures performed in 2019.[15] As nonsurgical facial and body contouring techniques continue to rise in popularity, practitioners should have a comprehensive knowledge of ATX-101 as a possible treatment option.

The on-label indication for ATX-101 injection is for the improvement of moderate-to-severe convexity associated with SMF. Submental convexity or fullness is a common area of aesthetic concern for males and females alike and can be resistant to reduction through standard diet and exercise as there are correlations between submental fullness and genetic predisposition.[25] Further, the accumulation of SMF is associated with negative social and psychological perceptions of oneself by both the patient and others.[17,18,19,20,21,22,23,38] Men, in particular, were found to consider submental fullness a significant aesthetic concern as they age.[17,24] With judicious patient selection and proper technique, ATX-101 injections can be used to reduce SMF, enhance jawline definition, and improve the cervicomental angle.

The off-label use of ATX-101 injections to treat adipose tissue in nonsubmental regions is common in clinical practice[29,30,31,32,33,34,35,36] and will be discussed in more detail in a later section (see section "Off-Label ATX-1").

22.4 Patient Selection

Prior to administering ATX-101, one should proceed with a detailed analysis of the area being evaluated. In general, the location should have good skin quality and palpable superficial fat.

22.4.1 Preoperative Considerations

In regard to the on-label use of ATX-101, a thorough analysis of the submental region should be performed. The preplatysmal fat should be isolated on examination by having the patient flex the platysma, which functions to separate the pre- and postplatysmal fat. This will also identify platysmal bands, which should be discussed with the patient prior to administering treatment with ATX-101. Platysmal bands may become more prominent following the reduction of SMF. Patients should also be made aware of prominent submandibular glands that may be contributing to submental fullness and cannot be altered with ATX-101. Evaluation of hyoid position is also key in obtaining optimal results. A low, anterior hyoid will remain in place in spite of treatment of preplatysmal fat, and this anatomic marker should be pointed out to the patient. Some patients also have a bulky digastric muscle, which is best seen in the lateral view, when the patient pushes their tongue to the roof of the month, creating submental fullness that cannot be altered. Patients with these anatomic characteristics may still show aesthetic improvement; however, it is important to have a thorough discussion about each patient's unique anatomy and the individual factors contributing to submental fullness prior to treatment. Notably, ATX-101 is safe for use in all skin types when administered properly.

Off-label applications of ATX-101 have been described in various anatomic regions from periaxillary fat to the posterior upper torso to the lower extremities. When considering the use of ATX-101 in nonsubmental regions, extensive knowledge of the anatomic area, including the underlying and adjacent neurovascular structures, is imperative to ensuring patient safety. A pinch test can be used to verify that intended treatment area consists of a superficial fat compartment.

22.4.2 Contraindications

The only absolute contraindication to the use of ATX-101 is an area with an active infection. Relative contraindications where practitioners should proceed with caution are (1) regions with moderate-to-severe skin laxity, (2) areas of skin redundancy, (3) regions with minimal adipose tissue, and (4) areas with compromised skin quality and/or dermal thinning (e.g., striae distensae). Massive weight loss patients should be screened for malnutrition prior to treatment as vitamin deficiencies can lead to interruptions in collagen synthesis. Because the outcome of ATX-101 injection depends on pathways related to dermal thickening and neocollagenesis, immunosuppressants (such as steroids or immunotherapy) should be discontinued if possible as these medications affect the wound-healing pathway and may impact the results of ATX-101. Additionally, patients with collagen vascular disorders will have deficiencies in their collagen synthesis pathway, which may lead to suboptimal results.

22.5 On-Label Technique

Most standard markings for submental ATX-101 injections limit treatment to a small central region of the submentum. This approach often undertreats patients

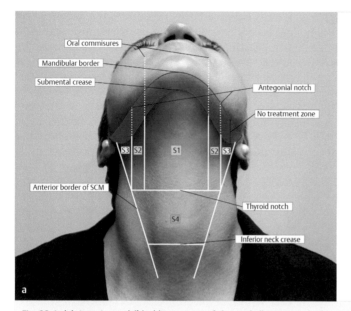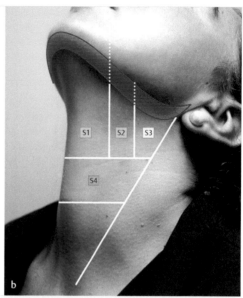

Fig. 22.1 **(a)** Anterior and **(b)** oblique views of the neck illustrating the key external anatomic landmarks, pretreatment markings, and safe zones for submental ATX-101 injections. Potential treatment zones (safe zones 1–4) are marked as S1, S2, S3, and S4. Zone borders are defined by the submental crease, thyroid notch, inferior neck crease, caudal continuation of the oral commissures, caudal continuation of the antegonial notch, anterior border of the sternocleidomastoid (SCM) muscle, and inferior border of the no treatment zone (NTZ). The *red* shaded region represents the NTZ, corresponding to the location of the marginal mandibular nerve.

with adipose deposition beyond the central submental area. Based on insights from cadaveric dye studies of SMF compartments, the lead author has developed a method for safely expanding the standard centralized treatment area. The expanded safe zone (ESZ) technique describes topographical landmarks that correlate to discrete fat compartments within the preplatysmal fat and facilitates individualized treatment fitted to each patient's unique anatomy.[39] When using ATX-101 to treat the submental region, the authors recommend adhering to the protocol described in the following section.

22.5.1 Step 1: Pretreatment Markings

- With the patient in a seated and upright position, mark the submental region according to the following anatomic boundaries (▶ Fig. 22.1a, b):
  - ○ **No treatment zone (NTZ):** To avoid the marginal mandibular nerve (MMN), mark the region 4.5 cm anterior to the gonion and 2 cm inferior to the inferior border of the mandible.[40,41] No injections should be administered within this region (▶ Fig. 22.1a, b).
  - ○ **Safe zone 1 (S1):** S1 is bordered by the submental crease (superior border), the thyroid notch (inferior border), and the caudal continuation of the bilateral oral commissures (lateral borders; ▶ Fig. 22.1a, b).
  - ○ **Safe zone 2 (S2; bilateral):** S2 is bordered by the inferior edge of the *NTZ* (superior border), the lateral extension of thyroid notch (inferior border), the caudal continuation of oral commissure (medial

border), and the antegonial notch (lateral border). After marking one side of the neck, mark the contralateral side (▶ Fig. 22.1a, b).
  - ○ **Safe zone 3 (S3; bilateral):** S3 is bordered by the inferior edge of the *NTZ* (superior border), the lateral extension of thyroid notch (inferior border), the caudal continuation of antegonial notch (medial border), and the anterior border of the unilateral sternocleidomastoid muscle (lateral border). After marking one side of the neck, mark the contralateral side (▶ Fig. 22.1a, b).
  - ○ **Safe zone 4 (S4):** S4 is bordered by the thyroid notch (superior border), the neck crease (inferior border), and the anterior border of the bilateral sternocleidomastoid muscles (lateral borders; ▶ Fig. 22.1a, b).

22.5.2 Step 2: Identification of the Treatment Zone

- After marking the patient, assess all six delineated regions (S1, S2 [bilateral], S3 [bilateral], and S4) to determine the extent of fat deposition. Palpate the intended treatment area to ensure the presence of sufficient subcutaneous fat. There should be a minimum of 1.5 cm of pinchable subcutaneous fat in the treatment area.
- Of note, not all patients will require injections to all six regions of the ESZ system. Some patients, for example, may only have excess fat within S1, S2, and S3, in which case the treatment areas would include S1, S2, and S3, but not S4.

- Outline the confirmed treatment area with a surgical pen. Be sure to avoid the *NTZ*.

22.5.3 Step 3: Injection Pattern

- Prep the treatment area with hypochlorous acid.
- Apply the 1-cm injection grid to the entire treatment area to mark the injection sites.

22.5.4 Step 4: Administration of Local Anesthetic

- To enhance patient comfort, inject the treatment area with lidocaine (1 or 2%) with epinephrine 1:100,000. The volume of local anesthetic injection ranges from 3 to 6 mL depending on patient sensitivity and the surface area being treated.
- Apply ice packs to treatment area and allow 10 minutes for the local anesthetic to take effect.

22.5.5 Step 5: Administration of ATX-101

- Draw 1 mL of ATX-101 (10 mg/mL solution) into a sterile 1-mL syringe.
- Using a 32-gauge 0.5-inch needle, inject 0.2 mL of ATX-101 into the preplatysmal fat immediately adjacent to each 1-cm grid mark (area-adjusted dose: 2 mg/cm^2).
- Dosage should be consistent throughout the treatment area; do not taper dosage laterally.
- Injections are administered perpendicular to the skin surface with the needle advanced midway into the preplatysmal fat.
- Do not withdraw the needle during injection as superficial (intradermal) injections can result in dermal necrosis.
- Needle resistance indicates possible contact with nonadipose tissue and the needle must be repositioned to an appropriate depth before injection.
- To avoid injury to the MMN, do not inject within the region 4.5 cm anterior to the gonion and 2 cm below the mandibular border.[40,41]
- A maximum of 50 injections (up to 10-mL ATX-101) may be injected in a single treatment.[42]

22.5.6 Step 6: Postinjection Ice

- Immediately following treatment, apply ice packs to the injected area.

22.5.7 Step 7: Subsequent Treatment Sessions

- Most patients will require two to four treatments (at 6-week intervals) for optimal results.
- A maximum of six single treatments may be administered (at intervals no < 4 weeks apart) with a maximum of 10 mL per single treatment session.[42]

- The number of injections per treatment and the number of treatment sessions depend on the individual patient's fat distribution, anatomy, and treatment goals.
- Of note, patients will not necessarily require ATX-101 injections in all six zones of the ESZ system at every session. Rather, ATX-101 injections should only be administered in zones with excess SMF with the goal of treating to endpoint. Often, lateral regions of SMF (e.g., S2, S3) have a lower fat density and are first to resolve; thus, subsequent treatments would concentrate on S1 (▶ Fig. 22.2).

22.6 Off-Label ATX-101

Although ATX-101 is currently FDA approved for the reduction of excess SMF, nonsubmental applications of ATX-101 injection have been described in the scientific literature and are commonly performed in clinical practice. Systematic review of studies on the off-label use of ATX-101 demonstrate nonsubmental applications to have a similar safety profile, effectiveness, and overall patient satisfaction compared to the FDA-approved use for persistent SMF.[43] Furthermore, the findings of clinical studies performed by our lead author demonstrate ATX-101 injections to be effective and unaccompanied by significant adverse events (AEs) when used to treat excess subcutaneous fat in nonsubmental regions. Anatomic areas that have been successfully treated with ATX-101 include the jowls, arms, anterior periaxillary region, abdomen, thighs, and knees. Provided a thorough understanding of the germane anatomy, accurate isolation of the treatment area, and proper injection technique, nonsubmental areas can be safely and effectively treated with ATX-101 injection. It is important to note that although current evidence is promising, further clinical trials and large sample studies are warranted to establish standards of practice and to determine explicit indications (e.g., anatomically specific dosing, toxicity, injection site spacing, and safety) for nonsubmental applications of ATX-101.

The injection technique for off-label ATX-101 aligns with the step-by-step protocol previously described (refer to Section 24.5) and should include pretreatment markings, identifying the treatment zone, applying the injection grid, administering local anesthetic, administering ATX-101, and postinjection ice. In this section, we discuss supplemental considerations for maximizing patient safety and treatment efficacy when using ATX-101 off-label. Further, we will describe technical considerations for treating jowl fat and anterior periaxillary fat (APAF).

22.6.1 Supplemental Considerations for Off-Label ATX-101

Pretreatment Considerations

Prior to administering treatment, a thorough assessment of the intended treatment region should be performed to

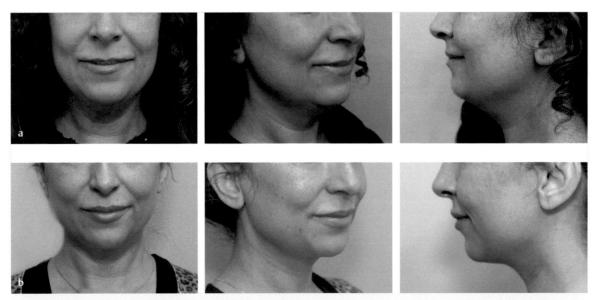

Fig. 22.2 (a, b) A 39-year-old female patient underwent two treatment sessions with ATX-101 (2 mg/cm^2) for the reduction of submental fullness. The submental region was treated with 8.0 and 5.0 mL of ATX-101 at treatment sessions 1 and 2, respectively. Patient is shown before treatment (baseline) and 12 months after her second treatment.

evaluate the extent of fat deposition and to identify the target treatment area. Clinicians should obtain a detailed medical history and caution should be practiced in patients with prior surgical or cosmetic procedures in the treatment area as anatomical changes or scar tissue may impact safe administration of ATX-101. Additionally, clinicians must consider the etiology of the fullness within the intended treatment area and screen for potential causes other than excess adipose tissue (e.g., malignancy, lymphadenopathy, accessory breast tissue, muscle hypertrophy). As with on-label treatment, patients should be counseled on the likelihood of needing two to four treatment sessions (at 6-week intervals) for optimal results.

Identifying the Treatment Zone

The planned treatment area should be outlined with a surgical pen, particularly avoiding any danger zones or underlying anatomic structures such as nerves or major blood vessels. Palpate the planned treatment area to ensure the presence of sufficient subcutaneous fat; there should be a minimum of 1.5 cm of pinchable subcutaneous fat within the treatment zone. Prior to applying the 1-cm injection grid, the grid can be trimmed to match the size and shape of the treatment area. If treating over a large surface area, multiple injection grids may be necessary.

Dosage of ATX-101

As with on-label treatment, off-label applications of ATX-101 injection should use an area-adjusted dose of 2 mg/cm^2. Dosage should be consistent throughout the treatment area and should not be tapered laterally or adjusted throughout the treatment area. When treating a large surface area, such as the abdomen, it is important not to exceed a maximum of 50 injections (with 0.2-mL ATX-101 per injection).[42] No more than 10-mL ATX-101 may be administered in a single treatment, regardless of the area being treated.

Treatment Cost

The use of ATX-101 for body contouring is, unquestionably, limited by cost—particularly in patients seeking treatment for excess fat in large regions of the body, such as the abdomen or thighs. To effectively target fat over a large surface area, a substantially greater volume of product is required than when treating relatively small areas such as the submental region. Accordingly, considering the current cost of product, favorable applications for nonsubmental ATX-101 injections involve small, localized deposits of adipose tissue (e.g., jowl fat, periaxillary fat).

22.6.2 Technical Considerations for Off-label ATX-101: Jowls and APAF

Jowl Fat

The loss of jawline definition is a characteristic feature of the aging face.[44] Excess jowl fat can contribute to reduced jawline definition and is an important component to address in patients seeking facial rejuvenation.

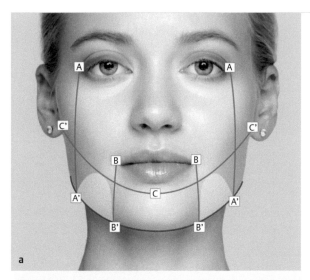
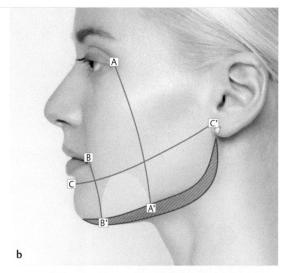

Fig. 22.3 (a, b) Facial markings used to isolate the jowl treatment area. A, lateral canthus; A', antegonial notch; B, oral commissure; B' prejowl sulcus; C, midline labiomental sulcus; C', ear lobule. *Yellow* shaded area is the inferior jowl fat pad. *Red* shaded region represents the zone of marginal mandibular nerve innervation at the inferior border of the mandible.

Patient Selection

Although ATX-101 injections can be an appropriate treatment for some patients presenting with jowl fat, careful assessment of the jowling mechanism is critical to determining the appropriate course of treatment. There are three principle mechanisms by which jowling occurs: (1) ptosis caused by compartment displacement, (2) atrophy of subcutaneous tissue, and (3) dehiscence of the mandibular septum allowing fat to flow over the mandible.[44] Only patients with jowling resultant of fat flow over the mandible should be considered for treatment with ATX-101. Conversely, patients with jowling due to superior compartment ptosis or subcutaneous tissue atrophy are not appropriate candidates for ATX-101 injection. Furthermore, eligible patients should have relatively minimal skin laxity as moderate-to-severe skin laxity of the jowl is a relative contraindication for ATX-101 treatment.[44]

Pretreatment Markings

With the patient in a seated and upright position, facial markings should be made to identify the jowl treatment area. The jowl fat can be consistently isolated by drawing four intersecting lines (▶ Fig. 22.3):
- Line 1 extends from the lateral canthus to the antegonial notch and forms the posterior border of the jowl treatment area (▶ Fig. 22.3).
- Line 2 extends from the oral commissure to the prejowl sulcus and forms the anterior border of the jowl treatment area (▶ Fig. 22.3).
- Line 3 extends from the labiomental sulcus to the ear lobule and forms the superior border of the jowl treatment area (▶ Fig. 22.3).

- Line 4 extends along the inferior border of the mandible, from prejowl sulcus to the ear lobule, and forms the inferior border of the jowl treatment area (▶ Fig. 22.3).

Injection Technique

- To optimize the injection angle and minimize risks, the jowl fat and skin should be pinched and pulled away from the underlying structures with the noninjecting hand. Pinching and retracting the tissue reduces the risk of MMN paresis as the terminal branches of the MMN occurring in the jowl region are deep to the subcutaneous fat.[44]
- Administer injections perpendicular to the surface of the skin and midway into the subcutaneous fat (to a depth of 6–10 mm) (▶ Fig. 22.4a,b).[44]

Anterior Periaxillary Fat

The presence of prominent or excess APAF is an area of concern for many patients. Excess APAF is a focal collection of fat that is often unrelated to a patient's body mass index (BMI) and is typically resistant to diet and exercise.[45] Traditionally, treatment options to reduce APAF have involved surgical approaches (e.g., excision, liposuction); however, ATX-101 injections can be an effective minimally invasive alternative for reducing APAF.

Patient Selection

A detailed medical history should be obtained for all patients considering treatment with ATX-101 for reducing APAF. Further, the clinician must consider the etiology of

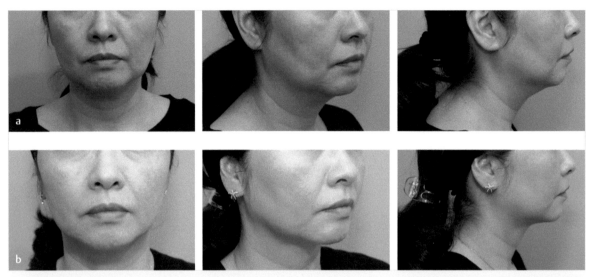

Fig. 22.4 (a, b) A 47-year-old woman underwent three treatment sessions with ATX-101 (2 mg/cm^2) for the reduction of submental fullness and jowl fat. The submental region was treated with 5, 4.8, and 1.6 mL of ATX-101 at treatment sessions 1, 2, and 3, respectively; the jowls were treated equally and bilaterally with 0.8, 0.6, and 1.2 mL at the three treatment sessions. The patient is shown before treatment (baseline) and 6 months after her third treatment.

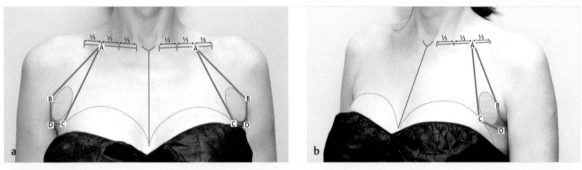

Fig. 22.5 (a, b) Diagram of markings used to identify the anterior periaxillary fat (APAF) treatment area. *A*, inner end of the lateral third of the clavicle; *B*, start of the anterior axillary fold; *C*, palpable junction of the breast upper outer quadrant and axillary skin; *D*, midaxillary line. The *yellow ellipses* represent the APAF treatment areas.

the fullness and rule out malignancy or accessory breast tissue. Patients reporting past or current pain and/or swelling in the anterior periaxillary region during their menstrual cycle, suggestive of the presence of accessory breast tissue, should not be treated.[45] A physical examination of the anterior periaxillary area should be performed in all patients. To ensure that periaxillary fullness is not secondary to hypertrophy of the pectoralis major muscle or tendons, patients should abduct their arms to activate the pectoralis major muscle.[45] A pinch test can further confirm the presence of subcutaneous fat. Supplemental screening diagnostic tests, specifically mammography or breast ultrasound, should be conducted in all patients who are suitable candidates due to risk factors and/or age.

Pretreatment Markings

The APAF treatment area lies within an ellipse in the right and left anterior periaxillary region.[45] With the patient in a standing and upright position, markings should be made to identify the appropriate treatment area. To isolate the treatment area and avoid breast tissue, delineate the lateral and medial borders of each treatment area according to the following protocol (▶ Fig. 22.5):

- Mark the jugular notch, clavicle, and midline of the chest (▶ Fig. 22.5).
- Demarcate the superior section of each breast with a dotted line (▶ Fig. 22.5).

- Mark the line along the clavicle into thirds. The inner end of the lateral third of the clavicle is designated as point A (▶ Fig. 22.5).
- Mark the start of the anterior axillary fold as point B (▶ Fig. 22.5).
- Draw a line connecting points A and B (▶ Fig. 22.5).
- Mark the palpable junction of the breast upper outer quadrant and axillary skin as point C (▶ Fig. 22.5).
- Draw a line connecting points A and C (▶ Fig. 22.5).
- Mark the midaxillary line as point D (▶ Fig. 22.5).
- Draw a line connecting points B and D, and a line from point C to point D (▶ Fig. 22.5).
- Fill in the treatment area with diagonal lines (▶ Fig. 22.5).

Injection Technique

- In contrast to on-label ATX-101 treatment, in which the MMN presents an "NTZ," there are no nerves or major blood vessels present in the anterior periaxillary region.[45]
- After marking the treatment area, place the patient in a relaxed, semi-reclined position, and apply the 1-cm injection grid. Trim the grid as needed to fit within the treatment zone.
- Administer injections perpendicular to the surface of the skin and midway into the subcutaneous fat (to a depth of 8–10 mm).
- Begin injections at the top lateral region of the treatment area and proceed vertically downward in columns across the area.
- Caution should be taken to avoid any visible striae distensae.

22.7 Posttreatment Instructions

Oral analgesics (i.e., acetaminophen) can be taken as needed posttreatment to avoid discomfort. Patients should be instructed to avoid lying down for a minimum of 4 to 5 hours following treatment. For the first 24 hours, cold compresses should be applied intermittently to the treatment area. Exercise, strenuous activity, alcohol, and salty foods are to be avoided for 48 hours. Patients should rest with their head elevated for 48 hours. For 1 to 2 weeks after the procedure, patients should avoid unnecessary exposure to heat, excessive cold, and excessive sun.

22.8 Potential Complications and Management

The safety of submental ATX-101 injections has been demonstrated in four phase 3 randomized controlled trials (RCTs).[40,46,47,48,49] The majority of AEs associated with ATX-101 treatment are transient, localized to the treated area, and mild or moderate in severity. Common injection-site AEs, such as tenderness, local edema, numbness, and bruising, can be effectively managed in clinical practice with several basic measures. To mitigate pain and bruising, oral analgesics (e.g., acetaminophen) can be administered 1 hour prior to treatment and lidocaine with epinephrine can be injected 10 minutes before treatment. Additionally, applying ice to the treatment area before and immediately after treatment can help reduce pain and swelling. To further manage swelling, patients should keep their head elevated, avoid exercise, and minimize salt and alcohol intake for 48 hours posttreatment. When possible, patients should discontinue medications and supplements that cause increased anticoagulant or antiplatelet activity 7 to 10 days before ATX-101 treatment to reduce the risk of bruising. Patients undergoing treatment with ATX-101 should expect tenderness, local edema, and numbness to last for approximately 3 to 4 days, 7 to 10 days, and approximately 4 weeks, respectively. Notably, in patients undergoing multiple ATX-101 treatments, the duration of injection-related AEs tends to decrease with subsequent treatment sessions.

Additional AEs associated with ATX-101 injection include transient injection-site alopecia, MMN paresis, and dermal ulceration. Mild-to-moderate transient alopecia at the injection site has been reported in up to 7% of male patients undergoing submental ATX-101 injections and typically resolves spontaneously within 4 months after the last treatment session.[39,50] It is hypothesized that temporary localized alopecia may be shock alopecia secondary to superficial injection or direct damage to the hair bulb.[51] Male patients in particular should be informed that temporary injection-site alopecia may occur following treatment.

MMN paresis was reported in approximately 2 to 4% of patients in RCTs[40,47,48,52] and clinical studies performed by our senior author demonstrate a similar incidence. Although all events of MMN paresis described in the literature resolved without sequelae, MMN injury results in significant cosmetic deformity. The marginal mandibular branch of the facial nerve supplies muscles of the lower lip, and injury results in distorted facial expressions, particularly on opening the mouth, smiling, and grimacing. A potential mechanism of MMN paresis after ATX-101 treatment is damage to the myelin sheath leading to temporary demyelination and a period of nerve inflammation.[50] It has also been proposed that asymmetric smile may be resultant of damage to the cervical branch of the facial nerve secondary to ATX-101 injection that is too deep, contacting the platysmal surface.[44] To avoid injuring the MMN, do not inject within the region 4.5 cm anterior to the gonion and approximately 2 cm below the inferior border of the mandible.[40,41] To avoid muscular injury and dysfunction, ensure that ATX-101 injections are within the subcutaneous fat.

Dermal ulceration following treatment with ATX-101 is an AE that results from inappropriate injection technique.

Although ATX-101 is a nonselective cytolytic agent, its cytolytic activity is lower in proteinaceous tissue compared to adipose tissue. Accordingly, subcutaneous fatty tissue is more susceptible to lysis by ATX-101 than protein-rich tissues, such as skin and muscle.[52] Skin ulceration can be evaded by placing ATX-101 injections midway into the subcutaneous fat, avoiding the dermis. The needle should not be withdrawn during injection as superficial injection increases the risk of dermal ulceration.

22.9 Pearls and Pitfalls

22.9.1 Pearls

- For maximal effectiveness, an area-adjusted dose of $2\,mg/cm^2$ should be used consistently throughout the treatment area. Dosage should not be tapered or modified, regardless of the area being treated.
- Treat the full surface area within the region of concern.
- Employ five measures to minimize AEs: ice aggressively, elevate the treated area, and avoid salty foods, exercise, and alcohol for the first 48 hours.
- The use of compression posttreatment is unnecessary.
- The use of local or systemic steroids for the purpose of minimizing the swelling should be avoided. Steroids are known to impede collagen formation and their use can inhibit skin retraction and wound healing.
- Results may continue to improve for 2 to 3 months following ATX-101 treatment.

22.9.2 Pitfalls

- *Inappropriate patient selection*: Poor aesthetic outcomes are often the result of improper patient selection. When treating excess SMF, patients should be screened for other potential causes of submental fullness (e.g., low hyoid position, enlarged or ptotic submandibular glands, thyromegaly, and/or cervical lymphadenopathy). Patients with excessive skin laxity and/or prominent platysmal bands are likely to be unsatisfied with ATX-101 treatment.
- *Miscalculating or misleading patient into thinking that they will require only one treatment*: The majority of patients will require multiple treatment sessions and patients should be counseled on the likelihood of needing two to four treatments for optimal results.
- *Downplaying the severity of edema*: Patients will experience significant swelling in response to ATX-101 as a result of adipocytolysis and induction of the local inflammatory response. Patients should be encouraged to embrace swelling as an indication of adipocyte breakdown.
- *A note on cost and pricing*: A common misconception is that treatment with ATX-101 is analogous to that of botulinum toxin or filler injection. Although these modalities do have some similarities, such as in-office procedure status, avoidance of time-consuming

treatment, and relatively short recovery period, the authors recommend considering the value and cost of ATX-101 as comparable to a surgical procedure due to inherent differences in these treatments. Whereas ATX-101, botulinum toxin, and fillers are all injectable interventions, botulinum toxin and filler treatments must be repeated periodically for maintenance of results, and the results of ATX-101 are permanent—similar to surgical intervention. Rather than pricing ATX-101 on a per-unit basis (as is often done with botulinum toxin and fillers), the authors recommend pricing ATX-101 treatment more similarly to that of surgery as well. For example, the addition of liposuction to an abdominoplasty procedure is quoted as less than liposuction alone, as liposuction does not incur significant time to the operating room or surgeon when added as an adjunct to the primary abdominoplasty procedure. Similarly, when one is treating the SMF region with ATX-101, the addition of the ESZ lateral prejowl region does not incur significant time. As such, we recommend additional vials of ATX-101 to treat the expanded prejowl region not be charged on a 1cost:1unit basis but rather as adjuncts to a primary SMF region procedure.

References

[1] Chia CT, Neinstein RM, Theodorou SJ. Evidence-based medicine: liposuction. Plast Reconstr Surg. 2017; 139(1):267e–274e

[2] Shridharani SM, Broyles JM, Matarasso A. Liposuction devices: technology update. Med Devices (Auckl). 2014; 7:241–251

[3] Bellini E, Grieco MP, Raposio E. A journey through liposuction and liposculture: Review. Ann Med Surg (Lond). 2017; 24:53–60

[4] Zocchi M. Ultrasonic liposculpturing. Aesthetic Plast Surg. 1992; 16 (4):287–298

[5] Apfelberg D. Laser-assisted liposuction may benefit surgeons, patients. Clin Laser Mon. 1992; 10(12):193–194

[6] Lee JC, Daniels MA, Roth MZ. Mesotherapy, microneedling, and chemical peels. Clin Plast Surg. 2016; 43(3):583–595

[7] FDA. Prescribing information. KYBELLA injection. Available from: http://www.accessdata.fda.gov/drugsatfda_docs/label/2015/206333Orig1s000lbl.pdf. Accessed November 16, 2017

[8] KYTHERA Biopharmaceuticals, Inc. KYTHERA Biopharmaceuticals Announces Health Canada Authorization of BELKYRA(TM), a Submental Contouring Injectable Drug(i). Available from: http://www.kythera.com/kythera-biopharmaceuticals-announces-health-canada-authorization-of-belkyra-a-submental-contouring-injectable-drug/. Accessed

[9] FDA. FDA Approves Treatment for Fat below the Chin. Available from: http://wayback.archive-it.org/7993/20171115021407/https://www.fda.gov/NewsEvents/Newsroom/PressAnnouncements/ucm444978.htm

[10] Cardis MA, DeKlotz CMC. Intralesional deoxycholic acid treatment for fibrofatty residua of involuted infantile hemangiomas: a novel therapeutic approach. JAMA Dermatol. 2018; 154(6):735–737

[11] Dubin DP, Farberg AS, Lin MJ, Khorasani H. Intralesional deoxycholic acid as neoadjuvant treatment of a large lipoma. Dermatol Surg. 2020; 46(5):715–717

[12] Fredriksen JH, Rosenqvist E, Wedege E, et al. Production, characterization and control of MenB-vaccine "Folkehelsa": an outer membrane vesicle vaccine against group B meningococcal disease. NIPH Ann. 1991; 14(2):67–79, discussion 79–80

[13] Yang J, Li ZH, Zhou JJ, et al. Preparation and antitumor effects of nanovaccines with MAGE-3 peptides in transplanted gastric cancer in mice. Chin J Cancer. 2010; 29(4):359–364

[14] Yuba E, Sakaguchi N, Kanda Y, Miyazaki M, Koiwai K. pH-responsive micelle-based cytoplasmic delivery system for induction of cellular immunity. Vaccines (Basel). 2017; 5(4):E41

[15] American Society for Aesthetic Plastic Surgery (ASAPS). Aesthetic Plastic Surgery National Data Bank Statistics. Available from: https://www.surgery.org/sites/default/files/Aesthetic-Society_Stats2019Book_FINAL.pdf Accessed June 25, 2020

[16] Center for Drug Evaluation and Research. Kybella Medical Review. Application number: 206333Orig1s000. Available from https://www.accessdata.fda.gov/drugsatfda_docs/nda/2015/206333Orig1s000MedR.pdf. Accessed June 25, 2020

[17] Shridharani SM, Behr KL. ATX-101 (deoxycholic acid injection) treatment in men: insights from our clinical experience. Dermatol Surg. 2017; 43 Suppl 2:S225–S230

[18] Ascher B, Hoffmann K, Walker P, Lippert S, Wollina U, Havlickova B. Efficacy, patient-reported outcomes and safety profile of ATX-101 (deoxycholic acid), an injectable drug for the reduction of unwanted submental fat: results from a phase III, randomized, placebo-controlled study. J Eur Acad Dermatol Venereol. 2014; 28(12):1707–1715

[19] Humphrey S, Sykes J, Kantor J, et al. ATX-101 for reduction of submental fat: a phase III randomized controlled trial. J Am Acad Dermatol. 2016; 75(4):788–797.e7

[20] Jones DH, Carruthers J, Joseph JH, et al. REFINE-1, a multicenter, randomized, double-blind, placebo-controlled, phase 3 trial with ATX-101, an injectable drug for submental fat reduction. Dermatol Surg. 2016; 42(1):38–49

[21] Rzany B, Griffiths T, Walker P, Lippert S, McDiarmid J, Havlickova B. Reduction of unwanted submental fat with ATX-101 (deoxycholic acid), an adipocytolytic injectable treatment: results from a phase III, randomized, placebo-controlled study. Br J Dermatol. 2014; 170(2):445–453

[22] Humphrey S, Dayan SH, Shridharani SM, et al. Personal and Social Impacts of Submental Fat in the US Population. Presented at Fall Clinical Dermatology Conference on Las Vegas, NV, October 20–23, 2016

[23] Humphrey S, Dayan SH, Shridharani SM, et al. Social Perceptions before and after Treatment with ATX-101 (Deoxycholic Acid Injection) for Reduction of Submental Fat. Presented at the American Academy of Dermatology Annual Meeting on Orlando, FL, March 3–7, 2017

[24] Jagdeo J, Keaney T, Narurkar V, Kolodziejczyk J, Gallagher CJ. Facial treatment preferences among aesthetically oriented men. Dermatol Surg. 2016; 42(10):1155–1163

[25] Raveendran SS, Anthony DJ, Ion L. An anatomic basis for volumetric evaluation of the neck. Aesthet Surg J. 2012; 32(6):685–691

[26] Hatef DA, Koshy JC, Sandoval SE, Echo AP, Izaddoost SA, Hollier LH. The submental fat compartment of the neck. Semin Plast Surg. 2009; 23(4):288–291

[27] Shridharani SM. Early experience in 100 consecutive patients with injection adipocytolysis for neck contouring with ATX-101 (deoxycholic acid). Dermatol Surg. 2017; 43(7):950–958

[28] Beer K, Donofrio L, Gross TM, Beddingfield FC III. Clinically Meaningful Reduction in Submental Fat during and after Treatment with ATX-101 in the US/CAN Phase 3 Trials, REFINE-1 and REFINE-2. Presented at American Academy of Dermatology Annual Meeting on San Francisco, CA, March 20–24, 2015

[29] Shridharani SM, Chandawarkar AA. Novel expanded safe zone for reduction of submental fullness with ATX-101 injection. Plast Reconstr Surg. 2019; 144(6):995e–1001e

[30] Shridharani SM. Injection of an adipocytolytic agent for reduction of excess periaxillary fat. Aesthet Surg J. 2019; 39(12):NP495–NP503

[31] Sykes JM, Allak A, Klink B. Future applications of deoxycholic acid in body contouring. J Drugs Dermatol. 2017; 16(1):43–46

[32] Verma KD, Somenek MT. Deoxycholic acid injection as an effective treatment for reduction of posterior upper torso brassiere strap adiposity. Plast Reconstr Surg. 2018; 141(1):200e–202e

[33] Jegasothy SM. Deoxycholic acid injections for bra-line lipolysis. Dermatol Surg. 2018; 44(5):757–760

[34] Asaadi M. Etiology and treatment of congenital festoons. Aesthetic Plast Surg. 2018; 42(4):1024–1032

[35] Newberry CI, Mccrary H, Thomas JR, Cerrati EW. updated management of malar edema, mounds, and festoons: a systematic review. Aesthet Surg J. 2020; 40(3):246–258

[36] Ascha M, Swanson MA, Massie JP, et al. Nonsurgical management of facial masculinization and feminization. Aesthet Surg J. 2019; 39(5):NP123–NP137

[37] Dover JS, Shridharani SM, Bloom JD, Somogyi C, Gallagher CJ. Reduction of submental fat continues beyond 28 days after ATX-101 treatment: results from a post hoc analysis. Dermatol Surg. 2018; 44(11):1477–1479

[38] Baumann L, Shridharani SM, Humphrey S, Gallagher CJ. Personal (self) perceptions of submental fat among adults in the United States. Dermatol Surg. 2019; 45(1):124–130

[39] Shridharani SM, Chandawarkar AA. Novel expanded safe zone for reduction of submental fullness with ATX-101 injection. Plast Reconstr Surg. 2019; 144(6):995e–1001e

[40] Jones DH, Carruthers J, Joseph JH, et al. REFINE-1, a multicenter, randomized, double-blind, placebo-controlled, phase 3 trial with ATX-101, an injectable drug for submental fat reduction. Dermatol Surg. 2016; 42(1):38–49

[41] Yang H-M, Kim HJ, Park HW, et al. Revisiting the topographic anatomy of the marginal mandibular branch of facial nerve relating to the surgical approach. Aesthet Surg J. 2016; 36(9):977–982

[42] Kythera Biopharmaceuticals, Inc. KYBELLA (deoxycholic acid) injection [prescribing information]. Available from: https://www.allergan.com/assets/pdf/kybella_pi. Accessed July 8, 2020

[43] Sung CT, Lee A, Choi F, Juhasz M, Mesinkovska NA. Non-submental applications of injectable deoxycholic acid: a systematic review. J Drugs Dermatol. 2019; 18(7):675–680

[44] Shridharani SM. Improvement in jowl fat following ATX-101 treatment: results from a single-site study. Plast Reconstr Surg. 2020; 145(4):929–935

[45] Shridharani SM. Injection of an adipocytolytic agent for reduction of excess periaxillary fat. Aesthet Surg J. 2019; 39(12):NP495–NP503

[46] Rzany B, Griffiths T, Walker P, Lippert S, McDiarmid J, Havlickova B. Reduction of unwanted submental fat with ATX-101 (deoxycholic acid), an adipocytolytic injectable treatment: results from a phase III, randomized, placebo-controlled study. Br J Dermatol. 2014; 170(2):445–453

[47] Ascher B, Hoffmann K, Walker P, Lippert S, Wollina U, Havlickova B. Efficacy, patient-reported outcomes and safety profile of ATX-101 (deoxycholic acid), an injectable drug for the reduction of unwanted submental fat: results from a phase III, randomized, placebo-controlled study. J Eur Acad Dermatol Venereol. 2014; 28(12):1707–1715

[48] McDiarmid J, Ruiz JB, Lee D, Lippert S, Hartisch C, Havlickova B. Results from a pooled analysis of two European, randomized, placebo-controlled, phase 3 studies of ATX-101 for the pharmacologic reduction of excess submental fat. Aesthetic Plast Surg. 2014; 38(5):849–860

[49] Dayan S, Jones DH, Carruthers J, et al. A pooled analysis of the safety and efficacy results of the multicenter, double-blind, randomized, placebo-controlled phase 3 REFINE-1 and REFINE-2 trials of ATX-101, a submental contouring injectable drug for the reduction of submental fat. Plast Reconstr Surg. 2014; 134:123

[50] Shridharani SM, Behr KL. ATX-101 (deoxycholic acid injection) treatment in men: insights from our clinical experience. Dermatol Surg. 2017; 43 Suppl 2:S225–S230

[51] Grady B, Porphirio F, Rokhsar C. Submental alopecia at deoxycholic acid injection site. Dermatol Surg. 2017; 43(8):1105–1108

[52] Shridharani SM. Early experience in 100 consecutive patients with injection adipocytolysis for neck contouring with ATX-101 (deoxycholic acid). Dermatol Surg. 2017; 43(7):950–958

23 High-Definition Body Contouring: Advancing Traditional Liposuction through Experience

Jason Emer and Michael B. Lipp

Summary

The desire for improvement in body shape has increased dramatically in recent years. This is mainly due to significant improvements in surgical techniques, reduced downtimes, and advances in nonsurgical approaches that not only reduce body fat but also tighten skin and improve cellulite. The demand for a "sculpted" and defined body over one that is just flat or improved has required surgeons to make advances in techniques and approaches to surgical body shaping that not only remove large volumes of fat in multiple locations at one time but also use this fat for muscular defining and body revolumizing while also addressing the desire for skin tightening and cellulite reduction. Newer adjunctive energy-based modalities such as lasers, ultrasound, radiofrequency (RF), and helium plasma allow surgeons to not only address the deep subcutaneous layers to remove bulk adipose but also work in the superficial layers for greater tightening, definition, and tone, which has long been avoided due to increased complications and risk of irregularities. For a full-body transformation, more aggressive high-definition body contouring (HDBC) procedures can be combined with surgical implants and/or skin removal in a series of procedures to get an ultimate transformation. Postoperative care such as lymphatic massage, superficial RF and ultrasound, vibration/shock therapies, and close follow-up are essential to ensure long-term complications are minimal and results are life-changing. Future studies are needed to look at the importance of noninvasive devices in the postoperative healing phase as well as how to further improve contour, cellulite, and skin-tightening results in conjunction with HDBC surgical techniques. Herein, we describe techniques for advanced body contouring procedures and demonstrate the results of these procedures.

Keywords: body contour, body shaping, cellulite, skin tightening, liposuction, body shaping, high definition body contouring, ultrasound, laser, radiofrequency, helium plasma, fat grafting, VASER, Thermitight, Bodytite, Renuvion

23.1 History and Evidence-Based Approaches

Over the past few decades, fat removal procedures have become increasingly popular, correlating with an increased desire for a smoother, contoured, lifted, and cellulite-free body. Increased social awareness of "healthy" and "organic" lifestyles with an importance on health and beauty has popularized surgical and nonsurgical body contouring procedures. In 2018, liposuction was the second most common plastic surgical procedure performed.[1]

A decade ago, liposuction was the only option for fat removal and/or reduction and more so the only option for body contouring beyond having a truly invasive skin removal surgery.[2,3] Today, the results obtained with traditional surgical liposuction methods almost match that of current nonsurgical options. For example, nonsurgical fat reduction (e.g., Coolsculpting) by "freezing the fat" has become a household name due to increased advertisement to consumers (brand awareness). Currently, there are several nonsurgical technologies that promise an array of options to target unwanted fat and cellulite as well as tighten skin such as trusculpt, Cutera (▶ Table 23.1). Many of these technologies in combination in a series of treatments can get results very close to traditional ("tumescent") liposuction (▶ Fig. 23.1).

Patient's expectations are tremendously higher than ever as fantastic results are now expected in the consumer-driven, competitive aesthetic environment glorifying procedures in these past years. Patients not only request improvements in fat removal but also expect body shaping and contouring, skin tightening and lifting, cellulite reduction, as well as improvements in the quality of the skin such as texture and tone. Now more than ever, they are demanding a visibly athletic toned body, one that is sculpted and contoured over one that is just flatter. These preconceived expectations require the body contouring surgeon to not only be technically skillful and meticulous but also artistic. This is not to say that traditional liposuction methods with a standard tumescent approach will not give good outcomes; it is just that the results obtained are typically more one dimensional compared to multidimensional HDBC, which addresses fat removal, skin tightening, and shaping more effectively.

Conventional liposuction can remove fat, mildly tighten skin, and improve body shape, it but cannot give the degree of improvement that HDBC can do in which multiple steps are used to remove fat, tighten skin, improve cellulite, and create definition and contour with etched lines. Alfredo Hoyos was the pioneer surgeon who initially defined and perfected this technique in which both deep and superficial layers of adipose tissue were treated. The technique has advanced into a process of debulking fat, creating definition, enhancing natural body lines and using harvested fat to reshape musculature. The current HDBC surgeon must combine science with art in order to get an aesthetically pleasing outcome, which makes this procedure extremely more challenging, but the only

Table 23.1 Noninvasive body contouring devices

Noninvasive cryolipolysis

- Coolsculpting (ZELTIQ Aesthetics, Inc., an Allergan affiliate. Allergan)

- Z Lipo (Zimmer Aesthetics)

Noninvasive laser lipolysis

- SculpSure (Cynosure, LLC., Hologic, Inc.)[a]

- Venus Bliss (Venus Concepts)[b]

Noninvasive radiofrequency

- BTL Vanquish ME (BTL Industries Inc.)

- Venus Legacy (Venus Concepts)[c]

- Exilis Ultra 360 (BTL Industries Inc.)[d]

- Forma Plus (Inmode)

- trusculpt ID (Cutera)

- trusculpt 3D (Cutera)

- Thermage FLX (Solta Medical)

Noninvasive ultrasound

- Ultrashape (Candela Corporation)

- Ultherapy (Merz Aesthetics)

Vibration/pressure/shock wave therapy for cellulite reduction

- eVive (Eclipse)

- Z Wave (Zimmer Aesthetics)

- Cellutone (BTL Industries Inc.)

- EMTone (BTL Industries Inc.)[e]

[a]1,060-nm wavelength.
[b]1,064-nm wavelength.
[c]Proprietary (MP)[2] technology (a combination of multipolar radiofrequency and pulsed electromagnetic fields).
[d]Combined radiofrequency and ultrasound.
[e]Combined monopolar radiofrequency and mechanical targeted pressure energy.

option for those patients desiring something transformative (▶ Fig. 23.2, ▶ Fig. 23.3). In the author's opinion (JE), even current traditional liposuction approaches combined with noninvasive fat reduction and noninvasive skin-tightening technologies are unable to give these types of life-altering body transformations (▶ Fig. 23.4).

Several advances in liposuction have been developed to assist the modern-day HDBC surgeon since the adoption of suction-assisted liposuction (SAL) was first introduced by Illuz in the early 1980s.[4] These technologies include water-assisted liposuction (WAL), ultrasound-assisted liposuction (UAL), power-assisted liposuction (PAL), laser-assisted liposuction (LAL), and radiofrequency-assisted liposuction (RFAL). In the author's opinion (JE), combining several of these technologies in a procedure gives superior results and is required for the social-savvy, athletic-conscious, current-day consumer.

WAL by body-jet (Human Med AG) is a technology that infiltrates subcutaneous fat with thin, targeted, fan-shaped jets of tumescent fluid prior to liposuction aspiration. It loosens fat cells during aspiration minimizing collateral damage of surrounding tissue and allowing for cleaner, more "pure" harvesting of adipocytes for fat grafting and stem cell therapies.

UAL transforms electrical energy into mechanical energy through an ultrasonic probe that vibrates at frequencies greater than 16 kHz. The oscillating sound waves produce pressures strong enough to overcome the molecular forces selectively within adipose tissues causing cavitation within the tumescent fluid and cellular fragmentation that can be used for fat grafting more effectively.[5] VASERlipo (Solta Medical) is the "gold standard" UAL technology that enables greater fragmentation of adipocytes at lower-energy settings by utilizing a pulsed rather than continuous energy.[6]

An increasing interest in combining liposuction with skin tightening has led to the development of RFAL. RF energy utilizes high-frequency oscillating electrical currents to create a thermal effect on surrounding tissues. Temperatures of 60 to 65 °C will cause shrinkage, denaturation of collagen fibrils, as well as neocollagenesis.[7] One of the first devices developed for internal skin tightening that can be used alone or with tumescent liposuction was ThermiTight (ThermiGen, in association with ARVATI).

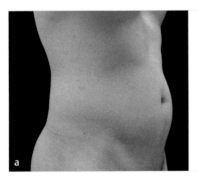 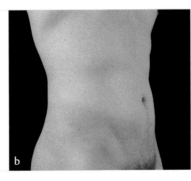

Fig. 23.1 Noninvasive body contouring with combination devices. **(a)** Male patient before Sculpsure and Vanquish treatment. **(b)** Six months after Sculpsure and Vanquish treatment.

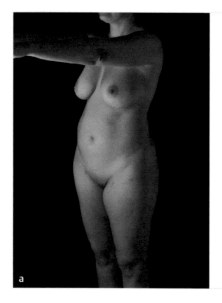
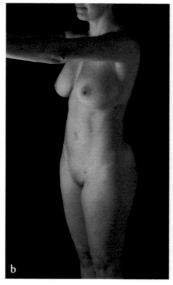

Fig. 23.2 Female high-definition body contouring (HDBC). **(a)** Before. **(b)** After (6 months postoperatively).

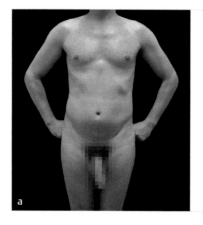
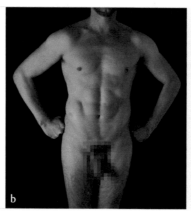

Fig. 23.3 Male high-definition body contouring (HDBC). **(a)** Before. **(b)** After (6 months postoperatively).

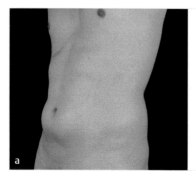
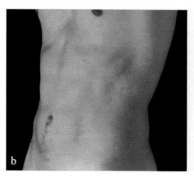

Fig. 23.4 Traditional liposuction and noninvasive body contouring. **(a)** Before. **(b)** After suction-assisted liposuction (SAL) followed by Vanquish.

The thermistor-controlled RF probe delivers precise controlled thermal energy that is inserted into the deep dermal and subdermal planes. An external infrared camera monitors skin surface temperature so as to not burn epidermal layers. By maintaining a temperature of 60 to 65 °C by the probe and keeping the skin surface temperature below 43 °C, the clinical effects of tightening and lifting of lax skin can be achieved.[7] However, this device (and all RF or internal heating devices) requires meticulous observation by the operator so as to not overheat the superficial skin.

Bodytite (InMode) is another RFAL device that delivers bipolar RF energy from the tip of a silicone-coated probe inserted below the skin. The RF current is monitored by an external electrode that glides along the surface of the skin in tandem with the internal electrode, closing the current. The external electrode also has a temperature-set (35–42 °C) thermal sensor that measures the skin surface temperature in real time allowing for uniform heating of the fibroseptal network in a more time-efficient and safe manner. Bodytite received its Food and Drug Administration (FDA) approval in 2016 for electrocoagulation of soft tissues. The RF energy emitted between the two electrodes coagulates fat, causes contraction of the fibroseptal network, and causes neocollagenesis in the long term.[8,9] Bodytite in combination with suction liposuction in one study reported a 34.5% reduction in skin surface area reduction compared to 8.4% reduction with SAL alone after 1 year.[10]

A newer internal tightening device is Renuvion (Apyx Medical), which works by internal contraction through conduction rather than bulk heating. This device creates a cold atmospheric microplasma (CAP) of helium powered by RF. Plasma can be created when gas is ionized. The probe of the Renuvion device is introduced through the subdermal plane delivering 85 °C heat for approximately 0.040 to 0.080 seconds, causing soft-tissue coagulation and instant contraction. With other devices, treating to 65 °C endpoint, the tissue being treated must be maintained at that temperature for greater than 120 seconds (or longer in most instances) for maximal contraction to occur.[11] As new structures are introduced to the tip of the probe, the plasma energy is constantly finding a new preferred path, quickly alternating between treating the different tissues within the fibroseptal network surrounding the tip of the device. This allows for the tissue surrounding the treatment site to remain at much cooler temperatures.

23.2 Surgical Criteria

Not all patients are candidates for HDBC. In fact, the majority are not good candidates and need to be guided toward the proper treatment plan with alternatives. Those with significant loose or lax skin, significant stretch marks, high body mass index (BMI) of > 30 or 10 lb over expected weight, poorly defined or toned underlying musculature, extreme cellulite, or stretch marks are not the best candidates. These patients must be directed to lose weight, improve muscle tone, and consider skin removal and lifting surgery with HDBC in the future. Even with full lifestyle modification, in some cases the results may be improved, but not a full-body transformation.

Conversely, a candidate who has an already low BMI, good muscular tone, and tight skin with little to no cellulite or stretch marks may be able to expect a chiseled and sculpted outcome from their HDBC. Expectations should be discussed with brute honesty of the anticipated results prior to any surgical intervention as to limit poor outcomes or unsatisfied patients Also, it must be explained

that lifelong maintenance of these results will require lifestyle modification with exercise, healthy eating, and external RF, and/or ultrasound skin-tightening procedures at the minimum.

23.3 High-Definition Body Contouring

23.3.1 Anatomy: Importance of Adipose Layers

An HDBC surgeon must have an expert knowledge of anatomy, body proportions, and features that define athletic beauty in both men and women. Without a deep understanding of the muscular structures creating anatomical lines and curves, it is impossible to create shape or contour.

The subcutaneous tissue is divided into three layers: the superficial adipose layer, the intermediate membranous layer (i.e., superficial fascia), and the deep adipose layer.[4,12] During conventional liposuction, fat is only removed from the deep adipose layer to debulk the body area. It is taught to most that removal of the superficial adipose layer is prohibited as there is a higher risk of postoperative irregularities, seromas, and worsening cellulite; thus, most surgeons avoid treating this layer, which is responsible for the visible muscular etched lines and body shapes created during HDBC. To treat the superficial layer, the author (JE) uses WAL with body-jet, UAL with VASER (probes), and PAL with PowerX (part of the VASER-lipo system, Solta Medical) or MicroAire (cannulas).

The water-assisted tumescence protects the superficial skin vasculature by pressurizing the epinephrine in the fluid. This allows the epinephrine to act quickly and with enhanced longevity and strength to limit bleeding and the potential for skin mottling after aggressive treatment. The hydrodissection of the water-assisted device creates a more defined and even plane to work in. It also hydrates the adipose with less use of total fluid as compared to traditional infiltration (e.g., Klein), so, more body areas can be treated at a given time with less swelling postoperatively.

The VASER technology is essential to "soften" (emulsify) the fatty layer prior to extraction, creating steam heat that tightens the skin more than power- and laser-assisted devices or hand extraction alone, as well as preparing the fat for transfer to areas that give the body contour such as buttock, breast/chest, shoulders, or calves.[13] With the multiringed grooved probes, the superficial layers can be treated evenly and softly with much less risk of irregularity in the right hands.

VASER produces sound resonance at frequencies that vibrate fat cells causing them to emulsify, whereas other tissue cells remain intact. Electrical energy in the VASER generator is converted to vibrational mechanical energy in the ultrasonic probes. Expanding microscopic air bubbles in the tumescent fluid implode, releasing energy that breaks down the structure of adipose tissue without damaging its structure ensuring that the fat is still suitable for grafting.[14] Bleeding is minimized and downtime is improved due to less surrounding tissue trauma.

Finally, traditional power-assisted devices (e.g., Micro-Aire, MicroAire Surgical Instruments) vibrate back and forth (i.e., similar mechanics to a jackhammer) and extract fat by creating tunnels. This increases the risk of irregularities and step-offs if larger cannulas are used and if the operator is "sloppy" or not very meticulous. Rotary power-assisted devices (e.g., PowerX) vibrate side to side in a rotational fashion physically shearing the tissue, allowing the surgeon to physically strip down on the thickness of the fat layer by layer without tunnels. The best comparison between these devices is creating a "Swiss-cheese" look to the fat layers with MicroAire versus "grating a block of cheese" with PowerX.

Liposculpting of the superficial layer is targeted in order to reveal the underlying musculature, to create the lines, and to further tighten skin in specific areas. It is an essential component to HDBC that differentiates it from traditional liposuction.

23.4 HDBC Key Steps

In order to perform HDBC, there are several key steps that are necessary in order to obtain symmetrical improvement and contouring (▶ Video 23.1). An important part of the surgery is addressing the superficial

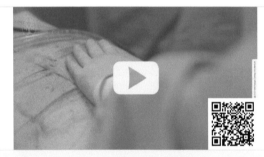

Video 23.1 Male body transformation surgery.

layers of fat after debulking the deeper layers. It is also paramount to have a thorough understanding of the underlying musculature in order to produce contouring, definition and etch lines.

23.4.1 Step 1: Marking and Placement of Port/Entrance Sites

Traditional approaches to fat reduction involved marking a large problem area of fat with concentric circles specifically identifying the area of most desired reduction. This type of approach, although logical for standard fat reduction in a localized area, makes it difficult to contour and reshape surrounding areas as the underlying anatomy is not taken into consideration (i.e., muscular lines and bony landmarks). With traditional liposuction, entrance sites are placed in areas around circularly identified bulk fat in order to allow the surgeon to address the area in a crisscross pattern. This method is thought to decrease the chance of irregularities. With hand cannulas or even traditional PAL, the back-and-forth nature of extraction can leave lines of fatty layers if not addressed evenly.

In HDBC, detailed markings of the underlying anatomical structures (i.e., muscular lines and bony landmarks) are mapped in pre-op to serve as a precise guide while in the operating room. Additionally, because this is a total torso and sometimes a total body procedure, most of the port access sites are placed within body folds such that scars are hidden or limited in discrete swimsuit-/bikini- or underwear-friendly areas. Using a combination approach of WAL, UAL, PAL, and internal tightening with RFAL or helium plasma, transformational results can be achieved and are seen best in nonstudio lighting (i.e., "selfies" or shadowed light to appreciate lines, definition, shaping, and contouring; ▶ Fig. 23.5, ▶ Fig. 23.6).

23.4.2 Step 2: Tumescent Anesthesia

In traditional liposuction approaches, true tumescent fluid (i.e., Klein formula) is infiltrated using a peristaltic pump to flood the fatty layers and prepare it for extraction. The original Klein tumescent formula was 1,000 mL of normal saline (0.9% NaCl), 50 mL 1% lidocaine, 1 mL of epinephrine 1:1,000, 12.5 mL of 8.4% sodium bicarbonate.

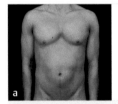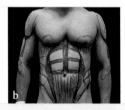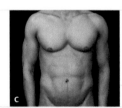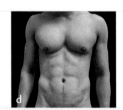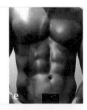

Fig. 23.5 Sequential timeline for high-definition body contouring (HDBC) in a male. (a) Before HDBC. (b) Preoperative markings. (c) Three days postoperatively. (d) One month postoperatively. (e) "Selfie" 6 months postoperatively showing his body transformation with enhanced muscular definition on the chest and stomach.

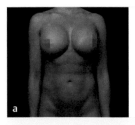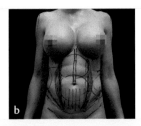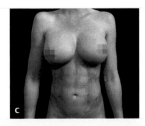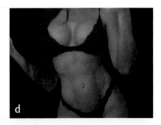

Fig. 23.6 Sequential timeline for high-definition body contouring (HDBC) in a female. **(a)** Before HDBC. **(b)** preoperative markings. **(c)** One day postoperatively. **(d)** "Selfie" photo 6 months postoperatively showing her body transformation with defined musculature, enhanced contours, and tight skin.

This technique also does not require general anesthesia. With HDBC, tumescent is used in a way that it hydrodissects tissue and provides a significant amount of vasoconstriction very quickly. The fluid is used not only for bulk reduction of fat but also to lift tissue, irregularities, and cellulite away from muscle and tendinous insertions so that superficial liposculpture can be performed after the deep fat extraction without risk of vascular plexus damage and irregularities. This also prepares the tissue for superficial etching, which is not possible when muscle insertions and adhesions are still present. Because HDBC is a more invasive procedure, general anesthesia is also used to keep the patient comfortable and for monitoring in most cases and is preferred by the main author.

23.4.3 Step 3: Energy-Based Treatment of Fat

As described earlier, VASER is essential for HDBC. The ultrasound technology breaks through scar tissue and adhesions and reduces fat without significant effort so that extraction of fat is simpler. Additionally, the steam heat generated from this technology provides significant skin tightening. The fat that is reduced with this technology can be safely used for fat harvesting, which is an essential component to the final outcome of HDBC. Typically, a two- or three-ringed probe, 1 minute for every 100 mL of tumescent anesthesia, is used; however, more time (i.e., 2–2.5x normal) should be used for significantly larger fatty areas or if more etching is going to be desired in the treated area. Risk of vascular plexus injury and seroma formation is a real concern with longer treatment times and higher vibrational amplitudes/resonance; so, postoperative care is essential (see later). For superficial treatment, the author prefers a five-ringed probe. For cellulite, fibrotic, and thick fatty layers, a two-ringed probe is preferred. The resonance is typically set at 50 to 70%, but if fat grafting is desired nothing above 60% should be used.

Finally, to enhance skin tightening in problem areas such as the arms, neck, inner thighs, buttock roll, or lower abdomen/mons pubis, internal skin tightening with Bodytite (▶ **Video 23.2**) or Renuvion (▶ **Video 23.3**) can be used to heat the dermis and enhance VASER results.

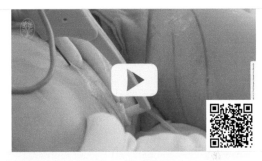

Video 23.2 Demonstration of BodyTite.

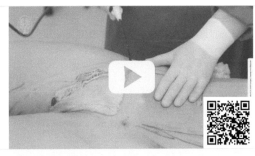

Video 23.3 Demonstration of Renuvion.

23.4.4 Step 4: Extraction and Fat Harvesting

Extraction of fat can be obtained through traditional SAL or more recently PAL, which have been shown to reduce operating times.[15] Many surgeons prefer PAL over traditional SAL as it is less labor intensive and the risk of irregularities is significantly less. In HDBC, bulk reduction is typically performed with one of two systems. PAL with the MicroAire (MicroAire Surgical Instruments) system uses an automatic, reciprocating, backward–forward 2-mm motion to the cannula to aid in penetration into the tissues. The other system is PowerX, part of the VASERlipo System, which uses rotary-powered action that can be adjusted from 90 to 720 degrees for deep and superficial liposuction. The superficial reduction and etching with

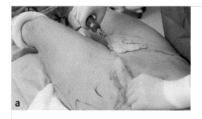
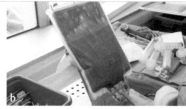
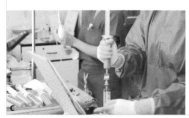
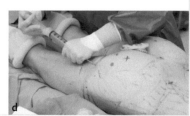

Fig. 23.7 Fat grafting procedure. **(a)** Fat extraction using power-assisted liposuction (PAL) with MicroAire. **(b)** Harvested fat is transferred to the Puregraft system before it is washed with lactated ringers for a more purified fat graft. The fat prior to washing is filled with blood contaminants and free-lipid oils. **(c)** Purified fat transferred to syringes for fat grafting. Note the significant change in color (*golden yellow*) of fat after the purification process. **(d)** Buttocks augmentation with fat grafting.

the PowerX device is described in the superficial muscular etching and defining section. Performing etching requires meticulous skill to avoid seromas and severe irregularities that are extremely difficult to repair. Extracted fat is used for grafting to complete HDBC and is an essential final component. Fat is grafted to areas that require more muscular definition such as the male chest (e.g., pectoralis major muscles), shoulders (e.g., deltoid muscles), and abdomen (e.g., rectus abdominis muscles) or areas that increase in size and projection such as the female buttock and breast.

In the author's practice (JE), fat is harvested into the Puregraft (Suneva Medical) filtration system that removes debris such as oil, connective tissue, and blood to get the purest fat for harvesting in an enclosed system leaving fat a yellow golden color theoretically increasing the long-term retention and better initial viability. With the Puregraft filtration system, the majority of contaminants are removed, making the fat much more pure for reinjection. Traditional decanting and centrifugation methods show higher contaminant levels (i.e., increasing the risk of inflammation and fibrosis) and the microscopic appearance of fat is less purified and less concentrated with viable adipocytes. With the Puregraft system, fat is injected easily and smoothly to chosen grafting sites with less risk of fat necrosis, fat cysts, inflammation, and calcification (▶ Fig. 23.7). Platelet-rich plasma (PRP) also is added to the fat in a 2 to 4:1 ratio to help survivability and longevity. Adding PRP to the fat cells may increase the longevity, but studies are needed to determine the appropriate ratios.

23.4.5 Step 5: Superficial Muscular Etching and Defining

After bulk reduction of fat is achieved through a combination of WAL, UAL, and PAL, the HDBC surgery proceeds with identifying important anatomical landmarks that will

be treated through superficial contouring in order to create shadows and lines. In the markings stage, certain sites such as the inferior and lateral chest wall, horizontal and vertical tendinous insertions of the abdominal rectus muscles, deltoid insertion of the shoulder, triceps insertions, and lower abdominal "V-taper" in males, and the lateral and midline vertical tendinous insertions of rectus muscles, anterosuperior iliac spine of the hip, lower back Venus (sacral) dimples, and deltoid insertion of the shoulders in females are key areas to address.

These areas require very meticulous sculpting through power-assisted rotary devices that scrape the dermis and cause significant skin retraction of the areas premarked for etched lines and definition (▶ Fig. 23.8). Essentially complete fat removal is performed intentionally in these areas so that there is controlled internal scarring pulling the skin down permanently. permanent lines or shapes that give definition and shadowing to make the body appear more athletic are the end result.

23.4.6 Step 6: Fat Grafting

In women, common areas of treatment include the breasts and buttocks, whereas in men, common areas are the chests, shoulders/arms, buttock, and calves. It may seem contradictory to remove fat for reduction but then reinsert the fat to a similar area, as is done in chest defining. However, to get definition and permanent reshaping of a certain area such as the chest in a male, you must remove all the fat completely along with the breast glands so the area is completely regular and flat and then rebuild the desired "squared-off" structure with fat to the muscle (▶ Fig. 23.9). Similarly, in women, when performing gluteal augmentation, you may liposuction part of the lower back, lateral thighs, and buttock roll to reduce bulk fat but then reimplant fat to the upper, middle, and lateral poles of the buttock to give projection and create a more "S-curve" shape of the hips/thighs

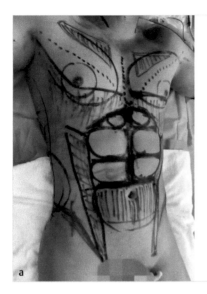
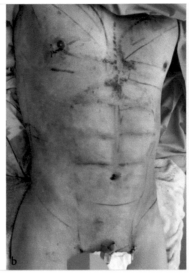

Fig. 23.8 Preoperative markings and superficial etching. **(a)** Premarked male patient with special attention to anatomical landmarks such as the abdominis rectus muscles to create "six-pack abs," external oblique and anterosuperior iliac spine to create a "V-taper," and serratus anterior muscles to create a defined masculine "squared-off" chest. **(b)** Immediate postoperatively from high-definition body contouring (HDBC). Areas of erythema can be appreciated where superficial etching plus internal radiofrequency was done to help contrast and emphasize masculine features.

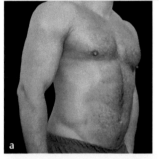
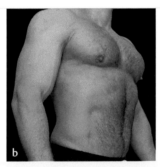
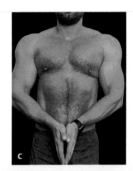
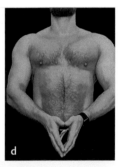

Fig. 23.9 Male chest augmentation with high-definition body contouring (HDBC). **(a)** Before. **(b)** After HDBC to chest. Internal heating to the lower and lateral border of the chest was performed with Renuvion. Fat was harvested and injected into the upper pole of the chest providing lift and adding volume to the pectoralis muscle. Injection behind the nipple also gives added projection. **(c)** Front view flexing chest (before). **(d)** Front view flexing chest (after).

(▶ Fig. 23.10). These body shape changes cannot be done without following this step-by-step approach and incorporating fat grafting.

23.5 Anatomy: Female versus Male

23.5.1 Female Physique

What defines a beautiful female body has always been a subject of much debate, and the perception of the ideal body shape has changed over time and still differs among cultures.[16] Nowadays a beautiful female body has several curves and chief lines that define it. The chief anterior line extends from the suprasternal notch along the midline of the linea alba to the umbilicus, whereas the chief posterior line is in the midline of the back between the erector spinae.[17] Additionally, in those females who truly desire a more athletic look, lateral rectus definition, hip contouring of the anterosuperior iliac spine, and lower sacral dimples can be created or enhanced using superficial liposuction techniques. It is not common for females to have horizontal lines at tendinous insertions of the rectus abdominis ("six-pack") as this is a more masculine feature and should be avoided unless the female is truly a candidate for this type of etching and desires a more "body-builder"-type look.

Fat of the thighs in females can present as major problem area and an area of extreme disproportion in some women. Excessive liposuction of the inner and outer thighs can give a smaller appearance, but also leaving one that is too flat or straight and may result in a manlier or more unattractive appearance. This area needs to be treated in a 360-degree fashion keeping lateral curves and some thickness to the anterior and inner thighs so that a proportionate leg shape is maintained.

The buttocks and lateral thighs are frequent areas requiring enhancement or contouring with fat transfer in order to create a smooth transition between the hip and leg. This is achieved by removing fat from the upper buttocks/lower back and inner thighs and adding fat volume

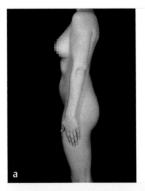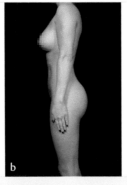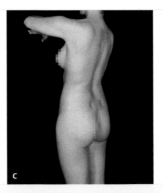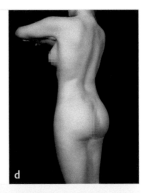

Fig. 23.10 Female buttocks augmentation with high-definition body contouring (HDBC). **(a)** Side profile before fat grafting to the buttocks. **(b)** After fat grafting to the buttocks. **(c)** Oblique angle before fat grafting to the buttocks. **(d)** After fat grafting to the buttocks.

to the lateral buttock and thigh. This technique gives the buttock a rounder appearance and further enhances the "S-curve" that is created when sculpting of the abdominals, flanks/sides, and lower back. Even without any leg contouring, the buttock and hips will look shapelier by fat reduction and skin tightening of the lower back and flanks/sides. It is important to recognize differences among cultures and ethnicities when performing an HDBC. Caucasian and Asian patients often desire a less defined and curvy thigh with much less laterally projected buttock, whereas Latin/Hispanic and African American patients desire much more prominent lateral thighs, larger buttocks, and very thin waists, often giving a less proportionate appearance or "snatched" look.

Other considerations include addressing cellulite with combination approaches such as motorized subcision with Cellfina (Merz Aesthetics), internal skin tightening with RF (e.g., Bodytite or ThermiTight), or helium plasma (e.g., Renuvion). Maintenance treatments can be kept up with external heating devices (e.g., Exilis Ultra 360, Venus Legacy, or Forma Plus). Injectable collagen stimulation with Sculptra aesthetic (Galderma), active ingredient poly-L-lactic acid (PLLA), can be for those who do not have enough fat reserves for fat grafting. Another option is the "bellalift" procedure, which is a blending of Sculptra aesthetic with Bellafill (Suneva Medical), active ingredient polymethyl methacrylate (PMMA), to synergistically build collagen and immediately provide lift. This is achieved by dividing the buttock into four quadrants and injecting a hyperdiluted mix of the two products together (20–50% PMMA:PLLA) into each quadrant to give a fuller more contoured shape to the buttocks. Several vials are needed in each session and several sessions may be needed to achieve the desired effect.

23.5.2 Male Physique

In contrast to a smooth, soft, and curved female body, a male body is more squared, tight, and defined by the muscles underlying the skin. Almost universally to all cultures, a broader and wider upper body as compared to lower abdominals with defined muscles and minimal fat is desired and found to be uniformly attractive. HDBC is successful upon complete fat removal in the deep adipose layer (debulking), followed by very meticulous removal in the superficial layers over the tendinous insertions of the muscles beneath.

Decreasing fat in an even linear fashion is extremely important so that retraction of the skin is symmetric over the underlying muscle and displays a true etched appearance. Inexperienced surgeons nervous to fully reduce the superficial layers may end up only partially doing so, leaving an irregular appearance and one that shows an initial improved appearance but is not maintained long term. In another scenario, someone nervous or less experienced in working through the superficial layers can cause uncontrolled (vs. controlled scarring for muscular defining) fibrosis/scarring that leads to fibrous banding, irregularities, incomplete contouring, and damage to the superficial vascularity, leading to skin discoloration. For a permanent body change with defined lines, fascial adhesions must be created by aggressive superficial fat removal. The best aesthetic outcome is with a complete understanding of anatomy so that the surgical markings of the fat layers, underlying musculature, and adhesion zones (i.e., proposed defined lines) are defined and addressed through the surgery.

Abdominal etching includes aggressive removal of the deep fat layers of the torso, superficial etching of the linea alba (i.e., the vertical crease above the umbilicus), the linea semilunaris (i.e., the lateral or outside edge of the rectus muscle), the horizontal lines across the tendinous insertions of the rectus abdominis muscle to get a "six-pack," and hip sculpting of the anterosuperior iliac spine (i.e., "V"-taper). Slight irregularities need to be integrated in a defined pattern to ensure a natural look of the abdomen after the etching. It is imperative not to forget liposuction of the mons pubis.

Chest and chest wall, upper back, sacral, and arm/shoulder areas need to be addressed to complete the body transformation. Most surgeons will forgo these areas due to the increased surgical and recovery times as well as inexperience in creating definition of these areas. In men, it is essential to create a more athletic shape by using harvested fat for muscular defining of the chest and shoulders/arms to give a broad upper body appearance.[18] The harvested fat is infused with PRP as described earlier in a 2 to 4:1 ratio to help survivability and longevity. Finally, the male breast glands (gynecomastia) should be removed if they are evident after lipocontouring of the breast and fat injection into the muscle.[19]

Case 1: Poor Planning and Anatomical Consideration in a Male Stomach with HDBC

To create an abdominal six-pack or "V-taper" in a male desiring a more contoured stomach, it is essential to identify all the tendinous insertions of the rectus muscles and aggressively define these areas but leave a small amount of fat over the muscle belly themselves. Improper placement of presurgical markings can lead to an incomplete abdominal six-pack shape and uneven resection of the superficial adipose layer can lead to fibrotic bands in the wrong location causing superficial irregularities often seen best during flexion/extension (▶ Fig. 23.11).

Case 2: Planning and Anatomical Consideration in a Male Chest Revision Surgery

The male chest requires at least five steps to get the best contouring: (1) UAL with VASERlipo, (2) both Stand PAL with Microaire and Rotary PAL with PowerX, (3) internal heating to the lower and lateral chest wall, (4) male breast gland removal, (5) fat grafting with PRP injected into the chest musculature. Patients who have only traditional liposuction to the chest with over-resection of the male breast gland can lead to a "flat" appearance without contour (▶ Fig. 23.12). A sixth step is sometimes necessary for those who have looser skin, which is a "nipple-lift" and helps give a chest lift without outside scars as all the scars are contained around the areola (areolar mastopexy; ▶ Fig. 23.13).

To repair this, HDBC of the chest and chest wall can be performed in the superficial layer to define a new lower and lateral border of the chest. Fat harvested and injected into the upper pole of the chest provides lift and volume to the pectoralis muscle. Injection behind the nipple gives added projection. Fat was also injected into the shoulders to give the upper body a broader appearance.

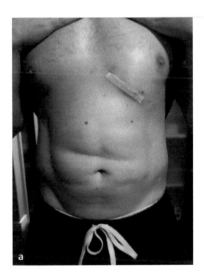
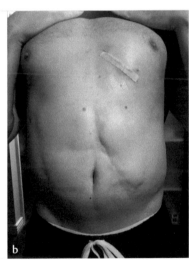

Fig. 23.11 Poor outcome from high-definition body contouring (HDBC). **(a)** Resting position. Improper placement of presurgical markings can lead to an incomplete abdominal six-pack, irregularities, and indentations. **(b)** Extension position. Uneven resection of the superficial adipose layer can lead to fibrotic bands in the wrong location causing superficial irregularities and loss of true anatomic muscular shaping.

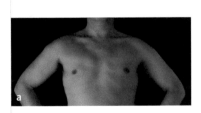
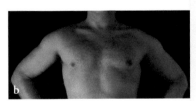

Fig. 23.12 Revision of male chest liposuction. **(a)** Excessive suction-assisted liposuction (SAL) performed to male breast tissue leaving behind a deflated appearance without contour. **(b)** Revision of male chest with high-definition body contouring (HDBC) defining lower and lateral borders. Fat grafting into the pectoralis muscles and below the nipple to provide volume and more muscular tone to the chest.

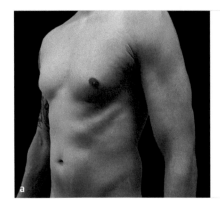
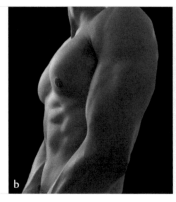

Fig. 23.13 Male areolar mastopexy. **(a)** Liposuction and breast gland removal to the chest area in this patient would leave excessive loose skin that cannot be corrected with internal heating alone. **(b)** Areolar mastopexy 6 months postoperatively.

Table 23.2 Tumescent fluid for high-definition body contouring (HDBC)

1 L normal saline or lactated Ringer's solution

10 mL of 2% (20 mg/mL) lidocaine hydrochloride[a]

2 ampules of 1:1,000 (1 mg/mL) epinephrine

1 mL (10 mg) of triamcinolone acetonide (Kenalog 10)

12.5 mL of 8.4% (1 mEq/mL) sodium bicarbonate

[a]For local tumescent cases that are not HDBC, dose increases to 50 mL/1 L of fluid.

23.6 Surgical Planning and Staging of Procedures

Full-body shaping requires significant downtime and discreet surgical planning. If numerous areas of the body are to be reduced in size and contoured, for safety reasons, the surgeries need to be staged. In some instances, surgical cutting/skin removal and/or permanent implants are needed for the best outcome and recovery time is needed between procedures.

In both males and females, the procedures are staged to keep each procedure less than 5 L in fat removal. These procedures are done under general anesthesia. Local tumescent approaches make it almost impossible to get an adequate amount of fat removed and body contours created without significant pain. Also, limitations in the amount of "caine" anesthetic require patients to undergo general anesthesia with a variation in the traditional tumescent fluid to limit toxicity (▶ Table 23.2).[20]

23.6.1 Typical Staging of a Female Full-Body Contouring Procedure (without Skin Cutting)

- Procedure 1: Calf/ankle and forearm.
- Procedure 2: Circumferential torso, upper arm, buttock (at least 3 days after the first procedure).

- Procedure 3: Circumferential thigh (at least 7 days after the second procedure).

In any of these procedures, the surgeon can add neck and face liposuction, fat transfer, cellulite release (i.e., Cellfina), and/or skin tightening (i.e., Facetite for the face and Bodytite and/or Renuvion for the body). Implants and skin removal surgery are best during the last procedure for the purposes of easier healing and simpler postoperative recovery. However, the procedures are tailored to the individual patient. Those with lipedema (i.e., larger amounts of disproportion fat) may require a more than a fourth surgery that addresses sections of the buttock or thigh that could not be addressed in the previous procedures and/or touchup of other areas to get more fat removal.

In some patients, you can address the full body in one longer surgery without increasing risk and fitting within the guidelines of acceptable safe amounts of fat removal if the patient is more athletic and require more contouring and shaping than large-volume fat removal. Fat transfer is typical in the breast, buttock, and thighs to give a more "S-curve" and projected buttock and hip for women. A typical expectation for improvement on the breast is 0.5 to 1.5 cup size. However, to maintain fat viability in this area, a series of future fat injection touchup procedures may be needed. Facial augmentation with any additional fat can give great improvement in facial contours.[21]

23.6.2 Typical Staging of a Male Full-Body Contouring Procedure (without Skin Removal)

- Procedure 1: circumferential torso, chest, and arms with male breast gland removal (gynecomastia), fat transfer ± nipple lift.
- Procedure 2: circumferential thighs and partial calves.

In the male athletic patient, the majority of all the work desired can be done in a single procedure (even sections of the thigh and calves). The length of the procedure is extended if the patient requires significant skin removal. If the patient is larger and significant debulking of fat is necessary, this should be done in a process as shown earlier in the female section. Three months to 6 months should be waited until HDBC (i.e., etching, sculpting, fat transfer) is performed.

In any of the neck, face, and calf liposuction procedures, fat transfer and skin tightening (i.e., Facetite for the face and Renuvion and/or Bodytite for the body) can be performed at the same time. The face and neck should be in the last procedure. If a significant amount of skin removal is needed for full-body lifting, the procedures are staged, but liposuction is performed at the same time immediately before the skin removal to "debulk" the area and later to contour and shape. Fat injections are completed at the end and typical locations include the buttock, chest, shoulders/arms, and calves. Chest, buttock, shoulder, or calf implants are placed concurrently with the liposuction procedure but staged so that healing times are appropriate. For example, a total HDBC in a male wanting "six-pack abs" with chest and buttock contouring but requiring implants for the best improvement would have full upper body liposuction with fat harvesting and injection to the chest and buttocks and only the chest implant placed. A healing time of 4 to 12 weeks would be allowed before addressing other implants such as the buttock to allow for easier postoperative recovery and less body stress.

23.7 Postoperative Aftercare and Follow-Up

In HDBC, the follow-up care and postoperative healing is essential to prevent complications (▶ Table 23.3).[22,23,24] High-definition procedures are much more aggressive than traditional tumescent approaches due to the increased number of areas treated in a single procedure, a larger amount of total fat removal as compared to standard small-volume cases, as well as the superficial nature of etching. This can lead to more significant dehydration requiring intravenous fluid replacement starting 12 to 24 hours after the procedure, the development of postoperative anemia requiring hyperbaric oxygen therapy (HBO), and a higher risk of infection due to the insertion of drainage tubes requiring antibiotics to cover both staph and strep species. There is an increased risk of seroma formation even with proper double compression, lymphatic and facial massage, as well as the development of fibrotic banding that requires RF and/or ultrasound manipulation of tissue immediately after the procedure and long term for 3 to 6 months.

It is essential that in the preoperative evaluation and consenting process, there is complete discussion over

Table 23.3 Complications of high-definition body contouring (HDBC)

Short-term expected	Short-term unexpected	Long-term unexpected
Pain	Seroma	Permanent indentations or asymmetry
Swelling	Hematoma	Worsening cellulite
Bruising	Infection	Fat necrosis
Bleeding	Allergic reaction (i.e., tape or compression bandage)	Fat calcification
Numbness	Inflammatory reaction (i.e., fat injection area)	Skin necrosis and scarring
	Contour irregularity (i.e., fibrous bands)	Skin discoloration (i.e., erythema ab liposuction)
	Burns	
	Pulmonary embolism or fat embolism	

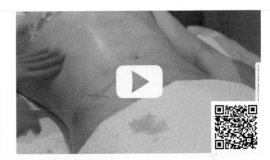

Video 23.4 Demonstration of lymphatic massage technique.

the postprocedural healing process with HDBC, as this is extremely different (i.e., much longer and more difficult) than a traditional liposuction and requires a significant number of steps after to ensure proper healing and an ultimate outcome that is permanent.

23.7.1 Lymphatic Massage

Also called lymphatic drainage or manual lymph drainage, lymphatic massage is a technique developed for the treatment of lymphedema, an accumulation of fluid that can occur after surgery. Stagnant lymphatic flow can cause increased swelling and chronic inflammation, as well as increased seromas and fibrotic tissue after aggressive surgery. Therapy should be started no more than 24 hours postprocedure to facilitate tissue healing and a more rapid recovery (▶ **Video 23.4**).

23.7.2 Hyperbaric Oxygen

HBO allows a patient to breathe concentrated oxygen at pressures greater than normal atmospheric pressure, helping the concentrated blood cells to speed up the healing process. It has been documented that with surgical cutting procedures HBO can decrease the rate of complications such as seromas, hematomas, and scarring.[25,26] Increasing the blood flow and oxygenation to tissue also helps increase the functional mobility of the body, which in turn helps patients return to activities much more quickly after an extreme procedure. Daily treatments for 2 weeks are essential for HDBC, especially if implants are placed and/or skin removal surgery is performed.

23.7.3 Ultrasound and Radiofrequency Devices

Similar to lymphatic massage, manipulation of tissue through mechanical stimulation as well as heat increases the ability for the skin to heal properly as well as decrease swelling. In one study, superficial PAL combined with external ultrasound with or without postoperative deep tissue massage/suction (Endermologie) was seen to decrease the overall complication rate, contour irregularity, and skin necrosis. There were no statistical differences regarding other complications.[24] In the author's (JE) practice, superficial RF (e.g., Exilis Ultra 360, Venus Legacy or Forma Plus) starting no more than 7 days after the procedure, continuing twice weekly for 3 to 6 months after HDBC, is performed. External ultrasound can begin the day after the procedure in conjunction with lymphatic and fascial massage.

23.7.4 Surgical Drainage Tubes

Placements of surgical drains are necessary in procedures that have large volume reduction and aggressive superficial skin manipulation. In traditional liposuction, port sites are left open to drain, but they often close within 24 to 72 hours in most instances and can leave fluid to build up increasing the rate of seroma, chronic inflammation, and hematoma. When superficial liposuction is performed, drainage can occur for weeks and tube placement ensures fluid movement out of the body during the initial 1 to 2 weeks, after which the tubes are removed and sites sutured closed if needed (for cosmetic purposes). If progressive tension suturing is used for the abdominoplasty, drains may not be required when liposuction is concurrently performed.[27,28,29]

23.8 Conclusion

HDBC is as much a science as it is an art. The demand for a more sculpted and defined body has required surgeons to make advances in techniques and approaches to surgical body shaping that not only removes large volumes of fat in multiple locations but also uses harvested fat for muscular defining and body shaping. Newer energy-based modalities have allowed surgeons to not only address the deep subcutaneous layers to remove bulk fat but also work in the superficial layers for etching and muscular shaping that has long been avoided. For more aggressive HDBC, surgical implants and/or skin removal in a series of procedures can be performed to get an ultimate transformation.

Postoperative care and follow-up are essential to ensure long-term complications are minimal and results are life-changing. Future studies will look at the importance of noninvasive devices in the postoperative healing phase as well as how to further improve contour, cellulite, and skin-tightening results in conjunction with HDBC surgical techniques.

References

[1] American Society of Plastic Surgeons. Plastic Surgery Statistics Report 2018. Arlington Height, IL: American Society of Plastic Surgeons; 2018

[2] Almutairi K, Gusenoff JA, Rubin JP. Body contouring. Plast Reconstr Surg. 2016; 137(3):586e–602e

[3] Mordon S, Plot E. Laser lipolysis versus traditional liposuction for fat removal. Expert Rev Med Devices. 2009; 6(6):677–688

[4] Stephan PJ, Kenkel JM. Updates and advances in liposuction. Aesthet Surg J. 2010; 30(1):83–97, quiz 98–100

[5] Zocchi ML. Ultrasonic assisted lipoplasty. Technical refinements and clinical evaluations. Clin Plast Surg. 1996; 23(4):575–598

[6] Jewell ML, Fodor PB, de Souza Pinto EB, Al Shammari MA. Clinical application of VASER: assisted lipoplasty—a pilot clinical study. Aesthet Surg J. 2002; 22(2):131–146

[7] Wu DC, Liolios A, Mahoney L, Guiha I, Goldman MP. Subdermal radiofrequency for skin tightening of the posterior upper arms. Dermatol Surg. 2016; 42(9):1089–1093

[8] Paul M, Mulholland RS. A new approach for adipose tissue treatment and body contouring using radiofrequency-assisted liposuction. Aesthetic Plast Surg. 2009; 33(5):687–694

[9] Paul M, Blugerman G, Kreindel M, Mulholland RS. Three-dimensional radiofrequency tissue tightening: a proposed mechanism and applications for body contouring. Aesthetic Plast Surg. 2011; 35(1): 87–95

[10] Irvine Duncan D. Nonexcisional tissue tightening: creating skin surface area reduction during abdominal liposuction by adding radiofrequency heating. Aesthet Surg J. 2013; 33(8):1154–1166

[11] Chen SS, Wright NT, Humphrey JD. Heat-induced changes in the mechanics of a collagenous tissue: isothermal free shrinkage. J Biomech Eng. 1997; 119(4):372–378

[12] Sterodimas A, Boriani F, Magarakis E, Nicaretta B, Pereira LH, Illouz YG. Thirtyfour years of liposuction: past, present and future. Eur Rev Med Pharmacol Sci. 2012; 16(3):393–406

[13] Leclère FM, Moreno-Moraga J, Mordon S, et al. Laser-assisted lipolysis for cankle remodelling: a prospective study in 30 patients. Lasers Med Sci. 2014; 29(1):131–136

[14] Duscher D, Atashroo D, Maan ZN, et al. Ultrasound-assisted liposuction does not compromise the regenerative potential of adipose-derived stem cells. Stem Cells Transl Med. 2016; 5(2):248–257

[15] Scuderi N, Tenna S, Spalvieri C, De Gado F. Power-assisted lipoplasty versus traditional suction-assisted lipoplasty: comparative evaluation and analysis of output. Aesthetic Plast Surg. 2005; 29(1): 49–52

[16] Singh D. Female judgment of male attractiveness and desirability for relationships: role of waist-to-hip ratio and financial status. J Pers Soc Psychol. 1995; 69(6):1089–1101

[17] Hoyos A, Prendergast P. High Definition Body Sculpting: Art and Advanced Lipoplasty Techniques. Vol. 1. Berlin: Springer; 2014

[18] Hoyos A, Perez M. Dynamic-definition male pectoral reshaping and enhancement in slim, athletic, obese, and gynecomastic patients through selective fat removal and grafting. Aesthetic Plast Surg. 2012; 36(5):1066–1077

[19] Pilanci O, Basaran K, Aydin HU, Cortuk O, Kuvat SV. Autologous fat injection into the pectoralis major as an adjunct to surgical correction of gynecomastia. Aesthet Surg J. 2015; 35(3):NP54–NP61

[20] Ostad A, Kageyama N, Moy RL. Tumescent anesthesia with a lidocaine dose of 55 mg/kg is safe for liposuction. Dermatol Surg. 1996; 22(11):921–927

[21] Rusciani Scorza A, Rusciani Scorza L, Troccola A, Micci DM, Rauso R, Curinga G. Autologous fat transfer for face rejuvenation with tumescent technique fat harvesting and saline washing: a report of 215 cases. Dermatology. 2012; 224(3):244–250

[22] El-Ali KM, Gourlay T. Assessment of the risk of systemic fat mobilization and fat embolism as a consequence of liposuction: ex vivo study. Plast Reconstr Surg. 2006; 117(7):2269–2276

[23] Kubota T, Ebina T, Tonosaki M, Ishihara H, Matsuki A. Rapid improvement of respiratory symptoms associated with fat embolism by high-dose methylpredonisolone: a case report. J Anesth. 2003; 17(3):186–189

[24] Kim YH, Cha SM, Naidu S, Hwang WJ. Analysis of postoperative complications for superficial liposuction: a review of 2398 cases. Plast Reconstr Surg. 2011; 127(2):863–871

[25] Stong BC, Jacono AA. Effect of perioperative hyperbaric oxygen on bruising in face-lifts. Arch Facial Plast Surg. 2010; 12(5):356–358

[26] Fulton JE, Jr. The use of hyperbaric oxygen (HBO) to accelerate wound healing. Dermatol Surg. 2000; 26(12):1170–1172

[27] Pollock TA, Pollock H. Progressive tension sutures in abdominoplasty: a review of 597 consecutive cases. Aesthet Surg J. 2012; 32(6):729–742

[28] Quaba AA, Conlin S, Quaba O. The no-drain, no-quilt abdominoplasty: a single-surgeon series of 271 patients. Plast Reconstr Surg. 2015; 135(3):751–760

[29] Epstein S, Epstein MA, Gutowski KA. Lipoabdominoplasty without drains or progressive tension sutures: an analysis of 100 consecutive patients. Aesthet Surg J. 2015; 35(4):434–440

24 Fat Transfer

Wilfred Brown and Amanda Fazzalari

Summary

Autologous fat grafting has become a routinely utilized technique that is considered safe and effective. It is used for both for augmenting soft-tissue volume and improving contour. This chapter describes the rationale and associated techniques for both employing and optimizing results from this effective procedure.

Keywords: soft-tissue augmentation, improved wound healing, body contouring, fat transfer, fat grafting, facial rejuvination

24.1 Introduction

Autologous fat transfer has become an increasingly popular treatment modality in recent years. The scope of its use has broadened as techniques have become more refined and standardized. Fat grafting is routinely utilized for soft-tissue augmentation, reconstruction for both congenital and acquired conditions, radiation injury, scarring, and rejuvenation of aged or damaged tissues.[1] This chapter reviews the history of fat transfer, principles of techniques, individual considerations, clinical applications, as well as pearls and pitfalls for the practice of fat transfer.

24.2 Background of Fat Transfer

The first "fat grafting" procedure dates back to the late 19th century, when a German plastic surgeon, Gustav Neuber (1850–1932), a German plastic surgeon, transferred fat from the arm to the orbital region to correct scars formed from osteomyelitis.[2] The first time fat transfer was performed for facial atrophy was in 1912.[3] In 1895, Dr. Viktor Czerny (1842–1916) transferred a lipoma to the breast to establish symmetry following a unilateral partial mastectomy.[4]

In 1912, Eugene Hollander described a technique of using a "broth" composed of a combination of human and ram fat to correct facial depressions and postmastectomy adherent scars. Results were inconsistent.[3]

Fat grafting had trouble gaining widespread acceptance over the next 100 years due to the unreliability of the long-term success associated with the procedure. Modern liposuction techniques had not yet been refined, and the viability of the aspirated fat was variable. Attempts at grafting aspirated fat often yielded inconsistent results.

In the 1990s, Coleman published techniques describing standardized procedures for fat extraction, processing, and injection. Since then, autologous fat grafting has gained in popularity and has now become a workhorse for soft-tissue augmentation throughout the body for both aesthetic and reconstructive indications,[5] as well as an increasingly relied-on technique for rejuvenation of damaged tissues.

Fat is abundant and easily accessible, and therefore, it is often considered preferential over the commercially available fillers. Unlike many synthetic fillers, viable fat remains soft and is durable. Since adipocytes that have been successfully transferred are viable, their behavior is dynamic. They respond to environmental stimuli such as changes in caloric intake, exercise, and alterations in hormonal milieu. Thus, living transferred fat changes size in proportion to the patient's weight gain and loss.

Fat transfer in the form of fat grafting has become a commonly used technique. According to the American Society of Plastic Surgeons, there were over 85,000 fat grafting procedures performed in the United States in 2017, up 8% from 2016 and 31% from 2000.[6]

24.3 Principles of Fat Grafting

Over 90% of adipose tissue volume consists of adipocytes, but nearly 50% of the in vivo adipose tissue total cell number consists of stromal stem cells, fibroblasts, endothelial cells, and pericytes in an extravascular matrix.[7] Many studies have demonstrated the regenerative potential of autologous fat transfer. This includes angiogenesis,[8] peripheral nerve regeneration,[9] enhancement of dermal thickness, and elasticity.[10]

Multiple factors have been identified that influence the success rate of fat transfer. These include, first, the method of harvest, second, the processing of the harvested fat, and, finally, the technique of placement of the graft into the recipient area.[1] Steps of the procedure are described below and summarized in ▶ Table 24.1.

24.3.1 Method of Harvest

A variety of techniques are currently used to aspirate fat from the donor area. These include the use of syringe aspiration or suction-assisted lipectomy using a mechanical vacuum generator. For smaller volumes, syringe aspiration of the fat is often thought to be more precise, while when larger volumes of fat are needed, liposuction machines with a catchment filter are utilized. Multiple studies have examined cell viability following harvest. No one technique appears superior to another when the tumescent technique is being employed. Usually the anterior abdomen or the flanks are utilized for fat harvest because of the availability of fat in these areas; however, other areas can be used if fat is available. No one area has been demonstrated to be superior in terms of long-term fat viability. Often patients request simultaneous liposuction

Table 24.1 Steps of procedure

Patient positioned appropriately for fat harvest and injection

Donor and recipient areas prepped with chlorhexidine or povidone-iodine

Donor area injected with tumescent solution (see below) recipient area anesthetized either with lidocaine 1% with epinephrine or tumescent solution

Suction lipectomy performed from donor area using either syringe or vacuum-assisted technique

Fat processed according to preferred technique

Fat transferred to appropriately sized syringes for injection

Fat injected using threading technique. Fat should be injected as deeply as possible so as to minimize visibility of the graft

Dressings placed on donor and recipient areas

Table 24.2 Tumescent solution for anesthesia

Ingredient	Action
1 L normal saline	Diluent
50 mL lidocaine 1%	Anesthesia
1 mL 1:1,000 epinephrine	Vasoconstriction
10 mL 8.4% sodium bicarbonate	Reduces acidity, and therefore discomfort when injecting

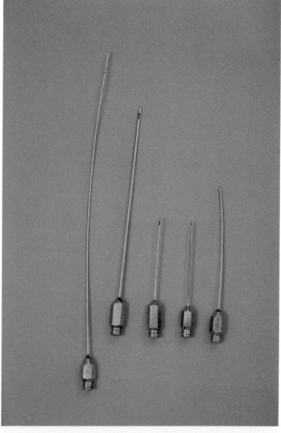

Fig. 24.1 Typical instrumentation required for fat harvesting and reinjection. This kit consists of an infuser for tumescent or local anesthesia, 2-mm suction cannula, and three injection cannulas of varying width and length.

of a particular area combined with fat transfer to another anatomically separate area. This should be discussed in detail with the patient in the preoperative consultation. Harvesting of fat for use in fat transfer is performed using tumescent anesthesia (▶ Table 24.2). Benefits of tumescent anesthesia include decreased discomfort, diminished blood loss, and improved ease of fat removal.[11,12] Tumescent anesthesia can be supplemented with either sedation or general anesthesia. Individual situations will dictate the type of anesthesia used. The use of lidocaine as a local anesthetic has not been demonstrated to have an adverse effect on the viability of adipocytes.[13]

24.3.2 Cannula

Cannulas that are specifically designed for harvest of fat should be used since they minimize sheer forces on the adipocytes (▶ Fig. 24.1). There is some evidence that larger diameter harvesting cannulas have improved yield of viable adipocytes; however, this remains controversial. Additionally, low-pressure suction systems such as syringe aspiration are believed to be less traumatic on the harvested tissue (▶ Fig. 24.1).

24.3.3 Time

Fat transfer should be performed as soon as possible after harvesting. Adipocyte viability decreases soon after harvesting, whereas stem cells can be harvested from the specimen up to 4 hours after harvest at room temperature, and up to 24 hours at 4 °C.[14] Storage of the harvested fat is not recommended since the viability of the adipocytes drops significantly, which may decrease graft efficacy. It is currently recommended that fat be used fresh.

24.3.4 Processing

Once harvested, a variety of techniques exist to process the aspirate to maximize viability of the grafted fat (▶ Table 24.3). These include cotton gauze processing (▶ Fig. 24.2). centrifugation (▶ Fig. 24.3), gravity separation, filtration, and washing (▶ Fig. 24.2). Retention of the highest number of viable stromal vascular fraction cells and stem cells are thought to maximize graft survival (▶ Table 24.3). Cotton gauze processing involves

Table 24.3 Techniques of fat processing

Cotton gauze processing

Filtration

Centrifugation

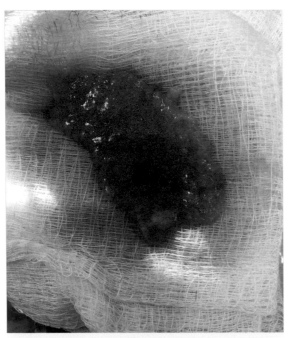

Fig. 24.2 Appearance of aspirated fat that has been placed on cotton gauze to allow for wicking of liquid component of the aspirate. The fat is often washed with normal saline or Ringer's lactate to further remove undesirable components of the aspirate.

placing the harvested fat on cotton gauze and allowing the oil and aqueous fraction to wick off by capillary action. The retained fat is then washed either with Ringer's lactate or normal saline before reinjection (▶ Fig. 24.2). Centrifugation exposes the graft to centrifugal forces, which separate the specimen into the injectable fraction and the fraction that is discarded (▶ Fig. 24.3).[15] The oil and tumescent layers are discarded, whereas the low- and high-density fat layers are retained. The high-density layer yields the highest density of viable cells. Histologically, the high-density layer also contained the largest proportion of endothelial cells and associated angiogenic factors.[16] Variation in centrifugal speeds have not been conclusively shown to affect cell viability; however, some evidence exists that forces higher than 3,000 rpm may cause increased cellular damage.[17] Gravity separation is usually performed at room temperature for up to 20 minutes. Once separation has occurred, the oil component is wicked off and the aqueous component is drained. Filtration and washing of the harvested fat can be performed either with a sieve or in a closed system.

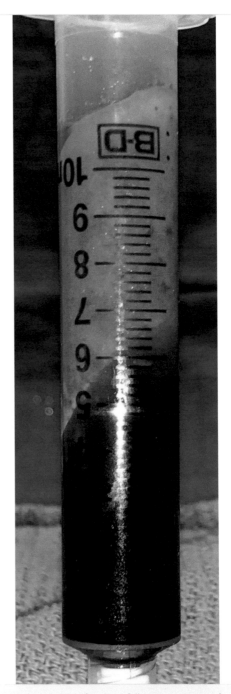

Fig. 24.3 Appearance of aspirate following 3 minutes of centrifuge. The fat is retained for injection.

A variety of commercially available closed filtration and washing systems are available. There is no conclusive evidence that one technique is superior to another.

24.3.5 Injection

Injection of the fat graft should be performed carefully and methodically. Usually, a 14- to 21-gauge fat injection cannula is used (▶ Fig. 24.1). The cannulas are usually blunt tipped so as to minimize trauma to the recipient site. Fat is carefully and slowly injected as the cannula is being withdrawn. The surgeon should constantly be aware of the location of the distal opening in the cannula. Fat grafts should be placed in areas that will have maximal survival and therefore ensure integration in the recipient bed. Smaller syringe (▶ Fig. 24.4) use leads to greater precision of placement. Volumes of less than 0.5 mL per pass of the syringe result in thin "strings" of fat being placed. Fat should be injected in a three-dimensional

fashion while minimizing repeat injections to the same site. It is often beneficial to insert the injection cannula through two or more stab incisions so that the grafted fat creates a matrix in a three-dimensional fashion in the recipient area. Once injected, only fat droplets smaller than 1.6 mm will reliably revascularize. Beneath the superficial 1.6-mm zone is the regenerative zone, where stem cells survive. These stem cells then regenerate a new adipocyte population. Ideally, this zone is 3 mm in width. Droplets or ribbons with diameters greater than 3 mm will inevitably develop a central area of necrosis.[18] Careful attention should, therefore, be paid not to allow coalescing of ribbon or droplet grafts.

The technique of placing "strings" of fat in the area to be augmented is similar to the techniques used for synthetic fillers; however, filling is achieved by placing layers of strings of fat, often approaching the recipient area from different angles to achieve smoothness of the overlying skin.

24.3.6 Recipient Site

There is no conclusive evidence that variables in the recipient site influence success of the graft (▶ Fig. 24.5, ▶ Fig. 24.6, ▶ Fig. 24.7, ▶ Fig. 24.8, ▶ Fig. 24.9, ▶ Fig. 24.10, ▶ Table 24.4). Increased vascularity of the recipient site may be beneficial such as is seen in muscle; however, tissues that have more mobility may negatively affect revascularization of the grafted tissue. Advancing age, presence of scar tissue, and large defect size have been shown to diminish success of the graft (▶ Table 24.1).

24.3.7 Additional Considerations

Supplementing fat grafts with supplemental stromal vascular fraction and adipose-derived stem cells has been shown to increase success of the graft. This has been attributed to the increased angiogenic and wound-healing capacity of the graft.[19,20] Enhancement of graft survival in heavily scarred or burned areas is observed when serial grafts are undertaken.

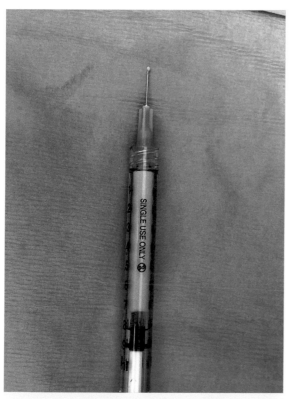

Fig. 24.4 Appearance of filtered fat prior to injection.

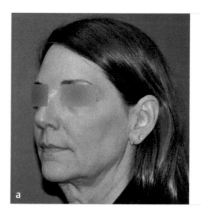
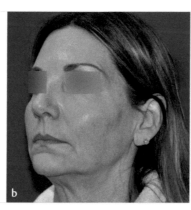

Fig. 24.5 Fat injection into malar regions of the face. Eight milliliters were injected superficial to the zygomatic process per side.

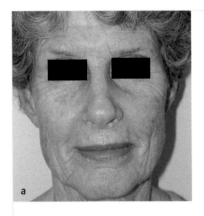

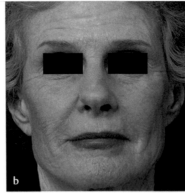

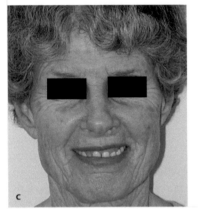

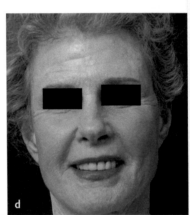

Fig. 24.6 (a–d) Fat grafting to the midface: postoperative photo taken 1 year postinjection.

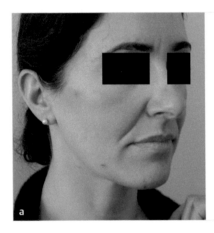

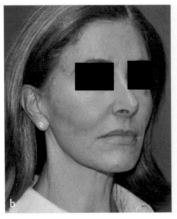

Fig. 24.7 (a, b) Ten milliliters of fat were injected per side to the midface resulting in significant volume augmentation.

24.4 Individual Considerations

24.4.1 Medical History

A thorough and complete medical history is important in all patients being considered for fat grafting. Many over-the-counter dietary supplements and vitamins are associated with an increased risk of bleeding.[21] Medications that interfere with the normal coagulation pathways or platelet function such as aspirin and nonsteroidal anti-inflammatory drugs should be discontinued prior to surgery. Congenital or acquired coagulation disorders will also increase the risk of postoperative bleeding and may need to be addressed prior to surgery. Any active infection, either local or distant, should be addressed and fully resolved before proceeding. Other contraindications include disorders of lipid metabolism, severe chronic disease, and acute organ failure. Lack of a donor site for fat harvest in thin patients may result in inadequate quantities

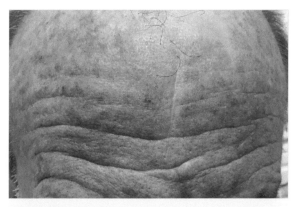

Fig. 24.8 Forehead scar prior to deep dermal and subcutaneous injection of fat.

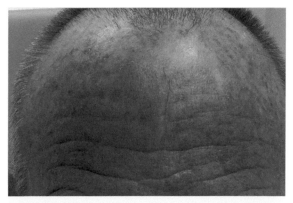

Fig. 24.10 Appearance of scar 6 months following fat injection.

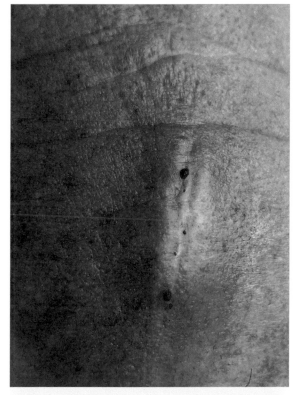

Fig. 24.9 Appearance of scar immediately following injection of fat.

Table 24.4 Recipient site variables that affect graft success

Improved success	Decreased success
Increased vascularity such as muscle	Decreased vascularity such as scar, fibrotic tissue
Smaller defect	Significant structural defect
Fixed tissue such as the malar and lateral cheek region	Mobile tissues such as lips and glabella
Younger patient	Advanced age
Prepared or preconditioned recipient site such as pre-expanded breast skin performed for 3 wk prior to grafting	Trauma to the overlying skin or severe burns

of fat harvest and also cause a contour issue in the area of harvest.

Since lidocaine is metabolized in the liver, caution should be exercised in patients with underlying hepatic disease. Cessation of smoking at least 4 weeks prior to the procedure has been demonstrated to decrease risk of wound-healing complications.[22] Significant compromise in the revascularization of the grafted fat has been demonstrated in patients who are actively smoking at the time of the procedure. Well-controlled glucose levels in patients with diabetes mellitus have been demonstrated to diminish the risk of wound infection.[23,24]

24.4.2 Physical Examination

A complete physical examination should be performed in all patients. Particular attention should be paid to potential areas for fat harvest as well as examination of the intended recipient area. The presence of hernias in the truncal area should be noted so as to minimize the risk of bowel injury. Usually areas targeted for fat donation are areas where perceived excess is noted by the patient and the surgeon. A detailed consultation should be conducted with the patient regarding the suitability of various donor areas. Commonly utilized areas are the abdomen, flanks, and thighs. Currently, there does not appear to be any difference in adipocyte viability or volume retention among different donor sites.[25,26,27,28]

24.4.3 Informed Consent

Counselling the patient prior to the procedure is extremely important. The patient should be fully informed of the risks of both the harvest of the fat and the injection of the graft. Potential risks and complications should be discussed in detail (see below). Patients should be made aware that the grafted fat consists of viable cells, which may change in volume just as regular fat does. The changes in volume may occur in response to increased caloric intake, exercise, and changes in the hormonal milieu.

Alternative treatment options such as synthetic fillers should be discussed. Patients should be allowed ample time to review the consent forms as well as to have any questions or concerns addressed. The technique of fat grating, including the anticipated area where the fat will be harvested from, processing technique, and location of injections should be discussed in detail. It is difficult to accurately quantify the percentage of graft that is retained long term; however, results are generally reported as excellent or good. Initial overcorrection is generally utilized to compensate for initial resorption or necrosis.[29]

24.4.4 Photography

Accurate pre- and postoperative photographic documentation is essential on all patients. Both the donor and recipient areas should be photographed. Comparable lighting and position of the patient is essential.

24.5 Clinical Applications

The volume of fat harvested for grafting is dictated by the anticipated volume that will be needed for injection. Smaller volumes such as 1 to 2 mL are required for minor filling, whereas larger volumes, often greater than 500 mL, are injected where larger volumes are needed.

24.5.1 Tissue Augmentation/Filling

Breast

Fat grafting as a means to correct both congenital and acquired deformities of the breast is a routine technique utilized by both reconstructive and aesthetic surgeons. Initial concerns regarding difficulties in differentiating areas of microcalcifications associated with fat grafts and potentially suspicious premalignant or malignant changes have largely been discounted. Areas of fat necrosis may mimic tumors; therefore, any new breast mass should always be assessed. Congenital conditions that have successfully been treated with fat grafts include Poland syndrome, micromastia, and tuberous breast deformity. Acquired deformities of the breast such as defects following lumpectomy or partial mastectomy are often ideally suited to volume augmentation with fat grafts.

Augmentation of the breast with fat grafts in the aesthetic patient can be performed as the sole augmentation procedure, or fat can be placed selectively in deficient areas in conjunction with a prosthetic implant.

Gluteal Region

Augmentation of the gluteal region has gained increased popularity in recent years. Large-volume fat grafts are injected into the subcutaneous tissues. Fat grafts provide a precise means to augment the buttock region while providing a more rapid recovery than implants. There is considerable risk associated with deeper injections of fat into this region, with fat embolism being the most serious complication observed. High fatality rates have been observed following this complication. thus, careful attention should be paid to the location of the cannula tip, which should remain superficial at all times.

Face

Aesthetic

Restoration of volume is considered a mainstay of facial rejuvenation (▶ Fig. 24.5, ▶ Fig. 24.6, ▶ Fig. 24.7). As the face ages, underlying soft tissues atrophy, and skeletal structures change. Loss of dentition in the older patient leads to profound skeletal changes in the mid and lower face. Adding fat to critical areas of the face restores lost volume, leading to a more youthful appearance. Specific deep and superficial fat compartments have been identified in the face. Specifically placing fat grafts into these compartments has been suggested to lead to a more natural rejuvenated appearance.[30]

Reconstructive

Fat grafting to the face has also successfully been used for a variety of reconstructive purposes including following craniofacial surgery, Romberg's disease, and HIV-related facial atrophy.

Hand

Hands are often the first areas to show signs of aging, which leads many patients to seek rejuvenation of the dorsum. The goal of fat grafting to the dorsum of the hand is to create slight subcutaneous fullness with decreased, but not obliterated, visibility of the veins and tendons. Placement of small aliquots of fat in the subcutaneous plane minimizes the risk of injury to deeper structures.

Genital

In females, fat grafts can be used to add volume to the labia majora or vulval areas. In addition, scars from previous surgery can be improved with fat grafts. The rich blood supply to this area results in a favorable success rate.

Iatrogenic Deformities Following Liposuction

Deformities following liposuction such as contour depressions are a common complaint of patients following liposuction procedures. The use of fat grafts is ideally suited to correct these deformities. Often scarring associated with the initial procedure is encountered and requires release prior to grafting. Small aliquots of fat are then placed in a three-dimensional fashion in and around the areas of depression.

Fibrosis and Scar Treatment

Stromal cells are abundant in adipose tissue. When fat is transferred, these cells and cytokines associated with them interact with the native tissues, resulting in a rejuvenating and regenerating effect (▶ Fig. 24.8, ▶ Fig. 24.9, ▶ Fig. 24.10). Adipose tissue has the highest percentage of stem cells found in the body.[31] The treatment of damaged tissue with fat and more specifically with adipose-derived stromal cells is very promising.[32] Adipose stromal cells have been demonstrated to secrete angiogenic factors that promote neovascularization into ischemic tissues.[33]

Difficult wounds and scars such as those observed post thermal injury or radiation therapy have consistently shown improvement following injection of fat into them. Often serial fat grafting is required to achieve the desired outcome because of the tenuous blood supply seen in such scars.

24.5.2 Risks and Complications of Fat Grafting

The generalized acceptance and widespread use of fat grafting as a standard surgical technique attests to the safety of the procedure. Risks that are common to all surgical procedures can occur with fat grafting, which include bleeding, infection, and injury to adjacent structures. Unique to fat grafting is the formation of oil cysts, calcification, fat necrosis, and fat embolism. As mentioned earlier, fat embolism is potentially the most catastrophic complication. Arterial emboli, particularly in the face, can lead to blindness, stroke, and skin necrosis. Venous emboli, which are most commonly seen following deep injection of fat grafts in the gluteal region, can be fatal. During this procedure, fat may inadvertently enter the gluteal veins and then embolize to the heart and lungs. Estimated fatality rates following gluteal fat grafting are 1 in 3,000, higher than for any other cosmetic procedure. Only surgeons who have an intimate knowledge of the relevant anatomy and are well versed with this procedure should perform it.

Theoretical risks such as fat grafts to the breast causing microcalcifications, which would cause ambiguous mammographic findings, have not been demonstrated to be valid. In addition, there is no evidence to suggest that grafted fat has an oncogenic potential.

24.6 Future

Applications of grafted fat continue to grow, not only when additional soft-tissue volume is desired but also in tissue repair. The fact that fat has the highest proportion of adult mesenchymal stem cells and adipose-derived stem cells presents exciting prospects for its use when differentiation into other tissue types is needed. The stromal vascular fraction of the lipoaspirate is rich in regenerative factors. Both of these findings have generated increased interest in the versatility of fat grafting.

24.7 Pearls and Pitfalls

24.7.1 Pearls

- Patient should be made aware that a less-than-expected outcome may occur.
- Always ensure that the area where the fat will be harvested from is inconspicuous and that no depression or scarring results.
- Treat the fat gently. Do not aspirate overly aggressively.
- When processing the fat, make sure that as much blood and oil are removed and washed away from the fat.
- Use blunt-tipped fat injection cannula when injecting.
- Place fat in "strings" by injecting slowly as the needle is being withdrawn.
- Fat should be placed in a gridlike pattern so as to create as smooth a contour as possible.
- Overfill areas requiring augmentation by 30 to 35%. Not all adipocytes will survive.
- Repeat procedures may be needed to achieve the volume augmentation needed.
- Fat should be injected as soon as possible after harvest to maximize cell viability.
- Inject the fat as deeply as possible to minimize the risk of contour issues.

24.7.2 Pitfalls

- It is difficult to accurately predict the amount of fat that will survive. Most injectors estimate that 70% of fat will survive in the long term.
- Do not place globules of fat on areas that are being filled—these often do not survive.
- Do not place needle entry points in conspicuous areas; use natural crease lines to hide these.
- Smokers have a higher rate of graft resorption, which can be unpredictable. Therefore, strongly encourage them to quit for at least 4 weeks prior to the procedure.
- Older patients do not do as well as younger ones.

References

[1] Gir P, Brown SA, Oni G, Kashefi N, Mojallal A, Rohrich RJ. Fat grafting: evidence-based review on autologous fat harvesting, processing, reinjection, and storage. Plast Reconstr Surg. 2012; 130 (1):249–258

[2] Neuber GA. Fettransplantation. Chir Kongr Verhandl Deutsche Gesellschaft fur Chirurgie. 1893; 22:66

[3] Hollander E. Die kosmetische Chirurgie (S.669–712, 45 Abb). In: Joseph M, ed. Handbuch der kosmetik. Leipzig: Verlagvan Veit; 1912:690–691

[4] Czerny V. Plastischer Ersatz der Brustdruse durch ein Lipom. Zentralbl Chir. 1895; 27:72

[5] Bucky LP, Kanchwala SK. The role of autologous fat and alternative fillers in the aging face. Plast Reconstr Surg. 2007; 120(6) Suppl: 89S–97S

[6] American Society of Plastic Surgeons. Survey of Plastic Surgery Procedures Performed in 2017. Available at: https://www.plasticsurgery.org/documents/News/Statistics/2017/plastic-surgery-statistics-full-report-2017.pdf

[7] Yoshimura K. Cell-assisted lipotransfer for breast augmentation: grafting of progenitor-enriched fat tissue. In: Shiffman M, ed. Autologous Fat Transfer. Heidelberg: Springer; 2010

[8] Rubina K, Kalinina N, Efimenko A, et al. Adipose stromal cells stimulate angiogenesis via promoting progenitor cell differentiation, secretion of angiogenic factors, and enhancing vessel maturation. Tissue Eng Part A. 2009; 15(8):2039–2050

[9] Walocko FM, Khouri RK, Jr, Urbanchek MG, Levi B, Cederna PS. The potential roles for adipose tissue in peripheral nerve regeneration. Microsurgery. 2016; 36(1):81–88

[10] Charles-de-Sá L, Gontijo-de-Amorim NF, Maeda Takiya C, et al. Antiaging treatment of the facial skin by fat graft and adipose-derived stem cells. Plast Reconstr Surg. 2015; 135(4):999–1009

[11] Klein JA. The tumescent technique for lipo-suction surgery. Am J Cosmet Surg. 1987; 4:1124–1132

[12] Klein JA. Tumescent technique for local anesthesia improves safety in large-volume liposuction. Plast Reconstr Surg. 1993; 92(6):1085–1098, discussion 1099–1100

[13] Kaufman MR, Bradley JP, Dickinson B, et al. Autologous fat transfer national consensus survey: trends in techniques for harvest, preparation, and application, and perception of short- and long-term results. Plast Reconstr Surg. 2007; 119(1):323–331

[14] Matsumoto D, Shigeura T, Sato K, et al. Influences of preservation at various temperatures on liposuction aspirates. Plast Reconstr Surg. 2007; 120(6):1510–1517

[15] Allen RJ, Jr, Canizares O, Jr, Scharf C, et al. Grading lipoaspirate: is there an optimal density for fat grafting? Plast Reconstr Surg. 2013; 131(1):38–45

[16] Butala P, Hazen A, Szpalski C, Sultan SM, Coleman SR, Warren SM. Endogenous stem cell therapy enhances fat graft survival. Plast Reconstr Surg. 2012; 130(2):293–306

[17] Kurita M, Matsumoto D, Shigeura T, et al. Influences of centrifugation on cells and tissues in liposuction aspirates: optimized centrifugation for lipotransfer and cell isolation. Plast Reconstr Surg. 2008; 121(3): 1033–1041, discussion 1042–1043

[18] Eto H, Kato H, Suga H, et al. The fate of adipocytes after nonvascularized fat grafting: evidence of early death and replacement of adipocytes. Plast Reconstr Surg. 2012; 129(5):1081–1092

[19] Khouri RK, Eisenmann-Klein M, Cardoso E, et al. Brava and autologous fat transfer is a safe and effective breast augmentation alternative: results of a 6-year, 81-patient, prospective multicenter study. Plast Reconstr Surg. 2012; 129(5):1173–1187

[20] Gentile P, De Angelis B, Pasin M, et al. Adipose-derived stromal vascular fraction cells and platelet-rich plasma: basic and clinical evaluation for cell-based therapies in patients with scars on the face. J Craniofac Surg. 2014; 25(1):267–272

[21] Broughton G, II, Crosby MA, Coleman J, Rohrich RJ. Use of herbal supplements and vitamins in plastic surgery: a practical review. Plast Reconstr Surg. 2007; 119(3):48e–66e

[22] Rinker B. The evils of nicotine: an evidence-based guide to smoking and plastic surgery. Ann Plast Surg. 2013; 70(5):599–605

[23] Van den Berghe G, Wilmer A, Milants I, et al. Intensive insulin therapy in mixed medical/surgical intensive care units: benefit versus harm. Diabetes. 2006; 55(11):3151–3159

[24] Liu J, Ludwig T, Ebraheim NA. Effect of the blood HbA1c level on surgical treatment outcomes of diabetics with ankle fractures. Orthop Surg. 2013; 5(3):203–208

[25] Rohrich RJ, Sorokin ES, Brown SA. In search of improved fat transfer viability: a quantitative analysis of the role of centrifugation and harvest site. Plast Reconstr Surg. 2004; 113(1):391–395, discussion 396–397

[26] Ullmann Y, Shoshani O, Fodor A, et al. Searching for the favorable donor site for fat injection: in vivo study using the nude mice model. Dermatol Surg. 2005; 31(10):1304–1307

[27] Li K, Gao J, Zhang Z, et al. Selection of donor site for fat grafting and cell isolation. Aesthetic Plast Surg. 2013; 37(1):153–158

[28] Small K, Choi M, Petruolo O, Lee C, Karp N. Is there an ideal donor site of fat for secondary breast reconstruction? Aesthet Surg J. 2014; 34 (4):545–550

[29] Gutowski KA, ASPS Fat Graft Task Force. Current applications and safety of autologous fat grafts: a report of the ASPS fat graft task force. Plast Reconstr Surg. 2009; 124(1):272–280

[30] Rohrich RJ, Afrooz PN. Finesse in face lifting: the role of facial fat compartment augmentation in facial rejuvenation. Plast Reconstr Surg. 2019; 143(1):98–101

[31] Strem BM, Hicok KC, Zhu M, et al. Multipotential differentiation of adipose tissue-derived stem cells. Keio J Med. 2005; 54(3): 132–141

[32] Klinger M, Lisa A, Klinger F, et al. Regenerative approach to scars, ulcers and related problems with fat grafting. Clin Plast Surg. 2015; 42(3):345–352, viii

[33] Rehman J, Traktuev D, Li J, et al. Secretion of angiogenic and antiapoptotic factors by human adipose stromal cells. Circulation. 2004; 109(10):1292–1298

Index

Note: Page numbers set **bold** or *italic* indicate headings or figures, respectively.